D1336970

Surgical
Emergencies

Surgical *Emergencies*

John Monson MD, FRCS
Academic Surgical Unit
The University of Hull
Castle Hill Hospital
Cottingham, North Humberside

Graeme Duthie MD (Hons), FRCS, FRCSEd
Academic Surgical Unit
The University of Hull
Castle Hill Hospital
Cottingham, North Humberside

Kevin O'Malley MCh, FRCSI
Department of Surgery
Mater Misericordiae Hospital
Dublin, Ireland

**Blackwell
Science**

© 1999 by
Blackwell Science Ltd
Editorial Offices:
Osney Mead, Oxford OX2 0EL
25 John Street, London WC1N 2BL
23 Ainslie Place, Edinburgh EH3 6AJ
350 Main Street, Malden
  MA 02148 5018, USA
54 University Street, Carlton
  Victoria 3053, Australia
10, rue Casimir Delavigne
  75006 Paris, France

Other Editorial Offices:
Blackwell Wissenschafts-Verlag GmbH
Kurfürstendamm 57
10707 Berlin, Germany

Blackwell Science KK
MG Kodenmacho Building
7–10 Kodenmacho Nihombashi
Chuo-ku, Tokyo 104, Japan

First published 1999

Set by Excel Typesetters Co., Hong Kong
Printed and bound in Italy by G. Canale & C. SpA, Turin

The Blackwell Science logo is a
trade mark of Blackwell Science Ltd,
registered at the United Kingdom
Trade Marks Registry

DISTRIBUTORS

Marston Book Services Ltd
PO Box 269
Abingdon, Oxon OX14 4YN
(*Orders*: Tel: 01235 465500
            Fax: 01235 465555)

USA
Blackwell Science, Inc.
Commerce Place
350 Main Street
Malden, MA 02148 5018
(*Orders*: Tel: 800 759 6102
            781 388 8250
            Fax: 781 388 8255)

Canada
Login Brothers Book Company
324 Saulteaux Crescent
Winnipeg, Manitoba R3J 3T2
(*Orders*: Tel: 204 837-2987)

Australia
Blackwell Science Pty Ltd
54 University Street
Carlton, Victoria 3053
(*Orders*: Tel: 3 9347 0300
            Fax: 3 9347 5001)

A catalogue record for this title
is available from the British Library

ISBN 0-632-05047-0

Library of Congress
Cataloging-in-publication Data

Surgical emergencies /
[edited by] John Monson, Graeme Duthie,
Kevin O'Malley.
      p.   cm.
   ISBN 0-632-05047-0
   1. Surgical emergencies.
   I. Monson, John R. T.   II. Duthie, Graeme.
   III. O'Malley, Kevin, MD.
   [DNLM: 1. Surgical Procedures, Operative.
   2. Emergencies. WO 700 S961   1998]
RD93.S86   1998
617′.026—dc21
DNLM/DLC
for Library of Congress   98-17789
                                       CIP

For further information on
Blackwell Science, visit our website:
www.blackwell-science.com

Contents

List of contributors

Daryll M. Baker PhD, FRCS (Gen)
Royal Free Hospital, Department of Surgery, Pond Street, London, NW3 2QG, UK

Michael P. Bannon MD
Department of Surgery, Mayo Clinic and Mayo Foundation, Rochester, Minnesota, USA

Aires A. B. Barros D'Sa MD, FRCS (Eng), FRCSEd
Vascular Surgery Unit, Royal Victoria Hospital, Belfast, BT12 6BA, UK

Sean R. Bennett FRCA
Department of Anaesthesia, Castle Hill Hospital, Cottingham, North Humberside, HU16 5JQ, UK

Dermot P. Byrnes FRCSI, FRCSEd
Department of Neurological Surgery, Royal Victoria Hospital, Belfast, BT12 6BA, UK

P. Declan Carey MCh, FRCSI, FCSHK
Department of Surgery, University of Wales College of Medicine, Heath Park, Cardiff, CF4 4XN, UK

Edmund G. Carton MD, FFARCSI
Department of Anaesthesia and Intensive Care, Mater Misericordiae Hospital, Eccles Street, Dublin 7, Ireland

Mary-Paula Colgan MD, FACA
Department of Vascular Surgery, St James's Hospital, Dublin 8, Ireland

Malachy Coughlan MD, MRCOG, FRCSEd
Department of Obstetrics and Gynaecology, Mater Misericordiae Hospital, Eccles Street, Dublin 7, Ireland

Neville Couse MD, FRCSI
Letterkenny General Hospital, County Donegal, Ireland

Ray J. Delicata MD, FRCSEd
Department of Surgery, University of Wales College of Medicine, Heath Park, Cardiff, CF4 4XN, UK

Deborah DeMarta MD
Department of Colorectal Surgery, Cleveland Clinic Florida, Fort Lauderdale, Florida, USA

Simon P. L. Dexter FRCS
The Centre for Digestive Diseases, The General Infirmary at Leeds, Great George Street, Leeds, LS1 3EX, UK

Philip J. Drew BSc, FRCSEd, FRCSEng, FRCS (Glasg)
Academic Surgical Unit, University of Hull, Castle Hill Hospital, Cottingham, North Humberside, HU16 5JQ, UK

Graeme S. Duthie MD, FRCSEd, FRCS
Academic Surgical Unit, University of Hull, Castle Hill Hospital, Cottingham, North Humberside, HU16 5JQ, UK

Ridzuan Farouk MCh, FRCSEd, FRCS (Glasg)
Royal Berkshire and Battle Hospitals, London Road, Reading, RG1 5AN, UK

John M. Fitzpatrick MCh, FRCSI
Mater Misericordiae Hospital, Eccles Street, Dublin 7, Ireland

O. James Garden MD, FRCSEd, FRCS (Glasg)
Department of Surgery, The University of Edinburgh, Royal Infirmary, Lauriston Place, Edinburgh, EH3 9YW, UK

Geoffrey Glazer MS, FRCS, FACS
Department of Surgery, St Mary's Hospital, Praed Street, Paddington, London W2

Roger M. Greenhalgh MA, MD, MChir, FRCS
Professor of Surgery, Imperial College School of Medicine, Charing Cross Hospital, Fulham Palace Road, London, W6 8RF, UK

Pierre J. Guillou BSc, MD, FRCS
Department of Surgery, St James's University Hospital, Leeds, LS9 7TF, UK

James Gunn FRCS
Academic Surgical Unit, University of Hull, Castle Hill Hospital, Cottingham, North Humberside, HU16 5JQ, UK

Thomas P. J. Hennessy MD, MCl, FRCS, FRCSI
Department of Clinical Surgery, Trinity Centre, St James's Hospital, Dublin 8, Ireland

Kevin Hickey MRCOG, FRCSEd, MMEdSc
The General Infirmary at Leeds, Great George Street, Leeds, LS1 3EX, UK

Michael J. Kerin MCh, FRCSI, FRCSEd, FRCS (Gen)
Academic Surgical Unit, University of Hull, Castle Hill Hospital, Cottingham, North Humberside, HU16 5JQ, UK

Andrew N. Kingsnorth BSc, MS, FRCS
Postgraduate Medical School, Level 7, Derriford Hospital, Plymouth, PL6 8DH, UK

Zygmunt H. Krukowski PhD, FRCS
Aberdeen Royal Infirmary, Foresterhill, Aberdeen, AB9 2ZB, UK

Thomas H. Lynch MMS, MCh, FRCS, FRCSI, FRCS (Urol)
Department of Urology, City Hospital, Belfast, BT9 7AB, Ireland

Iain M. C. Macintyre QHS, MD, FRCSE, FRCPE
Department of General Surgery, Western General Hospital, Crewe Road, Edinburgh, EH4 2XU

K. K. Madhavan MS, FRCSEd
Department of Surgery, The University of Edinburgh, Royal Infirmary, Lauriston Place, Edinburgh, EH3 9YW, UK

Anand Mahadevan
Department of Surgery, University of Wales College of Medicine, Heath Park, Cardiff, CF4 4XN, UK

Darren Mann MS, FRCS
Department of Surgery, St Mary's Hospital, Praed Street, Paddington, London W2

Averil O. Mansfield ChM, FRCS
Academic Surgical Unit, St Mary's Hospital Medical School, Queen Elizabeth Wing, South Wharf Road, Paddington, London, UK

Gerard P. McEntee MCh, FRCSI
Mater Misericordiae and St Vincent's Hospitals, Dublin 4, Ireland

Brendan McIlroy FRCS
Department of Surgery, Derbyshire Royal Infirmary, London Road, Derby DE1 2QY, UK

Peter McKenna MRGOG, MRCPS
Department of Obstetrics and Gynaecology, Mater Misericordiae Hospital, Eccles Street, Dublin 7, Ireland

Martin A. P. Milling MA, FRCSEd, FRCSEng
Department of Plastic Surgery, Morriston Hospital, Swansea, West Glamorgan, SA6 6NL, UK

John R. T. Monson MD, FRCS, FRCSI, FACS, FRCS (Glasg)
Academic Surgical Unit, University of Hull, Castle Hill Hospital, Cottingham, North Humberside, HU16 5JQ, UK

Dermot J. Moore MD, FRCSI
Department of Vascular Surgery, St James's Hospital, Dublin 8, Ireland

Colm O'Herlihy MD, FRCPI, FRCOG
Department of Obstetrics and Gynaecology, University College Dublin, National Maternity Hospital, Holles Street, Dublin 2, Ireland

Niall O'Higgins
Department of Surgery, University College Dublin, St Vincent's University Hospital, Dublin 4, Ireland

Terence J. O'Kelly MD, FRCS
Aberdeen Royal Infirmary, Foresterhill, Aberdeen, AB9 2ZB, UK

Kevin O'Malley MCh, FRCSI
Department of Surgery, Mater Misericordiae Hospital, Eccles Street, Dublin 7, Ireland

Simon Paterson-Brown MS, MPhil, FRCS
Department of Surgery, The University of Edinburgh, Royal Infirmary, Lauriston Place, Edinburgh, EH3 9YW, UK

Dermot M. Phelan FFICANZCA
Department of Anaesthesia and Intensive Care, Mater Misericordiae Hospital, Eccles Street, Dublin 7, Ireland

Akhtar Qureshi FRCSI
Academic Surgical Unit, University of Hull, Castle Hill Hospital, Cottingham, North Humberside, HU16 5JQ, UK

Manas K. Roy MS, FRCS (Glasg), FRCSEd
Department of Surgery, University of Wales College of Medicine, Heath Park, Cardiff, CF4 4XN, UK

Gregor D. Shanik MCh, FRCSI
Department of Vascular Surgery, St James's Hospital, Dublin 8, Ireland

Nicholas D. Stafford MB, FRCS
Department of Otolaryngology/Head and Neck Surgery, Academic Surgical Unit, University of Hull, Alderson House, Hull Royal Infirmary, Anlaby Road, Hull, HU3 2JZ, UK

Robert J. C. Steele MD, FRCS
Department of Surgery, University of Dundee, Ninewells Hospital and Medical School, Dundee, DD1 9SY, UK

William S. Walker MA, MB, BChir, FRCS
Department of Cardiothoracic Surgery, Royal Infirmary, Lauriston Place, Edinburgh, EH3 9YW, UK

Steven D. Wexner MD, FACS, FASCRS
Department of Colorectal Surgery, Cleveland Clinic Florida, 3000 West Cypress Creek Road, Fort Lauderdale, Florida, USA

Stephen J. Wigmore BSc, MD, FRCSEd
Department of Surgery, The University of Edinburgh, Royal Infirmary, Lauriston Place, Edinburgh, EH3 9YW, UK

Alastair C. J. Windsor MD, FRCS, FRCSEd
Department of Surgery, St James's University Hospital, Leeds, LS9 7TF, UK

Tonia Young-Fadok MBChB, FACS
E6A, Colon and Rectal Surgery, 200 First Street SW, Rochester, Minnesota 55905, USA

Preface

As we approach the millennium surgery is once again facing a series of changes and challenges. Increasingly, there is pressure to shorten the period of required training before a surgeon may embark upon a career of independent practice. Encouragingly this has resulted in a significant investment in improving the accountability of training programmes. The overall result is almost certainly that surgical trainees are offered the best opportunities to develop their skills than at any time in recent years. On the downside the shortening of the overall training period has inevitably reduced the total surgical experience in comparison to that seen by trainees of twenty years before. Comments such as these are true to a greater or lesser extent about surgical training in most countries worldwide.

No surgeon—trainee or consultant—will ever treat the surgical emergency as a trivial matter. Perhaps in no other area of surgical practice is there a greater number of possibilities and permutations facing the clinician. This text aims to provide a companion for the surgeon facing these challenges. We have specifically set out to avoid presenting the book as a discussion of emergency surgery for this is not truly how clinical practice works. Patients rarely present with an established diagnosis ready for surgery. Rather they present undiagnosed as a constellation of symptoms and signs in an acute setting—the surgical emergency. We have, therefore, attempted to reflect this scenario in the manner of presentation. For the more junior trainee there are chapters dealing with the commonly faced issues such as right iliac fossa pain and head injuries. However, for the more experienced clinician, along with the junior trainee, there are discussions relating to equally challenging and perhaps more life-threatening problems including aneurysm disease, large bowel obstruction and gastrointestinal bleeding. Although we have not attempted to present a true operative atlas or text there are instances throughout the book where descriptions of individual operations are provided in some detail. Every surgeon is familiar with the scenario of facing an ill patient, usually in the middle of the night and sometimes with less senior support than during daylight, and wanting to be reassured about some aspect of diagnosis or treatment. Sometimes the questions relate to simple issues of differential diagnosis or the most appropriate plan of investigation. On other occasions the concerns relate to treatment options or perhaps even the best approach to an operation. This book is for the surgeon facing these challenges.

The chapters generally follow a similar format allowing the reader the opportunity to dip into the text for quick reference. Each section has been compiled by surgeons with noted expertise in the field and is presented in a manner that allows the reader to retrieve information easily and (hopefully) quickly. The frequent use of illustrations is complemented by the regular appearance of highlighted boxes including practice points of special significance. No attempt has been made to exhaustively reference the text but suggestions for further reading appear throughout the text. We hope that this book will become a frequent and valued companion for any surgeon who is regularly faced with the surgical emergency.

John R. T. Monson
Graeme S. Duthie
Kevin O'Malley

CHAPTER 1

Emergency room treatment—the ATLS® philosophy

Niall O'Higgins

Introduction

Every student who has taken the Advanced Trauma Life Support (ATLS®) course knows the story of the orthopaedic surgeon who was in a private plane with his wife and four children when the plane crashed in a corn field in Nebraska. His wife was killed immediately, the surgeon and three of the children were seriously injured and one child had minor injuries. The surgeon considered that the standard of care given to him and his children was extremely poor and strongly recommended that the system of care following injury required radical change. This event stimulated a discussion amongst medical and educational bodies in Nebraska where the need for training in coping with trauma-related emergencies was identified and subsequently a programme of lectures with demonstrations of practical life-saving manoeuvres evolved to form the prototype ATLS® course.

The evolution of ATLS®

The evolution of the course was based on the simple assumption that the outcome after injury could be improved by early and appropriate care. Apparently self-evident, this assumption had not been demonstrated clearly at that time and became clear only after 1982 when the trimodal distribution of death from injury was described (Fig. 1.1). The *first peak* of deaths occurs within minutes of injury from brain or brain stem lacerations or major disruption of the heart or aorta. Because of the catastrophic severity of these injuries, no scope or potential exists to prevent deaths from these causes and efforts to reduce deaths from first peak injury are focused on accident prevention. The *second peak* occurs between minutes to hours after injury and relate usually to subdural or extradural haematomas, haemopneumothorax, internal abdominal injury caused by splenic or hepatic trauma, pelvic fractures or other major injuries associated with significant blood loss. ATLS® is concerned primarily with second peak deaths and a concept of avoidable or preventable deaths relates to the implementation of ATLS® principles in the pre-hospital or hospital setting. The *third peak* of death occurs days to weeks after injury and

results from sepsis or multiple organ failure. It is now clear that appropriate early resuscitation not only reduces deaths from second peak injury but also reduces the third peak deaths that usually occur in the intensive care unit. Thus, it is now understood that early appropriate primary care following multiple injuries has a distinct beneficial effect on long-term outcome both in survival and in reduction of long-term morbidity.

In design and conduct, the ATLS® course is authoritarian and doctrinaire, but it is also authoritative, since all statements and information are regularly subjected to critical analysis and review and are supported by convincing evidence in the medical literature. The ATLS® manual is reviewed regularly and rigorously. Originally, the course was intended for medical personnel who do not treat trauma frequently. It was appreciated that many factors render the provision of purposeful and appropriate care difficult for a medical person who encounters an accident, for example:

1 the instantaneous onset of the event;
2 the circumstances of the injury;
3 the variable nature of the severity and extent of the injury; and occasionally
4 the situation where many patients are involved.

If a doctor is not involved regularly and frequently in trauma care, it is unlikely that optimum care will be given in the first minutes or hours after injury unless clear, well-defined and highly specific directives are laid down. Without a systematic approach primary assessment is likely to be disorganized, resuscitation lacking in purpose, triage inappropriate and long-term morbidity increased. One of the reasons why the ATLS® programme is so authoritarian is to provide a valuable guide to the individual who has to deal with trauma occasionally but not regularly. However, so successful has ATLS® been throughout the world that the principles and techniques have become standard practice in most hospitals where trauma is dealt with, from the smallest to the largest trauma centre.

The ATLS® method

In conventional medical school training, students are taught basic sciences and biology before proceeding to understand-

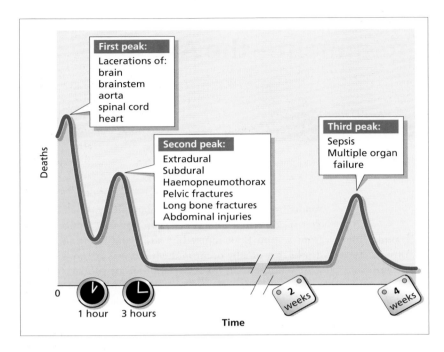

Fig. 1.1 Three peaks of trauma-related deaths.

ing the physiology, anatomy and pathology of the body. They then progress to clinical studies where the scientific principles are applied. The sequence of disciplines of history-taking, physical examination, clinical conclusion, investigation, diagnosis, treatment and rehabilitation are part of a continuum based on a logical evolution of deductive reasoning and investigation. In this system the idea of treatment preceding diagnosis would be anathema. Whilst ATLS® does not overturn the traditional method it requires that the approach to patients with trauma differs in the following three major ways.

1 The greatest threat to life is treated first.

2 Resuscitative treatment often precedes definitive diagnosis.

3 Early initial evaluation of an acutely injured patient does not necessarily require a detailed history.

These approaches lead to the evolution of the ABCD (A for airway with cervical spine control, B for breathing, C for circulation with arrest of haemorrhage and D for disability or neurological status). The ATLS® course teaches that loss of the airway kills a patient more quickly than does loss of the ability to breathe and inability to breathe kills more quickly than loss of circulating blood volume. The next most lethal condition is an expanding intracranial mass.

The ATLS® course is aimed at providing knowledge and skills for the immediate safe management of a patient following injury. The objectives are indicated in Table 1.1. One of the objectives of ATLS® is that at each step of the way the standard of care provided to the patient should not

Table 1.1 Objectives of the ATLS® course.

> **1** Rapid accurate primary assessment of the patient's condition.
> **2** A priority system of resuscitation and stabilization of a patient.
> **3** Ability to decide if patient's needs exceed the local capabilities, either in terms of personnel or other facilities.
> **4** A systematic approach to arranging inter-hospital transfer.
> **5** A system for ensuring that optimum care is provided at each step of the patient's management.

diminish during various phases of management. Thus, after primary evaluation and resuscitation, the care of the patient during transfer in the pre-hospital phase should never be less good than it was at the roadside and, in turn, the care given in the Accident and Emergency Department should be of a higher level than that provided in the pre-hospital situation.

ATLS® does not claim that its methodology and programme represent the only correct way of treating patients following trauma. It acknowledges that there are other ways and that details may be debated. It does claim, however, to be a safe, acceptable and practical method of primary assessment and resuscitation.

Development of ATLS® courses

By 1977, approximately one year after his plane had crashed, the orthopaedic surgeon approached medical and educational authorities and a critical care course for doctors, nurses and pre-hospital care personnel had been devised. A pilot course was conducted in Auburn, Nebraska in 1978, and in 1979 the Committee on Trauma of the American College of Surgeons approved the ATLS® programme, recognized trauma as a surgical disease and incorporated ATLS® as an educational activity of the College. The first American College of Surgeons' ATLS® course was conducted in January 1980 and the programme spread systematically across the United States during that year. In 1981 it expanded into Canada and during the next four years to Central and South America. In 1986 international training programmes were established with the Americas and a pilot study was started in Trinidad and Tobago. Over the next 10 years ATLS® has extended to Australia, New Zealand, the United Kingdom, Israel, Ireland, South Africa, Saudi Arabia, Singapore, Italy, Greece, Indonesia, Papua New Guinea and the Netherlands. In 1996 Taiwan, Sweden and Hong Kong were added to the list.

Three categories of courses are available:
1 Student
2 Student refresher courses
3 Instructor.

These courses range from a single day to an intensive 3-day programme. The ATLS® course activity for 1980 to 1997 is summarized on Table 1.2. Over 12 000 courses have been held and approximately 250 000 individuals have been trained in the system. For the year 1997 alone, 1354 courses have been held, 12 054 doctors have been trained and 739 retrained. The widespread enthusiastic acceptance of ATLS® throughout the world indicates the universal need for a system in trauma care in the early phase after injury.

A parallel-type course is the Pre-hospital Trauma Life Support (PHTLS) course sponsored by the National Association of Emergency Medical Technicians in the United States and is directed at emergency care technicians, paramedics and nurses who are involved in pre-hospital trauma care.

In order that ATLS® be brought to a country, the national surgical college or the national chapter of the American College of Surgeons must formally make a request to the Chairman of the ATLS® Sub-committee of the American College of Surgeons. Requests are directed to the American College of Surgeons, Committee on Trauma for approval by the Board of Regents. Once formal approval for the development of the course in any country has been obtained, the

Table 1.2 1980–1997 ATLS® course activity.

Course type	Total courses				Number trained				Number retrained				Others trained	
	COT³	IACS⁴	ISO⁵	Total	COT³	IACS⁴	ISO⁵	Total	COT	IACS¹	ISO⁵	Total	PEs²	Auditors
Instructor	1671	81	94	1792	21 434	546	1189	23 169						
Student	8733	1044	1114	10 891	169 771	14 157	17 765	201 693					[996]	[11 173]
Student/student refresher	1584	27		1611	25 000	1242		25 243	4766	20		4786		
Student refresher	403	7	11	421					4324	20	144	4488		
Instructor update	128	16		144	858	329		1187						
Independent operator	98			98	[3385]			[3385]						
Totals	12 563	1175	1219	14 957	217 063	16 274	18 954	251 292	9090	40	144	9274	996	[11 173]

1 Independent operators in the military are non-physician special forces medics who require training in advanced life support measures because of their military assignments.

2 PEs are defined as physician extenders (physician assistants or nurse practitioners who work in a rural emergency department or clinic at which there is no physician available).

3 COT; Canada, United States and Territories, Latin and South America countries that in 1995 will be considered separate international countries with an ACS Chapter (IACS): Argentina (1987); Bolivia (1990); Brazil (1987); Chile (1987); Colombia (1985); Mexico (1986); Peru (1992); Ecuador (not yet conducting ATLS Courses).

4 IACS; Countries that are conducting courses under the auspices of their ACS Chapter: Greece (1993); Italy (1994); Saudi Arabia (1991); Hong Kong (1996).

5 ISO; Countries that are conducting courses under the auspices of a recognized Surgical Organization: Australia (1988); Indonesia (1995); Ireland, Republic of (1991); Israel (1990); Papua New Guinea (1994 with Australia); New Zealand (1988); Singapore, Republic of (1992); South Africa, Republic of (1992); Sweden (1996); Taiwan (1996); The Netherlands (1995); Trinidad/Tobago (1990); United Kingdom (1988). Countries in which one-time-only courses have been conducted: Belgium (with the RCS of England; negotiations currently in progress to implement); Germany (US military site for doctors from the Baltic States); Switzerland (request to import forthcoming); Cyprus.

These tables were kindly prepared and sent by Irvene K. Hughes, RN, Manager, ATLS Division, American College of Surgeons.

Numbers for International Surgical Organizations (150) do not reflect courses conducted in 1997, only through 1996.

International ATLS® Course Director and the ATLS® Chairman plan the programme in conjunction with the local organizers. The initial course in a country consists of a National Faculty and members of the International ATLS® Committee. Details of the first course are closely supervised and controlled by the ATLS® Committee. Such close surveillance is considered essential in order to protect the high standard and integrity of the course from country to country. The organization, detailed planning and conduct of the course is scrutinized and inspected regularly to ensure the provision of a high quality. By 1997, 25 countries were actively participating in the ATLS® programme and to facilitate international dialogue, reciprocity of Instructors exists with qualified Instructors being accepted in each of the participating countries. The ATLS® Division of the American College of Surgeons maintains an international Instructor database so that the status and eligibility of all Instructors can be verified before they are assigned to teach on a course. The central concern in the widespread dissemination of the ATLS® course is the preservation of the core content and basic concepts of the programme and the maintenance of high quality.

Student course

The Student Course is run over two or two and a half days. It is highly intensive. A Course Director is responsible for the running of the course. Throughout the entire programme all instructors are in attendance, even at skill stations and lectures in which they are not directly involved. In this way both direct personal and close supervision of each student is ensured and also the integrated, collegial and mutually supportive teamwork approach is consolidated. A typical ATLS® course schedule is outlined in Fig. 1.2.

In advance of the course a manual is sent to each student. The manual contains the core content of each section of the course including the Initial Assessment and Management and subsequently the management of each system such as Airway and Ventilatory Management, Shock and trauma to chest, abdomen, head, spine and extremities. Special sections deal with injuries from burns and cold, and to trauma in children, trauma in pregnancy and ocular injury. A separate section deals with Stabilization and Transport. Associated with each chapter are the special skills required for primary resuscitation which are reinforced in the practical skill stations during the course. Thus, intubation, vascular access, thoracocentesis, pericardiocentesis, diagnostic peritoneal lavage, interpretation and management of radiographs of the cervical spine and techniques of immobilization and transport of patients are all described in detail.

Each student is expected to have read the manual carefully so that the lectures and the demonstrations at the skill stations continually reinforce existing knowledge. A simulated accident scenario, known as the 'Moulage' provides an approximation of a clinical problem in trauma. The student is tested on priorities of care during the examination component of the course. Whilst the course can be criticized for putting students under the particular stress of the simulated system of injury, the test is probably a valid reflection of the real-life pressure under which the clinician operates in situations of major injury. Once the student has read the manual several times, has had the core content reinforced by lectures, has been repeatedly exposed to the skill stations and is tested under stressful conditions, it is likely that the candidate will be confident and competent in the stepwise conduct of primary care of trauma.

Lectures

The formal lectures in the course are either 30 min or 45 min. The lecturer follows closely the details described in the manual in each section and utilizes specially prepared slides restricted for use at ATLS® courses. Each lecture ends with question time. During the lecture the Instructor deals sequentially with each of the items mentioned in the manual, emphasizing the salient messages in each case.

Practical skill stations

The practical skill stations utilize models and simulated systems so that they can be demonstrated repeatedly to the small group. During the skill stations each Instructor demonstrates the methods and each student in turn goes through the practical points by demonstrating them until each person is proficient. This system applies to all the skill stations including those dealing with airway and interpretation of spinal radiology (Fig. 1.3).

The Surgical Practicum

In the Surgical Practicum where the student deals with cricothyroidotomy, venous cut-down, peritoneal lavage, pericardiocentesis, needle thoracocentesis and tube thoracostomy, the arrangement depends on the local situation. In many circumstances, anaesthetized animal models are used whilst in other arrangements, simulated models or mannikins are employed. In each case, the technique of each method is demonstrated to the student and each student carries out the technique in rotation until proficiency is achieved.

Moulage

In each moulage scenario depicting severe injuries, the co-operation of volunteers is enlisted with appropriate make-up and acting skills. The moulage scenarios can be rendered most realistic. Students are involved in an interactive fashion in the management of a seriously injured

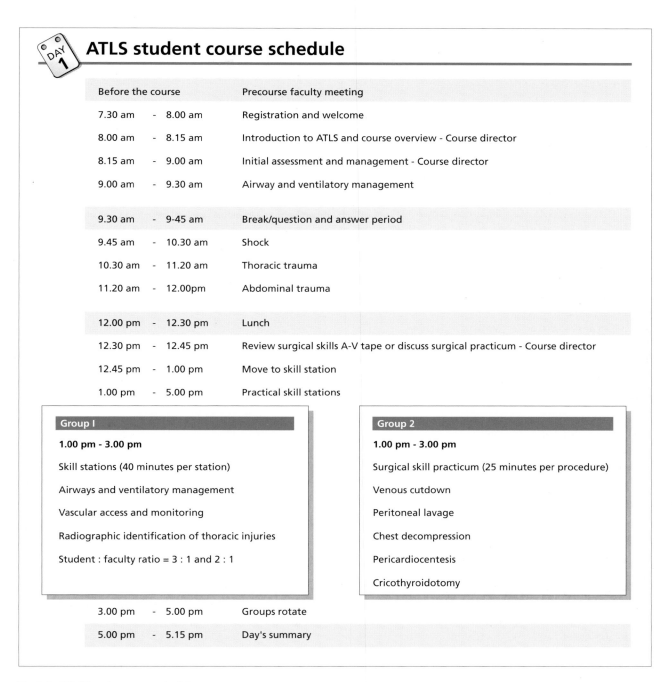

ATLS student course schedule

Before the course		Precourse faculty meeting
7.30 am	- 8.00 am	Registration and welcome
8.00 am	- 8.15 am	Introduction to ATLS and course overview - Course director
8.15 am	- 9.00 am	Initial assessment and management - Course director
9.00 am	- 9.30 am	Airway and ventilatory management
9.30 am	- 9-45 am	Break/question and answer period
9.45 am	- 10.30 am	Shock
10.30 am	- 11.20 am	Thoracic trauma
11.20 am	- 12.00pm	Abdominal trauma
12.00 pm	- 12.30 pm	Lunch
12.30 pm	- 12.45 pm	Review surgical skills A-V tape or discuss surgical practicum - Course director
12.45 pm	- 1.00 pm	Move to skill station
1.00 pm	- 5.00 pm	Practical skill stations

Group I

1.00 pm - 3.00 pm

Skill stations (40 minutes per station)

Airways and ventilatory management

Vascular access and monitoring

Radiographic identification of thoracic injuries

Student : faculty ratio = 3 : 1 and 2 : 1

Group 2

1.00 pm - 3.00 pm

Surgical skill practicum (25 minutes per procedure)

Venous cutdown

Peritoneal lavage

Chest decompression

Pericardiocentesis

Cricothyroidotomy

| 3.00 pm | - 5.00 pm | Groups rotate |
| 5.00 pm | - 5.15 pm | Day's summary |

Fig. 1.2 ATLS® student course schedule.

patient and must perform in accordance with the ATLS®-guided priorities. Fifteen minutes are spent at the first moulage after which another student carries out a critique on the performance. The student then moves to another station where he or she critiques another student. Finally the student moves to a third moulage scenario under test conditions during which assessment is made formally by two Instructors. A possibility of re-testing exists for candidates who do not satisfactorily complete the moulage test.

Students then are involved in discussion on a triage scenario where they are presented with situations involving many injured patients and triage management is discussed. Finally the students sit a post-test examination with multiple choice questionnaire format relating to the core content of the course.

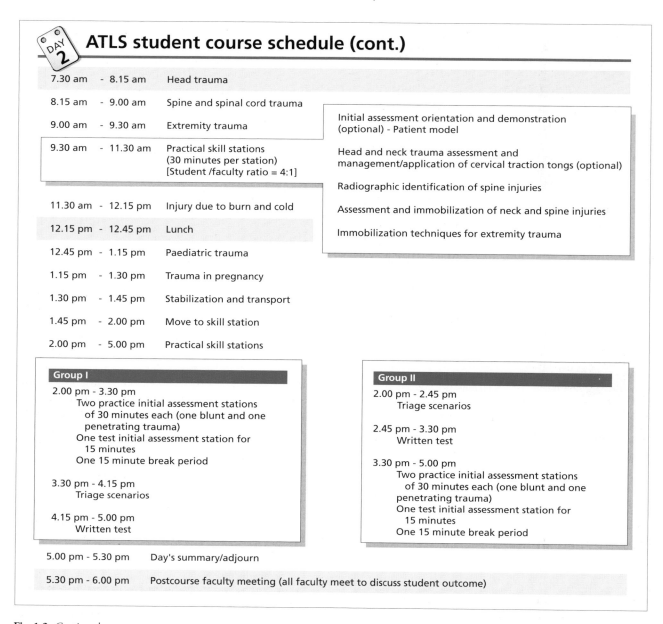

ATLS student course schedule (cont.)

DAY 2

7.30 am - 8.15 am	Head trauma
8.15 am - 9.00 am	Spine and spinal cord trauma
9.00 am - 9.30 am	Extremity trauma
9.30 am - 11.30 am	Practical skill stations (30 minutes per station) [Student /faculty ratio = 4:1]
11.30 am - 12.15 pm	Injury due to burn and cold
12.15 pm - 12.45 pm	Lunch
12.45 pm - 1.15 pm	Paediatric trauma
1.15 pm - 1.30 pm	Trauma in pregnancy
1.30 pm - 1.45 pm	Stabilization and transport
1.45 pm - 2.00 pm	Move to skill station
2.00 pm - 5.00 pm	Practical skill stations

Initial assessment orientation and demonstration (optional) - Patient model

Head and neck trauma assessment and management/application of cervical traction tongs (optional)

Radiographic identification of spine injuries

Assessment and immobilization of neck and spine injuries

Immobilization techniques for extremity trauma

Group I

2.00 pm - 3.30 pm
Two practice initial assessment stations of 30 minutes each (one blunt and one penetrating trauma)
One test initial assessment station for 15 minutes
One 15 minute break period

3.30 pm - 4.15 pm
Triage scenarios

4.15 pm - 5.00 pm
Written test

Group II

2.00 pm - 2.45 pm
Triage scenarios

2.45 pm - 3.30 pm
Written test

3.30 pm - 5.00 pm
Two practice initial assessment stations of 30 minutes each (one blunt and one penetrating trauma)
One test initial assessment station for 15 minutes
One 15 minute break period

5.00 pm - 5.30 pm	Day's summary/adjourn
5.30 pm - 6.00 pm	Postcourse faculty meeting (all faculty meet to discuss student outcome)

Fig. 1.2 *Continued.*

ATLS® provides a safe, simple, effective and didactic system of primary care capable of being followed by all medical practitioners. It is frequently noticed that specialist surgeons or anaesthetists argue about facets of the course. For instance, paediatric surgeons often claim that diagnostic peritoneal lavage has little or no role in the care of a child with suspected abdominal injury or chest surgeons may propose a method of chest tube insertion different from the ATLS® method. Treatment of a patient in a highly specialized centre, such as a paediatric or a chest unit, represents a different stage of care from the emergency primary care in the accident department. When patients come under the care of specialized teams they are then in the definitive care stage where specialist supervision is carried out in accordance with specialist protocols. In the emergency setting during the initial assessment and resuscitation, circumstances are quite different. It has been found worldwide that once this difference is appreciated by specialists they become enthusiastic defenders and protagonists of the ATLS® system.

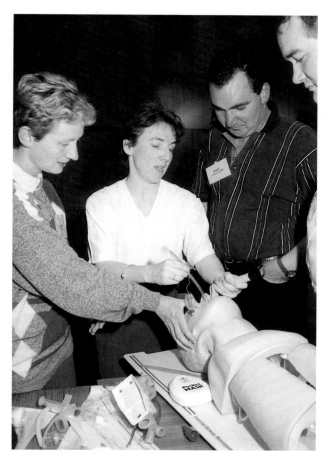

Fig. 1.3 A typical practical skill station.

Student refresher course

Each student who has successfully completed the ATLS® student course is given a card confirming this fact; this document is valid for 4 years. In order to maintain status in the ATLS® programme a refresher course of reverification is required. The refresher course usually consists of a half-day programme often carried out in conjunction with a regular scheduled ATLS® student course. Alternatively, the student may take the entire ATLS® student course again. Thus, the need for re-certification is built into the ATLS® philosophy and has always been accepted without question as an essential component of the programme. The manner in which ATLS® incorporates this renewal of skills after 4 years indicates an ideal and acceptable form of continuing medical education.

Instructor course

The high ratio of teachers to students on any one course indicates the intensity of the programme. The full-time involvement of each instructor requires an uncommon commitment to the principles of ATLS® and to faithful adherence to the course content and structure. It is a truism that not all good practitioners are good teachers, nor are all specialists good ATLS® Instructors. To be an ATLS® Instructor requires, above all, uncommon commitment to the programme, a keen enthusiasm to transmit the principles and the detail of the course, an ability to empathize with and guide students in a constructive directional fashion and also perhaps a sense of humour to lighten the intensity.

Potential Instructors are usually identified as those who have achieved high marks in the student course and who have sufficient enthusiasm to become involved. The identification of potential instructors is an important part of the final assessment in each student course. Before becoming an instructor, each potential instructor must take an Instructor Course and then teach on a student course as an 'Instructor candidate'. Having succeeded in these two tests, the individual becomes an ATLS® Instructor and is given the precious card to mark this achievement. An Instructor Course is a training programme designed to teach individuals how to instruct on an ATLS® programme. Instructor courses are required in each region from time to time in order to expand the cadre of teachers to meet the increasing training needs as ATLS® becomes more widely accepted. The Instructor Course is generally a one and a half-day programme, but may be incorporated in the student course or may be done in a single day. The purpose of the Instructor Course is therefore to allow the potential Instructor, who will have already graduated with distinction in a Student Course, to acquire and demonstrate teaching skills necessary to become an ATLS® Instructor. The course is divided into five primary sessions, each of which will be described briefly.

Session 1: Philosophies of learning and teaching

In the context of the course, learning is defined as being 'a relatively permanent change in behaviour that comes about as a result of a planned experience'. The 'change in behaviour' relates to knowledge, attitudes and skills. The Instructor Course provides guidance on identification of behaviour which requires change. The teaching session is conducted with this in mind and is followed by an evaluation of whether the change in behaviour has been achieved. The importance of motivation is stressed. The desire to learn must come from within the learner and all those involved as teachers on the Instructor Course are responsible, both separately and collectively, for creating an environment conducive to motivating the learner. The techniques of dialogue between teacher and student, the factors which enhance the formal lecture and the methods of improving presentation (including visual aids) are all dealt with in this session. Furthermore, psychomotor learning and the technique of teaching practical skills are analysed and developed.

A basic understanding of the teaching–learning process is provided and an ability to demonstrate and to teach at the skill stations is practised and refined. This session also stresses to the potential Instructor the importance of transmitting faithfully the course content to the student and emphasizes the need for a high level of commitment in all ATLS® Instructors.

Session 2: Group discussion

Methods of initiating, conducting and summarizing teacher–learner dialogue form part of the teaching process of group discussion. This section also deals with techniques of facilitating constructive discussion, controlling dissent, involving each member of the student group and dealing with 'difficult' students. Appropriate use of questioning techniques and guidelines for posing and evaluating questions to encourage dialogue are stressed. The difference between teacher-centred and learner-centred discussion is identified. In the teacher-centred format the Instructor poses a problem, the student responds and the teacher facilitates the discussion. In the learner-centred dialogue, the Instructor asks the leading question and the students discuss the issue in groups. The Instructor rotates among the groups but does not lead the dialogue. The advantages and disadvantages of group discussion as a teaching strategy are explained. Methods for directing and guiding these discussions are introduced.

Session 3: Skills teaching practice

The purpose of this session is to teach the skill stations and this involves the supervised demonstration that the potential Instructor outlines the steps in each practical skill station and then demonstrates the practical skills involved utilizing a teaching technique. There follows a critique by another potential Instructor who criticizes the performance both in terms of content and the mode of transmitting the information and the skill. In the skills-teaching session, airway and ventilatory management, assessment and management of head and neck trauma and radiological identification of spinal injuries are utilized.

Session 4: Microteaching

Session 4 is concerned with microteaching and during this part of the programme, each student is allowed the opportunity to practise lecturing techniques by conducting a 5-minute lecture after which a group discussion takes place. This is followed in turn by critique techniques. In this session the 5-minute lecture is videotaped and the group analyses the presentation with the Educator leading the group discussion. The mini-lecture is analysed and reviewed and critiqued. This system continues until each member of the group has presented a 5-minute lecture which is reviewed and analysed by all the other potential Instructors.

Session 5: Initial Assessment Skill Station

Session 5 in the Instructor Course aims at instructing the participant on the role and responsibility of each faculty member in teaching the Initial Assessment Skill Station of the ATLS® course. The purpose of the session is to enable the potential Instructor to describe the purpose of the Initial Assessment Skill Station and to state the steps involved in this process. He or she should also be able to define the roles of the student, the student Instructor and the faculty members at this Station and to demonstrate satisfactory methods for critiquing a student's performance.

Instructor cards are valid for 4 years from the date of successful completion of the teaching requirements for Instructor Candidates. An Instructor must teach four courses in 4 years if he wishes to retain active Instructor Status in the ATLS® programme. He or she also must be reverified every 4 years to retain certification.

The Course Director

The Course Director is a surgeon who has Instructor status. The Course Director is responsible for the supervision of the content and quality of the entire student course. These responsibilities include selection of the teaching faculty, the assignment of roles to each of the Instructors, the maintenance of time schedules for each part of the course and co-ordination of all assessments and reports during the course. Course Directors are therefore usually Instructors with very considerable ATLS® teaching experience who also have a thorough knowledge of the local arrangements on the course site.

The ATLS® Educator

Because the success of an ATLS® course depends largely on the quality of the teaching the role of a Medical Educator is crucial. The skilled and experienced Educator can transform Potential Instructors into highly effective communicators and teachers. Acquisition of teaching skills is relevant to all medical practitioners. The Instructor Course programme of ATLS® involves careful analysis of all the components involved in formal lecturing, small group dialogue and tuition in practical skills. The techniques involved are clearly spelt out in the Instructor manual and these are reinforced and enhanced by a committed Educator. In order to be a qualified Educator, an individual should have a doctorate degree in education, a proven ability to communicate effectively with medical personnel and must have proven abilities in lecturing and group discussion. The Educator should also have the ability to demonstrate both direct and indirect teaching styles and have experience in teaching workshops or continuing educational courses.

Recent changes in ATLS®

In 1987 the updated edition of the ATLS® programme introduced a new emphasis. It is now stressed that the ATLS® process is applicable to any trauma care environment from the most isolated rural areas to the most sophisticated trauma centre. Accordingly the content of the programme is expanded and more interaction with the students is encouraged so that some of the lectures are truly interactive discussions. All the skill stations now utilize a structured interactive format designed to explore cognitive as well as psychomotor skills. The change in the skill stations requires more intensive preparation on the part of the Instructors than heretofore. Major revisions in the course now requires that all Instructors, Educators and Coordinators take some refresher training before becoming involved in the new system. The Student Course Programme may involve extending the programme to two and a half days in most cases. This arrangement will inevitably pose additional strain, in terms of time, cost and good will, on all involved in ATLS® programmes. Such costs are considerable and may result in the lost of some experienced Instructors. On the other hand, the course is now more comprehensive and streamlined than previously.

Requirements for trauma care

A system of trauma care requires:
1 Rapid access to emergency care when an accident occurs;
2 Expeditious pre-hospital care;
3 a focused system of hospital care; and
4 an established programme of rehabilitation.
Although pre-hospital care and hospital care require both equipment and personnel, the most important element is the presence of highly-skilled personnel capable of providing advanced life support techniques. It is crucially important to recognize and insist that patients with multiple injuries should be transferred to the nearest appropriate centre capable of dealing with poly-trauma. Such patients with serious injuries should not be sent simply to the nearest hospital which may often lack personnel and facilities required (Table 1.3).

Trauma has been called the 'neglected disease'. It has been neglected in terms of research funding and in terms of organizational systems. It is also largely neglected in many surgi-

Table 1.3 Reasons for international acceptance of ATLS®.

1 The problem of serious injury is a concern in every country.
2 Recognition of the concept of preventable deaths after injury has led to recognition that patients with serious injuries are often treated inexpertly.
3 The need for a system of trauma care is accepted everywhere.
4 It has been demonstrated that expeditious appropriate primary care prevents 'second peak' and 'third peak' deaths following injury and probably reduces serious long-term disability.
5 A system of trauma care must focus on life-threatening problems and deal with these on a priority basis so that the greatest threat to life must be treated first.
6 The system must be highly directional, didactic, even doctrinaire, so that a rigid system can be followed in each case. Adherence to the system is accepted as being of great importance, particularly for practitioners who encounter seriously injured patients only occasionally.

cal training programmes where the inevitable drive towards specialization rarely involves a commitment or dedication to optimum primary care of the patient with multiple injuries. Yet trauma remains a surgical disease and all surgeons should be competent in orderly resuscitation following injury. All graduating doctors will be familiar with the theoretical sequences in such care but there seems little doubt that practical courses such as ATLS® are needed to translate the theory into practical action. The primary care of the patient with multiple injuries in the golden hour remains firmly the responsibility of the general surgeon. After initial primary survey and assessment of airway, breathing and circulation with immediate resuscitation there follows the secondary survey or total patient evaluation where all injuries are identified and assessed. After the patient's injuries have been identified, life-threatening problems have been managed, definitive care begins. Definitive care requires specialist involvement and frequently requires transfer of the patient to another institution.

Because the management of trauma is a problem for surgeons, the burden of commitment, training, education and quality assurance must fall on surgeons. Decisive and skilled primary care and competent definitive surgical treatment are needed for optimum care, yet current systems of training and practice in surgery often involve increasing specialization so that with seniority the surgeon becomes more and more remote from mainline primary care of the patient with multiple injuries. Thus, even in much-vaunted surgical rotation training programmes with a high degree of specialization, responsibility for emergency care may devolve to the most junior member of the team and management may become a travesty of good care. The report of the Working Party on the Management of Patients with Major Injuries established by the Royal College of Surgeons of England recognizes this anomalous situation. The report states that 'accidental injury is probably the most serious of all the major health problems facing mankind in the developed countries. Yet, with notable exceptions, it appears studiously to be ignored by governments, populations and professions alike'. Standards of care can now be evaluated by a variety of methodologies. The combination of the Trauma Score (TS) and the Injury Severity Score (ISS) is used to define the TRISS index. The Trauma Score is calculated from physiological variables (systolic blood pressure, capillary refill, respiratory rate and Glasgow Coma Score) observed at the time of admission and the Injury Severity Score based on assessment of injuries (major, moderate or severe) is calculated at the time of death or discharge. The patient's age is also considered. By plotting the TS and the ISS against each other in a scatter diagram a 50% probability of survival can be constructed. This type of methodology can be used to compare outcomes which can be used for internal audit and for external comparison. Evidence is accumulating that the introduction of the ATLS® system has been beneficial in improving outcome when assessed by such objective criteria.

Acknowledgement

It is a pleasure to acknowledge the considerable assistance provided by Irvene K. Hughes, RN, Manager, ATLS® Division of the American College of Surgeons, whose commitment, support and advice has been appreciated by everybody involved in the running of ATLS® courses.

Further reading

Ali, J. *et al.* (1993) Trauma outcome improves following the Advanced Trauma Life Support Program in a Developing Country. *Journal of Trauma* **34**(6) 890–899.

Boyd, C.R., Tolson M.A. & Copes, W.S. (1987) Evaluating Trauma Care: The Triss Method. *Journal of Trauma* **27**(4) 370–378.

Collicott, P.E. (1992). Advanced Trauma Life Support (ATLS): Past Present, Future, 16th Stone Lecture, American Trauma Society. *Journal of Trauma* **33**(5) 749–753.

Report of the Working Party on the Management of Patients with Major Injuries (1988) Commission on the Provision of Surgical Services–Royal College of Surgeons of England.

In: *Report by Task Force of the Committee on Trauma of the American College of Surgeons.* (1990) Resources for Optimal Care of the Injured Patient.

CHAPTER 2

Shock

P. Declan Carey, Manas K. Roy & Ray J. Delicata

Definition

Over the last century many authors have tried to offer a suitable definition for shock. In 1872, Gross described shock as 'rude unhinging of the machinery of life'. Blalock, in 1940, highlighted the importance of the heart, the vessels and circulating volume in maintaining homeostasis and recognized shock as a peripheral circulatory failure. This, he felt, resulted from a discrepancy in the size of the vascular bed and the volume of the intravascular fluid. Wiggers (1942) subsequently advanced the concept of effective circulating volume and that impairment of circulation leads to a state of irreversible circulatory failure.

Shock has also been concisely defined as a condition in which the metabolic needs of the body are not met because of inadequate cardiac output. Sepsis was subsequently recognized as another cause of shock, and as this is often associated with increased cardiac output it was time to broaden the definition of shock: 'inadequate blood flow to vital organs or the inability of the body cell mass to metabolise nutrients normally' (MacLean, 1977). This definition focused on two pathophysiological processes: inadequate blood flow and/or a defect in cellular metabolism, which are usually present in all forms of shock.

Classification

It is useful to classify shock into four broad aetiological categories: hypovolaemic, septic, cardiogenic and neurogenic (Table 2.1). A patient's initial cause of shock may fall into one of the above four categories, then, with continued progression, other forms of shock may simultaneously develop as a result of adverse consequences on organs and tissues such as the heart and endothelium (Fig. 2.1).

Hypovolaemic shock

Pathophysiology

Hypovolaemic shock is caused by loss to the vascular system of whole blood, plasma or extracellular fluid. This results in a decrease in the circulating (or effective) intravascular volume. In shock caused by whole blood loss there is also a deficit in the oxygen carrying capacity of the blood.

Cardiovascular response

A fall in systemic blood pressure leads to an immediate increase in the outflow of sympathetic activity from the central nervous system. This is mediated primarily by baroreceptors located in the wall of the aortic arch and in the carotid sinus. Hypotension decreases the stretch applied to the baroreceptors. This markedly decreases the number of receptor generated impulses which, under normal circumstances, exert an inhibitory control on the vasomotor centre.

The sympathetic outburst increases the cardiac output by: (a) causing venoconstriction, thereby increasing the venous return and hence the stroke volume; (b) increasing the myocardial contractility and the heart rate (which is further potentiated by circulating adrenaline released by adrenal medulla); and (c) causing vasoconstriction of the vascular beds of the skin, muscles, kidneys and splanchnic organs (this not only increases the blood pressure but also diverts the blood flow from these areas to the more important, but sparsely innervated, heart and the brain).

Renal response

Antidiuretic hormone (ADH) secreted by the posterior pituitary increases reabsorption of free water from distal tubules of the kidneys. The kidneys release renin in response to decreased renal blood flow. Renin cleaves circulating angiotensinogen (produced by the liver) to angiotensin I

Compensatory reflexes

- Venoconstriction increases venous return to the heart.
- Increased myocardial contractility augments cardiac output.
- Vasoconstriction in skin, muscles and splanchnic organs helps to divert blood flow to the heart and brain.
- Renal absorption of water (ADH) and sodium (aldosterone) helps to restore circulating volume.

Table 2.1 Various causes of shock.

Hypovolaemic shock	
Loss of blood	Crush injury
	Ruptured aortic aneurysm, etc.
Loss of plasma	Burns
Loss of extracellular fluid	Vomiting, as in intestinal obstruction
	Diarrhoea
	Uncontrolled diabetes
Septic shock	
Cardiac shock	
Cardiac compressive	Pneumothorax
	Pericardial tamponade
	Ascites
	Mechanical ventilation
Cardiogenic	Congenital defects
	Myocardial infarction
	Arrythmias
	Cardiomyopathies
Cardiac obstructive	Pulmonary embolism
	Mechanical ventilation
Neurogenic shock	Neurogenic
	Anaphylactic

which is subsequently converted to angiotensin II by the lung and kidney. Angiotensin II is not only a potent vasoconstrictor but also a powerful stimulator of aldosterone release from adrenal cortex. Aldosterone, in turn, leads to an increase in sodium reabsorption by the kidney. This coupled with the increase in free water retention induced by ADH leads to extracellular volume expansion (Fig. 2.2).

Microcirculatory changes

Normal movement of fluid across the microcirculation is governed by hydraulic and oncotic pressures (also known as Starling's forces) present within the lumen of the vessel and in the surrounding interstitium. Arteriolar constriction in response to hypotension decreases the capillary hydrostatic pressure downstream from the arteriole. The capillary colloid oncotic pressure thus becomes the predominating force and leads to net fluid reabsorption into the capillaries. This 'transcapillary refill' can lead to the infusion of fluid of up to 50–120 mL/h.

The capillary blood flow is dependent to a large extent on the viscosity of the blood which in turn is mainly determined by red cells, proteins and the flow rate. At low flow rates blood faces an increased resistance to deformation; this increases its viscosity dramatically, further impairing the compromised circulation in the capillary bed. During diminished microcirculatory flow the endothelial cells are

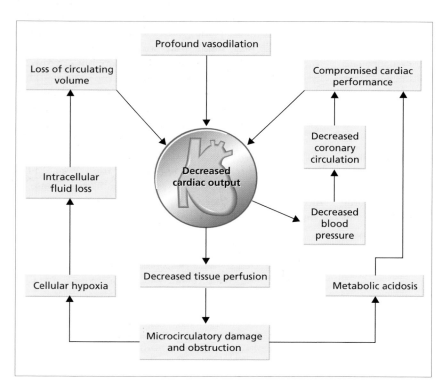

Fig. 2.1 Various causes of shock lead to a common self-perpetuating pathogenic cycle.

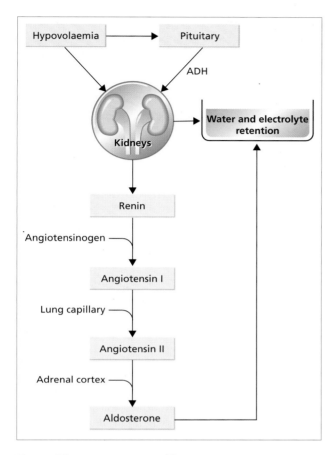

Fig. 2.2 The renin–angiotensin–aldosterone system.

no longer able to produce prostacycline (which normally prevents platelet aggregation). There is, thus, a tendency for microthrombi to develop.

Extracellular fluid response

Although the most common form of hypovolaemic shock results from external blood loss, marked internal redistribution of the extracellular fluid from the intravascular to the extracellular space can also result in a decrease in effective circulating blood volume. This 'third space' loss of fluid occurs in a variety of surgical illnesses, including burns, intestinal obstruction, peritonitis, crush injuries and pancreatitis.

Interesting changes have also been noted in extracellular fluid volume in haemorrhagic shock: there occurs an internal redistribution of extracellular fluid out of the interstitial space and is most likely caused by the isotonic movement of interstitial water and sodium into the neighbouring cell mass (see later). In animal models, this deficit could only be returned to control levels when balanced salt solution was infused in addition to whole blood.

Cellular response

With continued hypoperfusion progressive build-up of metabolic by-products occurs in the microcirculation; impairment of the ubiquitous ATPase-dependent $Na^+–K^+$ pump soon results. Consequently, K^+ leaves the cell and extracellular Na^+ enters the cell drawing with it the interstitial fluid. Replenishment of the depleted extracellular fluid (ECF) with balanced salt solutions helps in restoring the $Na^+–K^+$ pump and, hence, is an important feature of therapy in patients with hypovolaemic shock.

Finally, lack of oxygen leads to uncoupling of oxidative phosphorylation and anaerobic glycolysis then predominates in the intracellular organelles. The consequent intracellular acidosis and lysosomal damage causes spillage of various lysosomal enzymes leading to further breakdown of intracellular organelles and, eventually, cell death and organ dysfunction.

Organ response

Under resting conditions, the heart extracts 75% of oxygen delivered to it. In situations of excess demand the heart cannot extract more oxygen from haemoglobin because of the high affinity of haemoglobin for oxygen under conditions of low oxygen saturation. Furthermore, because increases in heart rate are achieved at the cost of decreased diastolic interval (during which maximum coronary flow occurs), a rapid heart rate further decreases myocardial perfusion. The situation is worse in patients with coronary artery disease because the flow fails to increase through stenosed atherosclerotic arteries. Finally, direct myocardial depression may result from cachectin/tumour necrosis factor (TNF) or other factors released into the circulation, perhaps from the hypoperfused gut.

The renal circulation is also affected by hypovolaemia. In addition to the decrease in total renal blood flow, there is an intrarenal shift of blood from the cortex to medulla (this coupled with renin–angiotensin–aldosterone system results

---

Effects of hypovolaemia

- Increased demand on the heart makes it particularly vulnerable to hypoxia.
- Transient ischaemia of the kidneys leads to non-oliguric failure while sustained hypotension causes tubular necrosis and oliguric renal failure.
- Splanchnic vasoconstriction renders the gut mucosa hypoxic while depression of hepatic metabolic capabilities is a late occurrence.
- Lungs are rarely affected by hypovolaemia.
- Sustained hypoperfusion disrupts cellular $Na^+–K^+$ pump allowing interstitial fluid to enter the cells; hence, some degree of extracellular fluid deficit usually accompanies haemorrhagic shock.

in increased tubular reabsorption of salt and water). Transient and less severe ischaemic insults primarily damage the cells of the thick ascending limb of Henlé. The subsequent decrease of NaCl transport into the medullary interstitium impairs the concentrating ability of the kidney. This defective solute reabsorption continues to produce large quantities of dilute urine leading to non-oliguric renal failure. With severe and/or sustained hypotension, tubular damage is more extensive leading to tubular destruction and backleak with the subsequent development of oliguric renal failure.

The compensatory splanchnic vasoconstriction in the defence of falling blood pressure may compromise gut barrier function. During hypotension, there is significant redistribution of blood favouring the mucosa and submucosa and the amount of blood flowing through mucosa may thereby be maintained. More villi are thus perfused, the vascular cross-sectional area increases and consequently the transit time of blood flowing through the mucosa is increased. The efficacy of the arteriole–venule countercurrent exchanger in villi thereby increases and the superficial part of mucosa becomes severely hypoxic. Reperfusion during resuscitation can also cause intestinal injury. All these factors contribute to increase the mural translocation of bacteria and endotoxin from the lumen into the systemic lymphatic or venous circulation and is believed to be a contributory factor for the eventual progression to multiple organ system failure.

Splanchnic vasoconstriction also affects the liver as portal blood flow is the major component of hepatic perfusion. Although frank ischaemic hepatic necrosis is unusual, ischaemic damage to the liver initially leads to a reduction in the level of ATP (or energy charge) which ultimately impairs the liver's overall metabolic and synthetic capabilities. Depression of reticulo-endothelial function finally ensues and contributes to the development of infection or further organ dysfunction after resuscitation from haemorrhagic shock.

The lung has easy access to the oxygen in the air in the alveoli and hypovolaemic shock on its own has little, if any, effect on lung structure or function. Patients who do develop acute respiratory failure (seen in 1–2% of cases) are those in whom haemorrhage is associated with either severe tissue damage or sepsis. It is due to damage to the alveolar–capillary interface with consequent leakage of proteinaceous fluid from the blood into the interstitial, and subsequently into alveolar, spaces. This results in hypoxia and produces a clinical picture ranging in severity from mild pulmonary dysfunction to progressive pulmonary failure (Fig. 2.3).

Traumatic shock

Traumatic shock is a more virulent form of hypovolaemic shock. Although it is characterized by external and/or inter-

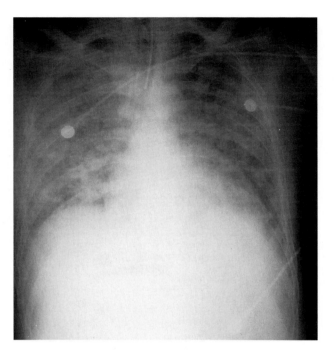

Fig. 2.3 Chest X-ray of a patient with adult respiratory distress syndrome.

nal loss of blood, the volume losses are made worse by extravasation of plasma into tissues. This is due to increase in systemic vascular permeability brought on by various chemical mediators such as: tumour necrosis factor (TFN), interleukin-1 (IL-1), O_2 radicals, kinins, serotonin, etc., released by white blood cells and platelets after being activated by tissue injury. These changes gradually worsen the pre-existing hypovolaemia and the major consequences of traumatic shock usually manifest fully 24–48 h following injury.

Clinical features

The clinical characteristics of hypovolaemic shock depend upon the degree of volume depletion, duration of shock and the body's compensatory reactions. The clinical findings tend to correlate with the organs that are compromised. Symptoms and signs may be: agitation, tachycardia, cool sweaty periphery, collapsed veins, hypotension, tachypnoea, low urinary output, and signs of myocardial ischaemia in ECG in the form of Q waves and depressed ST–T segments.

The normal estimated blood volume (EBV) is 6–8% of total body weight and in general, four categories of volume loss are recognized, based on the percentage loss of EBV (Fig. 2.4). This correlation tends to lose its relevance in patients with impaired cardiovascular function. The pulse rate does not consistently increase in response to hypovolaemia, especially in patients who are on beta-blockers,

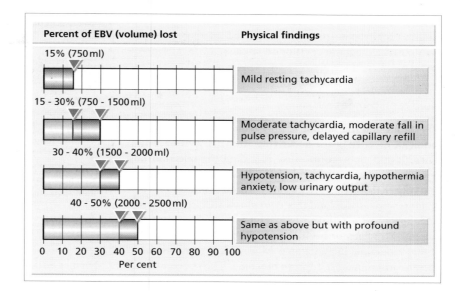

Percent of EBV (volume) lost   **Physical findings**

15% (750 ml) — Mild resting tachycardia

15 - 30% (750 - 1500 ml) — Moderate tachycardia, moderate fall in pulse pressure, delayed capillary refill

30 - 40% (1500 - 2000 ml) — Hypotension, tachycardia, hypothermia anxiety, low urinary output

40 - 50% (2000 - 2500 ml) — Same as above but with profound hypotension

0 10 20 30 40 50 60 70 80 90 100
Per cent

Fig. 2.4 Correlation between clinical signs and degree of hypovolaemia.

and in severely hypovolaemic patients bradycardia may reflect impending cardiac arrest.

Though impracticable in many surgical patients, postural changes in blood pressure are a simple and sensitive indicator of early shock. A systolic blood pressure fall of 20 mmHg, a diastolic blood pressure fall of 10 mmHg or a rise in pulse of 20 beats/min suggests early hypovolaemia. A low urinary output (defined as less than 0.5 ml/kg/h in the adult or less than 2.0 ml/kg/h in the infant) is also a sensitive indicator of early and progressing hypovolaemic shock. A fall in the haematocrit with intravenous administration of asanguineous fluid is another useful sign of continuing hypovolaemia.

These typical responses may be entirely blunted in the inebriated patient. High blood alcohol induces a generalized vasodilatation and also inhibits the secretion of ADH. Hypotension can thus be an early sign in these patients who may be warm and producing a good amount of urine.

In dealing with head injury patients who are also shocked, a diligent search should be made for any source of hypovolaemia as these patients may be hypotensive because of significant hypovolaemia. Normovolaemic patients with severe head injuries usually have a *high* blood pressure and a *low* pulse rate (Cushing's reflex).

Treatment

The therapy of hypovolaemic shock concentrates on detecting the causative mechanisms while providing support to the patient. Initial resuscitation should begin with ensuring adequate ventilation and oxygenation. In the unconscious patient, this is easily achieved by lowering the head with support of the jaw and administering supplemental oxygen.

In the presence of airway obstruction, the trachea should be intubated and mechanical ventilation initiated.

Haemorrhagic shock is best treated by identification and prompt control of the source of bleeding. External bleeding should be tamponaded by compression. In cases of internal haemorrhage, e.g. ruptured aortic aneurysm, stab wounds, etc., preparations must be made to transfer the patient to the operating theatre (informing the anaesthetist, theatre personnel, blood bank, etc.) as the initial resuscitation proceeds unabated.

Administration of intravenous fluids and/or blood remains the cornerstone of managing hypovolaemia and it requires a prompt access to the venous system. A percutaneously placed cannula in the upper extremity provides adequate access for management of cases of mild hypovolaemia. In severe cases two or three large-bore cannulae should be inserted. The best large-bore catheter is a length of intravenous tubing placed surgically into a saphenous vein at the ankle. A central venous catheter, though very useful to measure the right atrial pressure, is best placed semi-electively.

After obtaining venous access, blood samples must be withdrawn to estimate haematocrit, urea and electrolytes, glucose (as diabetic ketoacidosis may present with hypovolaemia while profound hypoglycaemia may mimic hypovolaemic shock) and for grouping and cross-matching.

A Foley catheter needs to be inserted and is only postponed (or replaced by suprapubic cystostomy) in cases suspected to have sustained injuries to urethra and urinary bladder. Passage of a nasogastric tube is essential in patients with abdominal catastrophe such as peritonitis or intestinal obstruction. Victims of trauma require X-rays of the cervical spine (with good views of C7), thorax, pelvis and specific sites of concern and due consideration should be given to tetanus prophylaxis. In cases of suspected internal abdominal injuries a diagnostic peritoneal lavage may be extremely useful.

Fluid replacement

The nature and the volume of fluid required during resuscitation are dictated by the underlying cause of hypovolaemia. There is still some controversy regarding the selection of crystalloid versus colloid solutions. Proponents of crystalloid believe that hypovolaemia affects both the intravascular and interstitial spaces and that crystalloids are distributed to both spaces in a ratio of 1:3. This is also important in patients with haemorrhagic hypovolaemia where alleviation of the reduction in functional ECF with crystalloids has been clearly shown to improve outcome. The concern that crystalloid infusion increases lung water has not been substantiated in experimental models. Those favouring colloidal solutions emphasize the urgency of expanding the intravascular volume; colloids produce a volume expansion greater than the transfused volume because of their osmotic properties. This advantage is transient as the molecules rapidly diffuse into the interstitial spaces. Also, in hypovolaemic shock associated with extensive tissue damage or sepsis (where the endothelium becomes leaky) they are less effective as plasma expanders, and in fact, may aggravate pulmonary oedema. Be that as it may, each case should be managed on its own merits depending on the nature and amount of fluid lost.

Ringer's lactate is the preferred crystalloid solution. It is isotonic, iso-ionic and the lactate buffers the hydrogen ion that is washed out of the ischaemic tissues. The lactic acid which is produced as a result requires enough liver function to convert the acid to water and carbon dioxide by the Kreb's cycle. The required amount of hepatic function is usually of no concern even if the patient is in deep shock. However, Ringer's lactate should preferably not be used in patients with severe pre-existing cirrhosis.

Hydroxyethyl starch, an amylopectin, and dextran, a polysaccharide are the most commonly used artificial colloid solutions. They are reasonably inexpensive and safe, although both have been associated with rare anaphylactoid reactions and ill-defined transient coagulopathies. These solutions have colloidal properties similar to albumin, which is rarely used for resuscitation today.

Hypertonic saline solutions (drawing water out of the cells) in combination with a synthetic colloid (retaining the recovered volume in the vascular space) have also been used. Current clinical data do not show an improvement in survival. They may have some role in prehospital settings where large volume resuscitation is impossible and skilled personnel unavailable. The greatest potential benefit may be in patients with head injury and hypovolaemic shock.

Treatment of hypovolaemic shock

- Restoration of circulating volume with crystalloids or colloids.
- Ringer's lactate is the preferred crystalloid: it is isotonic, iso-ionic and the lactate buffers the hydrogen ions derived from ischaemic tissues.
- Significant blood loss necessitates blood transfusion.
- A haematocrit of 30–35% provides adequate oxygen carrying capacity.
- Measurement of hourly urine output and CVP are simple aids to monitor fluid replacement.
- In patients with traumatic shock, fractures should be identified and stabilized.

Further management depends on the response of the patient to the fluid administered. Two to three litres of fluid given over 5–15 min resuscitates any patient whose haemorrhage has now stopped. Subsequent deterioration indicates ongoing bleeding and calls for prompt surgical control.

Blood administration

In haemorrhagic shock, blood transfusion should be limited to patients with uncontrolled bleeding and in whom the estimated blood loss is 30% or greater of expected blood volume (1500–2000 ml). If the patient can be operated on promptly, blood is best administrated after surgical control of bleeding is obtained. Initial resuscitation leads to release of products of anaerobic and catabolic metabolism into the systemic circulation. Transient myocardial dysfunction can thus result. This will be more pronounced if resuscitation begins with acidotic, cold bank blood with high potassium concentration. Administration of blood before surgical control of haemorrhage also means a waste of blood-bank reserves.

In patients with exsanguinating haemorrhage, blood may have to be given before surgical control of bleeding is obtained. If cross-matched units are not available, type specific blood can be administered. It has negligible risk for transfusion reaction as these patients have little of their own blood remaining in their vascular space after resuscitation. O negative blood can be given if type specific blood is not available; but this complicates typing of blood after the patient's initial resuscitation.

In deciding how much blood to transfuse it is important to recall that the microcirculatory flow is determined by viscosity of the blood which varies with the haematocrit levels. A haematocrit level of 30–35% will provide adequate O_2 carrying capacity without further impairing flow. This is the preferred limit of transfusion in patients with coronary heart disease while a young patient with a normal heart can tolerate haematocrit values as low as 15%, provided the circulating volume is kept normal.

Positioning

The traditional head-down position is no longer believed to be of value in treating hypovolaemic shock. It may transiently shift some blood from the limbs to the heart. In fact, in shocked patients, the peripheral venules and small veins are already empty from volume loss and vasoconstriction. The elevated extremities also place an added burden on the heart and in patients with chest trauma, the Trendelenburg position interferes with respiratory exchange. Finally, the effect of this posture on the cerebral circulation in the presence of hypovolaemia has not been clarified.

MAST garments

Military antishock trousers (MAST) may be of some value in immobilizing extremity fractures and minimizing blood loss. They, however, failed to live up to the expectation and to the belief that they increase venous return (see above). Over-inflation may jeopardize limb perfusion and hinder left ventricular emptying. Compression of the abdomen pushes the diaphragm into the chest, compresses the heart, and limits ventricular filling.

Pulmonary support

Oxygen saturation in the majority of patients with uncomplicated hypovolaemic shock is generally normal. However, in patients with pre-existing chronic obstructive lung disease, pneumothorax, pulmonary contusion, aspiration of gastric content, etc., it is essential to administer O_2 via a loosely fitting face mask.

Analgesics

It is important to administer analgesics in patients with shock if the causative injury produces severe pain as in victims of trauma, peritonitis, etc. Small doses of narcotics given intravenously serve the purpose well.

Antibiotics

Antibiotics are recommended in patients who have open or potentially contaminated wounds.

Steroids

Steroid depletion with hypovolaemic shock may possibly occur in the elderly patient or in patients who have specific adrenocortical diseases: Addison's disease, post-adrenalectomy patients or patients who have adrenal suppression with exogenous steroids. Intravenous administration of hydrocortisone is indicated in these situations.

Septic shock

Septic shock is currently the most common cause of death in non-coronary intensive care units. Septic shock is often a complication of opportunistic infection and is seen commonly in patients after major surgery, trauma, burns, advanced liver cirrhosis, diabetes mellitus, haematological and solid malignancies, renal failure or acquired immune deficiency syndrome (AIDS). Increasing use of intravascular and biliary devices, indwelling urinary catheter, prolonged endotracheal intubation, and also increasing numbers of patients receiving chemotherapy and immunosuppressive treatments have contributed to the greater number of victims of sepsis (Figs 2.5 and 2.6). Though all classes of organisms may cause sepsis, Gram-negative rod bacteria are by far the commonest.

It is well recognized that only half of the patients judged as septic have positive blood cultures and that patients with acute pancreatitis or trauma may have clinical signs of 'sepsis' *without* proven infection. Host response, hitherto believed to be passive, is now known to be responsible for the clinical expression of 'sepsis' in a variety of infectious and non-infectious situations.

It is believed that 'sepsis' is an evolving process. It has been recognized by the American College of Chest Physicians (Society of Critical Care Medicine Consensus Conference, 1991). Various stages of progression of septic state were outlined:

Systemic inflammatory response syndrome (SIRS)

SIRS implies a clinical response arising from a variety of insults and includes two or more of the following:
1 Temperature $> 38\,°C$ or $< 36\,°C$
2 Heart rate > 90 beats/min
3 Respiratory rate > 20 breaths/min
4 White blood cell count $> 12.0 \times 10^9\,L^{-1}$, $< 4.0 \times 10^9\,L^{-1}$ or > 0.10 immature forms (bands).

Sepsis

This state includes SIRS plus a documented infection (positive culture for organisms).

Severe sepsis

Sepsis associated with organ dysfunction, hypoperfusion abnormalities or hypotension is classed as severe. Hypoperfusion abnormalities include, but are not limited to,

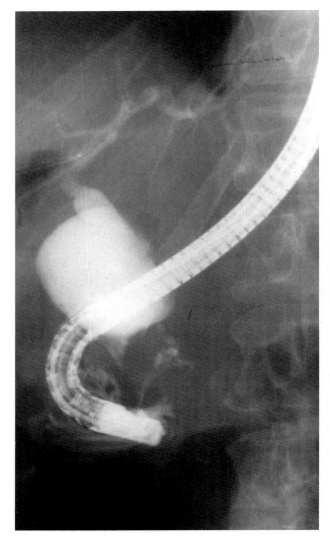

Fig. 2.5 Obstructed biliary system predisposes to cholangitis and bacteriaemia.

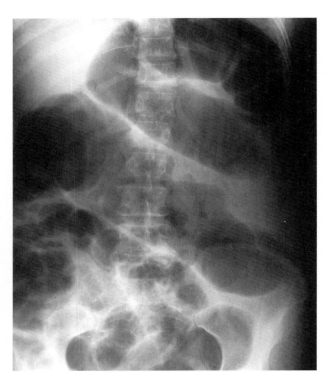

Fig. 2.6 Caecum may perforate during large bowel obstruction and cause fulminant faecal peritonitis.

lactic acidosis, oliguria or an acute alteration in mental status.

Septic shock

Septic shock is classed as sepsis-induced hypotension (despite fluid resuscitation) plus hypoperfusion abnormalities.

These stages are thought to represent a continuum of host response to infection and other inflammatory insults (see Fig. 2.7). Sepsis and its sequelae reflect increasing severity of the *systemic response* to infection and not increasing severity of infection. Bacterial infection and other acute insults

merely trigger an orchestra of chemical mediators which bring on the characteristic host response thereby precipitating a self perpetuating cascade.

Mediators of sepsis

The various mediators of sepsis are now briefly described followed by the possible mechanism of the sepsis cascade (Fig. 2.8).

Non-cytokine mediators

• *Endotoxin:* Lipopolysaccharide (LPS) component of the cell wall of Gram-negative bacteria, which is thought to start the process of sepsis.
• *Exotoxins: Staphylococcus aureus* (Gram-positive) toxin functions comparable to endotoxin.
• *Complements:* The well-studied complement cascade is activated by endotoxins, extensive soft tissue injury and also by interaction with the coagulation system. It is capable of producing vasodilatation and increased vascular permeability.
• *Coagulation factors:* The perturbation of coagulation, which is very common in sepsis, stems from activation of Factor XII by endotoxin. The most severe form of coagu-

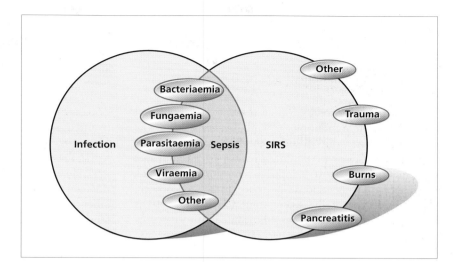

Fig. 2.7 Interrelationship between sepsis, SIRS and infection. (*Critical Care Medicine* 1992; 20: 865).

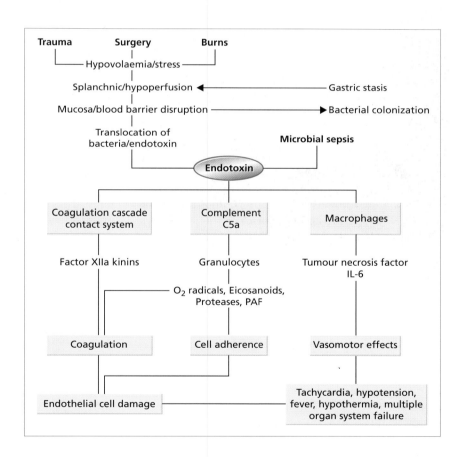

Fig. 2.8 Possible interactions leading to sepsis.

lopathy that it can cause is disseminated intravascular coagulation.

• *Arachidonic acid metabolites:* Priming of macrophages by LPS increases phospholipase-A$_2$ activity. Various pros-taglandins produced thereafter alter regional blood flow, enhance microvascular permeability, depress myocardial function and promote activation and chemotaxis of neutrophils.

• *Kallikrein–bradykinin system:* This is activated by Factor XII and leads to margination of leukocytes, smooth muscle relaxation and increased vascular permeability.

Cytokine mediators

The cytokines are produced in all organs of the body and establish a communication network between cells. The cytokines important in the pathogenesis of sepsis are:
• *Interleukins:* They are produced mainly by macrophages and endothelial cells. IL-1 induces a prothrombotic state, the degree of IL-6 response has been found to correlate with the severity of the septic condition while IL-10 is believed to downregulate major histocompatibility complex (MHC) Class II antigen expression on monocytes and T cells.
• *Tumour necrosis factor (TNF):* endotoxins release TNF from macrophages and many of the pathological sequelae of endotoxins are reproduced by infusion of exogenous TNF.
• *Interferons:* They are produced by lymphocytes and play a multifactorial role in the pathogenesis of sepsis. They are believed to increase production of IL-1 and also augment the production of complement.

Microcirculatory changes and the vascular endothelium

A large number of vascular abnormalities have been described in patients with septic shock; many vascular beds are dilated but some are also constricted. This results in maldistribution of blood flow. Aggregation of neutrophils and platelets and subsequent release of chemical mediators can cause direct endothelial damage and increased capillary permeability. This tilts the delicate balance between endothelial prostacyclin (inhibitor of platelet aggregation and vasodilatation) and platelet-generated thromboxane (platelet aggregator and vasoconstrictor) in favour of the latter.

The endothelium also produces nitric oxide; the inducible nitric oxide is thought to be responsible for causing profound vasodilatation and myocardial depression. Efforts are underway to see whether nitric oxide inhibition improves survival and whether its inhalation reduces pulmonary hypertension seen so often in acute respiratory distress syndrome (ARDS).

Cardiovascular abnormalities

Cardiac performance in sepsis is characterized by increased heart rate, increased cardiac output, normal stroke volume in the face of *reduced* ejection fraction and increased end diastolic and systolic volume. Endotoxin and TNF have been shown to be myocardial depressant and also, there is

poor β-adrenergic mediated stimulation of cAMP in the septic heart.

Marked vasodilatation and profound decrease of peripheral vascular resistance is another characteristic feature of septic shock. The consequent increase in blood flow, curiously, is excessive relative to the increased metabolic demands. This presumably is in response to oxygen debt incurred peripherally; a defect in oxygen and fuel substrate use is now considered to be the primary abnormality in sepsis. The cause of this decreased peripheral use of oxygen is not fully known. One possibility is the altered microcirculation (see above) leading to decreased tissue perfusion; the other hypothesis being abnormal cellular metabolism in sepsis. The relationship between O_2 delivery (Do_2) and consumption (Vo_2) is also abnormal in patients with septic shock: Vo_2 continues to increase (rather than plateau, as in normal subjects) as Do_2 increases. An effort, thus, must always be made to optimize oxygen delivery.

Gut in sepsis

The mechanisms regulating oxygenation of gut mucosa have been described earlier. Though splanchnic vasoconstriction is the normal response to hypotension, intestinal resistance in sepsis might be normal or decreased and then splanchnic blood flow will parallel changes in cardiac output.

Around 50% of patients with Gram-negative blood culture are endotoxaemic and this endotoxin is often *Escherichia coli*-derived. The gut is considered to be an important source of endotoxin in many patients. Impairment of gut barrier function, which facilitates translocation of bacteria and endotoxin, is in the majority of cases caused by mucosal hypoxia (rather than frank ischaemic necrosis) and measurement of gastric mucosal pH is believed to be a more reliable predictor of outcome than simple measurements of oxygen delivery.

Multiple organ dysfunction syndrome

Unabated progression of the septic state with worsening tissue perfusion and oxygenation leads to progressive deterioration in organ function: ARDS, circulatory instability, renal failure, liver dysfunction, disseminated intravascular coagulation, etc. gradually sets in. This pattern of multiple and progressive dysfunction of organ systems has been termed as multiple organ dysfunction syndrome (MODS).

Clinical manifestations

The patients with septic shock can be in a hyperdynamic or high flow state where the cardiac output is high and peripheral vascular resistance is low. The patient is warm and pink. Alternatively in the hypodynamic or low-flow form hypotension occurs in the setting of decreased cardiac output and a greatly increased vascular resistance. The extremities are cool, mottled and cyanotic, mainly caused by peripheral vasoconstriction brought on by increased sympathetic tone.

Response to sepsis is variable, with either the hyperdynamic or hypodynamic state predominating at a given point. The patient's transition between the two states depends on cardiovascular reserve and state of hydration. In general, during the early stages of septicaemia, the patient manifests confusion, fever, hyperventilation and is warm and dry with pink extremities, a bounding peripheral pulse and oliguria. Without adequate volume and cardiac resuscitation, the patient may then enter a state of hypodynamic septic shock. With fluid resuscitation, however, most patients will enter a state of hyperdynamic sepsis and will remain so until the infectious process is controlled or multisystem organ failure supervenes. As the cardiovascular reserve diminishes, the hypodynamic state usually predominates. A patient, however, with myocardial dysfunction or with diminished circulatory reserve (fluid loss from diarrhoea, vomiting, etc.) may be hypodynamic and hypotensive from the very beginning.

Management

The initial management is similar to that described in the section on hypovolaemic shock. The specific treatment plan is as follows:

Identification and eradication of sepsis

Using clinical wisdom and radiological techniques the septic focus needs to be promptly identified. Abscess cavities should be drained (surgically or percutaneously), the patient with cholangitis should have obstructing stones removed by endoscopic retrograde cholangiopancreatography (ERCP) and patient with peritonitis require urgent laparotomy etc. The use of specific antibiotics based on appropriate culture and sensitivity tests is desirable when possible. As the result may not be available for several days, a Gram stain of any aspirated material may be used instead. The third-generation cephalosporins continue to enjoy their popularity. Intra-abdominal infections also require the addition of metronidazole to cover the anaerobes. Ceftazidime or imipenem–cilastatin are acceptable single agents. As shock is an additional risk factor for aminoglycoside induced nephrotoxicity, many current regimens avoid the aminoglycosides.

Support of various organ systems

Patients with septic shock are frequently critically ill. They require close monitoring as regards their fluid balance, cardiac function, respiratory support, renal function, stress

---

Septic shock

- Patients with clinical signs of sepsis may not harbour an infective focus.
- Host response to chemical mediators released by infective or traumatic insults bring about the manifestations of sepsis.
- Marked vasodilatation and decreased peripheral vascular resistance is a characteristic feature.
- Impairment of gut mucosal integrity is a common occurrence: gut derived endotoxins are a frequent finding in the blood of patients with Gram-negative septicaemia.
- Depending on the cardiovascular reserve and the state of hydration, patients may either be hyperdynamic (warm phase) or hypodynamic (cool phase).
- Eradication of the infective focus constitutes the most important intervention.

---

ulcer prophylaxis, nutritional support, coagulation failure and are best managed in the intensive therapy unit (ITU) (see later).

Manipulation of inflammatory cascade

As an adjunct to the above mentioned antimicrobials, some promising research has suggested a role for immunomodulation of the 'sepsis' cascade. Monoclonal antibodies have been manufactured against components of endotoxin, TNF, interleukins and leucocyte adhesion receptors. Current clinical data is sparse and many trials are in progress. Though high dose steroids appear to reduce the release of lysosomal enzymes, data to date is disappointing in the clinical setting. Non-steroidal anti-inflammatory drugs (NSAIDs) have been shown to limit oxygen radical production by neutrophils, and hopefully, the future will lie in these exciting new treatments.

Cardiac shock

This form of shock is characterized by the inability of the heart to generate sufficient cardiac output in the face of adequate intravascular volume. It can be due to various causes (Table 2.1).

Diagnosis

In the appropriate clinical setting, it is not difficult to diagnose cardiac shock. Myocardial infarction classically presents with chest pain, palpitation and shock with crepts in the lung bases. Neck veins are usually distended; if flat a more thorough evaluation is necessary to exclude common causes of hypovolaemia. Although an ECG is extremely useful, hypovolaemia *per se* can induce ischaemic changes.

Cardiac tamponade is evident in patients who present with distended neck veins in addition to features of hypovolaemic shock. It is a useful clinical sign when confronted with an acutely injured patient with shock. Patients with a **tension pneumothorax** have a shift of the trachea to the uninvolved side, a hyper-resonant percussion note and diminished breath sounds on the involved side. A patient with muffled heart sound, enlarged cardiac shadow on the chest film with diminished voltage on the ECG is certainly suffering from **pericardial tamponade**. In a trauma victim if the chest film shows a double-air density in the left lower lung field, a blunted costophrenic angle and a nasogastric tube curled up in the chest **traumatic diaphragmatic herniation** has certainly occurred. Blunt trauma to the heart either produces an arrythmia or a cardiac rupture that is immediately fatal or produces no injury of any clinical consequence.

Treatment

The various therapeutic options available are tailored towards the underlying cause. A tension pneumothorax, diagnosed clinically, should be decompressed by the insertion of a 14 gauge needle in the second intercostal space in the midclavicular line followed by formal placement of a chest tube. The latter should be inserted into the fourth intercostal space (less chance of perforating the diaphragm) in the mid-axillary line (least muscular part of the thorax). Upon failing to reverse the haemodynamic abnormalities, a needle should be inserted in the opposite side as tension pneumothoraces can be difficult to lateralize in some patients. Acute pericardial tamponade in a stable patient is dealt with by pericardiocentesis with a needle inserted to the left of the xiphoid process directing it upwards and backwards at a 45° angle. Withdrawal of 50 ml of blood should return the vital signs to normal. Diaphragmatic lacerations are best dealt with prompt laparotomy and suture.

The initial treatment of cardiogenic shock begins with administration of oxygen, pain relief and strict monitoring of vital signs, ECG and hourly urinary output. Optimization of heart rate remains the first step in the treatment of cardiogenic shock and one suggested plan of management is as shown in the flow chart (Fig. 2.9).

Fluid management

It is important to optimize the ventricular end-diastolic volume and a decision needs to be made whether the patient needs fluid or a diuretic. If thought to be hypovolaemic, a fluid bolus of 250 mL should be given over a period of 10 min. Worsening of the patient's condition suggests pre-existing volume overload and a single intravenous dose of frusemide, 40 mg should be given. This important decision is simplified if a Swan–Ganz catheter is in place and fluid infusion guided by left atrial filling pressure.

Vasodilators

Reduction of the afterload with sodium nitroprusside can be of use in patients with low cardiac output despite high filling pressures. The consequent decrease in systemic vascular resistance augments ventricular emptying and increases tissue perfusion.

Inotropic agents

Dopamine and dobutamine are very useful inotropes. Dopamine in low doses (less than $5\,\mu g/kg/min$), not only increases myocardial contractility but also dilates renal vessels, thereby increasing renal blood flow. Only very occasionally they worsen the existing vasoconstriction.

Beta-blockers

These are indicated in those occasional patients with recent myocardial infarction and tachycardia. Decreasing myocardial contractility and heart rate decreases the myocardial oxygen requirement, thereby protecting the surrounding myocardium which has marginal viability.

Reperfusion strategies

Treatment modalities such as thrombolysis (streptokinase, tissue plasminogen activator (TPA)) and percutaneous transluminal coronary angioplasty have become popular in patients who have recently suffered myocardial infarction. The idea is to restore the patency of coronary arteries.

Mechanical support

In patients with severe left ventricular dysfunction, the inflation of the balloon of an intra-aortic balloon pump in

---

Cardiac shock

- Neck veins are usually distended.
- Shift of the trachea and a hyperresonant percussion note suggests tension pneumothorax.
- A 14-gauge needle is promptly inserted in the second intercostal space if tension pneumothorax is clinically suspected.
- Pericardial tamponade presents with muffled heart sounds and enlarged cardiac shadow on the chest radiograph; needle pericardiocentesis normalizes the haemodynamic status.
- Administration of oxygen, pain relief and optimization of heart rate are vital steps in the management of patients with myocardial infarction.

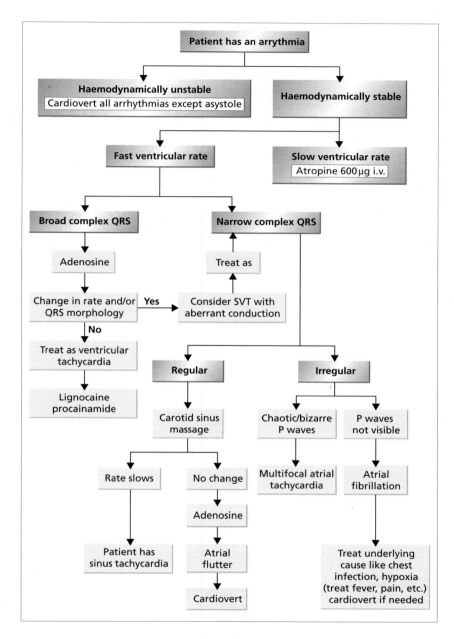

Fig. 2.9 An approach to a patient with acute arrythmia.

Neurogenic shock

This type of shock is a result of interruption of the autonomic innervation of the blood vessels. It is seen in patients with injury to the spinal cord or in those receiving high spinal anaesthesia. This is also the shock which occurs with sudden exposure to unpleasant events (e.g.

diastole (improving coronary filling) and deflation while in systole (augmenting ventricular contraction) can be of substantial value.

pain) and is commonly called syncope. Reflex interruption of nerve impulses also occurs with acute gastric dilatation.

Loss of vasomotor control expands the reservoir capacity in both arterioles and venules leading to peripheral pooling, inadequate ventricular filling and hypotension. Pulse rate may be slower if the adrenergic nerves to heart are blocked. Skin is usually dry, warm and pink. Heat loss is a major problem and the many patients are hypothermic. If not corrected at the right time, blood flow to major organs gradually becomes compromised.

Treatment

As in other forms of shock, treatment is directed towards the underlying cause. In syncopal attacks, simply removing the patient from the stimulus, relieving pain and elevating the legs may be all that is needed. The Trendelenburg position displaces the blood from the veins to the heart; in contrast to other forms of shock, as the vascular resistance is decreased, elevation of legs does not impede ventricular emptying.

Filling of the heart is also aided by intravenous fluid administration and several litres of fluid (in an adult) may be needed. Vasoconstrictors (e.g. phenylephedrine) are then added if blood pressure does not rise promptly. It is the only situation where a Swan–Ganz catheter may be omitted despite the patient being on vasoconstrictors. A word of caution is in order here: vasoconstrictors can excessively constrict vessels in organs with intact autonomic innervation.

Body temperature should be monitored and heating blankets should be used in patients who are hypothermic.

Further reading

Blalock, A. (1940) *Principles of Surgical Care, Shock and Other Problems.* C.V. Mosby, St Louis.

Gross, S.B. (1872) *A System of Surgery: pathological, diagnostic, therapeutic and operative.* Lea & Febiger, Philadelphia.

Kyle, J. & Carey, L.C. (eds) (1989) *Scientific Foundation of Surgery*, 4th edn. Heinemann Medical Books, Year Book Medical Publishers.

Maclean, L.D. (1972) Shock: causes and management of circulatory collapse. In: *Textbook of Surgery* (ed. D.C. Sabiston), Saunders, Philadelphia.

Morris, P.J. & Malt, R. (eds) (1994) *Oxford Textbook of Surgery.* Oxford University Press, Oxford.

Sabiston, D.C. Jr (ed.) (1991) *Textbook of Surgery. The Biological Basis of Modern Surgical Practice*, 14th edn. W.B. Saunders, Philadelphia.

Schwartz, S.I. (ed.) (1994) *Principles of Surgery*, 6th edn. McGraw-Hill, New York.

Society of Critical Care Medicine Consensus Conference 1991(1992) *Critical Care Medicine* **20**(6) 865.

Wiggers, C.J. (1942) Present status of shock problem. *Physiol Rev* **22** 74, 190.

CHAPTER 3

Response to surgical trauma

P. Declan Carey, Manas K. Roy, Ray J. Delicata & Anand Mahadevan

Introduction

Surgical patients often sustain major and rapid physiological changes from operative procedures performed either electively or as an emergency. Under these circumstances a number of adaptive responses are promptly set in motion. A rapid adaptation of circulatory mechanisms endeavours to restore blood pressure and volume. Clotting mechanisms are activated to reduce blood loss. The kidneys start to conserve water and electrolytes and in tandem with the lungs try to maintain acid–base neutrality. While these responses are readily apparent to the clinician, the less discernible, but equally important, adaptations of the metabolic and immunologic mechanisms are also set in motion at the very onset of trauma. The latter changes play an important role in the stability of the *milieu interieur*.

Surgical stress occurs before, during and after an operative procedure and is thus the end result of a variety of stimuli evoked by psychological stress, tissue injury, alterations in circulation, anaesthetic agents and postoperative complications. The ensuing adaptive host response encompasses three stress response systems: endocrine responses, sympathetic nervous system stimulation, and the acute phase response. The simultaneous activation of these axes and the consequent array of synergistic responses act in concert to return the host to a sustainable homeostatic plateau. In the following sections we will discuss the various causes which trigger the responses, how the stimuli are processed and finally some of the important host responses.

Stimuli for neuroendocrine reflexes

A number of stimuli are generated due to injury which are then conveyed by specialized receptors and nerves to the central nervous system (Fig. 3.1). The various stimuli are as follows:

Altered circulating blood volume

The loss of the effective circulating blood volume is perceived by the stretch receptors of the carotid arteries and aortic arch. Under normal conditions these receptors exert a tonic inhibitory influence on the central and autonomic nervous system. Diminution of the receptor stretch increases the secretion of adrenocorticotrophic hormone (ACTH), vasopressin, growth hormone (directly through central autonomic pathways) while the sympathetic nervous system releases catecholamines, glucagon, renin and increases cardiac contractility and causes peripheral vasoconstriction.

Pain

Painful stimuli are characteristic features of any injury and pain fibres provide the direct and quickest signals to the neuroendocrine axis. This is exemplified by the fact that both ACTH and growth hormone levels in the blood rise within 1 h of skin incision for a laparotomy and that paraplegics do not respond similarly to operations below the level of cord transection.

Altered blood composition

The chemoreceptors situated over the carotid and aortic bodies are activated by a decrease in blood concentration of oxygen and an increase in concentration of carbon dioxide and hydrogen ions. The stimulated chemoreceptors increase the cardiac sympathetic activity and stimulates the respiratory centre. Hypoglycaemia and changes in amino acid concentrations also stimulate the endocrine reflex.

Temperature changes

Core body temperature will change because of alterations in ambient temperature, loss of insulating barrier of skin (as in burns) or as a result of peripheral vasoconstriction (as in various shock states). The changes are sensed by the preoptic area of the hypothalamus and lead to adjustment in hormonal systems.

Wound

Inflammatory cells are invariably found in surgical wounds. Cytokines released from these cells spill over into the circulation to cause a generalized acute-phase response (*vide infra*).

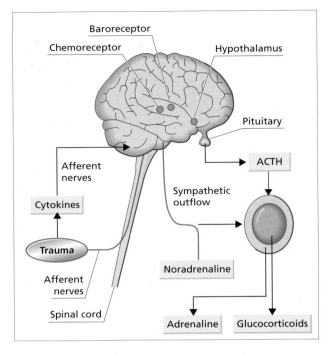

Fig. 3.1 The neuro-endocrine axis: its activation and response.

This response is intimately linked to the hypothalamic–pituitary–adrenal axis.

Stimuli integration

The afferent stimuli are processed in the hypothalamus. The posterior hypothalamus controls the release of ACTH from the pituitary which subsequently releases glucocorticoids from the adrenals. The paraventricular nucleus and supraoptic area of the hypothalamus secretes vasopressin (antidiuretic hormone; ADH). The sympathetic reflex activity which is generally regulated at the level of medulla and spinal cord is also partially coordinated by the posterior hypothalamus.

Because of the integration of different stimuli the response generated is not specific to a particular kind of stimulus. Furthermore, cytokines liberated by injured tissues have a profound influence on the hypothalamic–pituitary–adrenal axis and finally, concomitant disease and the physiological reserve of the individual alters the ultimate response.

Injury responses

As mentioned earlier, the injury response consists of three different arms: endocrine response, autonomic nervous system stimulation and acute phase response.

Injury responses

- Endocrine response
- Autonomic nervous system stimulation
- Acute phase response

Endocrine responses

The endocrine response is mediated through stimulation of hypothalamic–pituitary–adrenal axis (HPA). Alterations in the hormonal profile are characterized by a marked increase in ACTH, cortisol, growth hormone, glucagon, catecholamines, aldosterone and vasopressin. Thyroid-stimulating hormone (TSH), follicle-stimulating hormone (FSH) and leutinizing hormone (LH) change little during surgery.

CRH, ACTH and glucocorticoids

Afferent impulses increase the hypothalamic secretion of corticotrophin-releasing hormone (CRH). This stimulates the release of ACTH from the anterior pituitary, a process also facilitated by catecholamine and vasopressin. ACTH acts upon the adrenal cortex and induces the synthesis and release of glucocorticoids. The release of glucocorticoids is also increased by angiotensin, vasopressin and direct sympathetic stimulation of the adrenal cortex. Glucocorticoids have a global effect on homeostasis and feed back to the hypothalamus and pituitary to inhibit the release of CRH and ACTH; however, during prolonged stress high circulating levels of glucocorticoids *fail* to inhibit CRH and ACTH, which continue to be secreted at a high level.

Cortisol is the major human glucocorticoid and one of the earliest consequences of surgical incision is the rise in levels of circulating cortisol. The magnitude and duration of

---

Endocrine responses

- Marked increase in the secretion of cortisol, growth hormone, glucagon, catecholamines and aldosterone.
- Magnitude and duration of the increase in cortisol is proportional to the degree of surgical trauma and subsequent complications.
- Cortisol, growth hormone, glucagon and catecholamines tend to increase blood glucose by augmenting glycogenolysis, proteolysis and gluconeogenesis.
- In the initial phases increased level of glucose is not associated with a rise in the insulin; this spares the glucose to be utilized by vital organs like brain, red cells and renal medulla which are not dependent on insulin for glucose uptake.
- Aldosterone release increases sodium reabsorption while ADH assists the kidneys to conserve water.

the increase in circulating ACTH and cortisol correlates well with the degree of surgical trauma. The circadian rhythm of cortisol excretion is altered, but not abolished, after surgery and this promptly returns to normal once the traumatic insult is brought under control. Supervening infection, however, prolongs the duration of cortisol increase. In the elderly patient the initial surge of cortisol tends to decrease with time after the injury, suggesting that the endocrine response to trauma in the elderly may be attenuated.

Cortisol mobilizes amino acids from skeletal muscle and increases hepatic amino acid uptake. This increases gluconeogenesis which is also facilitated by elevated glucagon and adrenaline levels. Cortisol potentiates the hepatic action of glucagon and adrenaline and this is often referred to as permissive action of cortisol. As in liver, cortisol inhibits the action of insulin in peripheral tissues and decreases uptake and utilization of glucose. As a result, glucose is available for preferential utilization by tissues which are not dependent on insulin for glucose uptake, e.g. brain, red cells, renal medulla and peripheral nerves. Cortisol also stimulates lipolysis in adipose tissues and potentiates the action of other lipolytic hormones.

Glucagon and insulin

Glucagon and insulin are respectively synthesized by the α and β cells of the islets of Langerhans in the pancreas. In the initial phase of injury, insulin concentrations are low even in the presence of increased levels of glucose (under physiological conditions glucose is a potent stimulus of insulin release). This is caused by direct inhibition of insulin release by the α-adrenergic sympathetic nerves. During the later hypermetabolic phase, insulin concentrations are normal or increased. Its effect on peripheral tissue is blunted by the surge of cortisol, glucagon and catecholamines maintaining post-traumatic hyperglycaemia.

Glucagon is responsible for glycogenolysis, lipolysis and stimulation of hepatic gluconeogenesis; actions which tend to increase blood glucose. Initially plasma glucagon concentration may decrease transiently but later increases in all forms of major surgery and returns to baseline by 3 days.

Growth hormone (GH)

This polypeptide is secreted by the anterior pituitary. After injury, burns or surgery the rise of GH in the blood is in proportion to the degree of trauma. Its effect on tissues due to a direct action or secondary release of somatomedin or insulin-like growth factors I and II (IGF-I and IFG-II). During stress, GH promotes protein synthesis and enhances the breakdown of lipid and carbohydrate stores thereby contributing to glucose intolerance. Recombinant IFG-I decreases nitrogen loss in nonstressed human beings and may have therapeutic implications in future.

Renin–angiotensin–aldosterone

A sustained increase in renin activity is observed following surgical stress. Its release from the juxta-glomerular apparatus is enhanced by β-adrenergic stimulation, a decrease in renal perfusion pressure and when the macula densa receptors sense a decrease in tubular chloride concentration in the distal nephron. Renin converts angiotensinogen, produced by the liver, into angiotensin I which is converted to angiotensin II in the pulmonary circulation. Angiotensin II, a potent vasoconstrictor, stimulates heart rate and myocardial contractility and also increases the release of aldosterone and adrenaline from the adrenal glands.

Aldosterone is produced by the adrenal zona glomerulosa and its release is stimulated by angiotensin II and also by ACTH. Aldosterone increases sodium reabsorption in the distal convoluted tubule and early collecting tubule and thus is a major controller of extracellular fluid volume. Water reabsorption is also increased by enhanced release of antidiuretic hormone (ADH); the pressor receptors in the carotid artery and aortic arch and volume receptors in the left atrium initiate afferent signals which stimulate the release of ADH by the posterior pituitary. Atrial natriuretic peptide (ANP), secreted by the atria in response to atrial distension, is a potent inhibitor of aldosterone but its role in normal physiology and postinjury responses remains unclear.

Autonomic responses

The two arms of the autonomic nervous system (ANS) are the sympathetic and the parasympathetic systems. The sympathetic system is for the most part activated after stress and prepares the host to brave a 'fight or flight' situation. Embryologically the adrenal medulla is analogous to peripheral sympathetic ganglia, but in contrast, secrete adrenaline. The medulla encapsulated by the adrenal cortex offers a unique site for catecholamine–glucocorticoid interactions. The glucocorticoids synthesized in the zona fasciculata of the cortex reaches the medulla by way of an intraadrenal portal system. This glucocorticoid rich microenvironment stimulates the medullary cells to synthesize phenylethanolamine-N-methyltransferase (PNMT), an enzyme which increases the conversion of noradrenaline to adrenaline.

The ANS is stimulated under a variety of conditions: hypotension, injury, infection, hypoglycaemia, hypercarbia and also hyperthermia. During abdominal surgery the initial adrenergic activation occurs during the time of the actual surgery and not between the induction of anaesthesia and skin incision. The catecholamine level peaks at 24–48 h after injury following which it tends to decrease towards baseline. Catecholamines exert their diverse effects through transmembrane adrenergic receptors, which in the past have been simply classified into α and β subtypes; it is now apparent that there are at least nine distinct adrenoreceptors and a complete description is beyond the scope of this discussion. These receptors act via the intracellular second messengers, adenylate cyclase or phospholipase C. The number of adrenergic receptors in a given tissue is dynamic and the functional state is regulated by levels of catecholamine and other hormones like glucocorticoids. The ultimate outcome of catecholamine stimulation in a tissue is dictated by the presence and levels of specific adrenergic receptor subtypes. In general stimulation of α receptors results in vasoconstriction, $β_1$ stimulation increases heart rate and cardiac contractility while $β_2$ receptor stimulation is responsible for vasodilatation.

Catecholamines increase circulating glucose by stimulating glycogenolysis, gluconeogenesis and at higher concentration inhibit insulin thereby facilitating amino acid and fat mobilization. They also stimulate the secretion of glucagon, growth hormone and renin.

Acute phase response

The acute phase response (APR) is a systemic response to localized tissue damage (Fig. 3.2). This is a consequence of any traumatic insult but also occurs in response to infection and malignancy. It begins as a localized inflammatory process characterized by vasodilatation and increased vascular permeability. Mononuclear cells and granulocytes soon appear in the wound and together with fibroblasts and endothelial cells liberate cytokines (*vide infra*) into the peripheral circulation. Upon reaching the general circulation the cytokines produce a myriad of systemic effects: fever, leucocytosis, activation of immune system, stimulation of the HPA axis, activation of clotting cascade, etc. However, the most reproducible feature of APR is a change in serum levels of acute-phase reactants. These are proteins which are mainly secreted by the liver: $α_1$-antichymotrypsin, complement C3, ceruloplasmin, fibrinogen, haptoglobin and C-reactive protein (CRP) constitute the positive reactants whose levels rise during the acute

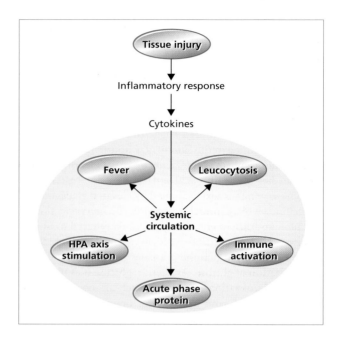

Fig. 3.2 The acute phase response.

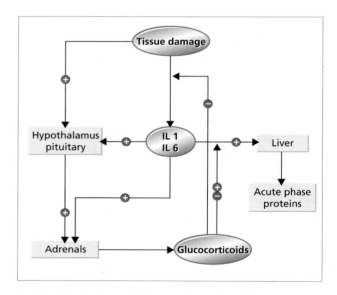

Fig. 3.3 Mutual relationship between glucocorticoids and cytokines.

phase response while the negative reactants are serum albumin and transferrin whose levels decline during the same period.

These reactants form an important component in the host defence mechanism; C3 and CRP are required by phagocytic cells for opsonization, fibrinogen is essential for blood coagulation while the proteases limit tissue destruction. The serum levels of these reactants rise during the first

---

Acute phase response

- Initiated by cytokines released by monocytes and neutrophils.
- Fever, leucocytosis, stimulation of HPA axis, activation of clotting cascade and changes in acute phase proteins characterize this universal response.
- Levels of $α_1$-antichymotrypsin, complement C3, ceruloplasmin, fibrinogen and C-reactive protein rise while synthesis of carrier proteins like albumin and transferrin decrease.
- Glucocorticoids facilitate cytokine mediated rise in the synthesis of acute phase proteins.

24–48 h after surgery; the actual rise, which is charateristic for a particular protein, is proportional to the severity of injury. The CRP level is most frequently used in clinical practice because it shows the greatest increase. The levels tend to come back to normal values after 48–96 h in patients with an uncomplicated postoperative course while the levels remain elevated in presence of sepsis or other complications.

The acute phase response and the HPA seem to interact bilaterally during stress (Fig. 3.3). The cytokines mediating APR are capable of stimulating the HPA axis. On the other hand, glucocorticoids facilitate the elaboration of the various acute phase proteins by the cytokines. Interestingly, the steroid hormones have also been shown to inhibit cytokine production. This paradoxical activity is caused by the dual role played by glucocortocoids: in a permissive fashion it initiates host response, and later if it remains elevated tends to attenuate the homeostatic responses.

Metabolic changes following injury

The metabolic changes following surgery are determined by the patient's health, nature and severity of injury, duration of subsequent starvation and presence or absence of complications like sepsis, prolonged ileus, etc. A brief resumé of the body composition in health and the changes during starvation are necessary for an understanding of the metabolic changes brought on by various traumatic insults.

Body composition and changes during fasting

The cells of the body and the supporting extracellular fluid, blood, body fat, bone and collagen matrix constitute a heterogeneous mass which is collectively known as lean body mass. The body cell mass refers to the metabolically active cells. These cells and adipose tissue represent a form of stored energy (Table 3.1). Fat is by far the main storehouse

> **Metabolic changes following injury**
>
> - Patients exhibit an increase in total energy requirement.
> - Excess demand for glucose, another unique feature, is due to avid use of glucose by inflammatory cells and fibroblasts in rapidly healing tissues.
> - Accelerated proteolysis becomes inevitable to sustain increased gluconeogenesis.
> - Glutamine acts as a carrier for inter-organ flux of nitrogen.
> - Intestinal mucosa avidly uses glutamine as fuel; this is inhibited during sepsis and this compromises mucosal integrity.
> - Although fatty acid degradation continues to provide the major metabolic fuel, interestingly, ketogenesis is not increased.

Table 3.1 Fuel composition of a normal 70 kg man.

Fuel	Weight (kg)	Calories
Tissues		
Fat	15	141 000
Protein	6	24 000
Glycogen (muscle)	0.150	600
Glycogen (liver)	0.075	300
Total		165 900
Circulating fuels		
Glucose (extracellular fluid)	0.020	80
Free fatty acids (plasma)	0.0003	3
Triglycerides (plasma)	0.003	30
Total		113

Adapted from Cahill, G.F., Jr. (1970) Starvation in man. *N Engl J Med*, **282**, 668.

> **Metabolic changes during fasting**
>
> - Glycogen stores are depleted within 24 hours of starvation.
> - Fat being a poor source of new glucose, enhanced proteolysis provides the vital amino acids for gluconeogenesis.
> - Body adapts to utilize ketone bodies; these are derived from acetyl CoA, an intermediate of lipolysis.
> - Ketone utilization halts the accelerated proteolysis and fat becomes the major source of calories.

of readily available energy and yields approximately 9 calories/g. Protein, the next largest substrate, is a relatively expensive source of energy. Although the calorific yield of protein is 4 calories/g, in reality the body protein merely yields 1 calorie/g. This is because the muscle protein is hydrated and contains three parts of water and one part of protein. This, coupled with the fact that loss of body protein is associated with loss of body function, makes protein an expensive source of energy. Glucose is a readily available source of energy but the major body source consist of only 75 g of glucose as hepatic glycogen.

As a result of starvation glycogen stores are depleted within 24 hours. This necessitates gluconeogenesis, because the brain, which has a very high metabolic rate, utilizes only glucose. Although fat is available in plenty, it is a poor source of new glucose. Only some glucose can be formed from glycerol and fatty acids cannot be transformed to glucose; this is because acetyl coenzyme A (CoA) cannot be converted to pyruvate (Fig. 3.4). This calls for proteolysis to sustain gluconeogenesis and there is a definite order in which various proteins are broken down. The digestive enzymes of the gastrointestinal tract and liver are the first to be sacrificed (hence, recommencement of oral intake after prolonged

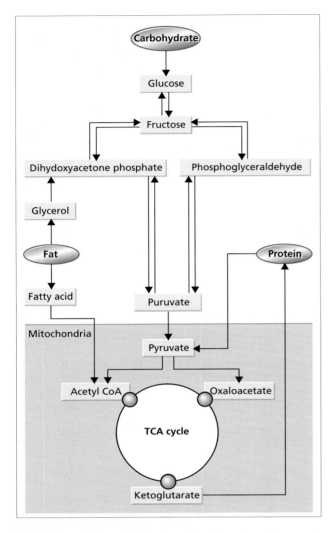

Fig. 3.4 Degradation of carbohydrate, fat and protein and the central role of the tricarboxylic acid (Kreb's) cycle.

preferentially participates in gluconeogenesis and is therefore relatively unavailable for acetyl CoA. This becomes the rate-limiting step and acetyl CoA is converted to ketone bodies. Subsequently these compounds are used as a source of energy by the heart, muscles, liver and kidney. The blood–brain barrier, which normally limits ketone transport, becomes more permeable to ketones and the brain starts to utilize ketones. The accelerated drive for gluconeogenesis is reduced, as is amino acid generation. Approximately 1 week from the outset, proteolysis diminishes to 20 g/day and fat becomes the major source of calories. These metabolic changes permit survival during prolonged periods of starvation. However, once the supply of fat has been consumed muscle protein is heavily drained to meet basal energy requirement. Impairment of overall body function does occur and loss of 30–40% of body proteins may prove fatal.

Metabolic responses to injury

The post-injury metabolic response is characterized by an early 'ebb phase', during which resting energy expenditure decreases. With the gradual increase in levels of stress hormones the metabolic rate begins to rise. This compensatory phase is associated with a rise of body temperature, increased glucose production, proteolysis and lipid breakdown and is termed the 'flow phase'. This catabolic response associated with hormonal alteration has also been termed the 'adrenergic–corticoid phase', which gradually merges into an anabolic phase if compensatory responses prevail over the acute insults. The transition phase between catabolism and anabolism (which usually starts 3–6 days after abdominal surgery) is characterized by a reduction in nitrogen excretion and spontaneous diuresis and often is termed as 'corticoid withdrawal phase'. During the late anabolic phase there is progressive reaccumulation of protein followed by deposition of fat in the adipose tissue. Various aspects of these changes are discussed in subsequent sections.

Increased metabolic rate

In contrast to simple starvation, surgical patients invariably exhibit a state of hypermetabolism and an increase in resting energy requirement. This is compensated for by a reduction in energy expended by physical activity (active metabolic energy) as a period of rest often accompanies surgery. Hence, the total energy requirement may not increase and patients with uneventful postoperative courses rarely increase their metabolic rate by more than 10–15% of the normal values. The total energy requirement, however, increases considerably following major resectional surgery, associated sepsis, multiple trauma and burns. This injury response upregulates the hypothalamic thermostat and patients develop a 1–2 °C rise in body temperature; this is probably mediated

starving often results in malabsorption and diarrhoea). The skeletal muscle proteins are next to be recruited and fasting individuals become weak and physically inactive, an important physiological adaptation which *decreases* the resting energy expenditure.

With prolonged fasting the body cannot afford to use glucose as the main fuel because of continued proteolysis. Hence, an important metabolic adjustment takes place and the body adapts to use ketones as an alternative fuel. The ketone bodies namely, aceto-acetates, acetone or β-hydroxy butyrate, are derived from acetyl CoA which is an intermediate of lipolysis. Under normal physiological conditions, acetyl CoA combines with oxaloacetate in the tricarboxylic acid cycle (Fig. 3.4). During starvation the latter compound

by interleukin-1. Fever *per se* increases the metabolic rate by approximately 7% for each degree Fahrenheit of fever. Healthy young adults with adequate muscle mass show marked increase in energy expenditure as compared to elderly patients with small body cell mass. This increase in metabolic activity is mainly caused by increased sympathetic activity and catecholamine release.

Changes in glucose metabolism

Injured victims exhibit excess demand for glucose, and whilst hyperglycaemia is not a common feature during simple starvation it is rather pronounced in injured patients. This occurs immediately after injury and continues into the flow phase. The increased demand is primarily because of the avid use of glucose by the inflammatory cells and fibroblasts. In rapidly healing tissues the metabolism of glucose to lactate probably provides the main energy source. Whereas the consumption of glucose by the kidneys increases twofold, the glucose consumed by the brain and spinal cord is approximately similar to that of a resting individual (120 g/day). Studies in injured victims have also shown that skeletal muscle can only utilize a fraction of available glucose. This 'insulin resistance' is believed to be caused by increased catecholamine, cortisol and glucagon release and is useful in a sense because important organs like brain and renal medulla can then preferentially utilize glucose, as they are not dependent on insulin for glucose metabolism.

In the initial period following injury, insulin concentration is depressed; presumably this is because of catecholamine-mediated reduction in β cell sensitivity to glucose. Later, in the flow phase there is persistent hyperglycaemia, insulin resistance and hyperinsulinaemia which is believed to be caused by an intracellular defect in glucose oxidation. This is a result of a reduction of skeletal muscle pyruvate dehydrogenase induced by trauma and sepsis with diminution of the conversion of glucose derived pyruvate to acetyl CoA which is normally destined to enter the tricarboxylic acid cycle. Under these circumstances pyruvate is converted to alanine and lactate. In rapidly healing tissues the metabolism of glucose to lactate provides the main energy source. Thus, the increased demand for glucose by the surgical patient can only be met by proteolysis and subsequent gluconeogenesis.

Changes in protein metabolism

The daily fecal and urinary excretion of nitrogen in a healthy young adult is 2–3 g and 13–20 g, respectively. Following injury the daily urinary losses increase two to three times signifying net proteolysis. Proteolysis, mediated by the stress hormones, primarily supply substrates to sustain the accelerated drive for gluconeogenesis. Only a minor amount of protein is utilized to supply calories. Patients who have undergone major operations rapidly suffer from wasting of skeletal muscles, suggesting that skeletal muscles are the principal sites of proteolysis and this is supported by the results of radiolabelled amino-acid incorporation studies. The magnitude of protein breakdown is related to the severity of surgery, sepsis, fever and also the physical build of the patient and is more pronounced in young, well-built individuals. Visceral organs such as liver respond in a different manner: synthesis of acute phase proteins namely fibrinogen, C-reactive protein, haptoglobin, ceruloplasmin, ferritin, etc. increase while synthesis of transferrin, albumin, retinols and prealbumin decrease.

Immediately after injury there is no or little change in total amino-acid concentration in the blood. The levels of alanine, however, increase in the early flow phase. Alanine and glutamine constitute over 50% of the circulating amino acids released after injury. Interestingly, they each constitute only 6% of the muscle protein. They therefore seem to be the principal carrier of nitrogen from skeletal muscles to the visceral tissues (Fig. 3.5). Upon being taken up by the kidneys, alanine is converted to urea and ammonium is released, a process which produces net loss of acids. Glutamine is avidly used up by gut mucosa as a fuel (mediated by glucocorticoids) and is metabolized to alanine and ammonia. On reaching the liver ammonia is converted to urea while the alanine, together with the alanine released from the skeletal muscles, is used by the liver for gluconeogenesis and

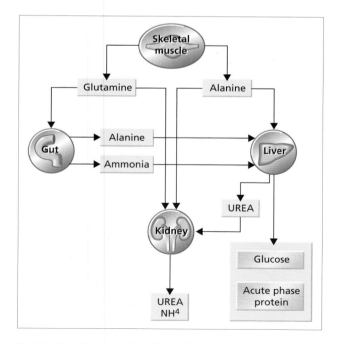

Fig. 3.5 Fate of amino acid residues of skeletal muscle proteolysis.

synthesis of acute phase proteins. However, during sepsis intestinal glutamine uptake falls and liver assumes the major role in glutamine consumption; this is believed to be cytokine mediated. Lack of glutamine has been shown to have a deleterious effect on mucosal integrity and administration of glutamine prevents gut atrophy. The increased requirement for glutamine by the gut mucosal cells is not met by the available enteral or parenteral preparations as there are inadequate amounts of glutamine in enteral feeds while glutamine is not added to parenteral preparations because it is unstable in solution and rapidly degrades to glutamate and ammonia. Considerable attention has also focused on the metabolism of arginine, which acts as an intermediate in the urea cycle, creatinine synthesis and has been shown to be the exclusive precursor of nitric oxide. Finally, because postinjury proteolysis is mainly stimulated to meet the increased demand for gluconeogenic precursors, administration of high-caloric nitrogen supplements either enterally or parenterally can reduce or revert the negative nitrogen balance. The role played by the various organs in glucose and protein metabolism is shown schematically in Fig. 3.6.

Changes in fat metabolism

The respiratory quotient of an injured victim is usually around 0.7 to 0.8 and this suggests that lipids are the *major* energy source for the stressed patient (Fig. 3.7). Lipolysis is stimulated by elevations of cortisol, catecholamine, glucagon and growth hormone levels. The lipase in the adipocyte is hormone sensitive and, hence, after injury, increased amounts of plasma free acids and glycerol are released into the circulation. The free fatty acids are oxidized by cardiac and skeletal muscles to produce energy, while glycerol contributes to gluconeogenesis. Lipoprotein lipase is another lipolytic enzyme which is bound to the capillary endothelium and is capable of hydrolysing triglycerides bound to very low density lipoproteins and chylomicrons. The fatty acids released are subsequently stored in adipocytes. Following trauma muscle lipoprotein lipase activity is increased while adipose tissue lipoprotein lipase activity is decreased by cytokines. This decreases the total body fat store.

In contrast to simple starvation and despite stimulated lipolysis, ketogenesis is not increased after major injury,

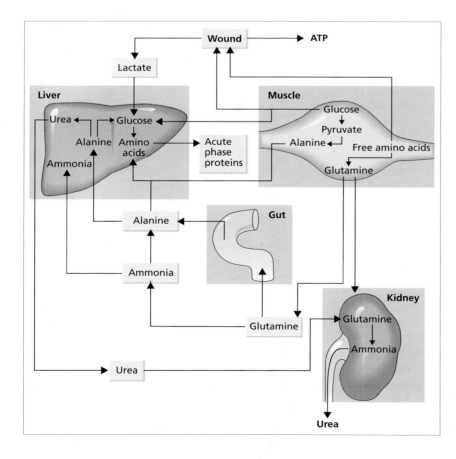

Fig. 3.6 Interorgan flow of metabolites in response to trauma. Adapted from Fischer, J.E. (1991) Metabolism in surgical patients. In: *Textbook of Surgery: The Biological Basis of Modern Surgical Practice* (ed. D.C. Sabiston). W.B. Saunders, Philadelphia.

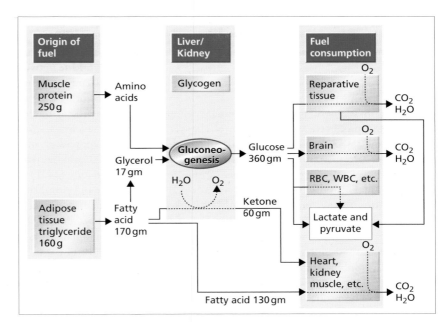

Fig. 3.7 A scheme of substrate flow in a traumatized individual. Despite the increased gluconeogenesis, fat still provides the bulk of calories. Adapted from: Cahill, G.F., *et al.* (1970) *Body Fluid Replacement in the Surgical Patient* (eds C.L. Fox Jr & G.G. Nahas), p. 286. Grune and Stratton, New York.

severe shock and sepsis. Ketones have been found to increase transiently during and immediately following surgery but return to normal after a few hours. The cause for reduced ketone formation has been ascribed to increased plasma levels of insulin, increase in other energy substrates such as alanine, glucose, and lactate, and increased uptake and oxidation of the free fatty acids.

Changes in water and electrolyte balance

All surgical procedures are associated with changes in water and electrolyte composition. Surgical dissection inevitably alters capillary permeability resulting in sequestration of fluid. This third space loss of fluid is actually derived from the functional extracellular fluid, the volume of which consequently contracts. This sequestered fluid in the third space, which can be quite significant in operations like gastrectomy or retroperitoneal dissections, is not available to expand circulating blood volume. Therefore, diuretics should not be routinely used in the postoperative patient in the absence of congestive heart failure. Diuretics worsen the situation by further contracting the functional extracellular fluid. Haemorrhagic shock also reduces the functional extracellular fluid; this however occurs because of the *intracellular* shift of water. The host response to normalize these alterations are mediated by the renin–angiotensin–aldosterone system (see above) with the kidneys playing a vital role during these changes. The increased release of aldosterone and ADH decreases water and electrolyte excretion and the postoperative patient passes a concentrated urine

despite adequate hydration. This water and electrolyte retention usually results in weight gain.

Operative procedures are often accompanied with varying degrees of hypovolaemia and hypotension. Although the formation of an ultrafiltrate at the glomerulus is governed by Starling's forces, the glomerular filtration remains unchanged despite a reduction in renal perfusion pressure to 80 mmHg. This autoregulation is caused by the capacity of individual nephron to sense the reduction in tubular fluid flow which then leads to an increase in the efferent arteriolar resistence (tubuloglomerular feedback). The fraction of glomerular blood which is filtered thereby increases. The resulting increase in the oncotic pressure of the peritubular blood increases the absorption of water, sodium and chloride from the proximal fluid. Consequently, the chloride delivered to the loop of Henle decreases and this decreases the sodium absorption, as sodium in the loop of Henle passively follows the chloride reabsorption. As a result, increased sodium is delivered to the distal tubule; this results in loss of potassium and hydrogen (mediated by aldosterone) causing metabolic alkalosis. This is the most common acid–base disturbance seen in the postoperative patient, while metabolic acidosis is commonly seen in situations of profound shock and renal failure. The most commonly seen electrolyte disturbance in postoperative patients is hyponatraemia with hyperkalaemia. Hyponatraemia is mainly dilutional, as an injury-related increase in ADH serves to increase water reabsorption in a patient who is often infused with non-solute containing fluids. Serum potassium may be elevated because catabolic reactions release potassium from cells; infusion of potassium-rich stored blood and reabsorption of blood from wound or peritoneum also contribute to this increase.

Other changes

Prostaglandin synthesis from cell membrane phopholipid increases and produce a wide spectrum of changes. While thromboxane (TXA$_2$) causes vasoconstriction and platelet aggregation, prostacyclin (PGI$_2$) mediates vasodilatation and inhibits platelet aggregation. The various forms of prostaglandin E (PGE) mimic the effects of ACTH and TSH by stimulating intracellular cAMP. Leukotrienes, amongst other actions, are responsible for neutrophil chemotaxis, activation and enzyme release. They also promote release of interferon (IFN) from lymphocytes while PGE$_2$ inhibits the T helper 1 (Th1) T lymphocytes (*vide infra*).

Synthesis of heat shock proteins constitute the most ubiquitous response to cellular stress. They are induced in response to a variety of stresses and are more appropriately termed as general stress response proteins. Their precise role is unknown but they are believed to act as chaperones in the process of assembly, disassembly, stabilization and internal transport of other intracellular proteins.

The wide expanse of the endothelial surface (approximately 400 m^2 in an adult) releases many factors as a result of injury. Prostaglandins play an important role in platelet aggregation and alterations of vessel calibre. Adhesion molecules such as intercellular-adhesion molecule (ICAM) and endothelial leucocyte adhesion molecule (ELAM) are expressed and various cytokines are synthesized and released. Cytokines (and endotoxins) stimulate inducible nitric oxide synthase (iNOS) in endothelium and vascular smooth muscles to produce nitric oxide (NO). NO is a potent vasodilator which is immediately inactivated by haemoglobin in the blood. Its precise role is still unclear, but has been implicated in maintenance of microvascular integrity.

Cytokine control of metabolism

Cytokines are soluble proteins synthesized by the body's own cells in response to an inflammatory stimulus. They are produced by a variety of cells: monocytes, macrophages, lymphocytes, epithelial and endothelial cells, fibroblasts and parenchymal cells of gastrointestinal viscera. Under normal circumstances the cytokines are either not functioning or functioning at a low level without disturbing homeostasis. Their production increases following an inflammatory stimulus. They are capable of amplifying their own production locally and also stimulating the production of other cytokines thereby initiating a cascade. When produced in excess the cytokines spill over into general circulation and then function like hormones. But unlike classic endocrine hormones they are produced by a variety of cell types and exert most of their tissue effects locally in a cell-to-cell paracrine fashion; this complex interaction is called **cytokine networking**. On one hand the cytokines appear to extend a helpful hand towards the host response while on the other they are potentially hazardous and are responsible for the systemic inflammatory response syndrome and the deleterious consequences of sepsis such as profound hypotension and mutiple organ failure (host tissue injury).

Cytokines can be classified broadly as tumour necrosis factors (TNF), interleukins (IL), interferons (IFN) and colony-stimulating factors (CSF). The ILs and TNFs mediate the various effects of sepsis and inflammation while IFNs and CSFs are primarily concerned with immune modulation. A variety of cytokines have been described; most of the metabolic responses are, however, mediated by TNF, IL-1, IL-6 and IFN-γ. Their relative contributions to the various substrate metabolism have already been referred to in the appropriate sections and a few salient features remain now to be discussed.

TNF is produced mainly by macrophages, lymphocyte, natural killer (NK) cells and Kupffer cells under the stimulus of injury, endotoxin and malignancy. It is believed to be the principle initial signal of the cytokine cascade and induces the synthesis of IL-1, IL-6 and IFN-γ and its levels have been correlated with severity and outcome in patients with sepsis. IFN-γ upregulates TNF receptors on various cell types and acts synergistically with TNF. In conjunction with IL-1, TNF upregulates the hypothalamic thermostat, thereby causing fever. It activates the HPA axis producing ACTH and cortisol. TNF is also an important mediator of skeletal muscle proteolysis, release of amino acid metabolites and cachexia. Concurrently, it also stimulates hepatic amino acid uptake and increases the synthesis of acute phase response proteins. This step is primarily mediated by IL-6, which is considered to be the end effector of the alteration in hepatocyte protein synthetic function. The alanine taken up by the liver cells is used for gluconeogenesis, a process facilitated by IL-1. IL-1 (with TNF) is also responsible for accelerated lipolysis during situations of stress. The decrease in body fat is caused in part by cytokine-mediated inhibition of lipoprotein lipase in the adipose tissue.

Immunological responses

The major impact of prophylactic antibiotics occurred about 10 years ago and, despite the introduction of new generations of antibiotics, the overall incidence of sepsis after elective surgery remains static in the region of 5–10%. Though technical factors may play a part this residual sepsis may be a reflection of perturbations of immune system due to surgical stress. While minor operations may stimulate the immune response, the predominant effect of major surgery on immune function is supressive. Because many major

Immunological changes

- Predominant effect of major surgery is immunodepression.
- Laparotomy downregulates MHC class II antigen on the monocytes; this is mediated by IL-10 released by the Th2 T cells.
- Defects in neutrophil chemotaxis, phagocytosis and lysosomal enzyme contents have been identified.
- Peri-operative blood transfusion also contributes to immunosuppression, but the underlying mechanism is largely unknown.

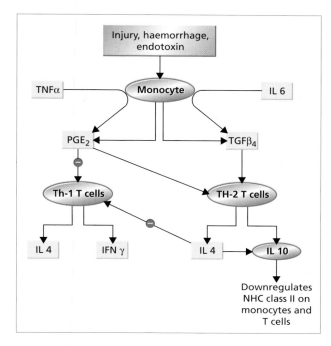

Fig. 3.8 Central role of monocytes in post-traumatic immune modulation.

operations are accompanied by haemorrhage, the postoperative immune depression may be caused in part by blood loss and cellular hypoxia rather than surgery. In fact haemorrhage, despite adequate crystalloid resuscitation, is sufficient to depress cell-mediated immunity. Interestingly enough, simple laparotomy without haemorrhage has also been shown to depress macrophage function.

A variety of impairments of immune function have been noted in postoperative patients. At least half of patients undergoing gastrointestinal surgery become anergic as assessed by hypersensitivity skin testing. Reduction of the ratio of T helper to T suppressor cells has also been noted as has been the lowering of the number of circulating NK cells. Defects in neutrophil chemotaxis, phagocytosis, lysosomal enzyme contents and depression of macrophage antigen presentation and macrophage phagocytosis have all been identified. This depression in immunity following surgery is most pronounced within 6–48 h of operation and, in most cases, appears to be transient.

The initial event in the generation of the immune response is uptake and degradation of foreign antigens by monocytes/macrophages. The antigens are then presented by the macrophages to the T helper cells. The T helper cells will only recognize the antigen when they are presented on macrophage cell surfaces in close proximity to major histocompatibility (MHC) class II antigens (HLA-DR in humans). In appropriate circumstances, T cells are activated with subsequent stimulation of B cells, leading to immunoglobulin production and enhanced phagocytosis of opsonized bacteria.

Thus, the monocyte with its HLA-DR antigen enjoys a central role in the generation of the immune cascade. Laparotomy and various other trauma downregulate the expression of HLA-DR on the monocyte surface. This is mediated by T cells, which are stimulated by factors released by monocytes activated by surgery, haemorrhage and endotoxin. The various steps in this complex mechanism are shown in Fig. 3.8.

It is evident how the monocytes play a key role in immune modulation following injury. The T cells have been subclassified into two types based on the pattern of cytokine release. Th 1 release IFN-γ and IL-2, which mediate cell-mediated responses. IL-4 inhibition of Th 1 cells explains the cutaneous anergy seen in postoperative patients. Th 2 cells liberate IL-4, IL-5, IL-6, and IL-10 which influence B-cell development. Prostaglandin (PGE$_2$) plays an important role as it stimulates the Th 2 T cells to produce IL-4 and IL-10; it also inhibits IL-1-mediated macrophage–T cell interaction. IL-10 downregulates the expression of vital HLA-DR antigen. Recent experimental evidence indicates that, following injury, there is upregulation of the mRNA for transforming growth factor (TGF)β$_4$ and IL-10 in the cells of the mononuclear phagocytic system and lymphocytes. Similar changes in the Kupffer cells decrease the phagocytosis of gut-derived bacteria during conditions of stress.

The downregulation of the macrophages after a traumatic insult may be beneficial in the early phase. During this phase, the devitalized tissue and bacteria are the targets of non-specific inflammation which is primarily mediated by neutrophils. This is generally a contained inflammatory process, the duration of which is dependent on the magnitude of the initial insult. The downregulation of the monocytes at this stage may be protective and may limit unnecessary and potentially autodestructive inflammation. In patients with significant trauma this downregulation appears to persist inappropriately and creates an immunocompromised host.

As mentioned previously postoperative immunosuppression may also be caused by haemorrhage. Significant intraoperative bleeding is usually compensated for by transfusion of allogeneic whole blood. Blood transfusion *per se* has been shown to contribute to immunosuppression. Blood transfusion decreases delayed hypersensitivity responses, IL-2 production and T-cell proliferation and also increases immunosuppressive PGE_2. The underlying mechanism of this immunosuppression is largely unknown. Leucocyte components such as tissue antigens (human leucocyte antigen, MHC) may induce alloimmunization, which may subsequently lead to immunosuppression. There is evidence that frozen washed red cells (which lack HLA antigens), filtered whole blood and buffy coat-depleted blood in artificial medium such as SAG-M (saline, adenine, glucose-mannitol) can be administered without inducing immunosuppression.

Patients who have had splenectomy undergo a different kind of immune alteration. These patients are more susceptible to infection with encapsulated bacteria like *Streptococcus pneumoniae*, and postsplenectomy sepsis has been reported up to 30 years after splenectomy. The spleen is normally concerned with removal of poorly opsonized bacteria (liver can only remove well-opsonized bacteria), parasites like malarial organisms and also with the production of two important opsonins: tuftsin, which promotes neutrophil phagocytosis and properdin, a vital component of alternative complement pathway. Splenic white pulp mounts the initial immunoglobulin M (IgM) antibody response after exposure to an antigen. Splenectomy deprives the host of these important immune responses. Children appear to be more vulnerable and the risk is enhanced if splenectomy is performed for conditions like thalassaemia and lymphoma. The most frightening aspect of postsplenectomy sepsis is fulminant bacteraemia (overwhelming postsplenectomy infection, OPSI) which is reported to occur in 0.9–6.9% of cases, with mortality exceeding 50%.

Further reading

Guillou, P.J. (1995) Adjuvant biological response modifiers after major surgery or trauma. *British Journal of Surgery* **82** 721–723.

Schwartz, S.I., Shires, G.T. & Spencer, F.C. (1994) *Principles of Surgery*, 6th edn. McGraw-Hill, Inc., New York.

Souba, W.W. (1994) Cytokine control of nutrition and metabolism during critical illness. *Current Problems in Surgery* **Vol xxxi, No. 7** 577–652.

CHAPTER 4

Peri-operative management of the emergency patient

Edmund G. Carton & Dermot M. Phelan

Introduction

The peri-operative care of emergency surgery patients places unique demands on a diverse group of health care professionals throughout the hospital. It is imperative that the particular expertise of individuals and services involved be co-ordinated efficiently to secure optimal patient outcome. The admitting surgical service adopts a pivotal role, not only in the surgical procedure itself, but also in the clinical assessment, laboratory investigation, and diagnostic imaging of patients for emergency surgery. The scope of this chapter reflects the wide spectrum of issues involved in the peri-operative care of these patients.

Pre-operative management

Initial assessment

The pre-operative phase is dominated by resuscitation and efforts to make the correct diagnosis based on the patient's history, physical examination, specific imaging and laboratory studies. Multiple concurrent issues need to be addressed in a timely and comprehensive manner. Throughout this process, it is essential that there is ongoing patient assessment to ensure that the patient has a patent airway, adequate respiratory effort, is haemodynamically stable, and remains in a satisfactory neurological state. Supplemental oxygen should be administered to all acutely ill patients during the early stages of assessment.

Surgical emergencies are frequently traumatic in nature, and the initial assessment and resuscitation principles are broadly similar for a wide variety of patients. In head injured patients, vigorous efforts must be made to avoid hypoxaemia, hypercarbia, and arterial hypotension, which may complicate and worsen the prognosis of the initial injury. If there is an acute deterioration in the level of consciousness, which may reflect an increase in intracranial pressure (ICP), hyperventilation, frusemide and mannitol are justified pending specific diagnosis and surgical intervention. Corticosteroids are indicated for an acute increase in ICP associated with an intracranial malignancy or abscess cavity.

Evidence of severe chest trauma (e.g. sternal or scapular fracture, multiple rib fractures, especially fracture of first or second ribs), should prompt the immediate exclusion of a significant aortic, tracheobronchial, or myocardial injury. In patients with a pneumothorax or haemothorax, urgent placement of chest tubes may avoid the need for tracheal intubation and should be considered prior to transport of the patient to the radiology suite or operating room. The position of these devices should be confirmed on a chest radiograph.

The classic constellation of abdominal signs, distension with rigidity, localized tenderness and loss of bowel sounds, is frequently obscured in the comatose or sedated patient requiring tracheal intubation. Interpretation of these abdominal signs is also difficult when there is concurrent pelvic injury. Peritoneal lavage and a computerized tomograph are useful supplementary tests, but frequently laparotomy is the safest option. Rectal examination is an essential part of the assessment of the acute abdomen. If the prostate is 'riding high' or there is blood at the tip of the urethra, suprapubic rather than urethral catheterization is indicated.

Long bone and pelvic fractures usually require intravenous opiate analgesia, but if there is a deterioration in neurological status associated with opiate-induced respiratory depression, tracheal intubation and ventilation may be required. Patients may require fracture immobilization and intravascular volume resuscitation to replace both overt and covert blood loss. Patency of peripheral pulses is checked with supracondylar or lower femoral fractures. Muscle compartments are examined especially with distal fractures of the upper and lower limb. Decompression and measures to minimize rhabdomyolytic acute tubular necrosis (e.g. volume expansion, mannitol, urinary alkalinization) may be indicated.

If sepsis is suspected, diagnostic cultures should be taken and therapeutic doses of appropriate antibiotic agents should be administered. Antibiotic therapy should be re-assessed after specific microbiologic culture and sensitivity information is available (see also Chapter 6).

> Tracheal intubation should be considered in head-injured patients with a Glasgow Coma Scale of 8 or less.

Airway and breathing management

In patients with head injury, tracheal intubation is recommended when the Glasgow Coma Scale (GCS) is 8 or less. Before tracheal intubation, a rapid clinical examination should be undertaken looking for lateralization of neurological signs, especially if sedation or neuromuscular blockers are to be used. Airway obstruction leading to hypoxia and hypercarbia will quickly compound a primary injury and must be treated immediately. Extensive facial trauma may cause airway obstruction especially if associated with bleeding and coma. Tachypnoea (> 30 breaths/min) or respiratory distress approaching exhaustion are indications for tracheal intubation. In the absence of a suspected cervical spine injury, the chin lift or jaw thrust manoeuvre, in addition to placement of a nasal or oral airway will open the airway in most patients. Foreign material should be removed from the upper airway. If these initial measures are unsuccessful, or if the patient has inadequate spontaneous ventilation despite a patent airway, tracheal intubation should be performed.

The importance of suspecting an injury to the cervical spine has been stressed by Advanced Trauma Life Support (ATLS) guidelines. Trainees with airway management skills may not always have to resort to a surgical approach to the airway as proposed by ATLS algorithms. However, substantial knowledge and experience is required for the safe use of short acting anaesthetic and neuromuscular blocking drugs used to facilitate tracheal intubation. When injury to the cervical spine is suspected, bimanual in-line stabilization applied during attempts to secure the airway should prevent both lateral flexion and anteroposterior flexion or extension of the cervical spine.

Tracheal intubation using standard cuffed tubes allows mechanical ventilation of the lungs and protects against aspiration of material into the lungs. Satisfactory placement of the tracheal tube is confirmed by auscultation of the chest and by detecting end-tidal carbon dioxide. The chest radiograph should be examined to confirm that the tube tip is 2.5–5.0 cm above the carina.

If it is anticipated that securing the airway will be difficult, tracheal intubation should be performed while the patient is still awake and breathing spontaneously. Awake intubation may be accomplished by blind nasal technique, using a laryngoscope and an intubating stylet, or a fibre-optic bronchoscope (Fig. 4.1). Nasotracheal intubation is contra-indicated in patients with suspected basal skull fractures. Whatever technique is chosen, the patient must be adequately prepared for awake intubation with regional or topical local anaesthetics, mucosal vasoconstrictors, and judicious use of sedative medication (see also Chapter 22).

Repeated unsuccessful attempts to intubate the trachea in the emergency setting may make the eventual placement of the tracheal tube increasingly difficult. Repeated manipulation of the airway also carries a substantial risk of vomiting or aspiration in an awake emergency surgery patient. At the same time, adequate ventilation of the lungs using a standard face mask may also become increasingly difficult. Although unconventional, a trial of the laryngeal mask airway may be justified under these circumstances.

When the lungs cannot be ventilated by face or laryngeal mask and the trachea cannot be intubated, emergency cricothyroidotomy and transtracheal jet ventilation may be life saving. It is imperative that the airway be at least partially open above the cricothyroid membrane with any technique

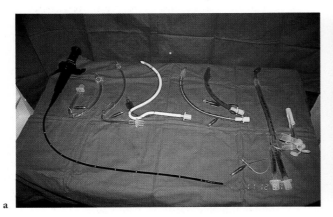

a

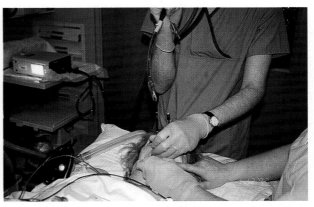

b

Fig. 4.1 (a) Bronchoscopic intubation. A full selection of endotracheal tubes should be available for all emergency intubation.

(b) Endotracheal tube is 'loaded' onto the bronchoscope. It is slid into place down the scope under direct vision.

of transtracheal jet ventilation, otherwise, dangerously high intrathoracic pressures may be generated. These measures may allow time for a more definitive airway to be secured. Even with optimal lighting and equipment, an emergency tracheostomy under local anaesthesia in a patient struggling for every breath may be extremely difficult.

The tracheal tube must be fixed securely without obstructing venous return from the head. Manual or mechanical ventilation of the lungs with a high fractional inspired oxygen concentration (F_iO_2) should be provided as required. In the majority of critically ill patients, the risk of arterial hypoxaemia is greater than the potential risks of oxygen toxicity or impaired hypoxic respiratory drive.

Circulatory management

Prompt recognition and treatment of circulatory shock is a fundamental part of the initial assessment of emergency surgical patients. Multiple, short, wide-bore intravenous cannulae will facilitate rapid fluid resuscitation in hypovolaemic shock, and there are several devices on the market which are capable of delivering high volumes of warmed intravenous fluid or blood to the patient (Fig. 4.2). If there is evidence of arterial hypotension, peripheral hypoperfusion, oliguria, or lactic acidosis, a 10–20 ml/kg crystalloid or 5–10 ml/kg colloid intravenous fluid bolus must be given immediately. Colloid containing regimens are more efficient in achieving a resuscitated state although there is no conclusive evidence of benefit of one fluid over another.

The volume of intravenous fluid required is determined on the basis of estimated deficit, ongoing maintenance, and replacement of losses. In hypovolaemic shock, fluid deficits may be up to 10–20% of total body fluid which represents 4–8 L in a 70 kg patient. This fluid deficit is usually replaced by normal saline, a litre given over 15–30 min, followed by a litre given over 30–60 min. Subsequent litres are titrated over 4–6 h depending on the response of the patient.

Hypovolaemia
• Colloids/crystalloids
• Red cell transfusions
• Blood substitutes
• Central venous pressure monitoring
• ? ICU

Ongoing blood loss is replaced with red cell transfusion and fluid loss from the gastrointestinal tract is usually replaced volume for volume with half normal saline.

If signs of circulatory shock persist despite intravenous fluid therapy as above, it is recommended to administer a monitored intravenous fluid challenge (as a bolus of crystalloid or colloid solution). In the emergency surgical patient it may be necessary to empirically titrate such bolus therapy at the bedside until normovolaemia is achieved. This is necessary not simply to compensate for inadequacies in the estimates made but also to facilitate the recognition of undiagnosed bleeding or of unanticipated losses (e.g. due to pancreatitis or sepsis).

If the patient remains hypotensive and oliguric despite apparently adequate volume resuscitation (central venous pressure of 14–17 mmHg), more sophisticated monitoring and interventions may be appropriate. Gravely ill patients may be referred to the intensive care unit (ICU) to expedite urgently required diagnostic and therapeutic manoeuvres such as invasive monitoring or mechanical ventilation. When an intensive care consultation is requested, there can often be an inclination to delay what had until then been considered an urgent need for surgery. It is imperative that the primary role of the surgical procedure is not obscured by the institution of supportive therapy in ICU.

In patients with advanced pulmonary disease or right ventricular failure, the central venous pressure (CVP) may falsely suggest adequate or even excessive left ventricular pressure. The relationship between left ventricular end diastolic pressure and volume may be unpredictable in patients with myocardial dysfunction (e.g. infarction, contusion, myocarditis, ventricular hypertrophy). In these situations, placement of a pulmonary artery catheter to estimate left ventricular end diastolic pressure may be indicated. However, the pulmonary artery catheter should not be considered a resuscitative tool and rapid intravascular volume replacement takes precedence over 'fine tuning' the cardiovascular system. If low ventricular compliance is problematic, it may be worth measuring ventricular volume by bedside echocardiography, or continuing the process of monitored volume loading in an attempt to identify the filling pressure and volume at which cardiac output or stroke volume is optimized.

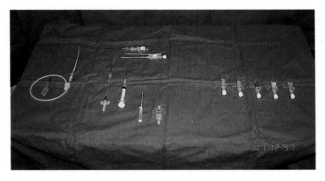

Fig. 4.2 For rapid access for high volume replacement, and for monitoring successful resuscitation, a central venous catheter is highly desirable.

Intra-operative management

Anaesthetic management

A secure patent airway, adequate ventilation of the lungs, and haemodynamic stability provide the framework for anaesthetic management. It is simplistic to assume that a regional anaesthetic is safer than general anaesthesia and it may be appropriate to use a combination of both techniques in an individual patient. The overall competence with which the anaesthetic is administered may have a more important bearing on patient outcome than the exact choice of technique.

Peri-operative physiological monitoring of emergency surgery patients may include electrocardiogram, invasive or noninvasive arterial blood pressure, pulse oximetry, end-tidal carbon dioxide, peripheral and core temperature, central venous pressure and urine output. Specialized monitoring (e.g. pulmonary artery catheterization, transoesophageal echocardiography, intracranial pressure and evoked potential monitoring) may be indicated in specific circumstances.

General anaesthetic agents may be administered intravenously (e.g. thiopentone, propofol, ketamine) or by inhalation (e.g. isoflurane, enflurane, sevoflurane, desflurane). The concentration of inhalational anaesthetic agents in the brain may be altered rapidly by changing the inspired concentration of these agents. Inhalational anaesthetics undergo minimal biotransformation, so that the anaesthetic may be excreted through the lungs at the conclusion of the surgery. Intravenous anaesthetic agents which are rapidly redistributed even after prolonged infusions (e.g. propofol) or are rapidly metabolized (e.g. by plasma cholinesterase) have become popular for total intravenous anaesthetic techniques. Variable rate infusion pumps which use available pharmacokinetic data in an attempt to achieve a constant drug concentration in the blood have recently become available.

> Anaesthetic agents cause myocardial depression and peripheral vasodilatation and may cause profound hypotension in the hypovolaemic patient.

Ideally, there should be resolution of arterial hypotension, peripheral hypoperfusion and lactic acidaemia before surgery and anaesthesia. With the exception of ketamine, intravenous and inhalational anaesthetic agents cause a variable degree of myocardial depression and peripheral vasodilatation. The abrupt introduction of these drugs at the time of induction of anaesthesia may cause profound arterial hypotension if the patient is hypovolaemic and dependent on high sympathetic tone to maintain an adequate perfusion pressure. Also, emergency surgical patients are at risk of intra-operative bleeding or bacteraemia associated with instrumentation of purulent collections. Therefore, it is desirable to have achieved normovolaemia or even hypervolaemia before starting anaesthesia and surgery.

Skeletal muscle paralysis is achieved when clinically indicated by non-depolarizing or depolarizing neuromuscular blocking drugs. Non-depolarizing neuromuscular blocking drugs (e.g. atracurium, pancuronium, vecuronium) are generally used to facilitate surgical access in the abdominal or thoracic cavity. Suxamethonium is used to provide profound short-lived muscle paralysis to facilitate tracheal intubation.

Emergency surgery patients are at risk of pulmonary aspiration during induction of anaesthesia and tracheal intubation. There may be a limited period of fasting and delayed gastric emptying due to pain, ethanol, and opioid medication. A rapid sequence induction/intubation technique should be considered in such patients. The technique consists of denitrogenation of the lungs, administration of an intravenous anaesthetic agent followed by suxamethonium and application of cricoid pressure.

Denitrogenation of the lungs or pre-oxygenation is achieved by up to 3 min spontaneous ventilation with 100% oxygen using a close-fitting face mask. Immediately after administration of an intravenous anaesthetic agent and suxamethonium, firm posterior pressure is applied to the cricoid cartilage (cricoid pressure or Sellick manoeuvre). Compression of the upper oesophagus between the cricoid cartilage and the vertebral column is used to prevent regurgitation of gastric contents into the pharynx before the airway is secured with a cuffed tracheal tube.

The most common predisposing factor for pulmonary aspiration is gastrointestinal obstruction. Other factors include difficulty in managing the airway, abdominal distension (e.g. ascites, obesity, pregnancy), depressed level of consciousness, recent food or alcohol intake, and diabetes mellitus. Inadequate anaesthesia or skeletal muscle paralysis, with coughing or straining during attempts at tracheal tube placement may also be associated with an increased risk of aspiration. If a nasogastric tube is already present, it is generally advised to leave it *in situ* as it may decompress the stomach during tracheal intubation.

Administration of suxamethonium in patients with crush or thermal injury, or with acute upper motor neurone lesions has been associated with a life threatening increase in serum potassium concentration. In susceptible patients, suxamethonium and inhalational anaesthetics are known

> **Rapid sequence induction technique**
>
> - Pre-oxygenation
> - IV anaesthetic induction agent
> - Suxamethonium
> - Cricoid pressure
> - Cuffed endotracheal tube

trigger agents for malignant hyperpyrexia. Suxamethonium is metabolized by plasma pseudocholinesterase. In patients with severe hepatic dysfunction and low concentrations of pseudocholinesterase, there may be a measurable but clinically unimportant prolongation of the duration of muscle paralysis with suxamethonium.

The ability of patients to ventilate their own lungs is lost with all neuromuscular blocking drugs, so that an inadvertent disconnection of the ventilator breathing system would lead to an immediate failure of ventilation. If these agents are used, it is imperative that the clinician has the ability to control the patient's airway and ventilate the lungs to achieve normal gas exchange. Detection of end-tidal carbon dioxide has become a standard monitor at all locations where neuromuscular blocking drugs are used. Low concentrations of anaesthetic agents may be administered to haemodynamically unstable emergency surgical patients. The risk of intra-operative awareness is a hazard when neuromuscular blocking drugs are used under these circumstances.

Narcotic analgesic agents may be administered by the systemic or spinal route. Intravenous narcotic administration in the intra-operative period may be continued into the postoperative period using patient controlled devices. Spinally applied narcotic analgesics have a specific local effect on pain transmission in the dorsal horn of the spinal cord. Respiratory depression is a potential hazard after any administration of narcotic analgesic agents and patients require prolonged careful observation for signs of hypoventilation and somnolence.

Non-steroidal anti-inflammatory agents have become a popular supplement to the analgesic effects of narcotics, although their use may be restricted in patients with renal impairment. The combination of narcotics, local anaesthetics, and non-steroidal agents may provide the most comprehensive approach to postoperative analgesia and facilitate early mobilization of the patient in the postoperative period.

Management of abnormal intra-operative bleeding

Recent advances in our understanding of the physiology of platelet aggregation and blood coagulation have led to a more rational approach to bleeding problems in emergency surgical patients. The starting point in the clotting process is the binding of circulating von Willebrand factor to exposed subendothelial collagen in damaged blood vessels. The subendothelial bound von Willebrand factor exposes multiple intrinsic binding sites for specific platelet membrane glycoprotein receptors (GPIb). Platelet adherence at the site of injury is essential for the subsequent steps in coagulation (platelet plug formation and fibrin deposition) and defective binding of platelet GPIb receptors to von Willebrand factor

may be of prime importance in acquired coagulopathies. Thrombin, adenosine diphosphate, and perhaps other activating stimuli act on bound platelets to enhance further platelet deposition and activation at the site of injury. These initial processes lead to the formation of a haemostatic platelet plug (Fig. 4.3).

The next step is the laying down of a fibrin mesh throughout the platelet plug. Activation of bound platelets leads to expression of further platelet binding sites (GPIIbIIIa and phosphatidylserine) which bind fibrinogen and serve as an essential surface for fibrin formation. A sequence of proenzymes and cofactors, present in trace amounts in plasma, are concentrated on the surface of activated platelets leading to an explosion of activity to generate thrombin. Fibrinogen is cleaved by thrombin to form fibrin.

At the same time as these procoagulant processes are being set in motion, the antithrombin and fibrinolytic systems are also being activated. The active fibrinolytic enzyme plasmin, is generated from plasminogen by the action of tissue plasminogen activator (TPA) which is released from damaged or ischaemic endothelial cells. Plasmin activity is estimated by measurement of plasma fibrinogen degradation products (from fibrin or fibrinogen) or D-dimer (from fibrin cross-linked by thrombin-activated factor XIII).

The classic division of the coagulation cascade into the intrinsic and extrinsic systems may owe more to *in vitro* coagulation studies than to an accurate description of what actually occurs *in vivo*. The standard tests of coagulation may be unable to detect subtle dynamic changes that may occur in the fully activated coagulation system and it is not surprising that many of the treatment strategies suggested for these acquired coagulopathies are empirical or controversial.

Massive transfusion is defined as replacement of the entire blood volume by stored homologous blood in less than 24 h. Severe tissue ischaemia or damage, hypovolaemic or septic shock, hypothermia, and excessive fibrinolysis contribute to the complex, acquired coagulopathy often seen in emergency surgical patients. Two separate mechanisms may contribute to the coagulopathy, dilution or consumption of platelets and soluble clotting factors. The coagulopathy is diagnosed by careful clinical observation of diffuse bleeding at the operative site and at the insertion site of intravascular catheters. The extent of the coagulopathy may be quantified by the standard tests of coagulation.

It is essential that hypovolaemic shock be treated aggressively with red blood cells and crystalloid or colloid solutions to restore circulating blood volume. After surgical control of major bleeding sites and active volume resuscitation, severe bleeding may be treated with 10–12 units of platelets, regardless of the actual platelet count. Fresh frozen plasma is transfused to replace labile factors V and VIII when the prothrombin time is greater than twice control.

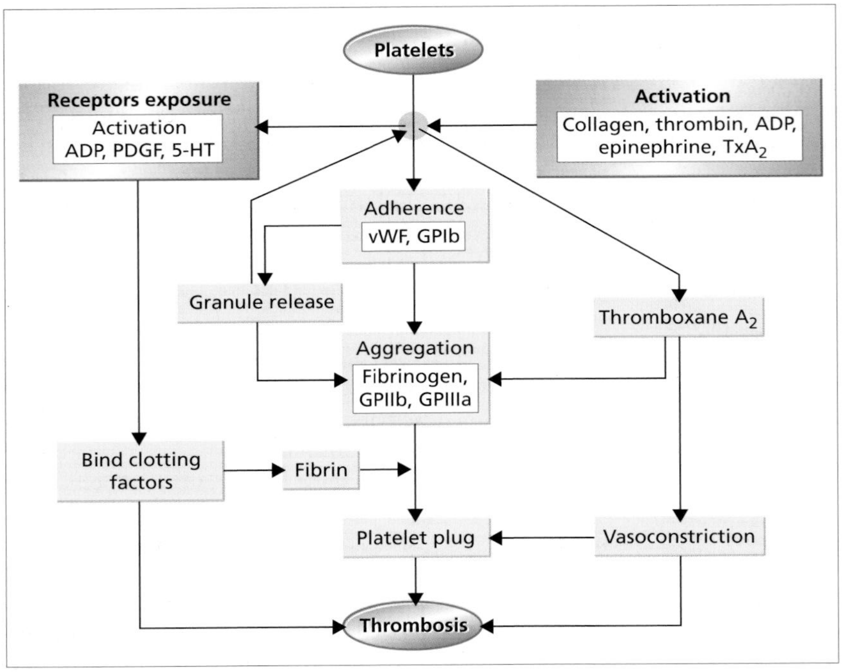

Fig. 4.3 Platelet aggregation and thrombus formation.

Cryoprecipitate contains high concentrations of factor VIII and fibrinogen and should be transfused if the fibrinogen concentration is less than 0.8 g/L. The effect of transfusion of these components should be monitored clinically and by laboratory testing. The prophylactic use of platelets or fresh frozen plasma in massive transfusion is not recommended in the absence of clinical evidence of coagulopathy.

After massive transfusion, the citrate in transfused blood products is metabolized rapidly. Chelation of calcium by citrate leading to symptomatic hypocalcaemia is rare and prophylactic calcium therapy is not recommended. Desmopressin has been used in uraemic patients with overt platelet dysfunction but its potential value in excessive perioperative bleeding is uncertain. The serine protease inhibitor aprotinin, in addition to an antifibrinolytic action, may enhance the binding of platelet GPIb receptors to bound von Willebrand factor. In management of excessive intra-operative bleeding, the use of aprotinin and synthetic antifibrinolytic agents (e.g. tranexamic acid, ε-aminocaproic acid) must be regarded as secondary to surgical expertise, volume resuscitation, and transfusion of platelets and clotting factors.

Postoperative management

Postoperative cardiovascular management

When peri-operative fluid loss has decreased and augmented maintenance requirements no longer pertain, it is usual to revert to predominantly water containing solutions (e.g. 0.18% sodium chloride and 4% glucose) for maintenance pending restoration of nutritional intake. Maintenance fluid requirements are 1–1.5 ml/kg/h and increased by 10% for each degree Celsius rise in body temperature.

If signs of circulatory shock persist despite adequate fluid loading, vasoactive medications to augment cardiac output and improve perfusion pressure may be indicated. Vasoactive medication is administered by accurate infusion pumps into dedicated central venous catheters. Positive inotropic agents (e.g. adrenaline, dobutamine) act directly or indirectly to improve cardiac contractility. If perfusion pressure is low despite adequate filling pressure and stroke volume, a vasoconstrictor agent may be indicated. Vasoconstrictors (e.g. noradrenaline, phenylephrine, metaraminol) act primarily on α-adrenergic receptors in the peripheral vasculature leading to an increase in arterial blood pressure.

Low concentrations of dopamine and dopexamine are active at dopaminergic receptors. The effect of these agents on renal and splanchnic blood flow has not been clearly defined in humans and the claimed improvements in regional perfusion may be secondary to global circulatory effects.

Amrinone, milrinone, and enoximone are noncatecholamine type III phosphodiesterase inhibitors. These agents inhibit the metabolic degradation of intracellular cAMP leading to an increase in intracellular calcium and a positive inotropic effect. In addition, phosphodiesterase inhibitors cause pulmonary and systemic vasodilatation without an increase in heart rate. Phosphodiesterase inhibitors have not gained broad acceptance and are generally used in conjunction with traditional inotropic agents.

The functional state of the cardiovascular system is assessed by repeated evaluation of volume status and ventricular performance. If we correctly predict the response to a particular haemodynamic manoeuvre, our confidence in the accuracy of the overall assessment is increased. Invasive haemodynamic monitoring is indicated when the aetiology of the haemodynamic crisis remains unexplained (e.g. pulmonary oedema with concurrent oliguria).

Goal-directed haemodynamic therapy involves the optimization of cardiac output and the manipulation of perfusion pressure to reverse organ dysfunction associated with major surgery, trauma, or other critical illness. The physiological basis for goal-directed therapy is the observed increase in cardiac output in response to major surgery or comparable states. Oxygen consumption-delivery relationships have been applied to single organs and to the whole body. Global oxygen consumption (Vo_2) is measured by analysis of the inspired and expired gases or calculated using the Fick equation. Oxygen delivery (Do_2) is derived from the product of arterial oxygen content and cardiac output.

Under normal conditions, an increase in Do_2 will not increase Vo_2, although mixed venous oxygen saturation may increase. This non-linear relationship between oxygen consumption and delivery (supply independence) reflects the reserve ability of the tissues to extract oxygen from the blood. Below a critical Do_2, oxygen consumption becomes supply dependent as oxygen extraction becomes inadequate to meet aerobic metabolic demands.

In pathological states, the relationship between oxygen supply and consumption may become more linear because of increased basal oxygen consumption or an inability to extract oxygen from the blood. There may be an elevated plateau or no plateau evident in the new relationship. During supply dependency, there will be progressive metabolic dysfunction with accumulation of lactate. A rapid increase in oxygen delivery that results in an increase in oxygen consumption has been considered as evidence of a supply dependent state.

> The only therapeutic measure to increase tissue perfusion in the critically ill patient is to increase cardiac output.

In critically ill patients, an increase in oxygen delivery may help meet increased tissue oxygen demands. As there is no agent capable of selectively increasing perfusion of specific tissues, the only therapeutic, although inefficient, method to ensure adequate oxygenation of underperfused tissues is to increase global cardiac output. Increased oxygen delivery to supranormal levels is achieved by red blood cell

transfusion and inotropic support. The effect of this strategy on patient outcome is not known. Improved hospital mortality has been demonstrated in non-septic surgical patients in whom supranormal levels of cardiac output, Do_2 and Vo_2 were achieved. This work has not been validated in patients with septic shock or adult respiratory distress syndrome. Indeed, there is evidence that the application of these haemodynamic goals to a heterogenous group of ICU patients may actually increase mortality.

Renal and gut vascular beds have limited reserve oxygen extraction, so that hypoperfusion of these organs is poorly tolerated. The proximity of arterioles to venules in the microcirculation of both organs may predispose to shunting of oxygen away from metabolically active cells. Gut hypoperfusion has become a central issue in sepsis and measurement of gastric mucosal pH by tonometry has been used to assess the adequacy of gut perfusion. A persistently low gastric mucosal pH is associated with increased morbidity and mortality in critically ill patients.

A global increase in oxygen consumption may not prevent covert tissue hypoxia or impaired oxygen extraction. Restoration of global oxygen delivery may be associated with persistent regional hypoperfusion states, e.g. gut mucosal perfusion may remain low despite near normal global gut perfusion. Local regulation of tissue perfusion is disrupted in patients with septic shock, so that achieving supranormal global Vo_2 and Do_2 may not assure satisfactory regional tissue perfusion.

There seems little doubt that higher cardiac index and oxygen delivery are associated with lower mortality. However, it may be that the haemodynamic pattern is merely a prognostic indicator and not directly responsible for a favourable outcome. Therefore, aggressive efforts to increase haemodynamic parameters to supranormal values in all critically ill patients may not be associated with an improvement in regional oxygen delivery or in overall prognosis.

Postoperative mechanical ventilation

In emergency surgery patients, postoperative ventilatory support is usually continued after a prolonged difficult intra-operative course complicated by excessive bleeding and hypothermia. Patients with pre-operative head injury, respiratory or cardiac failure, and septic shock may also benefit from the stability afforded by a short period of mechanical ventilation. Mechanical ventilation is provided to minimize the stress of respiratory dysfunction and is continued until the primary pathophysiological problems are controlled or resolving.

The commonly used mechanical ventilators can be classified in terms of achieving a specific airway pressure, tidal volume, or inspiratory flow rate in the respiratory cycle. The ventilator will switch from inspiration to expiration when one of these control variables reaches a preselected threshold value. The common patterns of adult ventilatory support are assist control, intermittent mandatory ventilation, and pressure support. Novel ventilatory modes are available on microprocessor-controlled mechanical ventilators, but it is not clear which patients will benefit from these new techniques. In most patients, a clear understanding of the advantages and limitations of the method employed may be more important than the actual mode of ventilatory support selected.

Ventilator settings are chosen based on the patient's size and clinical condition but may require careful adjustment based on repeated clinical examination and arterial blood gas analysis. When mechanical ventilation is initiated the fractional inspired oxygen concentration (F_iO_2) is set high to ensure adequate oxygenation. After 20 min, arterial blood gas analysis will dictate an appropriate F_iO_2. The usual goal is a P_aO_2 of 8.0 kPa or S_aO_2 of 90%, because higher values may not substantially enhance tissue oxygenation.

Careful adjustment of the ventilator will minimize incoordination between the patient's spontaneous respiratory effort and the ventilator. This is done by adjustment of the tidal volume, respiratory rate, ventilator sensitivity (degree of difficulty the patient has in initiating a ventilator-supported breath), inspiratory flow rate and positive end expiratory pressure (PEEP) to suit the patient.

Sedative or analgesic medication are carefully titrated to facilitate mechanical ventilation in the postoperative period. In the ICU, neuromuscular blocking agents are frequently used and should only be administered in conjunction with sedative medication. These agents expose the patient to the risk of life-threatening ventilatory failure in the event of an inadvertent airway disconnection. Patients with renal failure, hypomagnesaemia, and in whom high doses of corticosteroids and neuromuscular blockers were used are at risk of developing prolonged skeletal muscle weakness after neuromuscular blockers have been withdrawn. In critically ill mechanically ventilated patients, general care measures such as humidification of inspired gases, suctioning of tracheal secretions, oral hygiene, skin and wound care, should not be overlooked.

There has been a recent appreciation that high airway pressure during mechanical ventilation may aggravate lung parenchymal damage. It has been recommended that peak alveolar pressure, which may be estimated by end inspiratory plateau or pause pressure, should not exceed 35 cmH₂O. In patients who develop high airway pressures, a sudden decrease in dynamic compliance (tidal volume divided by peak airway pressure minus PEEP) with a relatively normal static compliance (tidal volume divided by plateau airway pressure minus PEEP) should prompt an immediate examination of the airways, in particular, the patency of the tracheal tube.

Complications associated with mechanical ventilation are generally related to the duration of ventilation. Problems associated with the airway include endobronchial intubation, tracheal ulceration and stenosis. A tracheostomy should be considered in patients who require more than 2 weeks of ventilatory support. In most patients, percutaneous tracheostomy guided by fibreoptic bronchoscopy can now be performed safely at the bedside; see also Chapter 22.

Between 10 and 50% of mechanically ventilated patients will develop pneumonia and the risk increases with the duration of ventilatory support at a rate of 1–3% per day. In the early hospital course, community-acquired pathogens (e.g. *H. influenzae* and *Strep. pneumonia*) may be responsible for nosocomial pneumonias. After a more protracted course, Gram negative or polymicrobial infections are common, with no pathogen identified in up to 20% of cases. The mortality rate from nosocomial pneumonia is 3%.

Discontinuation of mechanical ventilation is straightforward after short-term ventilatory support, but may be extremely difficult in patients on long-term support. There are numerous methods of weaning from mechanical ventilation which are often based on local in-house practices rather than scientific merit. Reversible factors should be dealt with in a co-ordinated fashion. As a general rule, the pulmonary process (e.g. infection, bronchospasm, sputum retention) should be stable or improving and there should be no evidence of haemodynamic instability. The ability of the patient to protect the upper airway and to cough effectively must be assessed. Optimal analgesia and adequate but not excessive nutritional support will facilitate the withdrawal of mechanical ventilatory support. If tracheal intubation was technically difficult, then extubation must be a planned and controlled procedure.

Peri-operative renal protection

Total renal blood flow has a wide range of physiological variation and may represent up to 20% of total cardiac output. Despite the high global renal oxygen delivery relative to its oxygen consumption, there is an oxygen gradient from the outer cortex to the inner medulla. The medullary thick ascending limb tubular cells have high metabolic demands, but operate in a relatively hypoxic environment. Even a small decrease in total renal blood flow could reduce the peritubular Po_2 to below the hypoxic threshold.

Post-operative mechanical ventilation—indications
• Prolonged surgery
• Excess bleeding, hypothermia
• Head injury
• Respiratory and/or cardiac failure
• Septic shock

A reduction in renal blood flow will stimulate the release of renin from the juxtaglomerular apparatus leading to generation of angiotensin II. Angiotensin II vasoconstricts the efferent arteriole and so preserves glomerular filtration in the face of reduced renal perfusion. The consequent increase in filtration fraction is associated with an increase in proximal tubular sodium reabsorption.

A reduction in the effective arterial or central blood volume due to hypovolaemia will be sensed by low-pressure or volume receptors in the atria and high-pressure receptors in the aortic arch and carotid arteries. These receptors regulate the sympathetic nervous outflow, the release of anti-diuretic hormone (ADH), and indirectly, the release of renin leading to increased retention of sodium and water. The peri-operative stress response will augment sodium and water reabsorption associated with reduction in effective arterial blood volume in order to preserve intravascular volume and perfusion of vital organs. Potassium concentration may be low due to excessive aldosterone activity.

Hypovolaemia → release of ADH
↓
↑ retention of sodium and water

After major surgery, ADH concentrations remain elevated for many days, whereas increased concentrations of renin, angiotensin, and aldosterone are short lived. Administration of glucose-containing intravenous solutions (dextrose 5%, 0.18% sodium chloride and 4% glucose) under these circumstances may lead to hyponatraemia. Abnormalities of sodium and water balance may be difficult to detect by physical examination alone. Pitting oedema may not become noticeable until there has been a weight gain of 5 kg. Arterial blood pressure may not decrease and heart rate increase until there has been a 10% reduction in extracellular fluid. Skin turgor is increasingly unreliable with advancing age and large intravascular volume changes may be associated with relatively minor changes in CVP. In conjunction with ongoing clinical assessment, serial body weights may be helpful.

Not uncommonly in the postoperative period, there may be reduced intravascular blood volume despite a marked increase in extracellular volume. Daily fluid management plans need to accommodate several divergent goals, e.g. preservation of renal perfusion, difficulty with oxygenation, intravenous nutritional support. Although renal blood flow may be better maintained in cardiogenic compared to hypovolaemic shock, excessive intravenous fluid administration may lead to interstitial fluid accumulation and progressive difficulty with oxygenation.

With active sodium and water retention, postoperative oliguria may not be always avoidable, but postoperative

acute renal failure should be. Under-replacement of fluid in the peri-operative period may lead to pre-renal impairment and acute tubular necrosis. In at-risk patients (e.g. jaundice, sepsis, pre-existing renal impairment), use of the CVP, core-to-peripheral temperature gradient, and body weight may help titrate appropriate volumes of intravenous fluid to avoid renal impairment. Even modest peri-operative fluid deficits should be corrected before surgery to limit activation of the neurohumoral mechanisms responsible for sodium and water reabsorption. With increasing age, the ability of the kidney to conserve sodium in the face of peri-operative fluid losses may be impaired.

In critically ill patients, a moderate ischaemic renal insult is often compounded by use of potentially nephrotoxic agents (e.g. contrast media, aminoglycoside antibiotics, amphotericin, cyclosporin and non-steroidal anti-inflammatory agents). Deposition of myoglobin in the renal tubules occurs in rhabdomyolisis. In patients with septic shock, renal vasoconstriction may be mediated by circulating endothelin, thromboxane, prostaglandin F_2, and leukotrienes. There is conflicting evidence for saline and osmotic diuretic administration in ameliorating the renal insult associated with nephrotoxins and aortic cross-clamping.

Patients should be euvolaemic and draining urine freely before intravenous diuretics are considered. High doses of frusemide have been used to convert oliguric to non-oliguric acute renal failure, although no difference in outcome has been demonstrated with this therapy. Once dialysis is required, frusemide probably does not alter the course of acute renal failure, and it is possible that patients who respond to frusemide have less renal impairment to begin with.

Use of low concentrations of dopamine to conserve renal blood flow and preserve urine output is a common practice. However, the renal effects of dopamine may be due to an inotropic and diuretic action rather than an intrinsic renal vasodilator effect. In some situations, dopamine may mask signs of renal ischaemia. The implication in humans is that the use of vasoactive drugs should not precede aggressive fluid resuscitation.

Administration of atrial naturetic peptide has been an exciting development in the management of acute renal failure. In animal and human studies, atrial naturetic peptide with or without diuretics has been shown to have a

---

Factors reducing renal function

- Ischaemia/hypovolaemia/hypotension
- Antibiotics (aminoglycosides, glycopeptides)
- Contrast media
- Myoglobin, bilirubin
- Inappropriate vasoactive or diuretic therapy

beneficial effect on ischaemic and nephrotoxic acute renal failure.

Postoperative gastrointestinal haemorrhage

The acute onset of painless upper gastrointestinal bleeding in critically ill patients may present within 2 weeks of admission to the ICU. The bleeding is rarely severe, being found in nasogastric aspirate in 50% of patients. Identified risk factors include thermal injuries, head injury, multiple trauma, sepsis, steroid therapy and renal failure. Upper gastrointestinal endoscopy demonstrates multiple small shallow ulcers with little induration or oedema most often in the proximal stomach. Preventive therapy includes antacids, H$_2$ receptor antagonists, sucralfate, and proton pump inhibitors. Prophylactic therapy has been recommended in all patients at risk of upper gastrointestinal bleeding in the ICU.

Although H$_2$ receptor antagonists do decrease the volume of gastric secretions, there has been concern about upper gastrointestinal tract bacterial colonization associated with the loss of gastric acidity. Bacterial overgrowth in the stomach may be followed by colonization of the oropharynx, with an increased risk of Gram-negative nosocomial pneumonia. Some clinicians believe that early enteral feeding will decrease the incidence of upper gastrointestinal bleeding in critically ill patients.

Severe upper or lower gastrointestinal bleeding may be the reason for admission to the ICU or it may complicate the care of patients already in the unit. Optimal management involves close co-ordination between the intensivist, the surgeon and gastroenterologist. Many patients stop bleeding spontaneously, but rebleeding is common. The first priority is to resuscitate the patient adequately and frequent estimations of the haematocrit may be useful to confirm stability. The site of bleeding may be difficult to define even after endoscopic examination, labelled red blood cell scanning and arteriography.

Upper gastrointestinal bleeding is usually managed endoscopically (e.g. heater probe, electrocoagulation, injection with adrenaline) and with H$_2$ receptor antagonists or similar agents. In patients with portal hypertension and bleeding oesophageal varices, transjugular intrahepatic portosystemic shunts (TIPS procedure) may decompress the high-pressure variceal system without jeopardizing the opportunity for subsequent liver transplantation.

Patients who fail to respond to endoscopic or invasive radiological measures or who bleed rapidly and excessively must be considered for surgery. In addition to their pre-existing problems, these patients may now be facing surgical exploration requiring constant blood transfusions and often without clear evidence of where the bleeding is coming from (see also Chapter 13).

Prevention of postoperative thrombotic disorders

Venous thrombo-embolism is an important cause of morbidity and mortality in postoperative surgical patients. The risk of venous thrombo-embolism is increased in immobilized, elderly, obese patients with heart failure, lower limb paralysis, or a previous history of thrombo-embolism. High-risk procedures would include lower limb amputation, major pelvic surgery for malignancy, or major orthopaedic lower limb or pelvic surgery.

Prophylaxis against venous thrombo-embolism has taken various forms. Low dose unfractionated heparin has been used widely although low molecular weight heparins are thought to be associated with less bleeding complications. Adjusted-dose heparin uses unfractionated heparin to increase activated partial thromboplastin time (aPTT) by 2–3 fold, but requires careful laboratory monitoring. Warfarin has been used for prophylaxis against venous thrombo-embolism, but it again requires laboratory monitoring and in an acute situation the anticoagulant effects of warfarin are more difficult to reverse than those of heparin. Dextrans reduce platelet aggregation, improve blood flow and may facilitate fibrinolysis. Intravenous administration may be associated with allergic reactions. Aspirin alone has not been shown to reduce the incidence of postoperative deep venous thrombo-embolism (DVT). Mechanical methods such as elastic compression stockings and intermittent pneumatic calf compression have also been described. The use of anticoagulants is a particular concern in patients after craniotomy and spinal surgery. Mechanical methods may be best, with anticoagulants avoided for the first 5 postoperative days.

Risk factors for haematemesis
• Burns
• Head injuries
• Trauma
• Shock
• Renal failure

Pharmalogical agents used in DVT prophylaxis
• Low-dose heparin
• Low molecular-weight heparin
• Unfractionated heparin
• Warfarin
• Dextran
• Aspirin

Regional anaesthesia, although not often used in emergency surgical patients, may contribute to a lower incidence of venous thrombo-embolism by peripheral vasodilatation and the reduction in viscosity as a result of fluid loading. There may be reduced activation of clotting factors and fibrinolysis, in addition to decreased platelet adhesion and aggregation.

Peri-operative nutritional support

The principles of peri-operative nutritional support include avoiding starvation in all patients, using the enteral route if possible, and recognizing specific nutritional deficiencies which may require treatment. A detailed history of dietary intake and excessive losses is a vital step in the nutritional assessment because most of the indices of nutritional status are non-specific. Although weight loss is well recognized to be associated with increased mortality, weight loss itself may be due to malnutrition, accelerated protein catabolism, or sodium and water depletion. Decreased serum albumin concentration in the critically ill patient more often reflects increased albumin consumption by the acute phase response and loss into the extravascular space rather than nutritional deficiency. Diminished anthropometric measurement or decreased functional capacity (hand grip strength) may represent an ongoing catabolic process. Specific nutritional deficiencies must be recognized in the peri-operative setting. In patients with alcohol abuse, potassium, magnesium, thiamine and folate deficiency may be evident. Neurological deterioration may progress if thiamin-deficient patients are given dextrose.

Pre-operative intravenous nutritional support will only benefit severely depleted patients in whom the gastrointestinal tract is unavailable. In general, the complications of preoperative intravenous nutrition outweigh the benefits. The intra-operative period is a relatively insulin-resistant state, and intravenous feeding is associated with hyperglycaemia and is probably superfluous.

> Intravenous nutrition is only of benefit prior to surgery in a severely malnourished patient with a non-functioning gastrointestinal tract.

In the first postoperative days, the emphasis is on correction of electrolyte, water source, vitamin, and zinc deficiencies. Many surgical patients incur major gastrointestinal potassium, magnesium, and zinc losses. The refeeding syndrome refers to early over-enthusiastic caloric support aggravating hypokalaemia, hypomagnesaemia, and hypophosphataemia, and leading to clinically apparent skeletal muscle weakness, lethargy and respiratory failure. This is probably best avoided by a cautious increase in calorie intake to 20–40 kcal/kg/day and meticulous attention to electrolyte needs, especially in patients with protracted losses or following a period of relative starvation. It is worth emphasizing that water soluble vitamins (B and C) are lost inexorably via the urine, and that thiamine deficiency in particular may aggravate cardiac, neurological and metabolic dysfunction. Early replenishment of thiamine and other water soluble vitamins may be very important in individual critically ill patients.

The role of protein catabolism in critical illness may necessitate a higher nitrogen input (1.5–3 g protein/kg/day). Daily protein losses can be measured, but the delay in getting the results back may limit the usefulness of this process in altering the prescription. Furthermore, there may be inaccuracies in the estimates of stool losses and urinary losses in severely oliguric or anuric patients. Caloric requirements may be more precisely estimated by oxygen consumption measurements in relatively stable ventilated patients in whom a low F_iO_2 is being used, but the application of this approach is limited.

Recombinant growth hormone has been used to supplement artificial nutrition postoperatively with improved nitrogen balance, weight gain, wound healing, and shortening of hospital stay. It appears that growth hormone is more likely to benefit patients who are moving clear of a septic or unstable period.

Enteral nutrition is more physiological, less expensive, and associated with fewer complications than intravenous nutrition. Enteral nutrition may also be associated with decreased bacterial and endotoxin translocation from the bowel, leading to a decreased incidence of pneumonia and improved patient survival.

> Enteral nutrition should be used before intravenous nutrition wherever possible.

In practical terms, enteral nutrition is commenced early in the postoperative course when nasogastric losses are less than 300 ml/day and without waiting for bowel sounds to be heard. Some clinicians start enteral nutrition in the immediate postoperative period. Our practice is to commence full concentration feed (1 cal/ml) at 20 ml/h and increase to 80 ml/h over 3–4 days if the residual volume is less than 200 ml 4 h after stopping the feed. Continuous enteral feeding may minimize vomiting and gastrointestinal hold up. Indeed, early enteral nutrition may replace the requirement for antacid and H_2 receptor antagonists. However, there is some evidence that stopping the feeding overnight may decrease the incidence of nosocomial pneumonia due to restoration of a starvation-associated low gastric pH.

A common limitation to early enteral nutrition seems to be gastroduodenal holdup or gastric atony. This may be overcome by nasoduodenal or nasojejunal intubation under fluoroscopic control, or at the time of surgery if gastric atony is anticipated. A formal jejunostomy tube may also be used, and there is some evidence that oligopeptides may be of benefit in these feeds. Addition of prokinetic agents (e.g. cisapride, metoclopramide, domperidone, erythromycin) has been claimed to improve the success rate of enteral feeding regimens.

Mental status changes in the postoperative period

Postoperative agitation is a constant source of frustration for ICU personnel. Patients may dislodge intravascular devices, chest and abdominal drains, nasogastric or tracheal tubes, they may injure themselves or staff members. For many patients in the postoperative period, sleep may be impossible, day and night cycles are disrupted, and there may be constant light, noise, and activity around the patient. Discussions with the patient's family may identify important pre-morbid factors, such as a history of mental illness or substance abuse. Elderly patients are most vulnerable after extensive surgery and on multiple medications. Anger, depression, disorientation, or frank psychosis are not uncommon. It is vital to exclude organic causes for mental status changes, particularly the presence of infection, postoperative pain, or hypoxaemia.

There should be a constant attempt to orientate the patient to time and place. Postoperative pain is treated with a combination of systemic or spinal applied narcotics, local anaesthetics, and non-steroidal anti-inflammatory agents. Physical restraints may re-inforce psychotic feelings but may be necessary in some patients. There are a wide spectrum of pharmacological agents used to treat postoperative agitation, although none are entirely satisfactory. In general, it is preferable to gradually increase the dose of a limited number of agents, rather than using short trials of many different agents. We have used haloperidol in patients with psychotic symptoms, and benzodiazepines (e.g. chlordiazepoxide or midazolam) for agitation. A simple regimen is desirable as many of these agents are themselves associated with mental status changes.

Conclusion

The perioperative care of emergency surgery patients involves a concerted approach to all systems including the early recognition and therapy for intercurrent sepsis. Timely and focused multidisciplinary management should expedite recovery and discharge from the intensive care unit.

Further reading

Fiddian-Green, R.G. (1995) Gastric intramucosal pH, tissue oxygenation and acid base balance. *British Journal of Anaesthesia* **74** 591–606.

Hewitt, P.E. & Machin, S.J. (1990) Massive blood transfusion. *British Medical Journal* **300** 107–109.

Jeejeebhoy, K.N. (1995) Nutrition in critical illness. In: *Textbook of Critical Care* (eds W.C. Shoemaker, S.M. Ayres, A. Grenvik & P.R. Holbrook), pp. 1106–1115. W.B. Saunders Co, Philadelphia.

Murphy, W.G., Davies, M.J. & Eduardo, A. (1993) The haemostatic response to surgery and trauma. *British Journal of Anaesthesia* **70** 205–213.

Shackford, S.R. (1987) Initial management of patients with multiple injuries. In: *Problems in Critical Care: Trauma* (eds S.R. Shackford & A.Z. Pesel), pp. 550–558. J.B. Lippincott, Philadelphia, PA.

CHAPTER 5

Burns

Martin A. P. Milling

Incidence

Across the world burns are a major scourge for many people with an untold toll of death, disfigurement and disability. In the developed countries of northern Europe and North America the total incidence of burn injury, the number of recorded deaths and the number of major burns have declined steadily since the Second World War (Fig. 5.1).

In 1874, *The Illustrated London News* noted in an editorial that three women had been burned to death in London in one winter week. The cause was the fashion for wide hooped skirts which all too often came too close to an open fire with rapid and often fatal consequences.

In more recent times regulations have helped to make the home a relatively safer place. For instance the Heating Appliances Act, Fireguards Act 1952, the Oil Burner Standards Act 1960 and the Nightdresses for Children Act 1962 have all helped to reduce the incidence of injury. Changes in patterns of living and social customs have probably had a much larger influence than specific laws and regulations aimed at preventing burns.

For instance, most homes in the UK are now heated by central heating and not by the once ubiquitous open coal fire. The clean air acts of the 1950s were more influential in this than any burn prevention programme. Similarly, there has been a revolution in the clothing industry with the introduction of synthetic materials. Untreated cotton propagates flame but newer materials such as nylon tend to propagate flame slowly and melt instead of flaming. The damage caused to the person wearing the garment is, consequently, much less. Conversely, when the synthetic foam used in furniture manufacture burns the products of combustion are highly toxic. The new requirements for higher standards of furniture are most welcome.

Most burning accidents continue to occur at home. Children under five years are still the largest group to be admitted and most of them will have suffered scald injuries. The other group who are most at risk is the elderly. MacArthur used the phrase 'can't get out of the way fast enough' and it is the relative immobility of the young, the old and the infirm which makes them particularly prone to burn injury.

Organizations such as the Child Accident Prevention Trust and the Royal Society for the Prevention of Accidents play a major and constructive role in influencing design of domestic appliances and in legislation.

It is just as important that doctors who treat the burn-injured take every opportunity to influence public opinion so that it becomes unacceptable to sell or use a potentially dangerous item either at home or in the workplace. They should also realize that education must always be more important than any legislation and take every opportunity to raise awareness of any burn hazard. About half of all households in the UK now have a smoke alarm fitted to the premises, but it is often disappointing to find how few have a fire extinguisher or flame-proof blanket in the kitchen where most fires start. The aim of all burns surgeons is to be able to close their burn unit for lack of patients.

First aid

Airway management is mandatory. As soon as the injured person is in a place of safety the state of consciousness is assessed and the airway is secured. Assessment of the patient continues according to principles of ATLS®. See Chapter 1.

The source of heat is removed as quickly as possible:

1 *Extinguish all flames*: lie the person down and roll them in a blanket or carpet or use a fire extinguisher.

2 *Turn off the electricity*: in rare instances this will have to be done before the injured can be approached.

3 *Remove the scalding liquid*: most scalds are caused by spillage of hot water; apply copious cold water and remove any clothing.

4 *Chemical burns*: apply copious cold water.

Do not pick up the flaming cooking pan; turn off the heat and cover the pan with a wet towel or fire blanket.

First aid

- Cold water is the mainstay of first aid.
- Morphine is the best analgesic: do not be afraid to give enough.

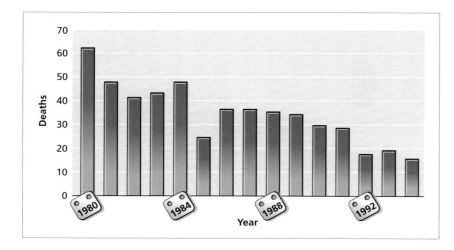

Fig. 5.1 There has been a steady decline in the number of burn related deaths in Wales (OPCS).

Do not go back into a burning building for the cat or anything else; you will be asphyxiated.

Do call the fire brigade.

Transport and admission to hospital
(Table 5.1)

The patient is evacuated from the scene of injury once he/she has been assessed and stabilized. Burned clothing may be left in place and the wound is wrapped in a clean sheet or towel until arrival at hospital. He or she must be kept warm at all times and pain relief must not be forgotten. Do not be afraid to give enough analgesia; small aliquots of intravenous opiate should be titrated against the analgesic effect.

Pathogenesis of burn shock (Fig. 5.2)

In the hours after burn injury the major considerations are the changes to the homeostasis of the separate components of blood: water, electrolytes, plasma proteins and red blood cells. It is the loss of these components from the circulation that induces 'burn shock'. Their loss is inevitably interlinked and they can be considered together. The loss of integrity of the skin which is damaged or destroyed is vitally important but, in addition, major changes occur in the tissues which lie deep to and around the burn itself. Damage in this zone is the cause of continuing losses.

Water, salt and protein are lost from the circulating blood volume by exudation onto the surface of the wound, by increased microvascular permeability and by increased interstitial osmotic pressure.

The rate of loss from the surface will be affected by external factors such as the ambient temperature and the method of treatment of the burn wound. For instance, burns treated by exposure in a high ambient temperature may lose consid-

erably more fluid by evaporation than those treated with occlusive dressings at a lower room temperature.

The increase in microvascular permeability is most marked at and near the site of injury, but will also be present distant from the wound. It will allow movement of large molecular weight proteins and water into the extracellular space with rapid accumulation of protein rich oedema. The abnormal capillary permeability will slowly return to normal within 36 h of injury. At the same time there is a great increase in intracellular osmolality; this is associated with large shifts of water and sodium into the damaged cells. The accumulation of oedema will be most marked in areas such as the face and the dorsum of the hand where the tissues are lax, but on the limbs and the palms of the hands it will be less obvious. However the hydrostatic pressures are just as great in these areas (Fig. 5.3).

The absolute quantities of fluid lost from the circulating blood volume will depend upon the size of the patient and the relative size of the burn. All calculations for replacement are based on the weight and the percentage of the body surface area (BSA) which is burned.

Estimation of area of burn

The average total BSA of an adult male is about 2 m². The estimation of fluid requirements is most accurate using an estimate of BSA injured in m². For most purposes it is sufficient to estimate the percentage BSA burned for the individual.

The charts shown in Fig. 5.4 have been used for many years. Note that the surface area of the head of a child represents a much higher percentage of the total than for an adult. The commonest mistake made by the beginner is to overestimate the BSA injured.

When estimating the area it is best to stay with the patient and draw the burned areas onto the chart. Remember the

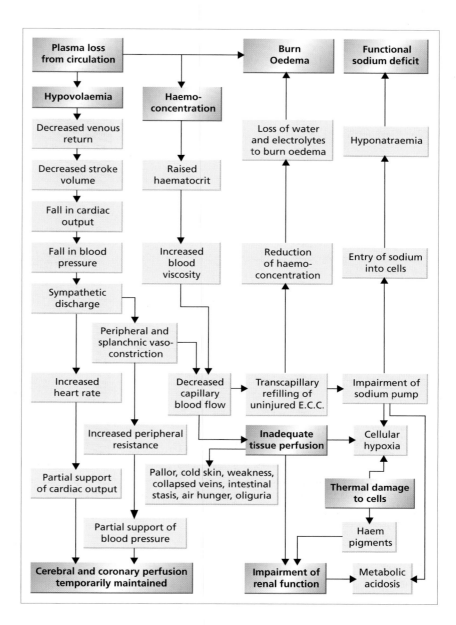

Fig. 5.2 Pathogenesis of burn shock. (Reproduced with permission from, Settle J.A.D. *Burns—The First Five Days*, Smith & Nephew Pharmaceuticals Ltd.)

three dimensions of the body are projected onto the chart. For instance it is easy to forget that the lateral side of the thorax extends to the mid-axillary line. Only the areas which are burned or blistered are included when estimating fluid requirements. The palm of the patient's outstretched hand and fingers is taken to be 1% of the body surface area of that patient. Patches of erythema without blistering are generally excluded from the sums although they should be noted.

Depth of burning

For practical purposes most skin burns can be classified as *partial thickness* or *full thickness*. The essential difference is that in full thickness skin injury all the layers which are capable of regeneration are destroyed, so that surgery will be required to close a wound of any significant size. Conversely, the partial thickness injury will heal without surgery.

If only the sweat glands remain the wound will still eventually heal. However, the slow progress of the deep, partial thickness injury will be associated with an unstable hypertrophic scar. For this reason, when the burn extends into the reticular dermis the term *deep partial thickness* is used. The depth of burn injury will have a major influence on subsequent management and every care should be taken to assess wounds accurately.

Table 5.1 Summary of action on admission of a burns patient.

History
Time of accident
Nature of accident: possibility of other injuries
Source of heat, time of exposure to heat (cold)
Age, sex, weight
Exposure to smoke, blast
First aid given
Past illnesses/accidents (including psychiatric)
Drug ingestion
Possibility of non-accidental injury?

Examination
Conscious level
Restlessness, pain
Pulse, blood pressure, respiratory rate, peripheral circulation
Soot in mouth, nostrils, sputum
Swelling of face, mouth, pharynx
Eardrums (if blast suspected)
Burn wound:
  %BSA
  depth $\left.\right\}$ Chart
Other injuries (head and trunk, spine, limbs)
Weight

Investigations
Hb, PCV, urea and electrolytes, calcium, glucose (SMAC)
Osmolality of blood and urine
Blood gases including pH
Carbon monoxide lactate
Chest X-ray

Monitor
Temperature: core and peripheral
Arterial blood pressure
Pulse oximetry
CVP (Swann–Ganz if necessary)

Treatment
Manage airway and institute CPR
Estimate fluid requirements and start IVI
Insert urinary catheter
Pain relief (intravenous?)
Dress wound
Treat other injuries
Assess tetanus immunization status
H_2 antagonist as prophylaxis against gastric erosion
Pass nasogastric tube and aspirate to pre-empt gastric dilatation.
  Start enteral feeding

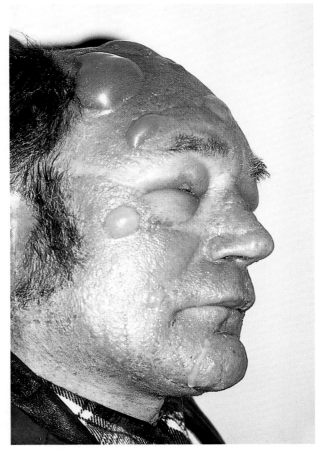

Fig. 5.3 Flash burn of face 24 h after injury to show accumulation of fluid as oedema, within blisters and on the surface of the skin.

Resuscitation

The circulating blood volume is maintained by the administration of sufficient quantities of water and salt. The calculation of the amount required varies between 2 ml/%/kg/h to 4 ml/%/kg/h. The largest part of the calculated volume is given in the first hours after injury.

In the UK the formula first described by Muir and Barclay (1987) using plasma is still most widely used (Fig. 5.5).

The first 24 hours after burning are divided into five periods: 3 or 4 h each in the first 12 h and 2 h in the subsequent 12 h. The amount of fluid to be given in each period is calculated by the formula:

$$\frac{\text{weight in kg} + \% \text{ BSA}}{2} = N\text{ml}$$

N ml are given in each period, with the first aliquot being started from the time of injury, not the time of arrival in hospital.

This formula is equivalent to giving 2.5 ml/%/kg. The most commonly used product for fluid replacement in the

Chart for estimating severity of burn wound

Name _____ Ward _____ Number _____ Date _____

Age _____ Admission weight _____

	Anterior	Posterior	

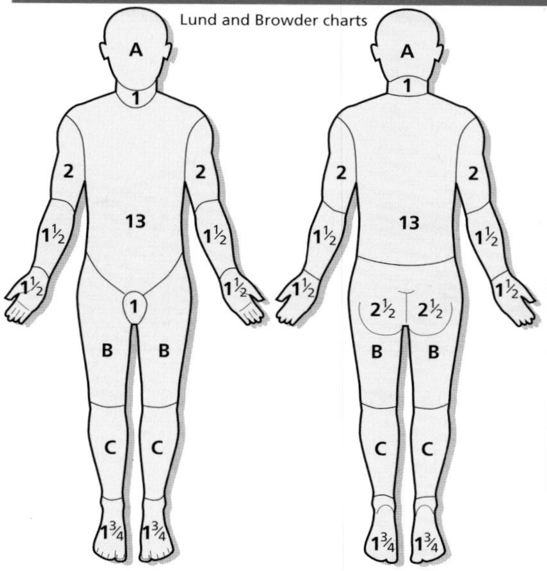

Lund and Browder charts

Ignore simple erythema

Partial thickness loss (PTL)

Full thickness loss (FTL)

Region	Ptl%	Ftl%
Head		
Neck		
Ant. trunk		
Post. trunk		
Right arm		
Left arm		
Buttocks		
Genitalia		
Right leg		
Left leg		
Total burn		
		%

Reflective percentage of body surface area affected by growth

Area	Age 0	Age 1	Age 5	Age 10	Age 15	Adult
A = ½ of head	9 ½	8 ½	6 ½	5 ½	4 ½	3 ½
B = ½ of one thigh	2 ¾	3 ¼	4	4 ½	4 ½	4 ¾
C = ½ of one leg	2 ½	2 ½	2 ¾	3	3 ¼	3 ½

Fig. 5.4 Lund and Browder Charts used for estimation of body surface area burned. Note the relatively large size of the head of the small child.

UK is human albumin solution (HAS) or its equivalent. This is manufactured from pooled plasma, but is treated to eliminate viruses and has a long shelf life. The solution contains proteins of molecular weight less than 80 000, and its value as a plasma expander is certainly less than plasma containing a full complement of high molecular weight proteins. The fluid requirements of many patients may exceed the amount calculated and extra HAS may need to be infused.

Resuscitation with crystalloid alone is widely used, particularly where plasma preparations are not available. Physiological solutions such as Ringer/lactate or Hartman's are cheap and readily available and they carry no fears about transmission of viruses. Fluid is given at the rate of 4 ml/%/kg for the first 24 h. There may be some advantage to using hypertonic saline if the total amounts given are carefully controlled. Other regimes may seek to introduce

Fluid resuscitation

Whatever the estimate of fluid requirements, keep going back to the patient to assess clinical response.

colloid when 12 h have elapsed and the worst phase of capillary leakage is beginning to resolve.

No trial has shown definitive benefits for any one 'formula' or regime. However, those who use colloid regimes continue to maintain that their use is associated with less oedema and fewer respiratory problems.

Whichever formula is used, regular assessment of the patient must be carried out at frequent intervals. The end of each period of the Muir and Barclay regime is a convenient and minimum interval for thought about continuing management.

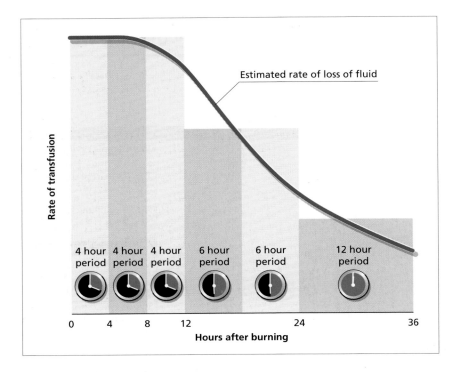

Fig. 5.5 Diagram to show how the rate of transfusion in the first 36 hours is calculated to match the estimated loss of fluid. (Reproduced with permission from Muir, I.F.K., Barclay, T.L. & Settle, J.A.D. (1987) *Burns and Their Treatment*, 3rd edn. Butterworth Heinemann, Oxford.)

Assessment during the shock phase

Observe
• General condition
• Urine output and osmolality of urine
• PCV and osmolality of blood
• Temperature: core and peripheral
• O_2 saturation (pulse oximeter)
• Serum electrolytes
• CVP ⎫
• Arterial blood gases. ⎬ as indicated
⎭
The general condition of the patient and the urine output are the foremost guides to progress. Restlessness and a failure to respond to analgesia may often point to inadequate hydration, particularly when dealing with children. The urine output should be maintained at about 0.5 to 1.0 ml/kg/h (50–70 ml/h in the adult).

Mortality

The mortality from burn injury has improved with active and aggressive treatment but it must be realized that some injuries are so severe that survival is impossible. The chances are closely related to age, pre-existing illness and the severity of the burn (Fig. 5.6).

Figure 5.6 shows the inexorable decline in the chances of survival with increasing age and the severity of injury. If significant smoke inhalation is present the chances of survival are greatly reduced.

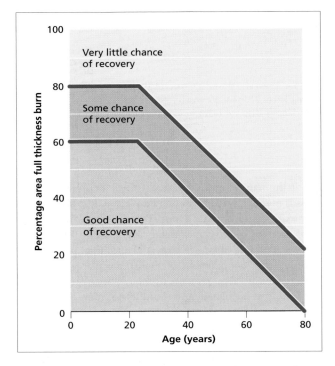

Fig. 5.6 Mortality probabilities. (Reproduced with permission from Muir, I.F.K., Barclay, T.L. & Settle, J.A.D. (1987) *Burns and Their Treatment*, 3rd edn. Butterworth Heinemann, Oxford.)

The surgeon may occasionally be faced with one of these tragic cases where he knows that attempts at treatment will only prolong life for a short period. He must make the difficult decision that resuscitation is not in the patient's interest. This can sometimes be extremely difficult, particularly as the injured person may be conscious, lucid and rational. Any decision should be made after consultation with a specialist burn surgeon, as well as the relatives and sometimes with the patient him or herself.

Treatment is directed to making the last hours as comfortable as possible.

Smoke inhalation

All UK burn units have seen a marked increase in numbers of patients admitted with smoke inhalation, although many of these cases will have comparatively minor burns. The change in admission patterns is related to different factors. First there is a true increase in incidence. Many cases are admitted from home where they have been exposed to the toxic fumes released by combustion of the polyurethane foam used for the manufacture of padded furniture.

Second, the training, skills and equipment of fire and ambulance crews have all improved dramatically. It is now possible for them to go into premises and rescue people from situations where once they would have been abandoned. Endotracheal intubation, ventilation and venous access at the site bring patients to hospital who would not previously have survived.

Injury is caused by four different factors: first, hypoxia as the available oxygen is consumed by fire. Second, the oxygen carrying-capacity of the blood is diminished by carbon monoxide. Third, carbon monoxide and cyanide reduces oxygen utilization at the cellular level. Cyanide poisoning is rarely seen in the absence of CO but if the CO level rises above 15% it may commonly be found. Fourth, irritant products of combustion affect gas exchange by direct damage to the all important alveolar lining.

Table 5.2 shows the range of toxic smoke compounds which may be released by combustion of different materials. These may be toxic in their own right but also potentiate the effects of the main agents carbon monoxide and cyanide.

Management of suspected smoke inhalation

The algorithm shown in Fig. 5.7 summarizes action in suspected cases. Although they will often co-exist, it is important to distinguish between burns of the upper respiratory tract and damage to the lower respiratory tract by inhalation of toxic products.

Smoke inhalation
The onset of clinical illness may be tomorrow.

Table 5.2 Toxic products of combustion of different materials.

Material	Location	Decomposition products
Cellulose	Wood, paper, cotton, jute	Aldehydes, acrolein
Wool, silk	Clothing, fabric, blankets, furniture	Hydrogen cyanide, ammonia, hydrogen sulphide
Rubber	Tyres	Sulphur dioxide, hydrogen sulphide
PVC	Upholstery material Wire/pipe coating Wall, floor, and furniture coverings	Hydrogen chloride, phosgene
Polyurethane	Insulation, upholstery material	Hydrogen cyanide, isocyanates, ammonia, acrylonitriles
Polyester	Clothing, fabric	Hydrogen chloride
Polypropylene	Upholstery material, carpeting	Acrolein
Polyacrylonitrile	Appliances, engineering plastics	Hydrogen cyanide
Polyamide (nylon)	Carpeting, clothing	Hydrogen cyanide, ammonia
Melamine resins	Household and kitchen goods	Hydrogen cyanide, ammonia formaldehyde
Acrylics	Aircraft windows, textiles, wall coverings	Acrolein

Reproduced with permission from Prien, T. & Traber, D.L. (1988) Toxic smoke compounds and inhalation injury: a review. *Burns* **14** 451–460.

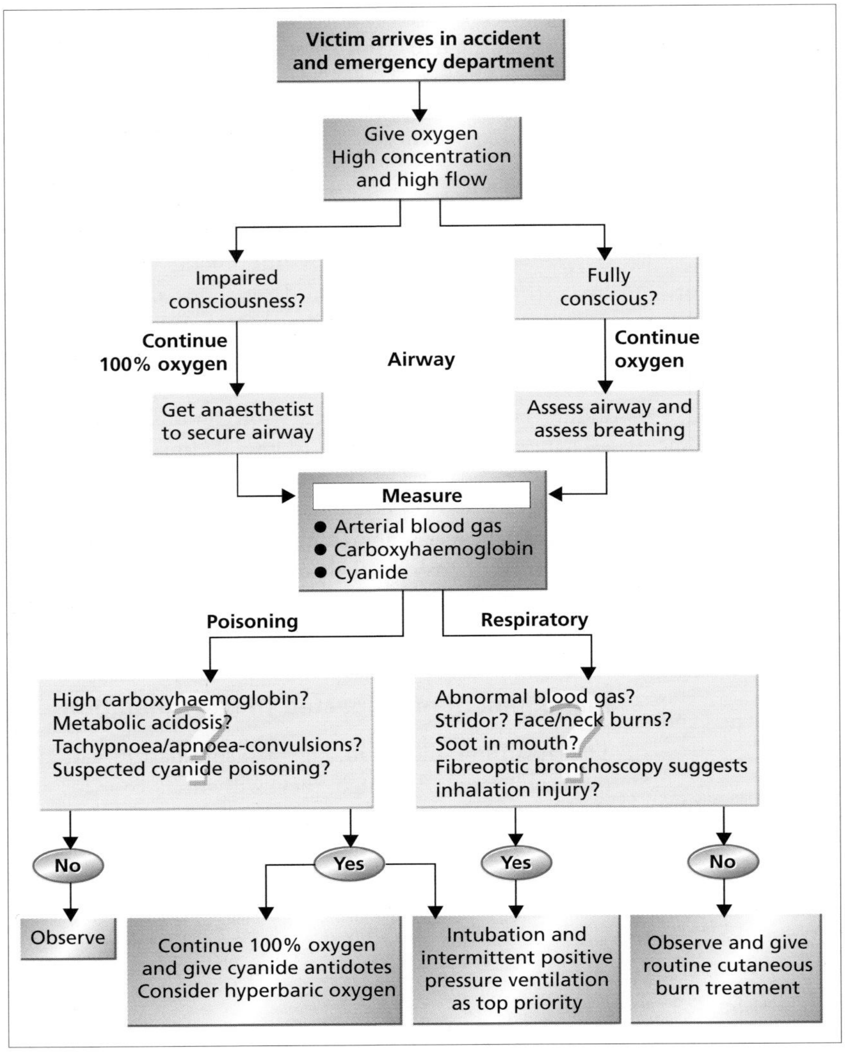

Fig. 5.7 Algorithm of action in case of suspected inhalation injury. (Reproduced with permission from Langford, R.M. & Armstrong, R.F. (1989) Algorithm for managing injury from smoke inhalation. *British Medical Journal* **299** 902.)

The history of the injury is crucial as there may often be little sign of smoke inhalation. Ask if the patient has been trapped with smoke in an enclosed space for any time at all. Direct damage to the respiratory tract by heat is less common. The inhalation of steam may be particularly dangerous because the high latent heat of water allows thermal energy to be carried into the lower respiratory tract. The direct inhalation of flame is uncommon but hot dry gases will cause extensive damage.

Enquiry must be made of any previous history of smoking and of cardiorespiratory disease.

All admissions with burns should be examined for signs of smoke inhalation: the lips and the inside of the mouth may be burned with blistering of the oral mucosa and the vibrissae of the nose are typically singed or coated with soot. The conscious level is also recorded.

Signs of cough, black deposits in the sputum, raised respiratory rate, irritation of the eyes, and clinical signs of upper airway obstruction may all be present. Auscultation of the chest and chest radiography may not be abnormal on presentation but will provide a baseline in the days ahead. Skin burns may make the classic signs of carbon monoxide poisoning difficult to see. Swelling of the tissues of the mouth, pharynx and larynx can be rapid and dramatic; occasionally the airway may be compromised and intubation must be carried out without delay. In the first instance this is preferable to tracheostomy, but tracheostomy is mandatory if the airway cannot be secured.

Investigation should include estimation of carbon monoxide as well as arterial blood gases. The initial level of carbon monoxide in the blood will often give a pointer to the likely course. This is partly because it is a marker for cyanide which is less easy to measure directly.

It is vital to realize that the effects of smoke inhalation may only manifest their full extent some days after the injury. In a typical case the patient will be admitted with a history suggestive of inhalation and little in the way of symptoms or signs. However, the condition will deteriorate over the succeeding day and within 3 days he may require assisted respiratory ventilation as a gross interstitial pneumonitis develops. In severe cases, 6 weeks may elapse before there is sufficient regeneration of the lining of the alveoli for normal gas exchange to occur again. During this time assisted ventilation, and all the facilities of the intensive care unit, should be available. The late onset of pulmonary signs is also seen in cases who have been subjected to blast in explosions.

Emergency surgery

The only surgery which may have to be done within a few hours of admission was set out by Maisels and is summarized by the triad

- To save a life: Tracheostomy
- To save a limb: Escharotomy
- To save an eye: Tarsorraphy

The need for tracheostomy is covered in the section on smoke inhalation above. The indications for its use have certainly diminished in recent years.

Escharotomy is a procedure which is frequently carried out in burn practice. When the skin is burned through its full thickness it loses its normal elasticity, and if the burn is circumferential it may then act as a constricting band. The leakage of fluid into the interstitial space deep to the burn is rapid and unstoppable. The combination of oedema and a tight band can result in ischaemia of the tissues both at, and distal to, the injury. Splitting of the eschar should be carried out without undue delay. In the UK specialist advice is usually available and no detriment will arise if the procedure is not done until the patient is in the care of the burn surgeon. A few hours can usually safely elapse during transfer, and during this time the peripheral circulation must be observed. It may be monitored by pulse oximetry, by measurement of skin temperature or by Doppler probe. However, if there is any doubt the inexperienced should not be afraid to split the eschar. The failure of pulses which have been monitored by doppler ultrasound is a indication to proceed without delay.

It is important to realize that circumferential burns of the chest (and abdomen in a small child) can cause respiratory embarrassment and difficulties with ventilatory support.

Escharotomy
Tight eschar can restrict respiration as well as the peripheral circulation.

Although the eschar is insensate and so may be cut without pain the escharotomy cut should extend into normal skin above and below the constriction. It is wise to have the services of a skilled anaesthetist on hand together with the full backup of an operating theatre. This will ensure best asepsis as well as the availability of diathermy for haemostasis. Most burns in civilian practice do not extend deeper than the fat immediately under the skin. The escharotomy should extend into this plane only; it is not a fasciotomy.

In rare cases there will be deeper tissue destruction; for instance, where the epileptic has fallen unconscious into an open fire or where the patient has come into direct contact with high voltage electricity. When it is clear that significant volumes of muscle are dead, the normal surgical principles of wide surgical toilet and fascial release must apply.

Immediate excision of large formic acid and chromic acid burns may rarely be needed to prevent systemic damage. Tarsorrhaphy may occasionally be needed if the eyelids are burned so badly that the cornea is exposed by ectropion of the lids. A simple stitch between the lids will suffice in an emergency. It is also possible to maintain the moisture of the cornea by frequent irrigation with normal saline or proprietary eyebath solutions.

Assessment of burn depth

History

Burns which will usually heal

- Sunburn
- Flash burns, including electrical
- Tea in a cup ⎫
- Bath water. ⎭ Prompt first aid may have an influence

Burns which will not usually heal

- Boiling water scalds
- Scalds where prolonged immersion has occurred
- Hot toffee
- Molten metal
- Clothes catching fire
- Contact electrical burns
- Prolonged contact with hot solid.

Examination

- Colour, consistency, smell
- Circulation
- Sensation: touch, pinprick
- Hair follicles
- Intact blisters usually conceal a superficial burn.

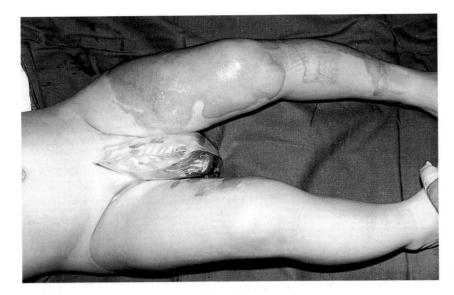

Fig. 5.8 Superficial scald caused by a cup of hot coffee. Note the pink exuding surface.

Tests

- Laser Doppler
- Ultrasound
- Vital dyes
- Thermography.

Superficial burns have an unmistakable pink moist appearance with excellent capillary return and a very tender surface (Fig. 5.8).

Scald injuries are notoriously difficult to diagnose correctly. An accurate history may often be the best clue: boiling water on the skin of a toddler will cause more damage than tea with added milk from a cup. Deep partial thickness wounds may be less sensitive and have a deeper red colour (Fig. 5.9).

It is sensible to review the status of the wound after 24 h. By this time assessment is more accurate and the prognosis for healing can be more confident. Topical antimicrobial agents will alter the appearance of the wound and should not be used until a decision about further management has been made.

Flame burns will usually cause deep injury. The skin has no visible circulation, it loses its normal elasticity and the surface may be white or charred. There will be no appreciation of pin-prick and sometimes the pungent smell of burning leaves little doubt (Fig. 5.10).

It is hoped that objective tests to estimate burn thickness such as those listed above may be developed into useful clinical tools. The burn surgeon wishes to know if the wound will heal in a reasonable time with a good scar. The tests are largely tests of blood flow and knowledge of blood flow will not necessarily answer this question: this is partly because the skin has itself a very variable thickness. At present clini-

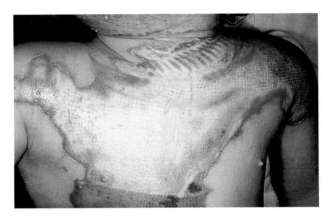

Fig. 5.9 This child pulled the flex of a boiling kettle. The wound is white and deep red at 24 h after injury. This injury is mixed deep and deep partial thickness.

cal observation combined with a careful history remains the mainstay of diagnosis.

Chemical burns

In common with other types of burn injury the incidence of chemical burns has diminished steadily. Admission of casualties from industrial processes is increasingly rare, but domestic accidents continue to occur. The commonest type of injuries are cement burns and burns caused by cleaning agents. Freshly mixed cement is alkaline and prolonged contact will cause deep burns. In common with other alkalis the tissue damage is progressive and the full extent of the damage may not be immediately apparent. Caustic soda

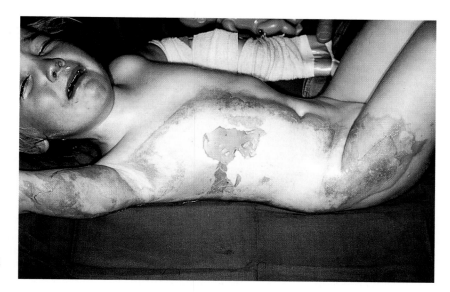

Fig. 5.10 This toddler's cotton shirt caught fire causing a deep burn. Note the charred and dead white areas.

(sodium hydroxide) is a common component of propriety brands of oven and drain cleaners. The manufacturers' directions are usually good, but misuse, particularly by children, can result in significant injuries.

The use of chemicals as weapons has filled man with special dread for centuries. Personal attacks are rare but can be very damaging. Suicide by swallowing corrosives is also uncommon, although small children may swallow domestic agents such as bleach.

Although chemical warfare is outlawed by international convention, the Gulf War of 1991 showed its lethal potential. Mustard gas (chlorine) and phosgene are the burning agents implicated.

Chemicals cause direct damage to the skin, but remember that they may be absorbed to cause injury to the subdermal structures and to distant organs: renal and hepatic failure are seen with chromic and formic acids as well as with organic compounds such as cresols, phenols and methyl bromide. They may also damage the mucosal surfaces of the eyes, respiratory and digestive tracts. The essentials of treatment are as follows:

Water in large quantities

Remove any contaminated clothing. It is important that those who help the injured are not themselves hurt. They should wear suitable protection such as plastic gloves. Continue irrigation until the patient notices lessening of the pain.

Identify the agent; further treatment will depend on the chemical. Most chemicals will be inactivated by water but it is easy to overlook the progressive nature of the injury, particularly in the case of alkalis. Specific measures may be indicated. Calcium gluconate gel is widely prescribed as a topical

application for hydrofluroric acid burns, and calcium gluconate may be injected under the burn to neutralize the acid to try to stop progression. The local poisons centre will give advise on specific chemicals.

In rare instances immediate surgical excision of large areas may be indicated. *Continue to apply water.*

Metabolic requirements

The severity and duration of the catabolic response seen in the severely burned patient continues to surprise even the most experienced observer. This uncontrolled expenditure of energy is related to the severity of the injury and must be met by an adequate supply of nutrition. If the patient becomes septic the catabolic rate increases still further. It is essential that early steps are taken to prevent and control infection and that wound healing is achieved as quickly as possible. Until the burn is healed the catabolism will inexorably proceed and as the body mass continues to be lost the mortality and morbidity will rise.

At one time it was hoped that it would be possible to reverse the response by controlled hyperalimentation; however, this promising approach foundered on the difficulties which itself produced. The large calorie load places a considerable burden on the respiratory reserve, which may already be compromised. Burke *et al.* showed in 1979 that the maximum calories that could be utilized by the body was approximately twice the basal metabolic rate (BMR).

Calculations of energy expenditure are related to the predicted BMR which may be derived from a standard nomogram or by the Harris–Benedict equations as follows:

BMR males

$$BMR \ (kcal/day) = (13.7 \times weight(kg))$$
$$+ (5.08 \times height(cm))$$
$$+ 66 - (6.8 \times age(years))$$

BMR females

$$BMR \ (kcal/day) = (9.6 \times weight(kg))$$
$$+ (1.7 \times height(cm))$$
$$+ 65 - (4.7 \times age(years))$$

Laitung and Settle (1989) have independently shown that the amount of increase of the BMR can be positively related to the depth and size of burn, and negatively related to the day post-burn. They have produced a formula for predicting the percentage increase in resting energy expenditure (REE) above that of the BMR obtained by the Harris–Benedict formula for normal individuals.

$$REE \ (kcal/day) = predicted \ normal \ BMR$$
$$+ \% \ increase \ in \ BMR$$

$$\% \ increase \ in \ BMR = 32 + (0.3 \times \%FT \ burn)$$
$$- (0.4 \times days \ post\text{-}burn)$$
$$+ 34 \ (if \ septic)$$

For example, a 25-year-old man (70 kg, 180 cm) with a 50% full thickness (FT) burn has a normal BMR of 1755 kcal/day. The percentage increase in BMR will be 78.2% if septic on day 7 (total 3127 kcal) and will be 33% on day 35 if no longer septic (total 2334 kcal).

Children

$$TEE = 1.3 \times predicted \ BMR \ (Goran \ et \ al.)$$

This will provide the foundation for adequate nutrition in the child and is a departure from the widely used formulae of Sutherland and Curreri which tended to suggest calorie loads which were much greater. Once the total energy expenditure (TEE) has been calculated it becomes possible to provide a measured amount of diet to the patient.

Calculation of protein and non-protein calories

The recommended proportions of carbohydrate, fat and protein are as follows:
- CHO   52%
- Fat   28%
- Protein 20%

This provides a non-protein calorie-to-nitrogen ratio of 100 : 1.

For example, a 20-year-old man with 60% FT burns requiring 3130 kcal/day would receive 407 g (1628 kcal) of carbohydrate, 97 g (876 kcal) of fat and 156 g (626 kcal) of protein.

Management of the burn wound

Once the size and depth of the burn wound has been assessed and the general condition has been determined and stabilized treatment of the burn wound can begin. This will be either as an out-patient or an in-patient.

Burns which should be admitted to hospital include:
1 Burns >10% BSA (often less in children).
2 Special sites: hand, face.
3 Suspected non-accidental injury.
4 For nursing care, e.g. perineal burns, the elderly and infirm.
5 Social difficulties.

The majority of burns will be treated as out-patients. Aseptic conditions are essential.

The wound is cleaned with an aqueous solution of mild antiseptic such as povidone–iodine or chlorhexidine. Blisters are probably best removed with sharp scissors and the wound is dressed with a non-adherent dressing, covered with a layer of absorbent material such as 'gamgee'. The whole is secured with a conforming bandage. The initial assessment of the wound determines subsequent management.

Superficial burns can be expected to lose large amounts of fluid for the first 2 days. After this time fluid loss will diminish. It is sensible to change the dressing after one or two days. This will give an opportunity to check that there is no sign of infection such as cellulitis. Thereafter, the dressing can be left intact for a further week. By then the wound should be well on the way to healing. Changing the dressing every day may disturb the progress of epithelialization as well as causing unnecessary pain to the patient. If the burn does not heal within 2 weeks it must be re-assessed as it can no longer be regarded as superficial. A decision should be made about the advisability of continuing with conservative treatment. Many small, deep or mixed depth burns where the deep area measures less than 2 cm across can be treated without resort to surgery. However, this should be a conscious plan of action by the doctor and not a sign of neglect. Any larger burn, or one affecting a special site such as the face or the hand, will often need earlier intervention and it is sensible to ask the advice of a burn surgeon. Topical antimicrobial agents such as silver sulphadiazine have a limited place in superficial burns but will help to prevent colonization and infection in deeper injuries.

Conservative treatment of the burn wound

The aims of treatment are: prevention of infection, relief of pain and the maintenance of function.

Measures to achieve these aims will often be much more rigorous for the patient and it is a mistake to think that conservative management of the wound is an easy or a gentle option as compared to early surgery.

Infection

It is crucial to distinguish between colonization and invasive infection of the burn wound. Colonization of the surface of the burn will occur within a few days from either the organisms carried by the patient in the gut, respiratory tract and skin or from carers and the surroundings. However careful the aseptic technique and however good the surroundings, nearly all wounds will be colonized by extrinsic organisms within 2 weeks of injury.

Invasive infection is primarily a clinical diagnosis. Cellulitis of the surrounding intact skin, fever and rigors are classic signs. Close inspection of the wound may show pus, and as an eschar separates pus may collect under it. Quantitative biopsy of tissue to measure the bacterial count per unit weight (g) is used as a research tool to make the diagnosis of invasive infection but has not been widely used in the routine clinical setting.

Severe infections may be difficult to diagnose in the patient who is already unwell. Collapse of the circulation, failure to adsorb food from the stomach, or an increased requirement for oxygen may all point to infection. This last may be seen as a fall in ventilatory reserve leading to the need for assisted ventilation, or as an increase in the requirement for oxygen to maintain peripheral oxygen tension in the patient who is already ventilated.

Systemic antibiotics have little or no place in prophylaxis; although a short (2-day) course of penicillin or erythromycin may be given to make sure that the β-haemolytic streptococcus is not introduced into the ward by a carrier.

Topical antimicrobial agents may be used to delay colonization and to minimize invasive infection. The most commonly used agent is silver sulphadiazine. It is active against Gram-negative bacteria and has few side effects. However, it does not penetrate into the eschar and is only active for less than 12 h after application. Absorption from the surface of a large wound may induce neutropenia which is unwelcome in the patient who is already immunocompromised.

Silver nitrate soaks are now not commonly used. The chemical is effective but the practical difficulties associated with its use are considerable. The soaks must be kept moist and inevitably the patient, the attendants and the bed all become stained with free silver.

Sulphamylon penetrates the eschar but its application may be very painful.

Trials are continuing with preparations containing a mixture of silver sulphadiazine and cerium nitrate.

Maintenance of function

The physiotherapist and the occupational therapist have a major role to play in achieving the best possible functional result. They will be involved with all respiratory problems and must start to work with the patient to maintain a full range of movements of the limbs as soon as possible after admission.

'When does rehabilitation start?' 'Now.'

The mainstays of treatment are elevation of the injured part (particularly hands), splintage and regular controlled movement.

Surgery

The management of significant areas of full thickness injury will include surgery to close the wound. This will usually mean spit skin grafting, although deeper injuries may require the full plastic surgical armamentarium to cover exposed deep structures. The timing of surgery will vary considerably depending on the circumstances and the general condition of the patient.

If the injury is large and potentially life threatening, surgical priorities will be different from the treatment of a smaller localized area of burn.

The majority of injuries are in the latter category, and the aim is then to provide optimum wound care consistent with the best possible long-term function and the least deformity from scarring.

Localized areas of deep burn are best excised and grafted as soon as practicable, usually within the first 5 days after injury.

The deep, partial thickness burn will present similar problems. Although these burns will heal by growth of epithelium from the depths of the skin, healing will be slow and the resulting scar will often be unstable and hypertrophic for many months. This has led to widespread early excision of deep partial thickness burns using a technique of tangential excision first described by Janzekowic in 1970 (Table 5.3). It is believed that careful surgery reduces scarring and will allow a speedy hospital stay, with less uncomfortable dressing changes. However, there are some disadvantages as well as the demonstrable advantages. Uncontrolled and unthinking early excision will extend the area of scarring and the unprepared will be surprised by the amount of rapid blood loss.

The majority of burns and scalds which are admitted to

hospital are of mixed depth with coexisting deep, deep partial and superficial thickness patches within the total wound area.

> **Burn surgery**
>
> Do not underestimate the amount of blood which will be lost.

The decision to operate early (within 5 days) should be made by an experienced surgeon after careful assessment of the general condition of the patient as well as the wound itself. This is best seen within 24 to 48 hours of the burn. Immediate assessment is often misleading, particularly with scalds, but examination at the later time will be reliable. If the wound has been treated with a topical antimicrobial such as silver sulphadiazine (Flamazine) it may be very difficult to gain good information from inspection of the wound itself, and if early surgery is likely it is best not to apply topical agents until a decision about surgery has been made.

Table 5.3 Tangential excision.

Advantages	Disadvantages
Early wound closure	More blood loss
Less infection	Surgery more difficult
Shorter hospital stay	Assessment of woun depth difficult
Less scarring	

Treatment of the major burn
(Figs 5.11 and 5.12)

The person who presents with a major life-threatening burn injury will tax the resources of the best equipped hospital as well as the mental and physical powers of the medical and nursing team, and those of the patient. Optimum results will only come with close co-operation and consultation between all members of the burn team. When planning to start treatment two factors are always present in the calculations:

1 Permanent skin cover can only be achieved with the patient's own skin (except for identical twins).

2 Multiple operations will be required before survival is assured.

The decisions to be made by the leader of the team will include answers to the following interlinked questions:

- Which members of the team need to be involved?
- Which supportive therapies are needed?
- When can surgery start?
- Which areas of the body should be tackled first?

- How much burn can be excised at each episode of surgery?
- Which technique of excision should be used?
- When and how often can we operate?
- How will skin cover be achieved?

Different members of the team will have a higher profile to the patient at different times. The nurses and surgeons may find that, as progress continues, the unglamorous duties of the psychologist or the school teacher may become the most important to the patient. Similarly, a well-organized pathology and blood transfusion service will only function at its peak if there are excellent communications between all members of staff.

The importance of nutrition is discussed in the section above. Enteral feeding is started as soon as possible partly to provide fuel and partly to protect the normal lining and flora of the gastrointestinal tract. H_2 antagonists are given as further prophylaxis against gastric erosion. Regular aspiration of the stomach must not be forgotten as acute gastric dilatation can otherwise go undetected. Its onset can be insidious, and if it does occur death from aspiration of stomach contents can be terrifyingly rapid.

It is customary to delay the first operation until the condition is stabilized after 24 or 48 hours have elapsed. However some surgeons think that with modern techniques of monitoring the circulation, there is no contraindication to beginning surgery within the first 24 hours.

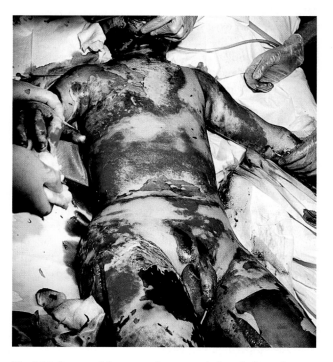

Fig. 5.11 Seventy-eight per cent burn caused when clothing of a 12-year-old caught fire.

If surgery is carried out within the first few days of injury before there is any hint of infection, the first skin grafts can be expected to survive and 'take' without difficulty. This first operation must be directed to reducing the burned area as much as possible. Only areas of definite full thickness burn should be tackled; deep partial thickness burns will heal, albeit slowly, and precious skin graft must not be wasted. If a large area of the back is burned the whole area can be excised at one sitting. If the front of the trunk is burned, it may be helpful to include the upper chest and root of the neck so that later insertion of subclavian lines can take place through healed skin grafts instead of burn eschar. Although it may be tempting to start with a 'critical area' such as the face or the hands, it is better to concentrate on reducing the size of the burn wound.

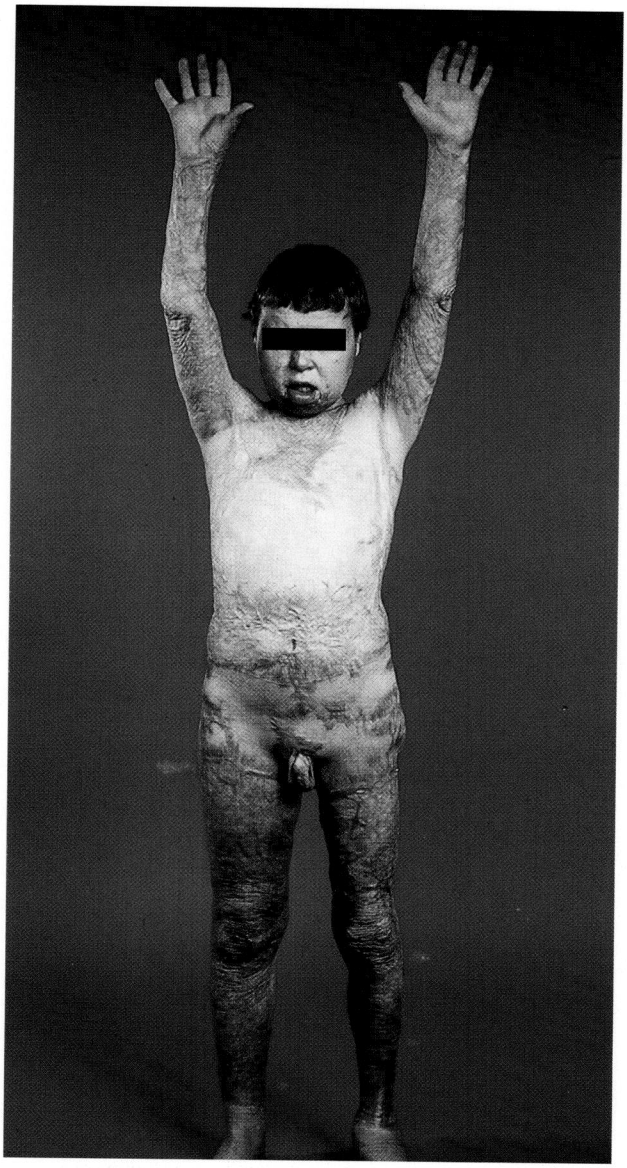

The amount of surgery which can be done at one sitting will be limited by the general condition of the patient and also by the amount of blood loss. When multiple procedures are inevitable, it is probably not wise to lose more than half the blood volume at each operation. More can be lost on the first occasion but the effects of repeated exchange transfusions will be detrimental. If a respiratory gas exchange 'shunt' is present it will often deteriorate by a further 5% after the transfusion of 2 L of stored blood. Special arrangements may have to be made to obtain fresh blood which is not generally available (Fig. 5.13a,b).

It is important to minimize blood loss during surgery. Selective use of tourniquets when excising burns of the limbs will save much blood. If grafts are then applied before the tourniquet is released the take is not reduced. Infiltration of the areas to be excised with dilute solutions of adrenaline is also helpful.

Tangential excision (sequential necrectomy) will cause more blood loss than excision of the eschar and the underlying fat down to the deep fascia. However, the take of grafts is no worse and the loss of otherwise viable fat compounds the eventual deformity.

The timing of recurrent operations will primarily depend on the condition of the patient. If the approach is too rapid the surgeon may lose the patient in his haste to remove all the burned tissue. However, if he is too slow, infection and progressive cachexia will have the same end point. After the first surgery the full support of all systems must be continued including active nutrition and intensive treatment of the burn wound. If there is insufficient donor site to provide autogenous cover, other types of temporary cover will be used until it is possible to recrop the available donor sites. Different methods may be used to extend split skin grafts (see Table 5.4).

Fig. 5.12 Same child as Fig. 5.11, 11 months later.

Table 5.4 Methods of extending skin grafts when donor sites are limited.

Alternating strips of autograft and homograft		
Mesh graft	1 : 1.5	(limited expansion)
	1 : 3	
Mesh graft	1 : 6	covered by homograft mesh 1 : 1.5
	1 : 3	
Micrografts under homograft		
Cultured keratinocytes can be used to provide skin cover		

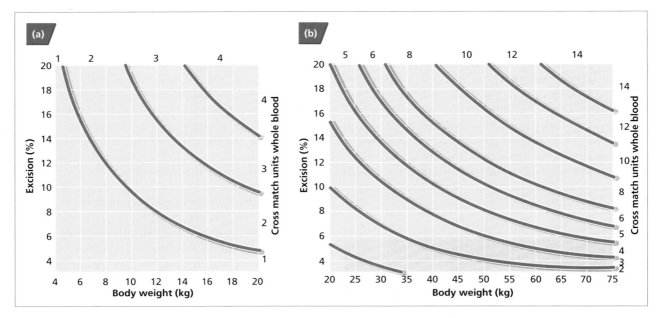

Fig. 5.13 Estimates of the amount of blood which should be available when excising burn wounds. (a) Children up to 20 kg weight; (b) Patients over 20 kg weight. (Reproduced with permission from Dye, D.J. (1993) Requirements for cross-matched blood in burns surgery *Burns* **19** 524–8.)

When used on their own, the usefulness of these methods is limited but when combined with an artificial dermis of collagen fibres their survival and durability are enhanced. The 'dermis' becomes vascularized and the keratinocytes are laid on to this collagen bed. The different combinations of collagen and keratinocytes which have been tried are outwith the scope of this chapter but the dream of a skin substitute which will be 'on the shelf' ready to use on the day of admission may soon help to shorten the long and difficult course which faces so many of the burn injured.

Further reading

Carvajal, H.F. & Parks, D.H. (1988) *Burns in Children: Paediatric Burn Management.* Year Book Medical Publishers, London.
Cason, J.S. (1981) *Treatment of Burns.* Chapman & Hall, London.
Davies, J.W.L. (1982) *Physiological Responses to Burning Injury.* Academic Press, London.
Herndon, D.N. (1995) *Total Burn Care.* W.B. Saunders, Philadelphia.
Langford, R.M. & Armstrong, R.F. (1989) Algorithm for managing injury from smoke inhalation. *British Medical Journal* **299** 902.
Muir, I.F.K., Barclay, T.L. & Settle, J.A.D. (1987) *Burns and their Treatment,* 3rd edn. Butterworth Heinemann, Oxford.
Settle, J.A.D. (1996) *Principles and Practice of Burns Management.* Churchill Livingstone, Edinburgh.

References

Burke, J.F., Wolfe, R.R., Mullaney, C.J. *et al.* (1979) Glucose requirements following burn injury. *Annals of Surgery* **190** 274–285.
Curreri, P.W. (1978) Nutritional support for burned patients *World Journal of Surgery* **2** 215–222.
Goran, M.I., Peters, E.J., Herndon, D.N. & Wolfe, R.R. (1990) Total energy expenditure in children using the doubly labeled water technique. *American Journal of Physiology* **259** E576–E585.
Janzekowic, Z. (1970) A new concept in the early excision and immediate grafting of burns. *Journal of Trauma* **10** 1103–1106.
Laitung, J.K.G. & Settle, J.A.D. (1989) Can the energy requirements of burned patients be accurately predicted? *British Journal of Surgery* (SRS abstract) **76** 644.
Maisels, D.O. & Saad, M.N. (1960) Early surgery in the treatment of burns. *British Journal of Plastic Surgery* **7** 26–43.
Muir, I.F.K., Barclay, T.L. & Settle, J.A.D. (1987) *Burns and their Treatment,* 3rd edn. Butterworth Heinemann, Oxford.
Sutherland A.B. & Batchelor A.D.R. (1996) Nitrogen balance in burned children. In: *Research in Burns* (ed. A.W. Wallace), pp. 147–158. Churchill Livingstone, Edinburgh.

CHAPTER 6

Life-threatening surgical infections

Michael P. Bannon

Introduction

Infectious problems are ubiquitous in surgical practice. Infections which require operation for cure may be primary problems or may arise as complications of surgical therapy. They are often of a life-threatening nature, and they require decisive intervention supported by aggressive critical care. Although mortality associated with surgical infections remains significant, even patients with infection complicated by severe organ dysfunction can often be returned to a normal lifestyle with vigilant management. For this reason, the care of patients with surgical infection is an extremely gratifying endeavour and remains a worthy challenge. This chapter will highlight infections general surgeons are likely to manage in an emergency room surgical practice. These include the necrotizing soft tissue infections, peritonitis, intra-abdominal abscess, fistula, biliary sepsis, and infected pancreatic necrosis. The adult respiratory distress syndrome will be reviewed as a complication of surgical infection.

Necrotizing soft tissue infection

Necrotizing soft tissue infection (NSTI) represents a true surgical emergency. Recognition demands immediate definitive operative intervention. This dictum places all types of necrotizing soft tissue infection under a single clinical umbrella. Attempts to subclassify necrotizing soft tissue infections on the basis of bacteriology, anatomic tissue level, and body region have created a confusing taxonomy of indistinct 'classic' syndromes. This plethora of syndromes is complicated and largely only of historic interest. The variations of necrotizing soft tissue infections are no longer felt to represent different disease processes. Rather, emphasis is now placed upon the shared pathophysiologic processes which involve a spectra of bacteriology, tissue levels, and body regions. Attempted pre-operative subclassification based upon these parameters is irrelevant and threatens dangerous delay of necessary operation. The various forms of NSTI share the qualities of rapid progression, life-threatening severity, and need for emergent, decisive operative care; thus they are best treated with a single common approach.

The recognition of advanced NSTI may be a fascinating exercise in physical diagnosis, but it is a diagnosis too late. The classic signs of fever, cutaneous necrosis, subcutaneous crepitance, and shock portend a grave prognosis that may be unalterable by aggressive surgical debridement. Diagnosis before these dramatic signs arise when NSTI still appears innocuous is the key to optimal management of NSTI. Thus, it is necessary for general practitioners and emergency room physicians, as well as surgeons, to be familiar with the early presentation of NSTI if mortality is to be minimized.

The eventual NSTI may demonstrate only the cutaneous erythema of simple cellulitis when the patient first seeks medical attention. Individuals with increased risk for NSTI must be recognized when they present with minor wounds and cutaneous infections so that they may be followed closely. These include patients with diabetes mellitus, chronic alcoholism, peripheral vascular disease, immuno-suppressed states, and need for steroid therapy. Patients with explicit risk of NSTI who present with contaminated wounds or apparent simple cellulitis and all patients with cellulitis-associated fever or leucocytosis must be admitted to hospital and re-examined within two to three hours. Other low-risk patients with apparent simple cellulitis in the absence of fever or leucocytosis may be treated on an ambulatory basis but must be instructed to return promptly to the treating physician if erythema advances. Rapid progression of erythema, ecchymotic cutaneous discoloration (Fig. 6.1), or appearance of more advanced and specific signs of NSTI demand surgical exploration. As has been emphasized by Lewis (1992), these signs include skin vesicles, crepitus, extension of oedema beyond the area of erythema, and an absence of lymphangitis and lymphadenitis.

Worrisome cutaneous changes demand that an incision be made to assess the viability of the underlying tissues. This exploration is usually best performed in the operating room. The first abnormality encountered may be scant bleeding from subcutaneous tissue which weeps a thin dirty fluid ('dishwater pus'). The subcutaneous tissue typically separates very easily from the underlying fascia. If involved, the fascia itself may be grey, green, or black in colour. The fascia should always be incised to allow inspection of underlying

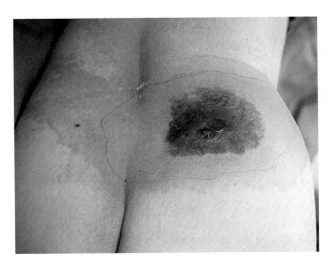

Fig. 6.1 Ecchymotic discoloration and surrounding progressive erythema developed at a bone marrow biopsy site in a 72-year-old woman with diffuse large cell lymphoma. Operative exploration revealed necrotic subcutaneous tissue which cultured *Escherichia coli*.

muscle. Involved muscle bleeds minimally, may be discoloured, and does not contract upon mechanical or electrical (cautery) stimulation.

If the appearance of a cutaneous lesion raises the possibility of a NSTI but this diagnosis is uncertain, a full-thickness biopsy of skin, subcutaneous tissue, and fascia should be performed under local anaesthesia. In the absence of grossly visible necrosis, the histology of the specimen should be examined immediately with the aid of frozen section to settle the issue of possible NSTI. Frozen section biopsy of early NSTI will reveal infiltration of tissue with polymor-

phonuclear leucocytes and bacteria along with necrosis, vasculitis, and thrombosis.

All non-viable tissue as described above must be widely excised. Some forethought should be given to the planning of eventual reconstructive flaps and cosmesis, but the complete excision of all necrotic and compromised tissue remains an inviolable principle. All wounds should be left open. Wounds should be reinspected in the operating room within 24 h of initial debridement and repeatedly thereafter as the condition of the wound dictates.

Several special circumstances deserve mention. Necrotizing soft tissue infections may develop in operative incisional wounds. Erythema on the day of operation suggests clostridial or streptococcal infection. Postoperative NSTI of the torso may develop as a result of underlying gastrointestinal perforation or leak (Fig. 6.2). Necrotizing perineal infection (Fig. 6.3) requires colostomy to prevent fecal contamination of the perineal wound. Colostomy is best deferred at the time of the initial debridement to allow expeditious return to the intensive therapy unit for resuscitation; it may be performed 24 h later during the second operative session. Perineal necrosis, often referred to as Fournier's gangrene, may be widespread, involve the external genitalia, and necessitate emasculation for adequate debridement (Fig. 6.4). Such lesions may develop from progression of neglected peri-anal abscess. Extensive loss of full thickness abdominal wall may accompany NSTI originating from intra-abdominal sepsis; the defect is best reconstructed acutely with an absorbable mesh panel (Fig. 6.5); once a healthy granulation bed develops, the wound can be closed with a split-thickness skin graft. The resulting ventral hernia may be closed in a delayed fashion either with prosthetic material or with autogenous tissue following soft tissue expansion or other plastic techniques. NSTI of an extremity

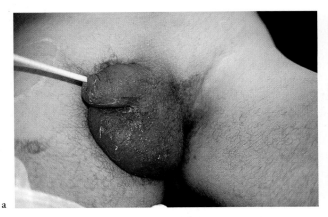

a

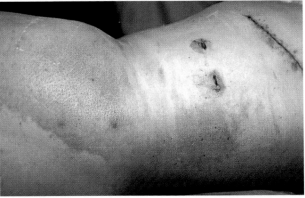

b

Fig. 6.2 (a) A 40-year-old man developed scrotal erythema 5 days following reoperative transthoracic gastric fundoplication. (b) Within 3 h, erythema developed on left flank. Note innocuous appearance of left thoracotomy and tube thoracostomy incisional wounds. Despite this appearance, intercostal musculature was necrotic at level of incision. (c, d, e, f) Computed tomography revealed gas within abdominal wall from costal margin to scrotum (arrows). (g) Necrotic external oblique muscle mobilized. (h) Torso wound following debridement. Source of necrotizing infection proved to be distal esophageal perforation. *Continued opposite.*

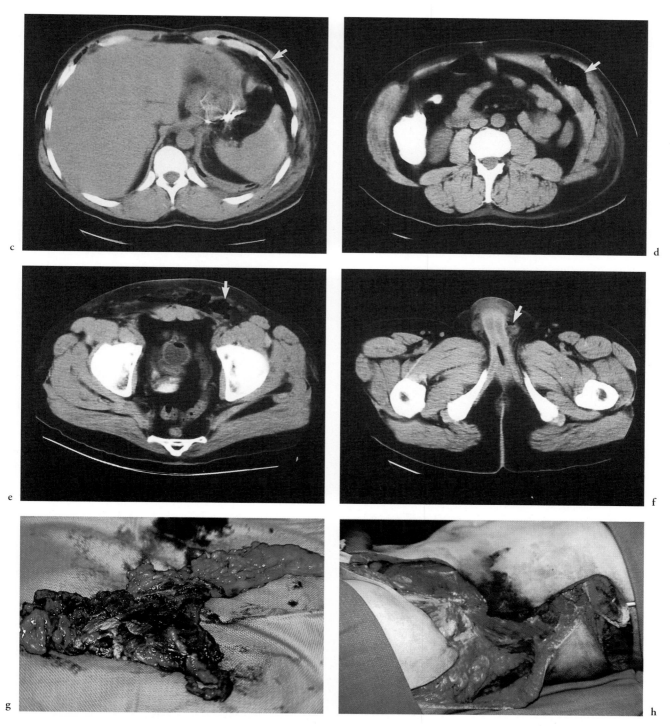

Fig. 6.2 *Continued.*

associated with muscle necrosis should be treated with prompt amputation.

Empiric antibiotic therapy directed to Gram-positive, Gram-negative, and anaerobic organisms should be initiated en route to the operating room for debridement. Continuous infusion of intravenous penicillin (20 million units over 24 h) combined with gentamicin and metronidazole is a rational empiric regimen. Alternatives are listed in Table 6.1. As alluded to previously, there is nothing to be gained from attempts to define the bacteriology of the lesion

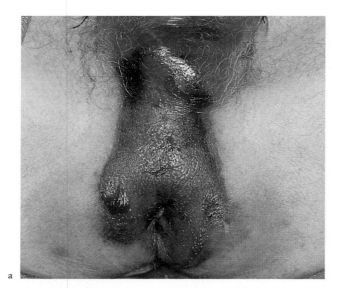

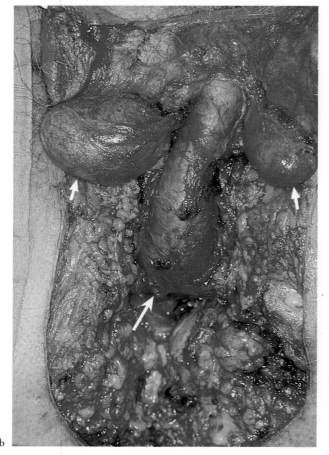

Fig. 6.3 (a) A 75-year-old man with Felty's syndrome developed perineal gangrene and necrosis of right colon and rectum following colonoscopic biopsies. Note deep erythema, vesicles, and ecchymotic discoloration of perineal skin. (b) Debridement exposed testicles (short arrows) and base of penis (long arrow).

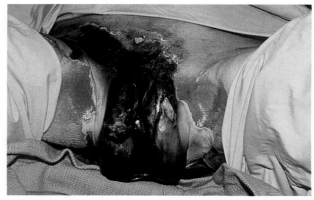

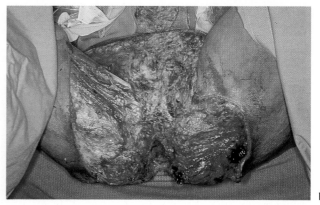

Fig. 6.4 (a) A 53-year-old man with long-standing diabetes and chronic renal failure developed a perianal abscess which was neglected and progressed to perineal gangrene with genital necrosis. (b) Debridement necessitated total emasculation.

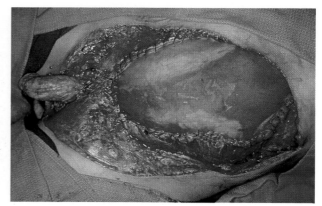

Fig. 6.5 Repeated debridements of necrotizing soft tissue infection resulted in full-thickness loss of abdominal wall which was reconstructed with vicryl mesh panel. Following granulation, the wound was closed with split-thickness skin graft.

Table 6.1 Empiric antibiotic regimens for necrotizing soft tissue infection.

Penicillin G (20 million units/day), aminoglycoside and metronidazole
Third generation cephalosporin and metronidazole
Aminoglycoside and clindamycin
Imipenem/cilastin

pre-operatively. Gram stain and culture of tissue obtained intraoperatively will identify aetiological bacteria. In general, one of three bacteriological situations will be found: pure streptococcal infection, mixed facultative Gram-negative aerobic and anaerobic infection, and clostridial infection. One should note that some infections will not easily fit any of these categories. Ultimate antibiotic therapy should be tailored to susceptibility data. Hyperbaric oxygen has not been shown to reduce mortality, and this potential adjunctive treatment must not be allowed to delay operative debridement.

Diffuse peritonitis

The clinical syndrome of peritonitis results from inflammation of the parietal peritoneum. In patients who are immunosuppressed, harbour ascites, and/or require an indwelling peritoneal catheter, inflammation may result from primary infection of the peritoneal cavity (primary peritonitis); this infection is usually monomicrobial and stems from a haematogenous source or ascending contamination along the intraperitoneal device. Treatment of primary peritonitis consists of antimicrobial therapy without operation. In contrast, secondary infection of the peritoneal cavity (secondary peritonitis) results from perforation or necrosis of the gastrointestinal tract; polymicrobial infection results and requires operative intervention. The salient symptom of peritonitis is abdominal pain exacerbated by movement. Although delineation of the initial and evolving characteristics of this pain may suggest an organ-specific aetiology, the diagnosis of peritonitis *per se* depends upon physical examination rather than clinical history. Exquisite abdominal tenderness heralds peritoneum rendered hyperirritable by an inflammatory process and is the essence of a diagnosis of peritonitis. In advanced cases, a rigid abdominal wall accompanies the tenderness.

Above all else, examination of the patient with possible peritonitis must be gentle. First, the patient's posture is observed. Patients with peritonitis will lie perfectly still to minimize discomfort. The presence or absence of abdominal distention should also be noted. The examination should then focus on soft percussion. Rather than immediately threatening the patient's tender abdomen, the examiner should demonstrate light percussion taps on the patient's shoulder or chest to help regain trust and abdominal relaxation lost to prior harsh examiners. Percussion should be initiated remote from the site of maximal pain. Initial percussion should be light. Its object is to send a gentle shockwave to the parietal peritoneum, and by careful observation of the patient's facial expression determine if this induces discomfort. If a grimace is elicited, no further stimulation of the peritoneum need be attempted; the patient has peritonitis. If no grimace appears, the intensity of percussion is slowly increased with continued careful observation. If percussion elicits no change in facies, the response to gentle palpation with the fingertips is sought. Palpation also allows detection of the involuntary guarding or board-like rigidity of diffuse peritonitis and the voluntary guarding associated with lesser stimuli. Under no circumstances should the abdominal wall be compressed and abruptly released in a search for rebound tenderness; this technique is both imprecise and painfully cruel. The incremental approach described above demonstrates concern for the patient and allows the examiner to grade the degree of peritoneal irritation by noting whether light percussion, stronger percussion, or palpation is necessary to induce objective tenderness. Following examination, fever and leucocytosis should be sought, as these are usually prominent in patients with clinical peritonitis.

Postoperative patients, the elderly, and the immunosuppressed may harbour diffuse intraperitoneal infection without clinical peritonitis. Abdominal tenderness, fever, and leucocytosis may be blunted; the need for emergent celiotomy may be difficult to recognize; and diagnostic adjuncts are thus useful in these situations. An upright chest X-ray may demonstrate pneumoperitoneum and prompt celiotomy. However, in the absence of this dramatic finding, complete evaluation of significant abdominal pain in patients with compromised physical examination may require computed tomography or ultrasound. These studies may demonstrate an organ-specific diagnosis, nonspecific signs of inflammation, or free intraperitoneal fluid. Free fluid should be aspirated for visual inspection, Gram stain, cell counts, and bacteriological culture. Bilious, feculent, or purulent fluid necessitates operation. Sanguinous fluid suggests intestinal ischaemia or necrosis. Diagnostic peritoneal lavage may help resolve some difficult diagnostic dilemmas; lavage fluid demonstrating 500 leucocytes/mm^3 or bacteria on Gram stain should prompt celiotomy.

Once diffuse secondary peritonitis is recognized, celiotomy should be undertaken expeditiously. Delay of operation exacerbates systemic effects of abdominal infection including fluid sequestration, acute lung injury, and multiple organ dysfunction/failure. Pre-operative imaging studies are not necessary for patients with frank clinical peritonitis; they are detrimental insofar as they postpone operation, and they also risk pulmonary aspiration of upper gastrointestinal contrast and, in the volume-depleted patient, renal toxicity from intravenous contrast. Pre-operative preparation should include volume resuscitation, nasogastric decompression, and empirical antibiotic administration. Intravenous hydration with lactated Ringer's solution should be promptly initiated and a urinary catheter placed. Flow of visually non-concentrated urine should be assured prior to induction of anaesthesia with a subsequent goal of 0.5 ml/kg/h urine output. Broad-spectrum antibiotics with activity against Gram-negative bacteria and anaerobes should be administered immediately and redosed intra-operatively if operative time is long.

Operation should begin with a midabdominal midline celiotomy. This can be extended superiorly for pathology in the supracolic compartment (i.e. perforated peptic ulcer) or inferiorly for pathology in the infracolic compartment (i.e. perforated diverticulitis). Although often immediately apparent after incision, the cause of peritonitis may remain occult after initial abdominal exploration, and the surgeon should be prepared to perform a meticulous intra-operative gastrointestinal examination to identify the site of perforation. For example, the patient presenting with peritonitis following recreational rectal instrumentation may provide no relevant history and may harbour a perforation of the anterior rectal wall hidden within the rectovesical fold; only purposeful exposure of the deep pelvis will expose such a lesion.

The first priority of operative management is to eliminate ongoing peritoneal contamination. The specific procedure performed depends not only upon the viscus perforated but also the degree of intraperitoneal infection and inflammation. In general, a perforated viscus may be primarily repaired, patched, or resected; diversion of the gastrointesti-

Table 6.2 Operative management of gastro-intestinal perforation.

Perforated viscus	Aetiology	Contamination mild–moderate	Severe
Stomach	Trauma	Debridement and primary closure	Patch closure
	Malignancy	Gastric resection with gastrojejunostomy	Patch closure
	Benign ulcer		
	Type I	Local excision and closure	Biopsy and patch closure
	Type II	Antrectomy with gastroduodenostomy or gastrojejunostomy	Biopsy and patch closure
	Type III	1 Vagotomy and pyloroplasty 2 Patch, vagotomy, and gastrojejunostomy	Patch closure
Duodenum	Peptic ulcer	1 Vagotomy and pyloroplasty 2 Patch, vagotomy, and gastrojejunostomy	Patch closure
	Trauma	1 Primary repair with/without tube duodenostomy 2 Closure with pyloric exclusion	1 Duodenal diverticulization* 2 Jejunal serosal patch†
Small intestine	Trauma	1 Primary closure 2 Resection and primary anastomosis	Resection with end enterostomy and mucous fistula
	Crohn's disease	Resection and primary anastomosis	Resection with end enterostomy and mucous fistula
Appendix	Appendicitis	Appendicectomy	1 Appendicectomy 2 Right hemicolectomy
Right colon	Trauma	1 Primary repair 2 Resection and ileocolostomy 3 Repair with proximal loop ileostomy	1 Repair with proximal loop ileostomy 2 Resection with end ileostomy
	Malignancy	Resection and ileocolostomy	Resection with end ileostomy
	Ulcerative colitis	Abdominal colectomy with end ileostomy	Abdominal colectomy with end ileostomy
Left colon‡	Trauma	1 Primary repair 2 Resection and colocolostomy	1 Repair with proximal diversion 2 Resection with end colostomy
	Malignancy	Resection with end colostomy	Resection with end colostomy
	Diverticulitis	Resection with end colostomy	Resection with end colostomy
	Ulcerative colitis	Abdominal colectomy with end ileostomy	Abdominal colectomy with end ileostomy

* if contamination localized; † if contamination diffuse; ‡ including intraperitoneal rectum.

nal stream should be a component of these procedures if inflammatory changes threaten the healing of potential suture lines. Inflamed friable tissue does not hold suture well and should not be closed primarily or incorporated into an anastomosis. Selected operative options for gastrointestinal perforation are outlined in Table 6.2.

Following control of the contaminating source, the next priority is to minimize the peritoneal bacterial load. This is accomplished by copious lavage with 10–20 L of saline. The peritoneal cavity must be suctioned completely dry following lavage so that peritoneal defence mechanisms are not impaired. The addition of antibiotic lavage has no proven efficacy, but seems innocuous. Also without proven benefit, but very labour intensive, are the adjuncts of intra-operative radical debridement of peritoneal fibrinous exudates and postoperative transcatheter lavage. The former procedure also carries risk of technical misadventure with possible consequent fistula.

If bacterial contamination at the time of initial operation is severe, repeated intestinal leaks occur, or operative intervention is inadequate, peritonitis may recur even after all leaks are ultimately controlled. Residual intraperitoneal bacteria lead to diffuse recurrence in these severe cases — instances of peritonitis begetting peritonitis. This devastating situation is best managed by treating the peritoneal cavity as an open wound. Planned repeated irrigations and pack changes are performed through the open abdominal incisional wound (laparostomy) in the operating room. In some cases, a fascial zipper may be utilized to maintain the peritoneal domain; however, the most advanced infections necessitate open packing until the peritoneal cavity develops healthy granulation, contracts, and allows eventual closure with a split-thickness skin graft applied directly to the peritoneal contents. Abdominal wall reconstruction may be performed electively 6 months to 1 year after the patient has convalesced in an anabolic state.

At the completion of celiotomy for peritonitis, the superficial wound should generally be left open. The wound may be closed in a delayed fashion after quantitative culture of a wound biopsy demonstrates less than 10^5 bacteria/g of tissue. In some cases with mild intraperitoneal contamination, the wound may be closed over a subcutaneous drain which is subsequently irrigated with antibiotic solution for 5 days; with this latter technique three-quarters of patients with mild peritoneal contamination should leave the hospital with a closed wound.

Multiple antibiotic regimens have efficacy for secondary peritonitis (Table 6.3). Although active against Gram-negative bacteria, aminoglycosides carry risk of renal toxicity and ototoxicity and require careful monitoring of dosing levels; less toxic alternatives should generally be chosen. The value of microbial culture and sensitivity data based upon intra-operative specimens is controversial. Most patients do well with unaltered empiric antibiotic regimens. Obtaining

Table 6.3 Empiric antibiotic regimens for peritonitis.

Imipenem-cilastin
Piperacillin-tazobactam
Third generation cephalosporin* and metronidazole†
Ciprofloxacin and metronidazole
Aminoglycoside‡ and metronidazole†
Aztreonam and clindamycin
Second-generation cephalosporin with antianaerobic activity§¶
Ticarcillin-clavulinic acid§
Ampicillin-Sulbactam§

* Cefotaxime or ceftizoxime.
† Clindamycin may be substituted for metronidazole.
‡ Relatively contraindicated in patients who are elderly, hypotensive, or have renal insufficiency.
§ Only appropriate for mild to moderately severe infections with low risk of resistant organisms.
¶ Cefoxitin, cefotetan, or cefmatazole.
Adapted from Bohnen *et al.* (1992) and Nathens & Rotstein (1996).

intra-operative specimens with the goal of tailoring postoperative antibiotics to sensitivity data is a reasonable practice for patients at high risk of harbouring resistant organisms, however. These patients include those who have hospital-acquired infections, postoperative infections, or have received prior courses of antibiotics. The role of anti-enterococcal therapy remains unclear. Anti-enterococcal therapy should be initiated for enterococcal bacteraemia and for intraperitoneal *Enterococcus* in patients who are not improving postoperatively. Empiric anti-enterococcal therapy appears unnecessary however. *Candida* will often be isolated from the peritoneal cavity after gastrointestinal perforation — especially if the perforation is proximal. *Candida* isolated only from the peritoneal cavity should be treated with an antifungal agent in immunosuppressed or critically ill patients; however, non-compromised patients do not require treatment. Postoperative antibiotics should be administered until fever, leucocytosis, and *bandaemia* have all resolved.

Localized peritonitis

Peritonitis can be localized to a single abdominal region. Localized peritonitis may be treated without operation in some circumstances. Localized peritonitis implies either contained or early perforation of a viscus or inflammation of an organ in contact with anterior parietal peritoneum.

A precise history detailing the sequence of events from the time the patient last felt well to the time of presentation should be elicited. The patient's abdominal pain should be characterized in terms of its onset (abrupt or crescendo), initial location, subsequent location, and radiation. Exacerbating and alleviating factors should be solicited. Presence or absence of associated nausea, emesis, change in

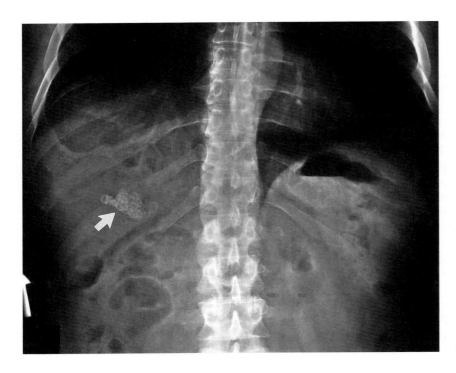

Fig. 6.6 Radio-opaque gallstones (arrow).

Table 6.4 Treatment options for localized peritonitis.

Aetiology	Treatment
Cholecystitis	Cholecystectomy
	Percutaneous cholecystostomy if non-gangrenous
Pancreatitis	Non-operative supportive care unless complicated
	Debridement of infected pancreatic necrosis
Contained perforated duodenal ulcer	Patch closure
	Resection with antrectomy/ gastrojejunostomy if size precludes patch
Appendicitis	Appendicectomy
Appendiceal abscess	Percutaneous drainage with/without interval appendicectomy
	Operative drainage with appendicectomy
Diverticulitis	Antibiotic therapy with interval colectomy if recurrent episode
Diverticular abscess	Percutaneous drainage with interval colectomy and primary anastomosis

bowel habit, fever, or chills must be noted. Abdominal examination, performed as described above for potential diffuse peritonitis, reveals localized percussion tenderness and possibly localized voluntary guarding. White blood count is assessed in all patients as it can be useful to gauge the severity of the inflammatory process. Serum bilirubin, hepatic transaminases, and amylase are measured in patients with epigastric or right upper quadrant pain in search of evidence for biliary obstruction, hepatitis, and pancreatitis respectively. Abdominal X-rays are helpful to confirm a diagnosis of small bowel obstruction and to detect calcific densities (Fig. 6.6). Additional imaging studies are chosen based upon the differential diagnosis generated by history and examination.

Aetiologies of localized peritonitis and treatment options are listed in Table 6.4. Whether operative or non-operative management is pursued depends upon the specific aetiology. Thus, unlike diffuse peritonitis which demands operation, localized peritonitis prompts evaluation to determine a precise aetiological diagnosis upon which decisions regarding operative versus non-operative interventions and their timing depend.

Intra-abdominal abscess

Intra-abdominal abscess may arise during the natural history of diffuse peritonitis, as a consequence of localized gastrointestinal perforation, or as a postceliotomy complication. Rarely, an abscess will arise from haematogenous bacterial seeding of vulnerable sites such as haematomas. In all cases, contaminating organisms persist, replicate, and incite a localized purulent fluid collection. Two general categories of intra-abdominal abscesses must be considered: those which communicate with the gastrointestinal tract and those which do not. Treatment of a communicating abscess requires not only drainage but also management of the subsequent fistula.

Abdominal abscess leads to fever, chills, and abdominal pain. Examination reveals localized tenderness and possibly a palpable mass. Overlying cutaneous erythema may be found in advanced cases. Pelvic abscess may be manifest as a tender fluctuance on rectal or vaginal examination; inflammatory irritation of the rectosigmoid may cause diarrhoea. In all cases, the patient should be carefully interviewed regarding initial symptoms which will have arisen days to weeks before the presentation of the abscess. The initial symptom complex will often elucidate the inciting pathology such as appendicitis or diverticulitis. For patients who have undergone recent operation, the history of the disease process leading to operation, operative events, and postoperative course must all be detailed. Postoperative abscesses typically become manifest between the fifth and tenth days after celiotomy. In addition to the general signs noted above, deep wound infection and fascial dehiscence should also prompt evaluation for postoperative abscess.

Computed tomography (CT) with intravenous and gastrointestinal contrast most expeditiously confirms the diagnosis of abscess and delineates its anatomic location. In order for CT to reliably differentiate a fluid-filled abscess cavity from fluid-filled bowel, the entirety of the gastrointestinal tract should contain contrast material; in some cases, this will most efficiently be accomplished by administration of contrast both per os and per rectum. CT may reveal contrast extravasation in instances of gastrointestinal tract perforation and thus define a communicating abscess and possibly delineate its source. CT identification of thickened bowel wall may also provide indirect evidence of the pathologic site giving rise to the abscess. Ultrasound provides less information about the potential source of an abscess and may be compromised by bowel distended with gas when ileus is present. Radionuclide studies are very non-specific and rarely useful. Undirected celiotomy is performed only in extenuating circumstances; celiotomy is rarely therapeutic when pre-operative CT is unrevealing. Diagnostic imaging performed prior to celiotomy for suspected abscess also allows the option of non-operative percutaneous drainage to be considered.

Unlike diffuse peritonitis which demands emergent celiotomy, intra-abdominal abscess must be treated urgently, not emergently. Drainage should be performed within 12 h of diagnosis, sooner if feasible. Indeed, patients critically ill with a severe systemic septic response require immediate drainage following initial hemodynamic and respiratory resuscitation.

CT or ultrasound-guided percutaneous drainage of abdominal abscesses has emerged as the procedure of choice in many circumstances. Unilocular abscesses abutting the anterolateral abdominal wall are most amenable to cure with non-operative drainage (Fig. 6.7). However, percutaneous techniques may also cure or provide valuable temporization for more complicated abscesses. An abscess situated deep in the abdomen or pelvis may be safely accessed percutaneously so long as a 'window' free of bowel and vascular structures extends from a potential abdominal wall puncture site to the fluid collection. The locules of multiloculated abscesses often communicate and in some instances may be effectively drained by a catheter placed into the primary cavity. If a secondary locule is not effectively drained, the initial catheter tract may be used to manipulate a guidewire and catheter into the undrained locule under fluoroscopic visualization. The septic response potentially associated with a communicating abscess may resolve with percutaneous drainage allowing more elective operative intervention for the resulting fistula. Reasons for failure of percutaneous drainage include the presence of locules which do not communicate adequately with the drainage catheter and semi-solid necrotic material which cannot be evacuated through the drainage catheter.

Operative drainage is necessary for those abdominal abscesses which are multiple (Fig. 6.8), are isolated but cannot safely be approached percutaneously, and/or are associated with systemic sepsis unresponsive to percutaneous drainage. Rarely, operation will be necessary to exclude malignancy (Fig. 6.9). There are two general operative approaches to abscess drainage: transperitoneal and extraperitoneal. Examples of the latter include a retroperitoneal iliac fossa approach to appendiceal abscess, bed of

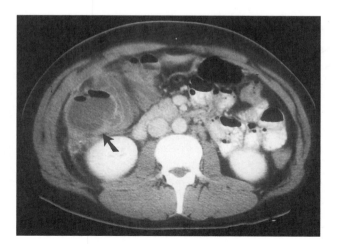

Fig. 6.7 Unilocular abscess (arrow) in proximity to anterolateral abdominal wall developed in an 18-year-old man 10 days following appendicectomy for perforated appendicitis. Abscess resolved with percutaneous drainage.

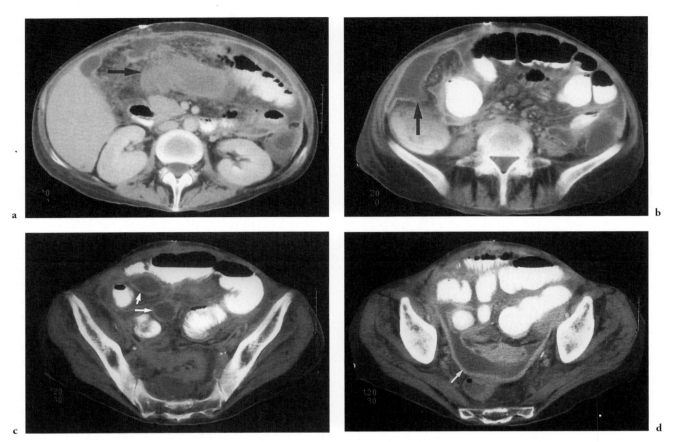

Fig. 6.8 Intra-abdominal *Candida* abscesses (arrows) developed in a 60-year-old woman referred for management of respiratory failure following right hemicolectomy for caecal perforation and subsequent cholecystectomy for perforated postoperative cholecystitis. Abscesses located in (a) lesser sac, (b) right anterior paracolic space, (c) between loops of small intestine, and (d) pelvis. Multiplicity of abscesses necessitated celiotomy.

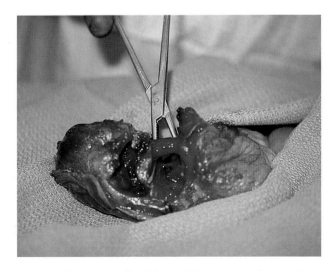

Fig. 6.9 Chronic appendiceal abscess/phlegmon (arrow) presenting as a palpable mobile mass in a 31-year-old stoic farmer with a 3-month history of fever, night sweats, tender adenopathy and weight loss. Note proximal appendix elevated on clamp.

12th rib approaches to subphrenic abscesses, and a transrectal approach to pelvic abscesses. Extraperitoneal approaches avoid the risk of contaminating uninvolved portions of the peritoneal cavity. Because many abscesses amenable to extraperitoneal drainage are also amenable to percutaneous drainage, extraperitoneal approaches are currently indicated infrequently. Transrectal drainage should be considered for simple pelvic abscesses however, because these are often bordered anterosuperiorly by bladder and bowel and thus lack a safe anterior 'window' of percutaneous approach. Although percutaneous approach to a pelvic abscess through the sciatic notch is technically possible, this risks injury to the internal iliac vasculature, necessitates that the patient lie on the drain site, and is recommended only in extenuating circumstances. The bed of 12th rib approach to a subphrenic abscess may be the only option feasible in complicated postoperative patients with an open peritoneal cavity obliterated by severe inflammation and semi-solid material filling the abscess cavity. Currently, abscesses drained operatively are those for which percutaneous drainage is not appropriate. As such, most abscesses coming to operation require a transperitoneal approach so that multiple abscesses may be drained, inter-loop abscesses may be exposed, and/or sources of associated gastrointestinal leaks may be repaired or resected.

Antibiotic treatment is an adjunct to drainage. *Escherichia coli* and *Bacteroides fragilis* are commonly encountered organisms. Initial empiric antibiotic therapy should have efficacy for Gram-negative bacilli and anaerobes. The empiric regimens and general approach to antibiotic therapy outlined for peritonitis are also appropriate for abscess. Antibiotics should be administered until fever, leucocytosis, and bandaemia resolve.

Communication of an abscess cavity with the gastrointestinal tract will become apparent by different means following percutaneous versus operative drainage of the abscess. The character of the effluent (for example bilious, enteric, or feculent) may indicate the presence of gastrointestinal communication after percutaneous drainage. When an abscess is drained operatively, an associated gastrointestinal perforation may be readily apparent and treated by repair with proximal diversion or resection and anastomosis as outlined above. However, within a chronically inflamed, largely obliterated peritoneal cavity, the perforation may not be accessible at celiotomy. Thus, even if the character of the abscess fluid clearly indicates the presence of active communication with the gastrointestinal tract, definitive management may not be technically possible. Operative placement of drainage catheters to control the resulting fistula may be the best immediate technical option; plans for definitive repair should be deferred in such cases until inflammatory changes subside to render the peritoneal contents technically accessible with greater safety.

Two commonly encountered types of abdominal abscesses are appendiceal and diverticular. Appendiceal abscesses encountered during appendicectomy for clinically uncomplicated appendicitis may be treated by transperitoneal drainage; appendicectomy may be performed if a safe stump closure can be effected. Appendicectomy can be safely accomplished with a severely inflamed appendiceal base by resecting a cuff of caecum with the appendix. This is easily accomplished by application of a linear stapling device across supple healthy caecum beneath the inflamed appendiceal base; however, care must be taken not to compromise the ileocaecal junction. An appendiceal abscess diagnosed pre-operatively is best approached by percutaneous drainage or extraperitoneal operative drainage. Interval appendicectomy may be considered, but is probably not always necessary. In many instances, the appendix is found to be replaced by a fibrosed cord which does not carry risk for recurrent appendicitis. It is the author's current practice to perform interval appendicectomy only if barium colon X-ray reveals a patent appendiceal lumen. If interval operation is not performed, it is important to exclude carcinoma in older patients by a barium study or colonoscopy.

Abscesses also arise as complications of acute diverticulitis. If feasible, non-operative percutaneous drainage should be performed. When successful, this procedure effects cure of the abscess, provides time for the acute inflammation of diverticulitis to resolve, sets the stage for resection with primary anastomosis, and thus allows the patient to be spared a colostomy and second operation for its reversal. When the abscess anatomy is too complex for percutaneous drainage or the patient's sepsis fails to respond to percutaneous drainage, celiotomy with abscess drainage, sigmoidectomy, end colostomy and closure of the proximal rectum (Hartmann-like procedure) should be performed.

Fistula

A fistula is an abnormal communication between two epithelial surfaces. Abdominal fistulas often arise from a septic process and always have the potential to create a septic process. They develop as a consequence of spontaneous perforation, injury, or anastomotic breakdown within the gastrointestinal tract. The breach in gastrointestinal integrity leads to a fluid collection or abscess which extends to the abdominal wall and subsequently communicates with the cutaneous surface spontaneously, through an existing postoperative drainage catheter, or through a drainage catheter placed percutaneously for treatment of abscess. Spontaneous fistulization through the abdominal wall (necessitans) most often occurs through an incisional wound or old drain tract. Fistulas may also develop by strangulation of bowel within a groin hernia or postoperative fascial defect with subsequent perforation and mucocutaneous communication.

The management of gastrointestinal fistulas must be organized and stepwise. Sequential management stages are outlined in Table 6.5. Because unreplaced volume losses through the fistula lead to hypovolaemia, assessment of volume status is the first priority in fistula management. Skin turgor, mucous membranes, orthostatic changes, and urine output must all be assessed. Invasive haemodynamic monitoring should be performed for patients with hypotension, a systemic septic response, or chronic cardiorespiratory

Table 6.5 Stages of fistula management.

Fluid and electrolyte resuscitation
Protection of the skin
Nutritional support
Delineation of anatomy
Drainage of associated abscesses
Resolution of intraperitoneal inflammation
Definitive operative management

compromise. Volume resuscitation with lactated Ringer's solution is appropriate for patients with acidemia associated with large bicarbonate losses from pancreatic or duodenal fistulas. Gastric fistulas lead to losses of hydrogen ion and consequent alkalemia; resuscitation with normal saline is best in these circumstances. Initial volume resuscitation should continue until the patient is normotensive without tachycardia and producing 0.5 ml of urine per kilogram per hour. Ongoing volume losses should be monitored and replaced. Hypokalaemia should be expected and repleted. Serum magnesium, calcium, and phosphorus should be monitored. In cases of severe electrolyte imbalance, measurement of electrolyte concentrations in the fistula effluent will guide appropriate choice of replacement fluids.

Skin surrounding the fistulous opening must be protected from the digestive effects of the effluent. This protection can often be provided with barrier devices and pastes such as karaya. Zinc oxide preparations will facilitate healing of excoriated skin. Control of a fistula to an open dehisced wound will challenge the resourcefulness of the most experienced surgeons and stomal therapists; intensive wound care with frequent (2 hourly) bedside irrigations may be all that can be performed to control fistula effluent (Fig. 6.10) until the fistula either closes spontaneously or can be resected at operation. Nutritional support must be provided early on; patients may be rendered hypermetabolic by inflammatory processes associated with the fistula. Parenteral nutrition is often necessary as enteral feeding may increase fistula output. In cases of distal small bowel or colonic fistulas, it may be possible to provide an elemental formula to the proximal bowel without exacerbating fistulous drainage.

Once the patient is so stablized, the anatomy of the fistula may be delineated. Computed tomography will identify pathological fluid collections which can then be sampled and possibly definitively drained percutaneously. The most efficacious means for identification of the fistula source is to observe injection of water soluble contrast through a well-formed fistula tract or a communicating drain under fluoroscopy (Fig. 6.11). Such a study is often referred to as a

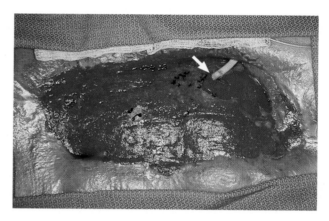

Fig. 6.10 Small bowel fistula manifest as mature enterotomy (intubated, arrow) within open abdomen. Granulation covers peritoneal contents.

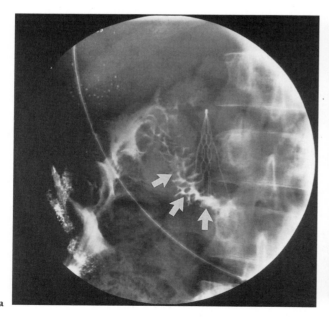

a

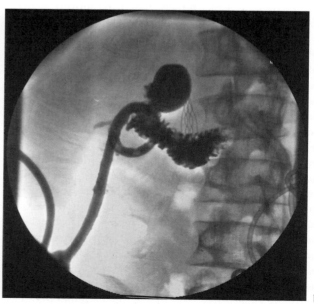

b

Fig. 6.11 Post-traumatic duodenal fistula necessitated to pin site of pelvic external fixator. (a) Contrast injection of cannulated tract demonstrates fistula manifest as contrast delineation of duodenal mucosa (arrows). (b) Tract subsequently controlled with locking loop catheter.

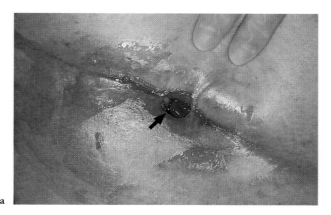
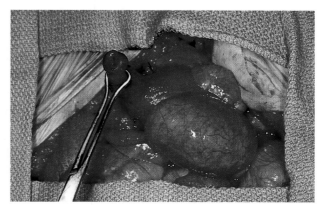

a
b

Fig. 6.12 (a) Visible mucosa (arrow) within 69-year-old appendectomy incisional scar of a 79-year-old woman. (b) Source of fistula proved to be residual appendix (within clamp).

fistulogram. Following identification of the fistulous source, the small intestine and colon should be examined with contrast studies in search of points of obstruction or other pathology. Abscesses identified with CT may be drained percutaneously.

Percutaneous drainage will potentially allow the inciting fistula to heal; even if the fistula persists, percutaneous drainage will often control the gastrointestinal leak, prevent sepsis and thus frequently allow definitive operation to be temporarily deferred. The value of temporizing percutaneous drainage arises from the need to allow acute intraperitoneal inflammation to resolve before definitive operation can be safely performed. Celiotomy and dissection in the face of dense vascular intraperitoneal adhesions risks enterotomies and additional fistulas. Indeed the most common technical complication of operation for fistula is another fistula. Anastomoses must be deferred in the face of purulence, gross contamination, or friable inflamed bowel. If resection must be performed under such conditions, stomas will be necessary. Thus, whenever possible, operative management should be deferred to allow acute intraperitoneal inflammation to resolve. As a rule of thumb, resolution of acute inflammation to allow safe operation requires a period of at least three months from the date of the last operation or other inflammatory insult. The interval may need to be longer in some instances. The exercise of patience prior to operation for fistula not only allows inflammation to resolve but also ensures that an adequate trial of non-operative management is undertaken.

If percutaneous drainage is not feasible or does not control the gastrointestinal leak, then early operative management will be necessary. If intraperitoneal inflammation is intense, the goal of operation should be to establish adequate drainage, prevent sepsis, and allow controlled fistula(s) to develop. Definitive operation with resection, diversion, and/or intestinal, biliary, or pancreatic anastomosis can then be performed after an appropriate interval. Antibiotics are

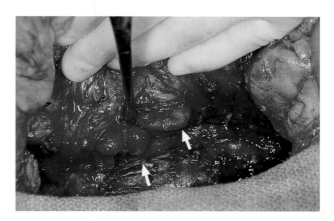

Fig. 6.13 Postoperative duodenal injury presented as fistula. Note two areas of pouting everted mucosa (arrows). Such mature enterotomies will not heal spontaneously. These lesions healed following debridement and primary closure protected by a tube duodenostomy.

indicated for fistula-associated abscess, cellulitis, deep wound infection, and/or systemic toxicity. However, a controlled fistula with a defined, well-drained tract or with direct mucocutaneous connection does not require antibiotic therapy.

Fistulas which should not be followed expectantly are those in which serosa is adherent to anterior parietal peritoneum rendering mucosa visible through the fistulous opening (Fig. 6.12) or those in which the mucosa of the underlying bowel has everted onto serosa and 'matured' to form a sort of pseudostoma; these will not heal without operative intervention (Fig. 6.13). Fistulas which can be expected to close without operation have a distinct tract between mucosa and skin but are not associated with epithelialization of the tract, retained foreign bodies, underlying malignancy, chronic inflammatory disease, or distal obstruction. The ability of octreotide, a somatostatin analogue, to hasten fistula closure remains unproven.

Infected pancreatic necrosis

Infected pancreatic necrosis represents an advanced retroperitoneal septic process arising from acute pancreatitis. Associated systemic toxicity is usually progressive and ultimately severe. The syndrome of epigastric pain, fever, leucocytosis, and hyperamylasaemia comprises acute pancreatitis. Abdominal examination may elicit mild localized epigastric tenderness or frank peritoneal irritation. CT will reveal a normal or edematous pancreas. Pancreatic necrosis should be suspected when pain continues to worsen beyond 72 h and is associated with high spiking fevers and rising leucocytosis. Dynamic bolus computed tomography should be performed in this setting to evaluate pancreatic microcirculation. Unenhanced areas of pancreas define necrosis (Fig. 6.14). Peripancreatic necrosis appears as mottled areas of heterogenous densities within the retroperitoneum (Figs 6.15 and 6.16). Necrotic areas containing air define gas-producing infection. Infection may also be diagnosed by fine needle aspiration and culture of peripancreatic fluid.

Infection manifest as either retroperitoneal air or culture-positive fine needle aspirate indicates the need for operative debridement. Patients with pancreatic necrosis without documented infection should be followed clinically and with weekly CT to screen for operative indications. A deteriorating clinical course in the setting of presumably sterile necrosis is also an indication for operation. Whenever apparent sterile necrosis causes respiratory failure, the author promptly proceeds to operative debridement. Some patients with sterile pancreatic/peripancreatic necrosis will improve

without operation; however, this is the exception rather than the rule, and the need for eventual operative debridement must be anticipated.

Operation for pancreatic necrosis is best performed through a midline celiotomy which allows exposure of the peripancreatic retroperitoneum and the retrocolic areas into which the necrotic process often extends (Fig. 6.17). The lesser sac should be entered through the gastrocolic omentum and its retroperitoneum explored. Pancreatic and peripancreatic necrosis will be evident as clay-like, malleable material which is green to black in colour (Fig. 6.18). All such necrotic material must be separated from surrounding viable tissue and removed. Blunt manual dissection is safest, but a purposeful conscious gentleness must be exercised to

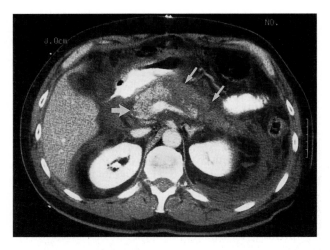

Fig. 6.14 Pancreatic necrosis. Pancreatic head (wide arrow) enhances with intravenous contrast whereas region of body and tail (narrow arrows) does not.

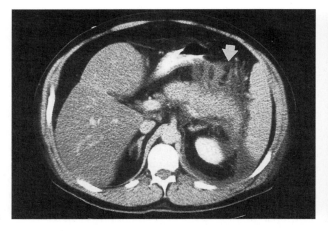

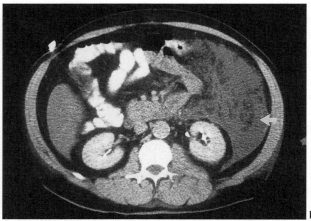

Fig. 6.15 Pancreatic necrosis. CT reveals (a) streaking densities (arrow) extending anteriorly from distal pancreas and (b) mottled densities (arrow) lateral to ligament of Treitz.

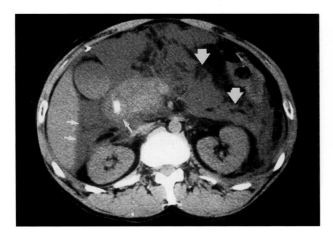

Fig. 6.16 Pancreatic necrosis. CT reveals mottled densities anterior to pancreas and kidney (wide arrows), oedematous duodenum (narrow arrow), fluid in hepatorenal space (double arrow).

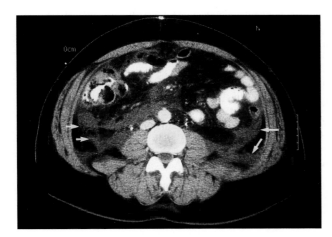

Fig. 6.17 Extension of peripancreatic inflammatory and necrotic changes posterior to right colon (long arrows) and left colon (short arrows).

avoid injury to retroperitoneal structures whose mechanical integrity may have been partially compromised by the digestive necrotic process. At particular risk are the splenic and middle colic vessels.

The tissues at the junction of necrosis and viability are inflamed, friable, and hypervascular. Disruption of such tissue can lead to significant capillary bleeding; although this can usually be controlled with pressure and/or packing, it is to be avoided nonetheless. Rather than risk haemorrhage from viable inflamed tissue at the initial debridement or leave necrotic tissue unresected, a course of multiple debridements at planned re-operations is often wisest.

Although progression to diffuse persistent peritonitis or

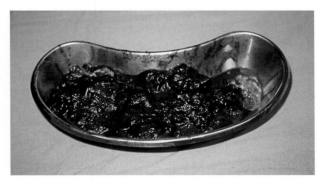

Fig. 6.18 Excised retroperitoneal tissue of peripancreatic necrosis.

development of severe intraperitoneal oedema may necessitate laparostomy with open packing or silo closure respectively, fascia can usually be closed with a zipper between debridements. Operative debridements are performed every 48 hours until ongoing necrosis has ceased and all necrotic tissue has been removed. At the final procedure, retroperitoneal drains are placed and definitive fascial closure is performed. Generally three to five debridements are necessary to control the retroperitoneal necrosis.

Biliary sepsis

The most common inflammatory conditions of the biliary tract seen in an emergency practice are acute cholecystitis and acute cholangitis; the former is encountered routinely and the latter infrequently.

Acute cholecystitis is usually an inflammatory—not an infectious—problem. Cystic duct obstruction leads to gall bladder distention, compromise of blood supply, consequent inflammation, and local peritoneal irritation. Patients present with constant right subcostal pain which may have initially been epigastric in location and often radiates to the back. Nausea and emesis are very common. Fever, leucocytosis, and hyperbilirubinaemia, if present, are mild. Ultrasound examination reveals cholelithiasis, gall bladder wall thickening, and possibly pericholecystic fluid; it also allows recognition of biliary dilatation suggestive of associated choledocholithiasis. Cholecystectomy within 24 to 48 hours of onset prevents progression of the disease process and can be performed safely via a laparoscopic approach in a majority of cases. If an uncontrolled exacerbation of chronic cardiorespiratory disease or other extenuating circumstance prevents early operation, the patient may be treated with analgesia, intravenous antibiotics, and interval cholecystectomy; percutaneous cholecystostomy will usually temporize those patients who do not initially respond to conservative measures.

If neglected, acute cholecystitis can progress from an

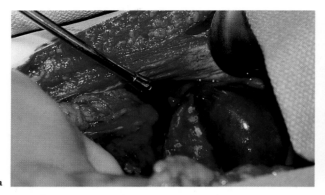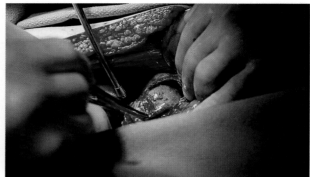

a   b

Fig. 6.19 (a) Punctate necrotic foci (arrow) on peritoneal gall bladder surface and (b) confluent necrosis of hepatic surface.

inflammatory condition to an infectious condition. Bile within the obstructed gall bladder can become infected, in essence creating an intracholecystic abscess. The gall bladder wall will develop focal (Fig. 6.19a) and subsequently confluent (Fig. 6.19b) areas of gangrene which threaten perforation and consequent intraperitoneal sepsis. Purulent and/or gangrenous cholecystitis can cause severe systemic sepsis with potential for acute lung injury and other secondary organ failures. When systemic sepsis is present, the best option is open cholecystectomy following volume resuscitation and control of respiratory failure if present. Percutaneous cholecystostomy can be considered but must be abandoned for open cholecystectomy if the patient does not rapidly improve. Percutaneous cholecystostomy will not prevent perforation of the already gangrenous gall bladder and will not resolve systemic sepsis if the gallbladder wall remains a source of proliferating micro-organisms.

In cases of uncomplicated acute cholecystitis, antibiotics should be administered pre-operatively and no longer than 24 h postoperatively; a first generation cephalosporin suffices. Antibiotic treatment for purulent, gangrenous, or septic cholecystitis should follow recommendations for cholangitis.

Acute cholangitis, bacterial infection of the bile ducts, is an intra-abdominal but extraperitoneal infection. Because it is an extraperitoneal process, abdominal pain will be both less predominant and less severe than that of conditions causing peritonitis. Bacterial contamination and obstruction of the biliary tree are both necessary preconditions for its development. Biliary obstruction may be caused by choledocholithiasis, benign stricture, or malignancy. Choledocholithiasis will be encountered most frequently. The proliferation of bacteria in the obstructed biliary tree raises intrabiliary pressures which can then drive bacteria and their products into the circulation. Thus, a profound life-threatening septic state may develop and demand urgent surgical attention.

Patients with cholangitis present with fever, right upper quadrant abdominal pain, and jaundice. The concurrent presentation of these findings comprises the classic triad of Charcot but does not occur in all patients. Fever is the most consistent finding, followed by jaundice, and finally abdominal pain. The addition of hypotension and altered mental status complete the pentad of Reynold and herald the need for emergent intervention.

Leucocytosis is present in the majority of patients and is more prominent than that associated with cholecystitis. Ultrasound examination of the right upper quadrant helps confirm a clinical diagnosis of cholangitis by demonstrating dilation of extrahepatic and intrahepatic bile ducts, cholelithiasis, and possibly choledocholithiasis. Computed tomography is less useful for identification of calculus disease but allows identification of ductal dilation, provides imaging of the pancreatic head for identification of tumour, and excludes intraperitoneal processes (Fig. 6.20).

Initial treatment consists of antibiotic therapy and volume resuscitation. Haemodynamic monitoring and, possibly, ventilatory support will be necessary for those patients with associated shock. Antibiotic therapy initiated immediately upon diagnosis should check the systemic progression of sepsis in most patients. If the patient does not respond to initial therapy, biliary decompression should be performed within 12 hours of presentation. However, patients in septic shock may require more emergent decompression to minimize mortality. The bacteria most commonly associated with cholangitis and complicated cholecystitis are *E. coli*, *Klebsiella*, and *Enterococcus*. The incidences of *Enterobacter* and *Pseudomonas* isolates are increasing with more frequent use of indwelling biliary catheters. *Bacteroides* and other anaerobes are isolated from a significant minority of patients. Initial therapy should thus have activity against Gram-negative aerobic organisms, *Enterococcus*, and anaerobes. An ureidopenicillin combined with metronidazaole is a rational empiric regimen with final antibiotic therapy

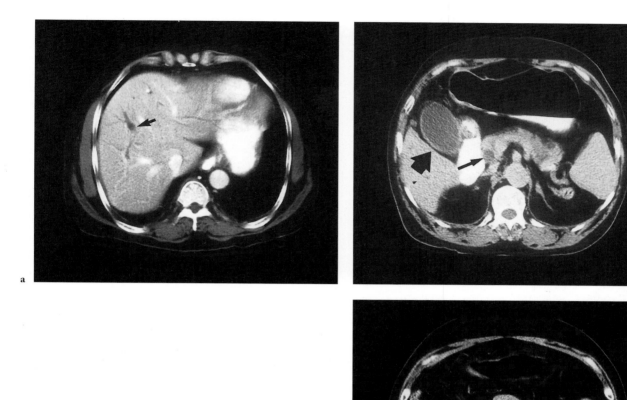

Fig. 6.20 CT of patient with choledocholithiasis and cholangitis reveals (a) intrahepatic and (b, c) extrahepatic ductal dilatation (narrow arrows). Note distended gall bladder in (b) (wide arrow).

determined by culture and sensitivity data. Intravenous antibiotics should be continued for a duration of 1–2 weeks — until fever and leucocytosis resolve.

The options for biliary decompression are endoscopic sphincterotomy, percutaneous transhepatic biliary catheter placement, and operative choledochotomy. Either endoscopic sphincterotomy (with or without placement of an endoscopic stent) or placement of a transhepatic biliary catheter (Fig. 6.21) are appropriate for cholangitis resulting from choledocholithiasis. These temporizing manoeuvres allow cholecystectomy and common bile duct exploration to be performed electively. For cholangitis resulting from proximal biliary obstruction or occurring in patients with biliary enteric anastomosis, the percutaneous transhepatic route will be necessary. Operative choledochotomy should be per-

formed urgently for sepsis only in the exceedingly rare circumstances that the two non-operative drainage procedures are technically impossible to perform, are unavailable, or fail to resolve the patient's acute sepsis.

Adult respiratory distress syndrome

Surgical infections may have far-reaching effects through the elaboration and systemic distribution of mediators which may incite inflammatory responses and damage organs distant from the focus of infection. Surgical infections are thus prominent among the aetiologies of the multiple organ failure syndrome. The organ to first manifest dysfunction is most often the lung, and indeed lung injury is an anticipated complication of severe surgical infection. This lung injury is

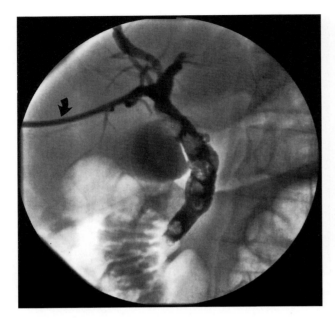

Fig. 6.21 Transhepatic catheter cholangiogram in a patient with choledocholithiasis and cholangitis. Catheter (arrow) enters right ductal system. Note multiple filling defects within common hepatic and common bile duct.

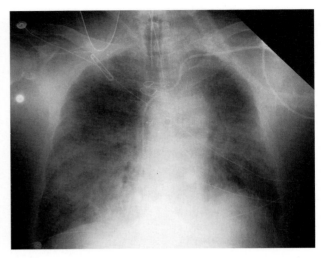

Fig. 6.22 Bilateral pulmonary infiltrates of ARDS arising postoperative day 5 in a 76-year-old man with a missed jejunotomy.

usually referred to as the adult respiratory distress syndrome (ARDS). Within the lung, the systemic mediators incite inflammatory responses which injure both the pulmonary endothelium and the pulmonary epithelium. Injury to the endothelium promotes interstitial oedema and eventually alveolar flooding. Injury to the epithelium leads to alveolar instability and ultimately alveolar collapse. Both mechanisms eventuate in obliteration of alveoli. Alveolar obliteration has two important pathophysiological manifestations. First, the lung becomes stiff; that is, its compliance diminishes. This means that the spontaneously breathing patient must work harder to move a given tidal volume of air. It is more efficient for such patients to move smaller tidal volumes rapidly than it is to move large tidal volumes slowly; hence, the rapid, shallow breathing pattern observed early in ARDS. Once the patient is mechanically ventilated, falling compliance means that a given tidal volume delivered by the ventilator results in a higher airway pressure. The second pathophysiological manifestation of alveolar obliteration is shunt. This allows a portion of desaturated mixed venous blood to pass to the systemic circulation without becoming oxygenated and is responsible for the refractory hypoxaemia of ARDS. The clinical manifestations of ARDS are thus: tachypnoea in the spontaneously breathing patient, high airway pressures in the mechanically ventilated patient, and hypoxaemia refractory to the administration of increasing concentrations of oxygen—all in the setting of non-cardiogenic pulmonary oedema. Specific criteria for ARDS

are a ratio of Po_2 to F_iO_2 (P/F ratio) of 200 or less, a pulmonary artery occlusion pressure of 18 mmHg or less, and diffuse bilateral infiltrates on chest X-ray (Fig. 6.22).

Mechanical ventilation supports the functions of the injured lung; it does not heal the lung. The management of ARDS is supportive, not curative. The respiratory support goals are to overcome poor pulmonary compliance for maintenance of ventilation and to overcome shunt for maintenance of tissue oxygenation.

Recent indirect evidence suggests that mechanical ventilation can exacerbate the lung injury seen in ARDS by traumatizing the non-compliant lung with high peak airway pressures and large tidal volumes. Thus current practice employs relatively small tidal volumes of 5–8 ml/kg and maintains peak airway pressures less than 35 cm H_2O. An increasingly popular technique to deal with decreased compliance is pressure control ventilation (PCV). With this mode, peak airway pressure is purposefully limited leaving tidal volume to vary directly with pulmonary compliance. Tidal volume is not guaranteed. Ventilation can be optimized by manipulation of the inspiratory flow waveform. However, minimization of peak airway pressure takes precedence over ventilation—even to the point of allowing Pco_2 to rise above normal levels. With this latter approach, referred to as permissive hypercapnia, Pco_2 is allowed to rise, and pH is controlled with buffers when necessary.

Shunt results in refractory hypoxaemia. To the extent that the lung injury of ARDS causes pure shunt (as opposed to V/Q mismatch), the associated hypoxaemia will not respond to increasing concentrations of oxygen (F_iO_2). High F_iO_2 damages the lung through generation of reactive oxygen metabolites. Thus, the use of high F_iO_2 is both inefficacious and detrimental. F_iO_2 should be kept at 0.4 or lower to minimize oxygen toxicity.

In the mechanically ventilated patient with ARDS, oxygenation is driven by *mean* airway pressure. Ventilator-induced lung injury seems to correlate with *peak* airway pressure. Traditional strategies employed high levels of positive end expiratory pressure (PEEP) to maintain oxygenation. PEEP increases mean airway pressure and thereby stabilizes alveoli and prevents their collapse. PEEP also facilitates expansion of alveoli in a slow, time-dependent process called alveolar recruitment. PEEP thus decreases shunt and improves oxygenation. However, PEEP directly increases the peak airway pressure generated by mechanical ventilation. Thus, PEEP is a source of ventilator induced lung trauma. Other strategies can maintain oxygenation by increasing mean airway pressure without increasing peak airway pressure.

The technique currently employed to achieve this latter goal inverts the inspiratory time to expiratory time ratio (I:E ratio). Normally, the I:E ratio is less than 1; that is, the expiratory phase is longer than the inspiratory phase. With inverse ratio techniques, the I:E ratio is increased above one so that the inspiratory phase is longer than the expiratory phase. This inverse ratio ventilation (IRV) increases mean airway pressure and thereby improves oxygenation. When combined with a pressure controlled ventilatory mode, peak airway pressures are not affected. Thus, pressure control–inverse ratio ventilation (PC–IRV) has become a popular mode for ventilating patients with ARDS in hopes of both maintaining oxygenation and minimizing ventilator associated lung injury.

ARDS occurring in the absence of primary pulmonary pathology should prompt the surgeon to search for inciting non-pulmonary processes which may require operative intervention. Such processes are very likely to be the surgical infections discussed in this chapter. When operation is necessary for control of an inciting course, it takes precedence over optimization of ventilatory management. Only by appropriate operation can the inflammatory source be eliminated and the respiratory failure cured. Thus, general surgeons need to be intimately involved in the management of postoperative respiratory failure because this complication may be a sign of incomplete control of the infectious source or a sign of recurrent infection. The appearance or persistence of ARDS may indicate the need for timely re-operation to afford the patient the greatest opportunity for survival (Fig. 6.23). Because ARDS is an anticipated complication of severe surgical infection, general surgeons should be facile with its diagnosis and treatment so that they can ensure optimal management for their patients.

Acknowledgement

The author wishes to extend his sincere thanks to Ms Karma Krumwiede's dedicated and expert assistance with manuscript preparation.

Further reading

Bohnen, J.M.A., Solomkin, J.S., Dellinger, E.P., Bjornson, H.S. & Page, C.P. (1992) Guidelines for clinical care: Anti-infective agents for intra-abdominal infection. *Archives of Surgery* **127**(1) 83–89.

Farnell, M.B., Worthington-Self, S., Mucha, P. Jr, Ilstrup, D.M. & McIlrath, D.C. (1986) Closure of abdominal incisions with subcutaneous catheters: a prospective randomized trial. *Archives of Surgery* **121**(6) 641–648.

Fildes, J., Bannon, M.P. & Barrett, J. (1991) Soft-tissue infections after trauma. *Surgical Clinics of North America* **71**(2) 371–384.

Foster, C.E. III & Lefor, A.T. (1996) General management of gastrointestinal fistulas: recognition, stabilization, and correction of fluid and electrolyte imbalances. *Surgical Clinics of North America* **76**(5) 1019–1033.

Gouma, D.J. & Obertop, H. (1992) Acute calculous cholecystitis: what is new in diagnosis and therapy? *HPB Surgery* **6**(2) 69–78.

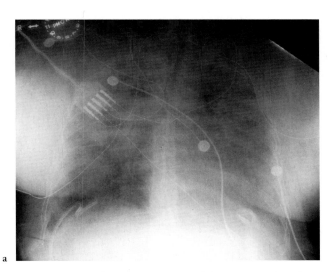

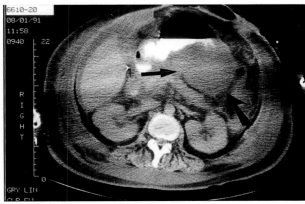

Fig. 6.23 (a) Severe bilateral infiltrates of ARDS in a 56-year-old woman did not improve following resection and diversion of leaking colocolostomy. (b) CT revealed a lesser sac abscess (arrow).

Krizek, T.J. & Robson, M.C. (1975) Evolution of quantitative bacteriology in wound management. *The American Journal of Surgery* **130**(11) 579–584.

Lewis, R.T. (1992) Necrotizing soft-tissue infections. *Surgical Infections* **6**(3) 693–703.

Lille, S.T., Sato, T.T., Engrav, L.H., Foy, H. & Jurkovich, G.J. (1996) Necrotizing soft tissue infections: Obstacles in diagnosis. *Journal of the American College of Surgeons* **182**(1) 7–11.

Marini, J.J. (1993) New options for the ventilatory management of acute lung injury. *New Horizons* **1**(4) 489–503.

Martineau, P., Shwed, J.A. & Denis, R. (1996) Is octreotide a new hope for enterocutaneous and external pancreatic fistulas closure? *The American Journal of Surgery* **172**(4) 386–395.

Morris, A.H. (1994) Adult respiratory distress syndrome and new modes of mechanical ventilation: Reducing the complications of high volume and high pressure (Review). *New Horizons* **2**(1) 19–33.

Nathens, A.B. & Rotstein, O.D. (1994) Therapeutic options in peritonitis. *Surgical Clinics of North America* **74**(3) 677–692.

Nathens, A.B. & Rotstein, O.D. (1996) Antimicrobial therapy for intraabdominal infection. *The American Journal of Surgery* **172**(Suppl 6A) 1S–6S.

Pissiotis, C.A. & Klimopoulos, S. (1993) Recent advances in the management of intra-abdominal infections. In: *Surgery Annual*, part 2/volume 25. (eds L.M. Nyhus), pp. 59–83. Appleton & Lange, East Norwalk, CT.

Ranson, J.H.C. (1995) The current management of acute pancreatitis. *Advances in Surgery* **28** 93–112.

Stamenkovic, I. & Lew, P.D. (1994) Early recognition of potentially fatal necrotizing fasciitis: The use of frozen-section biopsy. *Journal of Medicine* **310**(26) 1689–1693.

Stone, H.H., Bourneuf, A.A. & Stinson, L.D. (1985) Reliability of criteria for predicting persistent or recurrent sepsis. *Archives of Surgery* **120**(1) 17–20.

Sutherland, M.E. & Meyer, A.A. (1994) Necrotizing soft-tissue infections. *Surgical Clinics of North America* **74**(3) 591–607.

Wittmann, D.H., Schein, M. & Condon, R.E. (1996) Management of secondary peritonitis. *Annals of Surgery* **224**(1) 10–18.

CHAPTER 7

The acute abdomen and laparotomy

Terence J. O'Kelly & Zygmunt H. Krukowski

Introduction

There is no simple definition of the 'acute abdomen' other than a combination of signs and symptoms, including abdominal pain, which results in a patient being referred for an urgent general surgical opinion. The importance of the term is the risk to life of potential or actual infection or loss of effective circulating blood volume. The former most commonly arises as a result of release of gastrointestinal tract content into the peritoneal cavity and the latter by a variety of mechanisms varying from exsanguinating haemorrhage to rapid external fluid loss from a high small bowel obstruction. Commonly more than one mechanism for fluid loss operates.

Aetiology

The common causes of the acute abdomen in western societies and their relative incidence is shown in Table 7.1.

Pathophysiology

It is evident from Table 7.1 that in their various manifestations, both peritonitis and intestinal obstruction are important causes of the acute abdomen. The pathophysiology of these together with the pain they cause is considered here.

Peritonitis

The peritoneum consists of two layers, the visceral layer in direct contact with the underlying viscera and the parietal layer. The total surface area is similar to that of the body surface (approximately two square metres). The peritoneum behaves as a semipermeable membrane capable of rapid two-way transport of water and most solutes. The entire peritoneal surface participates in passive fluid transport but specialized lymphatic vessels concentrated in the muscular parts of the abdominal aspect of the diaphragm actively absorb both fluid and particles. Stomata between the peritoneal cells correspond with holes in the basement membrane and are believed to communicate directly with large lymphatic lacunae in the diaphragmatic muscle. In the normal peritoneum there is rapid movement of fluid, bacteria and deformable particles as large as leucocytes along well-defined pathways around the peritoneum, through the diaphragmatic lymphatics to the mediastinal lymphatics. The movement is facilitated by the fibrinolytic activity of the peritoneum derived from mesothelial cells and submesothelial blood vessels. This activity is lost after even minor peritoneal injury resulting in rapid adhesion between affected surfaces.

Peritonitis can occur with or without infection and when sepsis is present, pathogenic organisms reach the peritoneal cavity in the following ways.
1 Through perforation of the gastrointestinal or biliary tract
2 Through the female genital tract
3 By penetration of the abdominal parietes
4 By haematogenous spread.

Knowledge of the source of infection permits informed prediction of the organisms involved. Most cases of peritonitis are caused by organisms derived from the gastrointestinal tract although the bacteriology of established peritonitis is rather different from that of the intact gut lumen (Fig. 7.1). Only a few species of bacteria proliferate and many disappear spontaneously within a short time of inoculation. Infection is enhanced by synergy between organisms (aerobes, particularly *Escherischia coli*, reduce oxygen tension and facilitate growth of obligate anaerobes; Fig. 7.2) and by the presence of adjuvant substances such as faeces, bile or urine.

Although the peritoneum can eliminate experimentally inoculated bacteria very rapidly via the diaphragmatic lymphatics, peritoneal resistance to infection relies upon localization rather than dispersal of a contaminant. Inhibition of peritoneal fibrinolysis permits stabilization of fibrinous exudates and limits the spread of infection. The omentum and intraperitoneal viscera have a remarkable ability to confine infection. Generalized peritonitis represents failure of localization and occurs when:
1 Contamination develops too rapidly to permit effective localization;
2 Contamination persists or is repeated and overwhelms attempts to contain it;

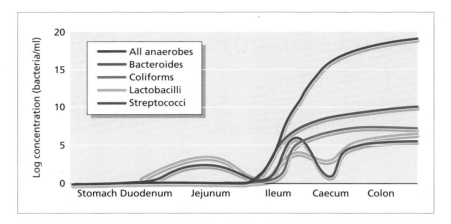

Fig. 7.1 Bacteriology of the normal gastrointestinal tract.

Table 7.1 Final diagnosis in adult patients admitted to hospital in Great Britain and Scandinavia with acute abdominal pain.

Diagnosis	%
Non-specific abdominal pain	30–45
Acute appendicitis	20–25
Acute cholecystitis and biliary colic	7–8
Peptic ulcer perforation and haemorrhage	4
Urinary retention	4
Acute pancreatitis	3
Small bowel obstruction	3
Renal and ureteric colic	3
Trauma	3
Malignant disease	2–4
Medical disorders	2–4
Acute diverticulitis	2
Large bowel obstruction	2
Vascular disorders	2
Gynaecological disease	1

From: Jones, P.F. (1987) *Emergency Abdominal Surgery*, 2nd edn. Blackwell Scientific, Oxford.

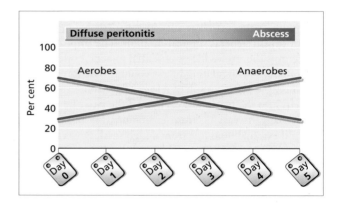

Fig. 7.2 The changes which occur in the bacterial population in peritonitis.

3 A localized abscess continues to expand and ruptures into the peritoneal cavity.

Because of its large surface area even sterile inflammation of the peritoneum may result in fluid loss sufficient to cause oligaemia and when infection is superimposed, the effects of oligaemia are compounded by the absorption of intact organisms and toxins.

Intestinal obstruction

Intestinal obstruction occurs from the presence of abnormalities:
1 In the lumen of the bowel (e.g. foreign bodies, gallstones);
2 In the bowel wall (e.g. inflammatory strictures, tumours);
3 Outside the bowel (e.g. adhesion bands, tumours, hernia sacs).

The bowel proximal to an obstruction dilates as food, gas and fluid accumulate. Gas is derived from swallowed air and the products of bacterial fermentation. Fluid isotonic with plasma collects because secretion continues above the obstruction and reabsorption ceases. Several litres of fluid can be sequestered within obstructed bowel loops and this is effectively lost from the system until the obstruction is resolved. Further fluid is lost through vomiting. The net result is reduction of extracellular fluid volume which affects both the intra- and extravascular compartments leading to dehydration and ultimately, circulatory collapse. In addition, gut distension opposed by contraction of smooth muscle in its wall leads to an increase in wall tension with consequent reduction in perfusion and ischaemia which can result in perforation.

Abdominal pain

Abdominal pain can be visceral, somatic or referred. These are not mutually exclusive and patients commonly present with a combination of pains. Visceral pain results from stimulation of pain receptors in smooth muscle which occurs as a consequence of ischaemia, distension or isometric contraction (increase in tension without shortening). The visceral peritoneum is insensitive to normally painful stimuli but some ill-defined mechanisms, for instance capsular stretching of solid viscera, may result in pain. Embryologically the gut is a midline structure which develops in three parts (fore-, mid- and hindgut), each with its segmental blood supply with which splanchnic sympathetic nerves run, accompanied by pain fibres. As a consequence, visceral pain is not well localized, is felt in the midline and occurs in the upper, central or lower abdomen depending upon whether the structure affected is derived from fore-, mid- or hindgut. Somatic abdominal pain results from stimulation of pain receptors in the parietal peritoneum or abdominal wall and these pass information centrally via segmental somatic sensory nerves. Somatic pain is therefore accurately localized but referred pain can occur, for instance shoulder-tip pain with diaphragmatic irritation (C4 innervates both). Abdominal pain may also be referred from above the diaphragm, most commonly as a result of pleural irritation.

Assessment

Making a definitive diagnosis of the cause of an acute abdomen should be attempted but it must be recognized that this is only part of the management of the patient and as such is not always the most pressing issue. Diagnosis is based upon history, examination and the results of investigations, which ultimately include inspection of the peritoneal cavity by laparotomy or laparoscopy when the combination of clinical concern and limited information from available investigations fail to define an alternative safe management policy.

Assessment
• Making a definitive diagnosis of the cause of an acute abdomen should be attempted but it must be recognized that this is only part of the management of the patient and as such it is not always the most pressing issue. • The characteristics of abdominal pain differentiate peritonitis from colic and the developing pattern of pain may provide useful clues to the progression of the underlying disease. • The general state of a patient commonly reflects the significance of the underlying abdominal condition and its haemodynamic consequences. • The convention of withholding analgesia until a diagnosis is made is inappropriate and inhumane.

History

The characteristics of abdominal pain differentiate peritonitis from colic and the developing pattern of pain may provide useful clues to the progression of the underlying disease. Colicky pain, with its characteristic 'waves' and 'spasms' often superimposed on a background of discomfort, makes patients restless and they typically describe a fruitless quest for a comfortable position to ease the pain. In contrast peritonitis causes continuous pain exacerbated by movement: coughing, bumps in the road on the journey to hospital and abdominal examination. The parietal inflammation in peritonitis leads to a severe, localized pain which over-rides the early visceral component and accounts for the classic shift of midline pain to the area of inflammation. Visceral pain is associated with malaise, nausea/vomiting and sweating, features which are often absent in purely somatic pain.

In addition to determining the type of pain, it is important to define its site (previous, present and radiation), speed of onset (sudden onset of peritonitis suggests perforation whereas rapid onset of colic suggests passage of a calculus or volvulus) and associated phenomena (appetite, nausea/vomiting, distension, bowel habit, etc.). A relevant previous medical and family history must be taken as well as an appropriate system enquiry. Correlating these features with the type of pain experienced will suggest possible diagnoses and subsequent management.

Because of the constraints of time it is not infrequently necessary to overlap history taking with examination and to concentrate attention on only the most relevant aspects of the presenting problem. In these circumstances it is necessary to adopt a pragmatic approach, gained through experience which allows a surgeon to discriminate between what is ideal and what is absolutely necessary in both history taking and examination. At the same time the surgeon must recognize that this introduces the possibility for error.

Examination

Examination begins as the patient is approached and continues as the history is taken. The general state of a patient commonly reflects the significance of the underlying abdominal condition and its haemodynamic consequences. A spectrum exists from the patient who looks well, is sitting up in bed and talking and moving freely to those who appear moribund, lie flat in bed, are cerebrally obtunded and cannot move without experiencing pain. It is important to determine where in this spectrum a patient lies and to institute appropriate resuscitation. In all cases reliable temperature, pulse and blood pressure (supine and erect if hypovolaemia suspected) should be recorded. The presence of fetor, jaundice and lymphadenopathy should be noted. Reduced skin turgor, sunken eyes and a dry mouth indicate severe dehydration but it is rare in contemporary practice to see the 'Hippocratic facies' of advanced peritonitis.

Abdominal examination begins with inspection. The presence of skin discoloration, prominent veins, scars, wounds and masses should be noted. In intestinal obstruction, peristalsis may be visible. If the abdomen is distended then this can provide an important clue to the cause of distension (i.e. ascitic fluid produces fullness in the flanks, whereas gas-filled obstructed loops of small bowel produce central distension). Respiratory excursion is diminished in peritonitis. The external genitalia in males and the hernial orifices in both sexes should be examined and this is routinely done after inspection and before palpation of the abdomen.

When palpation of the abdomen causes discomfort, patients should be asked to indicate where they experience pain and this area should be examined last. The convention of withholding analgesia until a diagnosis is made is inappropriate and inhumane. Apprehensive patients with diffuse pain are more profitably assessed after analgesia has been given and widespread tenderness often localizes to a particular area or quadrant of the abdomen. There is no evidence that serious pathology is more likely to be missed if analgesia is used appropriately.

Palpation which should be gentle initially, detects tenderness, masses and pulsation. When an abnormality is present it should be defined further. The site and extent of tenderness and guarding (reflex contraction of abdominal wall muscles in the presence of peritonitis) is assessed. Percussion of the abdomen indicates the degree of tenderness present and localizes the area of maximum discomfort when there is diffuse tenderness. Eliciting rebound tenderness by brisk removal of the examining hand is redundant if light percussion has already demonstrated the sign. In the presence of somatic pain, abdominal wall tenderness can be demonstrated by palpation of the symptomatic area as the patient contracts and relaxes the anterior abdominal wall musculature. Exacerbation of tenderness provoked by contraction (voluntary guarding) indicates that the pain arises in the parietes rather than the peritoneal cavity. The patient's facial appearance provides clues to the underlying problem and apprehension frequently accompanies peritonitis but this diagnosis is unlikely if the patient's eyes remain closed throughout the examination ('closed-eye sign').

In addition to localizing tenderness, percussion of the abdomen may reveal loss of liver dullness with free intraperitoneal gas and suprapubic dullness with urinary retention. Consideration should always be given to the possibility of a vascular catastrophe, particularly leaking or ruptured aortic aneurysms (see Chapters 22 and 24).

Auscultation of bowel sounds provides useful information if performed correctly. A brief application of the stethoscope may miss the rush of hyperactive sounds which are most readily heard during a bout of colic. Bowel sounds should be described as (i) present and normal, (ii) present and obstructed and (iii) absent. Transmitted and sometimes amplified heart sounds are typical of gross gaseous distension.

Digital rectal examination is 'routine' but it is not unreasonable to omit it particularly in young patients when a diagnosis and management plan have already been formulated which will not be affected by any information likely to accrue from this examination. When rectal examination is performed, particular note should be made of the presence of tenderness, a mass or abnormality of the accessible pelvic viscera. The presence of pus, excess mucous or faecal occult blood should be determined. Vaginal examination is required to confirm or refute possible gynaecological disorders.

Investigations

The range of investigations available for the assessment of an acute abdomen is extensive and their role and value are considered elsewhere under specific diagnostic headings. The ability to interpret routine haematological and biochemical tests, to read plain radiographs and to select appropriate contrast and other radiological studies are important skills which should be acquired. The value of any investigation is enhanced if it is performed to answer a specific question. Emergency laparotomy is a very direct method of corroborating or refuting the findings of investigations upon which a decision to operate has been based.

Making a diagnosis

Making a diagnosis in a patient with an acute abdomen is an imprecise discipline which requires experience and pragmatism. Some patients present with 'classic' symptoms and signs, but commonly the diagnosis will be uncertain. In these circumstances time and a period of 'active observation' (returning to the patient to repeat clinical assessment) can be very helpful but it is important to recognize that the only decision which may be necessary or indeed possible, is to determine whether or not an operation is required and if so, how urgently.

Not infrequently clinical assessment and the results of investigations will condense into a few key facts which

---

Examination

- Auscultation of bowel sounds can provide useful information but only if performed and interpreted correctly.
- Peritoneal irritation in patients with acute abdominal pain was traditionally considered to be an indication for an emergency operation, but if applied indiscriminately leads to unnecessary surgery.

reduce the possible options to one or two diagnoses. It is not in the character of surgeons to then conduct a meticulous systematic interrogation but deviation from familiar patterns, odd symptoms, inconsistent signs and uncertainty should always provoke a cautious approach. Most surgeons pride themselves on their diagnostic acumen but it is apparent that this is a skill which atrophies without constant practice.

Laparotomy

Decision to operate

Peritoneal irritation in-patients with acute abdominal pain is traditionally considered an indication for an emergency operation but if applied indiscriminately, leads to unnecessary surgery. Transmural inflammation of an abdominal viscus may produce considerable inflammatory exudation but even when there is a degree of bacterial contamination in the fluid, operative intervention may be avoidable. The results of conservative management of acute cholecystitis, diverticulitis and pelvic inflammatory disease bear witness to this. Sealed perforations which result in localized peritonitis can be managed conservatively. However, evidence of continuing leakage, generalized peritonitis and failure to respond to non-operative measures are all indications for surgery. The reason for proceeding to operation can only be that the balance of risk is less for the patient if an operation is performed than if the abdomen is not opened.

Pre-operative management

Except where surgery is required to stop exsanguinating haemorrhage, patients benefit from a period of resuscitation and stabilization. The priority is normally correction of hypovolaemia by administration of intravenous fluid. Crystalloid solutions (except dextrose) are generally satisfactory but colloid may be necessary if there has been considerable inflammatory exudation into the peritoneal cavity. The minimum of invasive procedures compatible with adequate resuscitation and monitoring are required. Clinical assessment of tissue perfusion, pulse and blood pressure may give sufficient information but when necessary, urine flow and central venous pressure should be recorded. Antibiotics effective against probable infecting pathogens must be given to those with peritonitis and all patients should receive appropriate peroperative antibiotic chemoprophylaxis.

> **Pre-operative management**
>
> Except where surgery is required to stop exsanguinating haemorrhage, most patients benefit from a period of resuscitation and stabilization.

Subcutaneous heparin and TED stockings are used where indicated. Informed consent should be obtained. Good communication with the family frequently reduces postoperative difficulties in the event of an adverse outcome.

Surgery

The objectives of surgery in the acute abdomen are:
1 To confirm or establish a diagnosis;
2 To correct the disease process (if possible); and
3 To prevent further complications.
Although the details of operative technique and treatment of specific problems are dealt with elsewhere in the text, a number of principles can be enumerated.

Incision

A midline incision is recommended except when the intention is to gain access to only one quadrant of the abdomen (e.g. for appendicectomy). This is rapidly made, relatively atraumatic and avascular, opens the minimum of tissue planes, can be extended in either direction easily and does not prejudice the placement of any stoma.

Wound protection

Contamination of the parietes cannot be avoided completely but the degree of soiling (for instance by intestinal content) can be minimized with appropriate wound protection involving plastic ring drapes.

Bacteriology

A specimen from intra-abdominal fluid should be sent immediately for culture and Gram stain of the fluid will give an indication of both the number and types of bacteria present. Absence of bacteria (as is frequently the case with peptic perforation) is an indication that a long course of antibiotics is not necessary.

Peritoneal debridement

All loose fluid and debris should be aspirated or mopped out. Adherent fibrin is removed when possible, but not if this traumatizes the underlying viscera.

Intestinal decompression

This greatly improves access and is best achieved by either retrograde stripping of the small intestine content for aspiration from the stomach or aspiration of colonic gas by insertion of a 22G intravenous needle through a convenient taenia.

Peritoneal lavage

Although there is debate about the value of adding anti-biotics to lavage fluid, our continuing favourable experience leads us to recommend a solution containing normal saline and tetracycline (1 mg/ml), used in sufficient volume to produce a clear return (Fig. 7.3). If there is gross peritoneal contamination lavage should be performed when the abdomen is opened and repeated prior to closure. The rationale behind the use of peroperative lavage is outlined in Table 7.2.

Laparotomy examination

The peritoneal cavity and retroperitoneum should be examined systematically to document causal, associated and incidental pathology. It is embarrassing, for example, to fail to remark on a large aortic aneurysm in the urgency of treating a duodenal perforation.

It is essential that surgical trainees develop a faultless and meticulous technique for laparotomies such that all areas and all organs in the abdomen are examined as part of a complete diagnostic exercise. If the initial approach does not give sufficient diagnostic access then the midline incision should be extended up to the xiphoid or down towards the symphysis, as appropriately directed by the suspected pathology. It may be necessary to enter the lesser sac in more difficult cases. It is also worthy of note that occasionally colonic perforations or duodenal perforations may occur into the retroperitoneum and the surgeons should therefore be conversant with mobilization of the retroperitoneal portions of the duodenum, right and left colon.

Management is based upon these findings and the accuracy in detection and documentation is crucial. It is not inappropriate to emphasize the need to extend the incision in cases of diagnostic difficulty.

Abdominal drainage

It is futile to attempt to drain the general peritoneal cavity. Drains are used only for specific indications: to aspirate bile or pancreatic fluid and, occasionally, blood and serum from a site of dissection. Small bore suction drains are satisfactory for short-term use but sump drains are recommended if prolonged drainage is envisaged.

Table 7.2 Peroperative antibiotic lavage.

Mechanically removes and dilutes peritoneal contamination
Abolishes growth of bacteria in peritoneal fluid
Permits safe radical surgery
Reduces the incidence of wound and intraperitoneal infection
Reduces the requirements for postoperative antibiotics

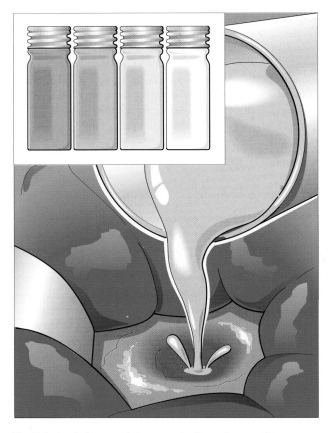

Fig. 7.3 A solution containing normal saline and tetracycline (1 mg/ml) is instilled into peritoneal cavity and then aspirated. This is repeated until the aspirate is clear. Sequential aspirates are shown in the inset.

Closure of the abdomen

The abdomen is closed with a continuous mass closure technique with a monofilament suture which obviates the need for tension sutures. The subcutaneous tissues are irrigated with a further aliquot of tetracycline solution and the wound closed with a subcuticular suture or interrupted monofilament sutures or staples if the operation is classed 'dirty'. Subcutaneous sutures are not used but a small-bore suction drain may be placed in the subcutaneous space in the obese. Delayed primary closure is not necessary if this regimen is followed.

Postoperative care

This will normally be determined by the findings and surgery but some general principles apply.

Postoperative oliguria

This is usually caused by inadequate renal blood flow secondary to low cardiac output and oligaemia. Maintenance of renal function is a priority and can normally be achieved through restoration of plasma volume.

Pain

Pain relief is important not only on humanitarian grounds but also because pain depresses respiratory function.

Nasogastric suction

Nasogastric intubation and aspiration is indicated in the presence of diffuse peritonitis and gross intestinal distension (even after operative decompression). It should be continued until either bowel sounds return to normal or, the volume of aspirate is negligible. In any event nasogastric tubes should be removed as rapidly as possible because of their adverse effect on pulmonary infection. Intravenous fluids are continued until adequate oral intake is assured. Parenteral nutrition is not normally required until at least 5 days have elapsed but should be instituted earlier if there is no prospect of early recovery of intestinal function.

Antibiotics

Postoperative antibiotic requirements are modified in the light of the operative findings, the Gram stain of the peritoneal fluid and the definitive bacteriology. The need for antibiotics beyond the third day should be questioned in all but the most serious infections. Generalized peritonitis should be treated with broad-spectrum antibiotics effective against anaerobes, coliform organisms and probably enterococci. Whilst some modern single agents achieve acceptable activity against these, no single agent is superior to a combination of intravenous metronidazole, gentamicin and an ampicillin derivative. Now that once daily administration

of high dose gentamicin (7 mg/kg) with once daily trough estimation has been established, this remains the favoured agent against Gram-negative aerobes.

Conclusions

Management of the acute abdomen can present a difficult clinical challenge. The history, examination, results of investigations and a period of active observation may provide a diagnosis and suggest an appropriate treatment. In some instances, however, the diagnosis is not clear and, based upon clinical findings, the only course is to perform a laparotomy. It is recognized that occasionally the laparotomy findings will suggest that a non-operative treatment would have been sufficient but this approach is reasonable as long as clinical assessment is sound and mortality and morbidity from surgery are kept to a minimum. Adherence to the principles enumerated above should ensure this is the case.

Further reading

Gallegos, N. & Hobsley, N. (1992) Abdominal pain: parietal or visceral. *Journal of the Royal Society of Medicine* **85** 379.

Gray, D.W.R. & Colin, J. (1987) Non-specific abdominal pain as a cause of acute admission to hospital. *British Journal of Surgery* **74** 239–242.

Jones, P.F. (1987) *Emergency Abdominal Surgery*, 2nd edn. Blackwell Scientific Publications, Oxford.

Krukowski, Z.H. & Matheson, N.A. (1983) The management of peritoneal and parietal contamination in abdominal surgery. *British Journal of Surgery* **70** 440–441.

Paterson-Brown, S. & Vipond, M.N. (1990) Modern aids to clinical decision making in the acute abdomen. *British Journal of Surgery* **77** 13–18.

Thomson, H.J. & Jones, P.F. (1986) Active observation in acute abdominal pain. *American Journal of Surgery* **132** 522–555.

CHAPTER 8

Laparoscopy in the acute abdomen

K. K. Madhavan & Simon Paterson-Brown

Introduction

Over the last few years the use of laparoscopy by general surgeons has undergone a tremendous change in both the elective and the emergency setting. Although some surgeons had been using laparoscopy as a diagnostic tool for many years to diagnose intra-abdominal conditions in both the acute abdomen and in the investigation of masses and malignancy, it has taken the recent introduction of videolaparoscopy and the associated development of therapeutic laparoscopic surgery for the undoubted benefits of laparoscopy to reach a much wider population of surgeons and patients.

Over the last 20 years or so great changes have taken place in the management of the acute abdomen with the introduction of many adjuvant techniques to aid the emergency surgeon in the decision-making process, in both the improvement of diagnostic accuracy and the reduction of inappropriate management decisions. These have included peritoneal lavage, peritoneal cytology, ultrasonography, computer-aided diagnosis, contrast radiology and diagnostic laparoscopy. With the subsequent development of therapeutic laparoscopy, the potential role of 'emergency laparascopy' now has major implications on the management of many patients with acute abdominal pain and abdominal trauma. This chapter will explore these implications further and discuss the relative indications and contra-indications of 'emergency' diagnostic and therapeutic laparoscopy.

Diagnostic laparoscopy in the acute abdomen

In the management of the acute abdomen patients can be classified into those with non-traumatic causes and those who have suffered abdominal trauma, either blunt or penetrating. Many studies have been reported over the last few years demonstrating the value of diagnostic laparoscopy in both these groups of patients. In any patient with an 'acute abdomen' making an accurate diagnosis is not as important as making the correct surgical decision; either to perform exploratory surgery or to observe the patient and perform additional non-invasive investigations as required. When at

Diagnostic laparoscopy in the acute abdomen
• Decision to operate uncertain
• Young females with suspected appendicitis
• Suspected intestinal ischaemia

laparotomy the pre-operative diagnosis is found to be incorrect but the decision to operate is correct, the patient's management will not have been detrimentally influenced. The same cannot be said when an incorrect decision to operate or not is made—both being associated with a (potentially) significant increase in morbidity and occasionally mortality. In the acute abdomen it is those patients in whom the decision to operate is uncertain who benefit most from diagnostic laparoscopy. Studies from St Mary's Hospital in London have demonstrated that the potential error rate in this difficult group of patients can be reduced from around 30% to almost zero using diagnostic laparoscopy. Similar figures are also true in abdominal trauma.

Indications for diagnostic laparoscopy in the non-traumatic acute abdomen

When the surgeon assesses a patient with acute abdominal pain he/she invariably, albeit often subconsciously, classifies them into one of three groups: definitely needs operation; definitely does not need operation; and need for operation uncertain. There is now good evidence to support the almost routine use of laparoscopy in this difficult third group of patients in whom the decision to operate is uncertain. Obviously in some patients additional non-invasive pre-operative investigations, such as ultrasound, contrast radiology and so on, may produce a definite diagnosis whereby the decision for surgery becomes clearer. However, it has also been shown that even in the group of patients in whom the surgeon's decision is 'definitely requires operation' errors still occur, particularly in young women with suspected appendicitis. In these patients, where the potential cause of the abdominal pain is multi-factorial (see Table 8.1), and national figures of up to 40% for the removal of a normal appendix are still reported, there is the most pressing argu-

Table 8.1 Differential diagnosis of right-sided lower abdominal pain in young women of child-bearing age.

Diagnosis	Laparoscopic intervention	Open surgery
Acute appendicitis	Possible	May be required
Pelvic inflammatory disease	Not required	Not required
Ruptured corpus luteum cyst	Possible	Not required
Ruptured ovarian follicle	Not required	Not required
Ruptured ectopic pregnancy	Possible	May be required
Retrograde menstruation	Not required	Not required
Endometriosis	Not required	Not required
Primary peritonitis	Possible	May be required
Twisted ovarian cyst	Possible	May be required

Diagnostic laparoscopy in blunt abdominal trauma

- Stable patient
- Equivocal signs/symptoms
- Positive lavage
- Multisystem injuries

ment for almost routine laparoscopy before appendicectomy. Although pre-operative pelvic ultrasonography can occasionally be of value in the demonstration of ovarian cysts, in the presence of lower abdominal 'peritonism' it is much easier to accept a diagnosis of ruptured ovarian cyst if it has been seen at laparoscopy and acute appendicitis has been excluded.

Another group of patients in whom diagnostic laparoscopy is particularly useful is the elderly patients, many of whom present with a vague history and inconclusive abdominal signs. Mesenteric infarction is easily identified at laparoscopy, and, in the case of acute diverticulitis, intraperitoneal perforation can be confirmed or refuted.

Diagnostic laparoscopy in penetrating abdominal trauma

- Stable patient
- Equivocal signs/symptoms
- Bloodstained lavage

Indications for diagnostic laparoscopy in abdominal trauma

As has already been discussed for the acute abdomen of non-traumatic origin, in the management of abdominal trauma the decision to operate or observe is of paramount importance and the accurate diagnosis of organ injury, although important, takes second place. Even in the presence of significant abdominal trauma which requires surgery, evaluation and decision-making is often obscured by other injuries, in addition to the reduced co-operation and consciousness which is so common in this group of patients. The more widespread use of peritoneal lavage, ultrasonography and more recently CT scanning, have all been of great benefit to the emergency surgeon, but there remains a small, but clinically significant group of patients in whom the decision to operate can be extremely difficult.

In the evaluation of blunt abdominal trauma persistent bleeding and visceral rupture are the two most pressing indications for surgery. Ultrasonography, CT scanning and peritoneal lavage are all excellent techniques, in skilled hands, to detect the former, but are less accurate in revealing the latter. Furthermore the presence of blood alone is no indication for surgery, and indeed many surgeons have performed laparotomy for a positive lavage only to find clinically insignificant lacerations to the liver, spleen and small bowel mesentery. It has been suggested that as many as one-third of patients

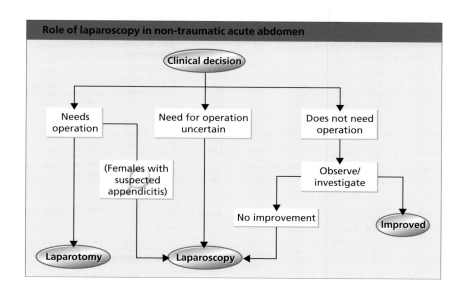

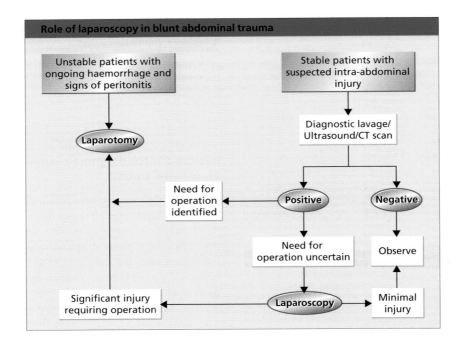

Role of laparoscopy in blunt abdominal trauma

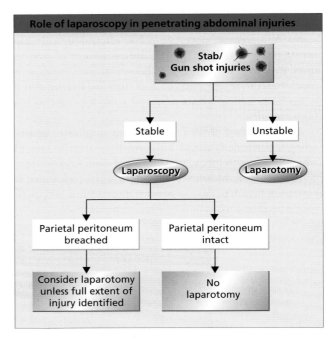

Role of laparoscopy in penetrating abdominal injuries

undergoing laparotomy for a positive lavage do not require any surgical intervention at operation. Although close clinical monitoring of these patients will reveal those with persistent blood loss and developing peritonitis from a perforated viscus, in the presence of multiple injuries—particularly in patients who require surgery for other systems (such as orthopaedic and head injuries)—a definitive diagnosis regarding the severity of the intra-abdominal injury is essential at an early stage in the overall management of the patient.

For these reasons diagnostic laparoscopy has begun to emerge as a useful technique in this group of patients, and although the majority of the difficult decisions fall into the category of blunt trauma, laparoscopy can also be of use in the assessment of penetrating trauma to both abdomen and, as studies from the United States have reported, the chest.

In blunt abdominal trauma the patients who are most likely to benefit from diagnostic laparoscopy are those with a positive peritoneal lavage who are cardiovascularly stable, particularly if there are associated injuries to other systems which may require surgery, transfer to another hospital, or both of these. In other words laparoscopy is being used instead of laparotomy to exclude injuries which require operative treatment. In addition, patients without a positive lavage but who demonstrate equivocal signs of peritoneal irritation, may benefit from laparoscopy if other investigations are unhelpful and signs do not settle after a short period of observation (4–6h). In these patients it is the detection of intestinal rupture which is difficult. In penetrating abdominal trauma laparoscopy can be used to demonstrate breach of peritoneum and any underlying injury. Reports from South Africa, where many hospitals have a

large experience in the treatment of penetrating injuries, have shown that initial observation appears a safe option if the patient is stable, progressing to laparotomy only if signs of peritonitis or ongoing haemorrhage develop. In some of these patients whose clinical signs are equivocal, laparoscopy can be used. The real role of laparoscopy in penetrating injuries is in tangential stab and gunshot wounds. The method provides an excellent view of the parietal peritoneal layer from within and if a breach in this lining can be ruled out an unnecessary laparotomy can be avoided. However, if the parietal peritoneum is breached, further dependence on laparoscopy to detect the exact nature and extent of injury and to attempt laparoscopic repair may not be the ideal step and a laparotomy is the procedure of choice. This is because of the often unpredictable route taken by the offending weapon or missile and constant movement of abdominal viscera making a full assessment of damage impossible without a full laparotomy.

Anaesthesia for diagnostic laparoscopy

Diagnostic laparoscopy may be safely performed under local anaesthesia with intravenous sedation. However, in the emergency setting, particularly if the decision to proceed to surgical intervention is anticipated, it is best performed in theatre under general anaesthesia with endotracheal intubation. If laparoscopy is being carried out under local anaesthesia, full monitoring is required with an anaesthetist on standby. After administration of intravenous sedation, a local anaesthetic agent is infiltrated into the skin in the infra-umbilical region, extending down to and through the linea alba. Thereafter, the open technique of laparoscopy is performed as described below, and further infiltration is carried out at the point where the second port is going to be inserted.

Surgical technique of laparoscopy

The open method of laparoscopy is the one the authors routinely perform and recommend. It removes the potential risk of injury during blind insertion of a Veress needle and first trocar, and in the presence of previous scars and bowel obstruction is mandatory. After preparation of the abdomen, the pit of the umbilicus is grasped with toothed artery forceps and everted. A short longitudinal incision is then made in the infra-umbical direction to expose the 'umbilical tube' (Fig. 8.1) which connects the pit of the umbilicus to the peritoneum through the linea alba. A small incision is made in this tube and forceps are then inserted through into the peritoneum. The laparoscopic port without the internal trocar is then inserted (Fig. 8.2) and a pneumoperitoneum created to a pressure of 10 mmHg. A port with a bevelled tip is easier for this purpose than one with a flat tip. The laparoscope is then inserted and full inspection of the peritoneal cavity performed. An additional port is almost always required to manipulate and grasp intra-abdominal structures to improve inspection, and can be inserted in any strategic position, taking care to avoid the epigastric vessels. Visibility may be further improved by tilting the patient. If required the lesser sac may be examined by passing the laparoscope through a window in the gastrocolic omentum. For adequate examination of the pelvic organs the patient should be placed in the Trendelenberg

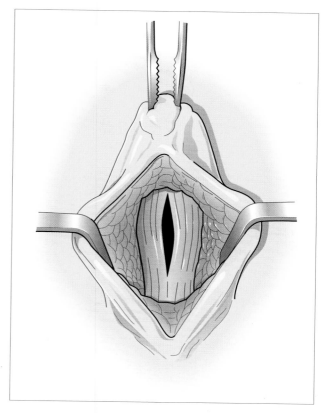

Fig. 8.1 Incision through the umbilical tube to access the peritoneal cavity (the umbilical skin has been firmly grasped and everted while two retractors ensure incision in the midline).

position and the uterus and ovaries identifed by manipulation with instruments inserted through the second port (Fig. 8.3). The authors often use the suction tube for this purpose. A retrocaecal appendix may only be seen by lifting up the caecal pole, and occasionally requires some caecal mobilization; this will be discussed in greater detail later under 'therapeutic laparoscopy'. Examination of the small bowel may require the introduction of atraumatic grasping forceps in order to identify the disease process.

When diagnostic laparoscopy is being performed for trauma additional factors need to be considered. Firstly, suction and irrigation will usually be required to fully evaluate any haemoperitoneum; secondly, if there is a stab wound this may require temporary closure during insufflation so as to prevent loss of the pneumoperitoneum; and thirdly, the surgeon must remain aware of possible retroperitoneal injury. If any doubt remains as to the integrity of the gastro-intestinal tract or the nature of persistent bleeding then the procedure should be converted to laparotomy. A haemoperitoneum observed at laparoscopy may be divided into three categories:

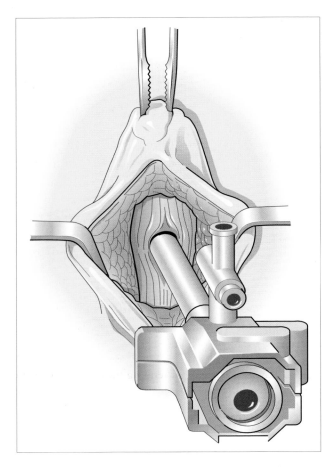

Fig. 8.2 Insertion of the first 10-mm port into the peritoneal cavity under direct vision using the open method (a cannula with a bevelled tip is very helpful in this procedure).

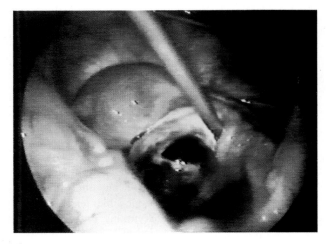

Fig. 8.3 Manipulation of uterus and adnexae through the second laparoscopic port. In this patient, the cause of pain is clearly revealed as a haemorrhagic cyst in her right ovary.

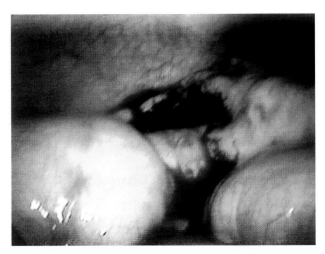

Fig. 8.4 Laparoscopic view of minimal haemoperitoneum in a patient with blunt abdominal trauma.

1 Minimal haemoperitoneum: a small volume of blood is seen in the paracolic gutters or streaking loops of intestine (Fig. 8.4). If, after irrigation and aspiration, no further blood is noted the laparoscopy may be terminated and the patient observed.

2 Moderate haemoperitoneum: a puddle of blood is seen in the paracolic gutters and once this is aspirated it recurs. If the bleeding site is found it may be treated laparoscopically if appropriate or by conversion to laparotomy.

3 Severe haemoperitoneum: this should be evident from the outset of laparoscopy, usually during initial cutdown, and laparotomy should follow immediately.

Although intra-abdominal injuries from stab wounds are relatively straightforward to detect at laparoscopy, the same is not true for missile injuries. Low-velocity missile injuries often follow unpredictable pathways around fascial planes and formal exploration should be considered in any case where the exact path of the bullet cannot be accurately seen and followed. Laparoscopy has almost no role to play in the assessment of high-velocity missile injuries, except perhaps in thoraco-abdominal wounds where laparoscopy or thoracoscopy can be used to exclude involvement of the peritoneal or pleural cavity. Gas embolization has been reported in the presence of major venous injuries, particularly if the central venous pressure is low. Pneumothorax can complicate laparoscopy if there has been a diaphragmatic tear, although if the insufflating pressure is kept below 10 mmHg this should not be a problem.

Therapeutic laparoscopy

As surgeons have mastered the techniques of laparoscopic cholecystectomy, so they have begun to attempt other surgical procedures including those for acute abdominal conditions and traumatic injuries. Great care must be taken in the selection of patients for this type of surgery, selecting the procedure performed and assessing the overall benefit which

> **Therapeutic laparoscopy**
>
> - Patient selection
> - Surgical experience
> - Appropriate condition
> - Low threshold for conversion

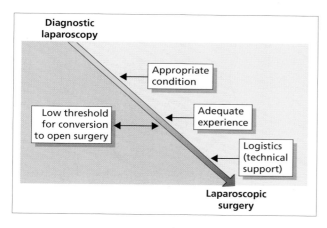

Fig. 8.5 Factors affecting the progression of diagnostic laparoscopy in acute abdomen to therapeautic laparoscopic surgery.

this provides for the patient (Fig. 8.5). The first, and most important dictum in emergency surgery is to ensure that the condition is treated safely and the patient makes a full and uneventful recovery where possible. Early discharge and return to normal activities, however desirable, must take a very distant second position. However, reduced wound pain and less postoperative ileus are attractive gains for both patient and surgeon. Thus there is undoubtedly a place for laparoscopic surgery in the management of the acute abdomen, mainly for non-traumatic causes, but occasionally for trauma, and these will now be discussed.

Therapeutic laparoscopy in the non-traumatic acute abdomen

A number of recognized procedures can now be performed laparoscopically for acute abdominal pain of non-traumatic origin. Each will be considered in turn, with a description of the technique.

Laparoscopic appendicectomy

As mentioned earlier, diagnostic laparoscopy has a major role to play in confirming or refuting the diagnosis of acute appendicitis in the presence of equivocal clinical signs, especially in women (Fig. 8.6). However, once the diagnosis has been confirmed the surgeon now has an option to proceed to laparoscopic appendicectomy. Although many series of laparoscopic appendicectomies have now been reported,

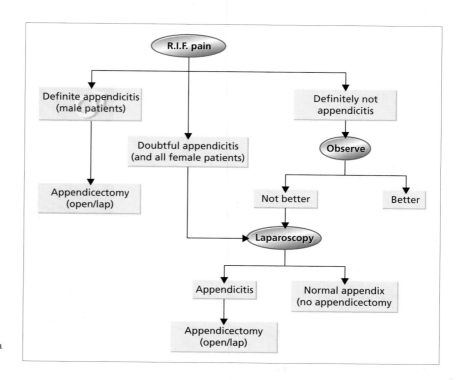

Fig. 8.6 Flow chart showing action-plan in a patient with suspected acute appendicitis.

there remains no strong evidence to support its widespread use in all patients with acute appendicitis. However, many of the studies which have tried to compare laparoscopic versus open appendicectomy in a controlled randomized fashion have included those with perforated appendices and have also gone on to remove a normal appendix if found, which may have masked any potential benefits of the laparoscopic procedure. Although, as yet there is no data to support this, we feel that it is the group of patients who have non-perforated appendicitis who might benefit most from laparoscopic appendicectomy, particularly if they are obese. Those patients with perforated appendicitis are often ill from the systemic disease and in our experience take longer to recover whichever technique is used.

A technique whereby diagnostic laparoscopy is performed, acute appendicitis confirmed and a small incision made directly over the appendix, which is then removed by conventional means, has been reported and certainly is attractive for its simplicity, especially if a surgeon with the skill for full laparoscopic appendicectomy is not available. Debate still rages as to what to do if a normal appendix is found and no other cause for the patient's symptoms revealed. We are quite clear on this matter and leave the appendix well alone. The argument that there may be some mucosal inflammation which the laparoscopist cannot see has not been a problem in our experience, and to proceed to an unnecessary appendicectomy, even using laparoscopic techniques, is removing much of the benefit of diagnostic laparoscopy. If there is doubt as to whether the appendix is inflamed, and sometimes the video camera needs to be removed so that the surgeon can inspect the appendix with his/her naked eye (in case the colour setting on the monitor alters the true picture) then the surgeon should proceed to appendicectomy. If the appendix is perforated we recommend conversion to open appendicectomy although laparoscopic appendicectomy is still feasible and safe in experienced hands.

Surgical technique

Under general anaesthesia the umbilical port (10 mm or 11 mm) is inserted using the open technique. Following pneumoperitoneum, the patient is placed in the Trendelenberg position to allow the small bowel to fall out of the pelvis. A further 10-mm port is introduced in the left iliac fossa and a 5 or 10-mm port on the right side (Fig. 8.7). The telescope may be introduced either through the umbilical port or the left iliac fossa port. Very often the caecum will have to be swept towards the midline to gain visibility of the appendix. The adhesions between the bowel and the parietal peritoneum of the anterior abdominal wall and also between the caecum, appendix and terminal ileum can often be separated easily by blunt dissection, sweeping with a blunt dissector or the suction cannula. The appendix is grasped with a toothed grasping forceps introduced through the right iliac

fossa port (Fig. 8.8). The authors then use a pair of dissecting scissors connected with diathermy introduced through the other lateral port and staying close to the wall of the appendix, dissect the appendix from the mesoappendix using diathermy to coagulate the small branches of the appendicular artery. Any bleeding branch not well controlled by diathermy may be secured using metal clips. In this way dissection is kept well away from the main appendicular artery and any undue haemorrhage avoided. Alternately the

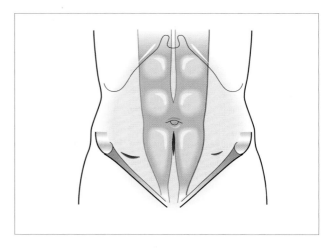

Fig. 8.7 Position of laparoscopic ports for appendicectomy. Alternately the right iliac fossa port may be replaced with a 5-mm port in the right hypochondrium to improve ease of manipulation.

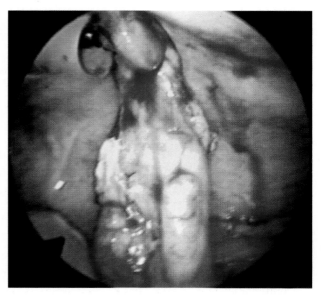

Fig. 8.8 Laparoscopic view of the inflamed appendix elevated using a grasping forceps introduced through a port in the right iliac fossa.

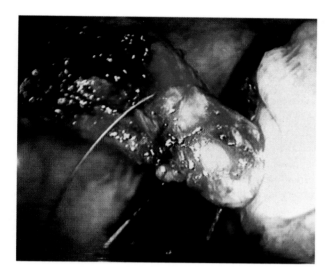

Fig. 8.9 The base of the appendix being secured using pre-tied catgut ligatures. The second ligature is about to be applied.

mesoappendix may be secured at its base using a stapling device. When using this the tips of the stapler should be clearly visible to avoid accidental application on adjacent viscera. The base of the appendix is then divided after securing with two pre-tied catgut ligatures using Roeder knots (Endoloop, Ethicon UK Ltd) (Fig. 8.9). If the base of the appendix is perforated a cuff of caecum may be stapled and excised with it. If the caecal attachment of the appendix is not clearly identified it is advisable to convert to open operation to avoid the possibility of a subtotal appendicectomy with a future risk of further appendicitis. The appendix is removed through one of the larger ports and the peritoneal cavity washed out with antibiotic solution. A drain may be left in through one of the port sites if indicated. If the appendix is too bulky to be removed intact through a large port, it can either be retrieved in a delivery bag or removed under vision through a right iliac fossa incision made directly over it (laparoscopic assisted appendicectomy). Alternately one of the port sites may be enlarged just sufficiently to remove the bag and contents from the abdominal cavity. Large series of laparoscopic appendicectomies reported in the literature suggest a conversion rate of less than 5%.

Laparoscopic closure of perforated peptic ulcer

There have recently been both experimental and clinical evidence suggesting that laparoscopic treatment of perforated duodenal ulcers is both possible and safe. Intracorporeal suturing, fibrin sealant or alternatively peroperative insertion of a Dormia basket endoscopically to pull a plug of omentum through the perforation have all been successfully used. Although not all perforated ulcers can be treated laparoscopically, in the frail and elderly patient, the sparing

of an upper abdominal incision should permit early mobilization with reduced postoperative complications.

Surgical technique

At laparoscopy, if there is evidence of spontaneous sealing of the perforation, all that may be required is a thorough peritonal toilet using normal saline with tetracycline (1 g/l). If the perforation is still leaking additional ports are inserted as shown in Fig. 8.10. The greater curve of the stomach is retracted downwards and towards the left using atraumatic bowel-grasping forceps. If the left lobe of the liver obscures the view then a retractor is inserted down the epigastric port (the sucker will do) to elevate the liver. Although surgeons have recently reported a number of ways to close the perforation including suturing, stapling, insertion of fibrin glue and using a gelatin plug, the authors recommend simple suture with omental patch as is normal practice at open surgery (Figs. 8.11 and 8.12). Two laparoscopically placed sutures are usually adequate and are tied with either intracorporeal or extracorporeal knots over an omental patch. This is facilitated by a suction cannula introduced through a 5-mm port and kept either in the perforation or in its close vicinity to suck away the constantly leaking duodenal contents. Thorough peritoneal lavage is then carried out. The decision to drain is left to the individual surgeon.

Laparoscopic cholecystectomy for acute cholecystitis

In many of the early series reporting experience with laparoscopic cholecystectomy, acute cholecystitis was considered a contra-indication to the procedure. However, as laparoscopic skills have developed more surgeons are now offering laparoscopic cholecystectomy for the majority of patients with acute cholecystitis. At laparoscopy there are two types

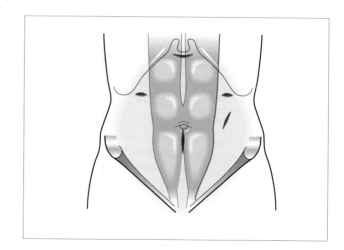

Fig. 8.10 Position of ports for laparoscopic closure of perforated duodenal ulcer.

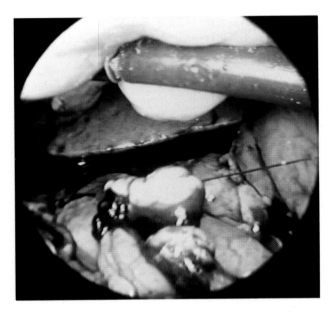

Fig. 8.11 Operative photograph of laparoscopic repair of a perforated duodenal ulcer. A piece of omental fat has been brought over the perforation and is being sutured using intracorporeal sutures.

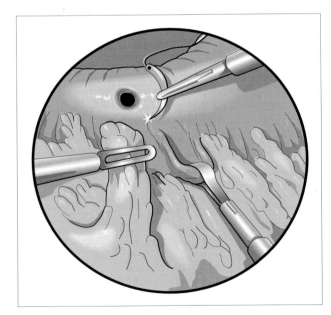

Fig. 8.12 Diagrammatic representation of omental patch repair of a perforated duodenal ulcer. The greater curve of stomach has been grasped and pulled down to reveal the perforation.

important to recognize these two different categories as the first is relatively straightforward to treat laparoscopically, whereas the second can present a formidable challenge to even the most experienced laparoscopist. The conversion rate in this latter group is correspondingly higher, and in our own experience reaches 25%, whereas the milder group can be treated laparoscopically in over 95% of cases.

If symptoms have been present for more than 5–7 days, and the patient improves quickly with non-operative treatment, delayed laparoscopic cholecystectomy should be performed after 6 weeks. If symptoms do not subside and surgery is required open operation will usually be required, although nothing is lost by initial laparoscopic assessment. Although laparoscopic cholecystostomy is easily performed, it is usually only indicated in the seriously ill, elderly patient, and can equally well be achieved under ultrasound guidance without recourse to any form of surgery.

Surgical technique

The approach to urgent laparoscopic cholecystectomy for acute cholecystitis is the same as for the elective operation with the exception that the gall bladder will often require decompression to facilitate grasping and further dissection (Fig. 8.13). This can be acheived by either direct puncture using one of the right upper quadrant trocar and ports, or by incising into the fundus with scissors. After the gall bladder has been decompressed the hole can be left or sutured depending on whether there are multiple stones which might spill out. Attempts to decompress the gall bladder with a percutaneous needle are rarely successful because of the viscosity of the contents.

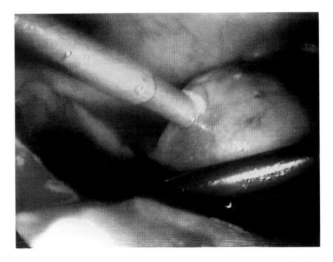

Fig. 8.13 Laparoscopic decompression of a tense and distended gall bladder prior to laparoscopic cholecystectomy. If cholecystectomy is not technically possible, a cholecystostomy may be performed laparoscopically.

of acute cholecystitis: the distended and slightly oedematous gall bladder of someone with a short history of acute, but relatively non-severe symptoms; and the patient who has a grossly inflamed and thickened gall bladder in association with systemic toxicity and severe clinical symptoms. It is

Once decompressed the gall bladder is grasped with toothed grasping forceps. If the wall is too thick to be grasped by the standard 5-mm grasping forceps, the 5-mm lateral right upper quadrant port should be replaced with a 10-mm port and the large toothed gall bladder retrieving forceps used to grasp the fundus of the gall bladder. Once Calot's triangle has been identified and the cystic duct dissected free an operative cholangiogram is performed if possible. In the acute situation this may be technically demanding, and if pre-operative liver function tests and ultrasonography have not suggested choledocholithiasis, the surgeon can abandon attempts at cystic duct cannulation if the likelihood of success is small, on the reasonable assumption that in the presence of acute obstruction of the cystic duct the chance of common bile duct stones being found is small. If laparoscopic ultrasonography is available then it can also be used to assess the biliary tree. If a cholangiogram demonstrates stones within the common bile duct the surgeon has three options, depending on the clinical situation and the surgical expertise available: firstly, to perform laparoscopic duct exploration; secondly, to convert the patient to open surgery and explore the common bile duct in the conventional fashion; or thirdly, to complete the operation and refer the patient for postoperative endoscopic removal. It is beyond the scope of this chapter to go into these options in more detail. Suffice to say that the decision should be made by the senior surgeon.

Laparoscopic division of band adhesions producing small bowel obstruction

Although intestinal obstruction is usually considered a contraindication to performing laparoscopy, those patients in whom the cause is thought to be due to a single band adhesion, such as might follow appendicectomy, can benefit from laparoscopic surgery (Fig. 8.14). It is essential that this is performed using the 'open' technique described earlier, and great care must be taken in grasping and manipulating the distended loops of bowel which are extremely easy to puncture. Once the band has been identified, and the surgeon must observe distal to the band to confirm that this is indeed the point of obstruction, it can be divided. Once divided, the remainder of the bowel rapidly fills up and further assessment becomes impossible.

Laparoscopic treatment of gynaecological emergencies

Gynaecological emergencies remain a common cause of admission to general surgical wards, and have been estimated to account for over 10% of acute surgical admissions. The rationale for using laparoscopy before laparotomy in the young female patient with lower abdominal pain has

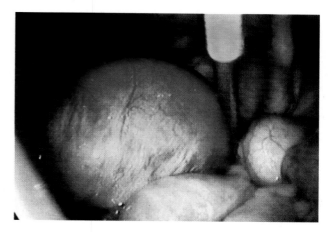

Fig. 8.14 Laparoscopic view in a patient with intestinal obstruction. Presence of some dilated and some collapsed loops of intestine is diagnostic.

already been discussed in detail. If acute gynaecological causes are detected the gynaecologist should be summoned to theatre to give an opinion. Many of the acute pelvic conditions can be treated without surgery, but it is always courteous to permit the gynaecologist to come and see for him/herself if they are going to be asked to treat the patient afterwards. Simple rupture of corpus luteal cysts do not require further treatment, but large ovarian cysts of dubious nature, tubal abnormalities and pelvic inflammatory disease often require a more specialist laparoscopic assessment than the general surgeon can provide. Video recording of the examination can always be carried out if the problem is uncomplicated and the gynaecologist is otherwise occupied.

Many gynaecologists are now performing laparoscopic excision of ovarian cysts and removal of ectopic pregnancies, and should therefore be given the option to do so when these conditions are inadvertently discovered by the general surgeon during diagnostic laparoscopy. In most instances pre-operative suspicion will allow laparoscopy to be undertaken in the presence of both surgeon and gynaecologist.

Therapeutic laparoscopy in trauma

Although some surgeons have reported repair of ruptured viscera using laparoscopic tchniques following both blunt and penetrating abdominal trauma, the role of therapeutic laparoscopy in this field is small. Laboratory studies using fibrin glue injection through the laparoscope shows promise in the management of solid organ injuries and may soon become clinical reality. However, at the present time the role of laparoscopy in trauma should be limited to diagnosis except in the very exceptional circumstance. The surgeon wishing to repair a perforated viscus laparoscopically must be certain that no other injury exists, and in the presence of an isolated injury, often with associated mesenteric haematomas and free blood, it is usually difficult to establish this fact with confidence.

Summary

Although laparoscopy and laparoscopic surgery have much to offer in the management of patients with acute abdominal pain, the emergency surgeon must ensure that adequate expertise and appropriate instrumentation are available. If realistic and safe decisions regarding the use of emergency laparoscopy are made, undoubted benefits will reach a much wider population.

Further reading

Alexander-Williams, J. (1994) Laparoscopy in abdominal trauma. *Injury* **25**(9) 585–586.

Fabian, T.C., Croce, M.A., Stewart, R.M. *et al.* (1993) A prospective analysis of diagnostic laparoscopy in trauma. *Annals of Surgery* **217**(5) 557–565.

Ivatury, R.R., Simon, R.J., Weksler, B. *et al.* (1992) Laparoscopy in the evaluation of the intrathoracic abdomen after penetrating injury. *The Journal of Trauma* **33**(1) 101–108.

Navez, B., d'Udekem, Y., Cambier, E. *et al.* (1995) Laparoscopy for management of Nontraumatic acute abdomen. *World Journal of Surgery* **19** 382–387.

Paterson-Brown, S. (1993) Emergency laparoscopic surgery. *British Journal of Surgery* **80** 279–283.

Tate, J.J.T., Chung, S.C.S., Dawson, J. *et al.* (1993) Conventional versus laparoscopic surgery for acute appendicitis. *British Journal of Surgery* **80** 761–764.

CHAPTER 9

Oesophageal emergencies

Thomas P. J. Hennessy

Introduction

Injuries to the oesophagus requiring emergency treatment can be categorized as follows.

1 Obstruction of the oesophageal lumen caused by a food bolus or a foreign body.

2 Perforation of the oesophageal wall caused by external injury, foreign body or some form of instrumentation.

3 Mucosal or transmucosal damage arising from ingestion of either liquid or solid state strong acid or alkali.

4 Bleeding from mucosal tears or oesophageal varices

Foreign body impaction

Impaction of a foreign body is the most frequently encountered oesophageal emergency. It is a common occurrence in children but is not infrequent in adults. It may cause no more than simple obstruction of the oesophagus or the foreign body may penetrate the oesophageal wall with consequent mediastinitis or the development of a tracheo-oesophageal or broncho-oesophageal fistula. Damage to the oesophagus may also occur during removal or attempted removal of a foreign body.

Spontaneous rupture

Spontaneous rupture of the oesophagus occurs mainly in adults although it has been known to occur in neonates, particularly premature infants. It is a life-threatening condition requiring prompt recognition and intervention.

Perforation

Traumatic perforation of the oesophagus is most commonly iatrogenically induced from instrumentation of the oesophagus. Less frequently, perforation may be caused by external penetrating trauma such as gunshot wound or stab wounds usually involving the cervical oesophagus (Sheely *et al.*, 1975).

Perforation of the oesophagus caused by the ingestion of strong acid or alkali solutions is relatively rare nowadays. It occurs mainly in children but may occur at any age. Caustic

liquid solutions pass rapidly through the pharynx and oesophagus and inflict most damage on the distal oesophagus and stomach. Solid state caustics cause extensive damage to the oral cavity, pharynx and upper oesophagus. Alkaline substances induce liquefaction necrosis with deep tissue penetration and later stricture formation. Acid ingestion produces a coagulation necrosis. Perforation may occur in the acute necrotic phase. Severe damage follows acid ingestion in more than 80% of cases with 38% developing stricture (Zargar *et al.*, 1989).

Perforation of the oesophagus may also occur as a result of underlying disease such as Barrett's ulcer or stress ulceration associated with extensive burns.

Mucosal tears

While spontaneous rupture is often the outcome of retching and vomiting, more often the damage from such straining is restricted to the oesophageal mucosa which sustains linear tears giving rise to haematemesis. About 10% of upper gastrointestinal bleeding is considered to be caused by mucosal tearing (Mallory–Weiss syndrome) (Bubrick *et al.*, 1980).

Operative injury

Damage to the oesophagus may occur, although rarely, during adjacent operative procedures such as vagotomy, fundoplication, etc., and unless recognized promptly may prove catastrophic.

Bleeding

Oesophageal varices which develop as a result of portal hypertension may bleed spontaneously or as a result of minor trauma during eating or from erosion of the overlying mucosa from acid reflux. Life-threatening haemorrhage may occur.

Foreign body in the oesophagus

This is usually an unmasticated bolus of meat or gristle. Sometimes the offending mass is a meat or fish bone. In

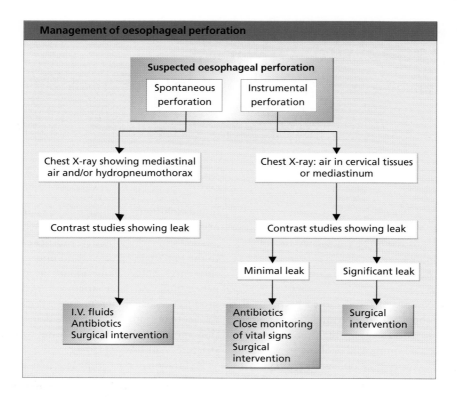

children, coins are commonly swallowed. Dental bridges and dentures are sometimes swallowed accidentally.

The patient is often very apprehensive. He or she gives a clear history of something getting stuck in the gullet. Pain and discomfort are often experienced and excessive salivation may occur.

Ideally, foreign bodies should be removed using large grasping forceps via the rigid oesophagoscope under general anaesthesia (Fig. 9.1). The flexible endoscope is not an ideal instrument because no forceps of adequate size can be used and the operator sometimes relies on pushing the bolus into the stomach. If the impacted object, e.g. bone, etc., has sharp edges this may result in the wall of the oesophagus being perforated. Patients who have had a foreign body removed should have nil orally for 6 h and only liquids for a further 12 h.

Technique

Passage of the rigid oesophagoscope is carried out under direct vision from beginning to end. The patient's neck should remain flexed while the rigid instrument is passed through the oropharynx and the upper oesophageal sphincter. When the instrument passes beyond the cricopharyngeal sphincter the neck is extended and the instrument is passed down the oesophagus under direct vision. When the impacted foreign body is located a large grasping forceps is passed down the lumen and the foreign body is firmly grasped. Oesophagoscope and forceps holding the foreign body are then withdrawn simultaneously.

Spontaneous rupture of the oesophagus

Spontaneous rupture of the oesophagus (Boerhaave's syndrome) is a relatively rare condition. It occurs after forceful vomiting and retching which abruptly raises the intra-abdominal and intra-oesophageal pressures. Although the classic case of Baron von Wassenaar, described by Boerhaave, involved excessive eating and drinking, such overindulgence is not a necessary prerequisite and the condition has been known to accompany convulsions, defecation and childbirth (Beal, 1949; Kennard, 1950; Conte, 1966). It is twice as common in males as it is in females and is most frequently observed in patients of middle age.

Many patients have a recent history of indigestion associated with duodenal ulcer or reflux oesophagitis.

In the classic presentation the retching and vomiting precedes the severe epigastric pain which may radiate to the left chest and shoulder. There is tenderness and guarding in the epigastrium and bowel sounds may be absent. It is accompanied by tachycardia, hypotension and dyspnoea. In the 60% of patients in whom this classic pattern is not observed the situation may be further confused by the central location of the chest pain, suggesting myocardial infarction or the location of the pain in the epigastrium accompanied by pleuritic pain and later pleural effusion suggesting

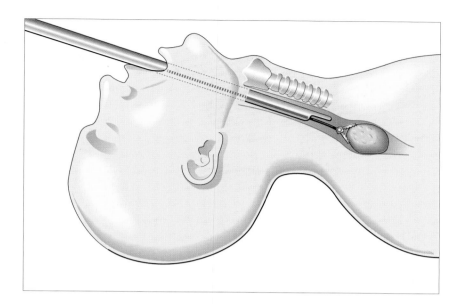

Fig. 9.1 Bolus extraction with rigid oesophagoscope.

pancreatitis. An initial wrong diagnosis may seriously worsen the prognosis.

Subcutaneous emphysema is a late manifestation and while it confirms the presence of a perforation, diagnosis should preferably precede its onset.

Because of an intrinsic weakness of the muscular wall of the left lower oesophagus most spontaneous perforations occur on the left side of the lower oesophagus above the diaphragm thus giving rise to a left-sided pleural effusion or hydropneumothorax. This is accompanied by dullness on percussion and the absence of breath sounds. Differential diagnosis includes myocardial infarction, acute pancreatitis, pneumonia, perforated peptic ulcer, strangulated intrathoracic hernia and dissecting abdominal aneurysm.

Plain films of the chest may show air in the mediastinum but contrast studies of the oesophagus are more reliable. A water soluble medium, such as Gastrografin, should be used rather than barium. Contrast studies are more effective in establishing the diagnosis than endoscopy.

Management of spontaneous perforation

Early perforation

A decision to intervene surgically should be taken as soon as the diagnosis is made. Broad-spectrum antibiotic therapy should be started immediately, oral intake should be suspended and intravenous nutrition commenced.

Unless there are indications that the perforation is at an unusual site (e.g. midoesophageal right-sided perforation) the surgical approach is through a left thoracotomy, excising the eighth rib. The associated pleural effusion is evacuated. The mediastinal pleura may already be ruptured over the oesophageal tear in which case the pleural cavity will be con-

taminated with gastric contents. Either way, the mediastinal pleura is opened widely to provide adequate mediastinal drainage.

After mobilizing the involved segment of the oesophagus and identifying the extent of the tear the latter is closed in layers (mucosal and muscular) using unabsorbable interrupted sutures. While simple suture in early perforation can be expected to be successful the addition of a pleural–intercostal flap or a diaphragmatic flap confers added security.

Pleural–intercostal flap

The pleural–intercostal flap is based medially and is sutured over the repaired defect with a 1-cm margin to spare on all sides (Middleton & Foster 1972). The extent of the tear may, therefore, limit the use of this flap (Fig. 9.2).

Diaphragmatic flap

Alternatively, a diaphragmatic flap may be used (Rao *et al.* 1974). This involves raising a full thickness flap of diaphragm centrally based and measuring 12 × 6 cm. The diaphragmatic defect thus created is closed by interrupted non-absorbable sutures and the raised flap is sutured to the oesophageal wall with interrupted sutures over the closed tear (Fig. 9.3a, b).

At the conclusion of the procedure pleural lavage is performed and the thoracotomy incision closed in layers. The chest cavity is drained via a large-bore intercostal tube attached to an underwater seal drain.

In the postoperative period parenteral feeding is maintained until oesophageal integrity can be confirmed by Gastrografin swallow. Meanwhile an empty stomach is maintained by nasogastric suction.

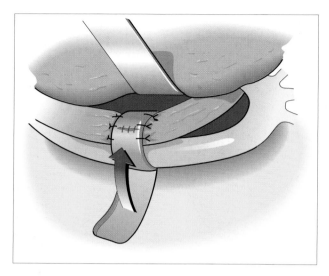

Fig. 9.2 Pleural–intercostal flap sutured over oesophageal tear.

Late perforation

Reference has already been made to some of the difficulties in diagnosis and not infrequently 24 hours or more may have elapsed before the nature of the condition becomes apparent. As already mentioned, the pathognomonic sign of surgical (subcutaneous) emphysema is a late presentation.

In these circumstances the extensive oedema in the oesophageal wall makes direct suture impossible and closure of the defect is achieved by use of the diaphragmatic flap already described applied and sutured over the unclosed tear (Fig. 9.4). Drainage of the mediastinum and long-term drainage (several days) of the pleural cavity are essential.

With late perforations suspension of oral intake and parenteral feeding may have to be maintained for 3 or 4 weeks. If healing of the perforation has not been confirmed

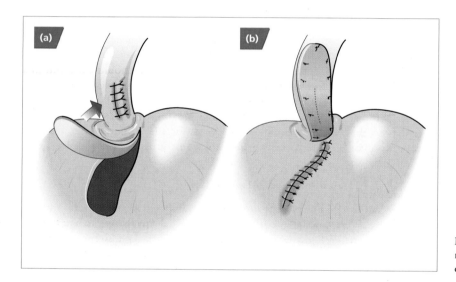

Fig. 9.3 (a) Suture of oesophageal tear and raising of diaphragmatic flap. (b) Buttressing of a sutured tear with diaphragmatic flap.

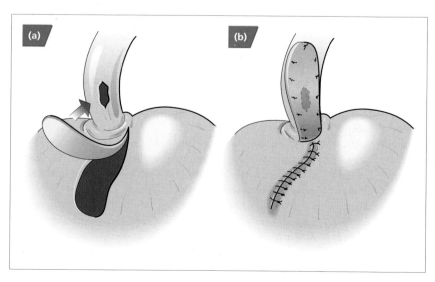

Fig. 9.4 Closure of late perforation with diaphragmatic flap.

by then consideration should be given to the establishment of a feeding jejunostomy.

Conservative measures with antibiotic cover, nasogastric suction, intravenous nutrition and drainage of the chest cavity have sometimes been successful in dealing with late perforations, but unless the patient's general condition makes operative intervention too hazardous it is preferable to try to close the perforation.

Indirect approaches such as oesophageal diversion have also been used and will be described later under the heading of late traumatic perforations.

Traumatic perforations

Instrumental

Instrumental perforation of the oesophagus is the most common form of oesophageal perforation. Perforation from flexible endoscopy is extremely rare but can occur with oesophageal stricture or in the presence of an unrecognized pharyngeal or other diverticulum (Flynn *et al.*, 1989). Perforation is more common with the nowadays rare use of the rigid oesophagoscope or in association with bougie dilatation of benign or malignant strictures. Pneumatic dilatation for achalasia may also cause perforation, and penetration of the oesophageal wall may occur during laser treatment.

Penetrating injuries

These occur most commonly in the cervical oesophagus. Gunshot injuries are usually associated with other injuries such as damage to the trachea or larynx, spinal cord or carotid artery. Stab wounds to the neck may also cause isolated oesophageal injury or include damage to other regional structures.

Blunt injury

As a source of external traumatic injury, blunt injury is very rare but has been recorded in association with high speed road traffic accidents.

Diagnosis of traumatic perforation

Instrumental perforation may be recognized or suspected at the time of occurrence as may perforation from external penetrating trauma. Perforation from blunt trauma is more likely to lead to delay in diagnosis.

The signs and symptoms of oesophageal perforation have already been described and consist of tachycardia, fever, fall in blood pressure, dyspnoea and thirst, followed by the appearance of a pleural effusion and the radiological signs of hydropneumothorax.

Systemic signs and symptoms are less severe with cervical perforation but surgical emphysema may appear early rather than late and there may be a mucous discharge from the wound after external penetrating injury.

Management of traumatic perforations

Cervical perforations

Conservative management

A conservative approach is permissable when there is no underlying oesophageal pathology, and the leakage is minimal and confined to the neck. Evidence of sepsis should be minimal with absence of tachycardia and fever. Surgical emphysema should not be evident in the mediastinum on chest radiograph. The leakage track in contrast studies should be confined within the cervical structures and should not extend into the mediastinum.

The patient should be monitored carefully for evidence of sepsis. Persistent pain and tenderness in the neck with pyrexia and tachycardia are indications for surgical intervention. Broad-spectrum antibiotics should be given and intravenous nutrition commenced. More than half the patients will require drainage of a cervical abscess ultimately.

If a fistula develops at that time it should close within a few days. Evidence of extension into the mediastinum, namely, mediastinal emphysema on chest X-ray, tracking of contrast medium into the mediastinum is an indication for prompt surgical intervention with closure of the tear and drainage of the mediastinum and cervical area.

Surgical treatment

The approach to an injury of the cervical oesophagus is along the anterior border of the left sternomastoid muscle. After division of the cervical fascia the omohyoid is identified and divided and also the middle thyroid vein. The carotid sheath and its contents are retracted laterally and the thyroid gland medially. After identification of the recurrent laryngeal nerve the oesophagus is mobilized and the perforation is identified. Repair is carried out in two layers with interrupted unabsorbable sutures. Suction drainage is applied and the incision closed in layers.

Thoracic perforations

Conservative management

There is a place for conservative management of instrumental perforation of the intrathoracic oesophagus. Such a management approach is indicated where a minor injury results from maladroit use of a guide wire or small calibre bougie. It may also be employed when splitting of the oesophageal wall occurs in the process of dilating an oesophageal carcinoma. Because the patient is fasting and the oesophagus and stomach are empty and the perforation is small, contamination is relatively slight and very often the perforation is contained within the mediastinum without breach of the visceral pleura. The situation is quite unlike the gross contamination that occurs with spontaneous rupture when the contents of a full stomach are expelled forcefully through the perforation. Symptoms are relatively mild and the patient's condition is stable.

Once the diagnosis has been established by administration of water-soluble contrast medium antibiotics are given and multiple suction drainage is established. This consists of drainage of the oesophagus via a naso-oesophageal tube; drainage of the stomach via a gastrostomy tube and drainage of the extra oesophageal cavity via an oesophageal tube passed from the oesophageal lumen through the perforation into the peri-oesophageal cavity. Drainage of the pleural space is included if there is a pleural effusion. Good results have been reported for this technique (Erwall *et al.*, 1984). Conservative treatment should be abandoned in favour of surgery if the patient's clinical condition deteriorates.

Surgical management of early perforation

The surgical approach is dictated by the position of the perforation and whether it is located on the right or left side of the oesophagus. The seventh or eighth intercostal space is appropriate for left thoracotomy when a left-sided perforation is located below the arch of the aorta. Right thoracotomy should be through the sixth intercostal space and will allow access to any part of the intrathoracic oesophagus. An adjacent rib may be removed if additional space is required for access.

After dividing the visceral pleura, and mobilizing the relevant segment of the oesophagus the perforation is identified and repaired in layers using interrupted unabsorbable sutures and the chest closed with underwater seal drainage. When carried out within 24 hours of the injury the results of primary repair are excellent (Bladergroen *et al.*, 1986). Buttressing with a pleural–intercostal or diaphragmatic flap may be added for extra security. In the author's view the diaphragmatic flap is superior to the pleural–intercostal flap.

Surgical management of late perforation

Late perforations can be managed using one of the techniques already described for late spontaneous rupture; namely closure of the perforation with a pedicled flap of diaphragm and drainage of the pleural cavity. This, of course, is only feasible if the perforation is in the lower region of the oesophagus. An alternative in that situation, or in perforation of the abdominal oesophagus, is the use of a fundal patch reinforced by fundoplication, i.e. the gastric fundus is sutured around the margins of the perforation and kept in place by using the remainder of the gastric fundus as a fundoplication.

Oesophageal diversion and exclusion loop

Oesophagotomy of the cervical oesophagus, where the opened cervical oesophagus is sutured to the skin, does not achieve complete diversion of oesophageal content. An alternative technique in which a 1.5-cm wide Dacron tape is passed round the distal cervical oesophagus and sutured around it in such a fashion as to occlude the oesophageal lumen has been described (Ergin *et al.*, 1980). Above or proximal to the occluded oesophagus a stab wound is made in the oesophagus through which a DePezzer or Malecot catheter is inserted (Fig. 9.5). The catheter is brought out through a separate stab wound in the cervical skin. The long ends of the occluding Dacron tape are brought out through the lower end of the sutured cervical incision. Two/o catgut is used to anchor the catheter in the oesophagus. The catheter can be removed at a later stage when a track to the exterior is established. The occluding tape can be removed after dividing its occluding sutures through a small incision at the lower end of the cervical skin incision.

In addition to the cervical oesophageal diversion, lower oesophageal exclusion can be carried out via a thoracotomy with closure of the lower oesophagus by a Teflon band. Alternatively the abdominal oesophagus may be banded and gastrostomy carried out. In either case underwater seal drainage of the pleural cavity is required. In due course the

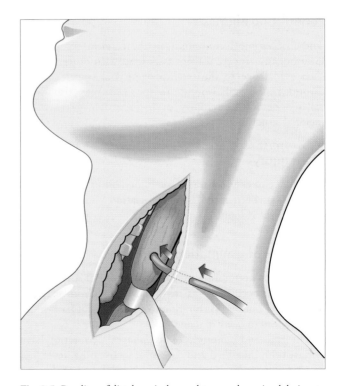

Fig. 9.5 Banding of distal cervical oesophagus and proximal drainage with DePezzer catheter.

proximal band is removed along with the catheter and subsequently the distal oesophageal band is removed. This technique involves complicated procedures and is only recommended if alternatives are not available or possible.

Excision of the oesophagus

If repair or spontaneous healing of the oesophagus after diversion and exclusion are regarded as unlikely, excision of the oesophagus may be considered if the patient is fit enough to withstand the procedure. Transhiatal excision is the technique usually chosen. Excision of the oesophagus may be accompanied by immediate cervical anastomosis or if the situation is more critical a cervical oesophagotomy may be established with closure of the cardia and gastrostomy (for subsequent enteral nutrition) and anastomosis deferred until sepsis has subsided and adequate nutrition has been established via the gastrostomy.

Intubation

One of the simplest ways of dealing with a difficult oesophageal perforation is to occlude the leak site by passing either an Atkinson or a Celestin tube.

An alternative method of intubation is the use of an intraluminal T-tube around which the oesophageal tear is loosely sutured. A mediastinal drain is also placed (Fig. 9.6) in addition to conventional underwater seal drainage of the pleural space. Feeding is established through a gastrostomy. The T-tube is removed when an exteriorized track is established and the pleural and mediastinal drainage is discontinued when water soluble contrast material demonstrates that there is no longer an oesophageal leak (Cuschieri & Hennessy, 1992).

Perforation associated with oesophageal disease or irreparable injury

Injury

External penetrating injuries such as gunshot wounds may damage the oesophagus to such an extent that the only viable option is resection. Associated injuries to other vital organs in the region may make it inappropriate to carry out immediate reconstruction. In these circumstances the cardia should be closed following resection and the proximal oesophagus brought to the surface as a cervical oesophagostomy. Reconstruction may be undertaken at a later date.

Underlying disease

When perforation occurs during pneumatic dilatation for achalasia a myotomy should be carried out at a different site on the oesophageal circumference from the tear. The latter

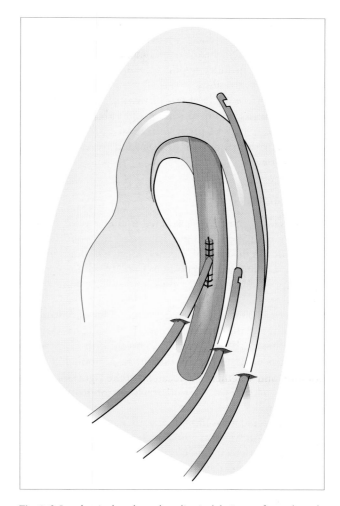

Fig. 9.6 Intraluminal t-tube and mediastinal drainage of oesophageal perforation.

should be sutured in layers. A fundal wrap or a diaphragmatic flap may be added as a buttress.

Perforation of a Barrett's ulcer may occur into the aorta with rapid exsanguination and death (Gillen & Hennessy, 1989). Perforation into the mediastinum warrants resection of the thoracic oesophagus. If there has been a delay and severe mediastinitis is present the mediastinum and thoracic cavity are drained, the cardia closed and a cervical oesophagotomy established. Reconstruction and an anastomosis via the posterior mediastinum or the retrosternal route is carried out at a later date.

Oesophageal bleeding

Mallory–Weiss syndrome

This is a common condition encountered in from 5–10% of patients undergoing endoscopy for haematemesis (Bubrick *et al.*, 1980). The clinical presentation is one of painless haematemesis associated with retching and vomiting often but not invariably induced by over-indulgence in alcohol. There is a high incidence of associated upper gastrointestinal disease which includes peptic ulceration, gastritis, hiatus hernia and oesophagitis.

The lesion is a mucosal tear of varying length from 1 to 4 cm on the gastric side of the oesophagogastric junction. Multiple tears may be present. In most cases the bleeding stops spontaneously but can be sufficiently severe to warrant intervention.

Management

The diagnosis should be suspected if after a prior bout of vomiting the patient becomes nauseated and vomits bright red blood. A history of alcohol ingestion need not be present. Differential diagnosis is from bleeding oesophageal varices. About 30% of patients will require blood transfusion.

After resuscitation upper gastrointestinal endoscopy is carried out and the lesion identified. If bleeding has stopped the patient may be treated conservatively with H_2 receptor antagonists or proton pump inhibitors. A number of alternatives including photocoagulation with the laser, electrocoagulation or the use of the heater probe may be used endoscopically.

If endoscopic measures fail or if there is recurrent bleeding surgical intervention is undertaken. At laparotomy a gastrotomy is carried out and bleeding controlled by a running catgut suture along the extent of the tear. The gastrotomy is closed in layers.

Corrosive injury to the oesophagus

A multiplicity of caustic agents which are readily available for domestic or commercial use have caused serious damage to the oesophagus when ingested accidentally or with suicidal intent. The agents most frequently encountered are strong alkalis such as sodium or potassium hydroxide and concentrated acids, e.g. sulphuric acid, hydrochloric acid and phosphoric acid. Other agents include ammonia, potassium permanganate, sodium hypochlorite and potassium dichlorate.

Extent of damage

Strong alkalis such as lye tend to adhere to mucosal surfaces so that most damage is caused in the pharynx and proximal oesophagus. Concentrated acids cause burns to the oesophagus and stomach. Bleaches and detergents containing sodium hydrochlorite cause less damage usually producing mucosal oedema only. If the amount and concentration of the caustic substance is sufficiently severe full thickness necrosis of the oesophageal or gastric wall may occur with perforation and mediastinitis or peritonitis. Destruction of the mucosa and damage to the muscular layer will give rise to stricture formation later on.

Symptoms

Initially there is likely to be a burning sensation in the lips and tongue and face. Chest pain and epigastric pain are common. If the damage is severe, fever and tachycardia are present and shock may supervene. Haematemesis is of grave import. If perforation occurs there is evidence of mediastinitis or peritonitis.

Treatment

General measures

Other than cleansing the oral cavity of any residual substance in children, there is no effective immediate treatment. Emetics should not be given. Patients with supraglottic oedema may require tracheostomy. Pulmonary oedema is a rare complication but may follow aspiration of the ingested agent.

The administration of steroids formerly recommended is not now regarded as beneficial. Early endoscopy is advocated to assess the degree of damage. The use of the paediatric endoscope is obviously mandatory in children but is also the instrument of choice in adults.

If there is severe necrosis present it is advisable not to pass the endoscope beyond the site of injury, but where damage is less it is permissable to carry out a full endoscopic examination of the oesophagus and stomach.

Intravenous fluids are necessary in the early period of treatment but the majority of patients are able to resume oral fluids after a few days. Stenting of the oesophagus to maintain a lumen has been advocated but its value is debatable. Dilatation of strictures should commence from between 10 days and 3 weeks depending on the severity of the stricture.

Specific treatment

The severity of the damage can be usefully graded into three categories for the purpose of management and treatment (Bremner & Wright, 1992).

In Grade I burns the injury is limited to the superficial layers of the mucosa giving rise to hyperaemia, oedema and superficial erosions. Sedation, analgesia and antacids are administered. A short course of antibiotics and an antifungal agent such as nystatin should be used. Stricture is extremely unlikely but check endoscopy should be carried out some weeks after discharge.

In Grade II burns there is also mucosal oedema and reactive hyperaemia. Deeper ulceration occurs but is limited to the mucosa and submucosa. Pain may be more difficult to control. Antibiotics and antifungal agents should be given for the first 10 days. Intravenous fluids should be maintained until the mucosal oedema subsides and the patient can swallow saliva. Cautious oral feeding can then be commenced. If a stricture develops dilatation should be commenced early at 3 or 4 weeks.

Grade III patients may be shocked on admission. Immediate measures include intravenous fluids, analgesia, antibiotics followed by careful clinical and radiological evaluation.

Clinical evidence of peritonitis is an indication for laparotomy. Total gastrectomy is required if the stomach is necrotic. If the abdominal oesophagus is also necrotic oesophagogastrectomy is indicated. Cervical oesophagostomy and feeding jejunostomy are established. Reconstruction with colon is carried out at a later date.

Chest pain, fever, tachycardia and inability to swallow saliva may accompany necrosis and perforation of the oesophagus. Radiological evidence includes widening of the mediastinum, air in the mediastinum, a soft tissue mass or pneumothorax. Emergency oesophagectomy with cervical oesophagostomy is indicated, but carries a high mortality.

Early endoscopy should be carried out in most cases. However, if damage is severe the endoscope should not be passed beyond the injured area. If oesophageal or gastric necrosis does not occur full endoscopy may be carried out some weeks later. Dense strictures develop as a result of Grade III injury and dilatation should be commenced at about three weeks.

Acute variceal haemorrhage

Acute bleeding from oesophageal varices may be of alarming proportions and there should be a clearly defined protocol for its management.
• After initial rapid assessment of the patient's condition, infusion of vasopressin should be begun. It is our practice to give 20 units as a bolus over 20 min followed by 0.4 units/min for 12 h.
• Blood losses should be replaced as early as possible.
• A nasogastric tube should be passed and gastric lavage carried out in preparation for endoscopy.
Even if oesophageal varices are identified a full upper gastrointestinal examination should be carried out. Rarely the bleeding may be coming from gastric erosions or a gastric or duodenal ulcer. If the bleeding is from gastric varices the location may be difficult to identify even with a J-manoeuvre.

If bleeding has stopped by the time of endoscopy no more needs to be done until arrangements can be made for injection sclerotherapy or variceal banding.

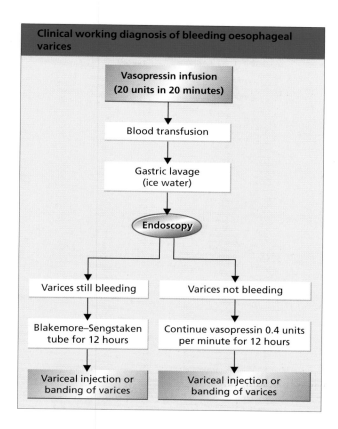

Blakemore–Sengstaken tube

If bleeding persists and visibility at endoscopy is limited a Blakemore–Sengstaken tube should be placed as illustrated (Fig. 9.7) and maintained in place for 12 h. Most models now have four channels so that the oesophagus above the longitudinal oesophageal balloon can be aspirated. If this is not the case a separate catheter for aspiration is placed in the proximal oesophagus.

Injection sclerotherapy

Once the bleeding has been controlled by infusion of intravenous vasopressin or a combination of vasopressin and balloon compression injection sclerotherapy should be undertaken. This is effective in the short term, and also in the long term in controlling and preventing bleeding. A more detailed description of endoscopic techniques for oesophageal varices is contained in Chapter 17.

Gastric varices

Gastric varices may continue to bleed despite conservative measures and are generally not amenable to injection. In these circumstances laparotomy may be required when the varices are obliterated with a running catgut suture after gastrotomy.

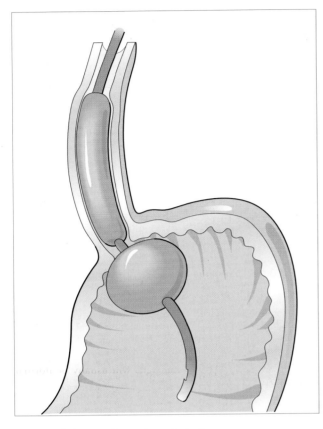

Fig. 9.7 Blackemore–Sengstaken tube *in situ.*

Surgical intervention

Although bleeding can be controlled by sclerotherapy in more than 90% of cases (Spence *et al.*, 1985) occasionally life-threatening haemorrhage may persist despite all conservative measures. Despite the grim mortality associated with emergency surgery for variceal haemorrhage no other option may be available.

Oesophageal transection using the circular stapler is probably the best option although Johnson recorded a 30% mortality for the procedure (Johnson, 1981).

Emergency portacaval shunting may carry an even higher mortality and should only be resorted to if everything else fails (Orloff *et al.*, 1977).

References

Beal, J.M. (1949) Spontaneous rupture of the esophagus. *Annals of Surgery* **129** 512–516.

Bladergroen, M.R., Lowe, J.E. & Postlethwaite, R.W. (1986) Diagnosis and recommended management of oesophageal perforation and rupture. *Annals of Thoracic Surgery* **42** 235–239.

Bremner, C.G. & Wright, N.C. (1992) Corrosive and non-reflux oesophagitis. In: *Surgery of the Oesophagus*, 2nd edn, (eds T.P.J. Hennessy & A. Cuschieri), p. 230. Butterworth Heinemann Ltd., Oxford.

Bubrick, M.P., Lindeen, J.W., Onstad, G.R. *et al.* (1980) Mallory–Weiss syndrome: analysis of 59 cases. *Surgery* **88** 400–405.

Conte, B.A. (1966) Oesophageal rupture in the absence of vomiting. *Journal of Thoracic and Cardiovascular Surgery* **51** 137–142.

Cuschieri, A. & Hennessy, T.P.J. (1992) Oesophageal perforations. In: *Surgery of the Oesophagus*, 2nd edn (eds T.P.J. Hennessy & A. Cuschieri), Chapter 4, pp. 104–105. Butterworth Heinemann Ltd., Oxford.

Ergin, M.A., Wetstein, L. & Giepp, R.B. (1980) Temporary diverting cervical esophagostomy. *Surgery Gynecology and Obstetrics* **151** 97–99.

Erwall, C., Ejerbald, S., Lindholm, C.E. *et al.* (1984) Perforation of the oesophagus. A comparison between surgical and medical treatment. *Acta Otolarnygologica* (*Stockholm*) **97** 185–192.

Flynn, A.E., Verrier, E.D., Lawrence L.W. *et al.* (1989) Oesophageal perforation. *Archives of Surgery* **124** 1211–1215.

Gillen, P. & Hennessy, T.P.J. (1989) Barrett's oesophagus. In: *Reflux Oesophagitis* (eds T.P.J. Hennessy, A. Cuschieri & J.R. Bennett), Chapter 4, p. 106. Butterworth & Co., London.

Johnson, G.W. (1981) Bleeding oesophageal varices: the management of shunt rejects. *Annals of the Royal College of Surgeons of England* **63** 3–8.

Kennard, H.W.H. (1950) Ruptures of the esophagus during childbirth. *British Medical Journal* **1** 417.

Middleton, C.J. & Foster, J.H. (1972) Visceral pleural patch for oesophageal anastomosis. *Archives of Surgery* **104** 87.

Orloff, M.J., Duguay, L.R. & Kosta, L.D. (1977) Criteria for selection of patients for emergency portacaval shunt. *American Journal of Surgery* **134** 146–152.

Rao, K.V., Mir, M. & Coghill, C.L. (1974) Management of perforation of the thoracic esophagus. A new technique utilizing a pedicle flap of diaphragm. *American Journal of Surgery* **127** 609–612.

Sheely, C.J., Mattox, K.I., Beall, A.C. Jr *et al.* (1975) Penetrating wounds of the cervical esophagus. *American Journal of Surgery* **130** 707–711.

Spence, R.A.J., Anderson, J.R. & Johnston, G.W. (1985) Twenty-five years of injection sclerotherapy for bleeding varices. *British Journal of Surgery* **72** 195–198.

Zargar, S.A., Kochkar R., Naqi, B. *et al.* (1989) Ingestion of corrosive acids. Spectrum of injury to upper gastrointestinal tract and natural history. *Gastroenterology* **97** 720–727.

CHAPTER 10

Acute peptic ulcer disease

Iain M. C. Macintyre

The incidence of peptic ulcer disease throughout the world continues to decline. It has been described as 'a disease of the 20th century', the suggestion being that it may have all but disappeared by the millennium. Elective operations for peptic ulcer disease have indeed virtually disappeared in the developed world. Despite this the incidence of peptic ulcer perforation has remained remarkably constant. It remains a common surgical emergency and all the more important because of the changing demography of the disease. Whilst in the first half of this century it was predominantly a disease of young men it has become, in the latter half of the century, predominantly a disease of older females. The incidence of perforated peptic ulcer in females over the age of 65 continues to increase (Fig. 10.1). Perforated peptic ulcer now occurs predominantly in a more vulnerable population and this carries a higher morbidity and mortality. Indeed the mortality rate which was 10% in the 1930s and 1940s, remains 10% or higher as the century draws to a close, despite the advances which have resulted in safer anesthesia and surgery and more effective intensive care. The disappearance of elective duodenal ulcer surgery has meant that the surgeons currently dealing with these older high risk patients have had little or no experience of elective peptic ulcer procedures.

Bleeding from duodenal ulcer has also declined. The surgeons' exposure to such patients has been further reduced by advances in therapeutic endoscopy. Thus the modern emergency surgeon is increasingly dealing with patients with massive or recurrent haemorrhage—less severe bleeds having been selected and treated by therapeutic endoscopy which has almost inevitably delayed the surgical treatment. The challenge for the surgeon dealing with a bleeding or perforated peptic ulcer far from diminishing continues to increase.

The differential diagnosis of acute upper abdominal pain

Acute upper abdominal pain remains one of the most common diagnostic problems amongst emergency surgical admissions. Improvements in imaging techniques which have facilitated the diagnosis of many surgical conditions

have with the exception of ultrasound had little impact on improving the diagnosis of acute upper abdominal pain. The diagnosis, which must be made with some degree of urgency, remains essentially a clinical one.

Acute gastritis

Acute gastritis can present with severe epigastric pain often accompanied by nausea and anorexia. The patient may have a history of previous attacks or recent ingestion of an agent known to cause mucosal injury. It is unusual for the patient to be systemically upset. Vital signs will usually be normal (Fig. 10.2).

Acute duodenitis

Acute duodenitis is generally regarded as a less aggressive form of acute duodenal ulcer disease and may often be a precursor to ulceration. The pain tends to be localized, epigastric with possible radiation. There are no systemic features. Abdominal examination shows tenderness localized to the epigastrium. It can usually only be distinguished from acute duodenal ulceration by upper gastrointestinal endoscopy (Fig. 10.3).

Acute duodenal ulcer

The pain of acute duodenal ulceration or an acute exacerbation of a chronic duodenal ulcer is characteristically highly localized in the epigastrium. With a posterior ulcer the pain may radiate through to the back. Relief by food and antacid is characteristic as is the cyclical nature of the pain which frequently wakes the patient at 2.00 or 3.00 a.m. Epigastric tenderness may be accompanied by guarding. The remainder of the abdomen is not tender, bowel sounds are present normally and pyrexia is uncommon.

Biliary colic

Biliary colic is severe upper abdominal pain which may be felt either in the right upper quadrant or in the epigastrium. Radiation to the back is common and radiation to the tip of

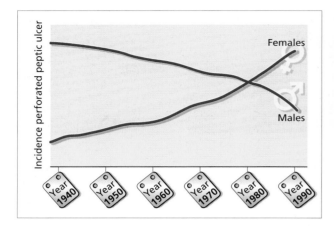

Fig. 10.1 Changing demography of perforated peptic ulcer over 50 years.

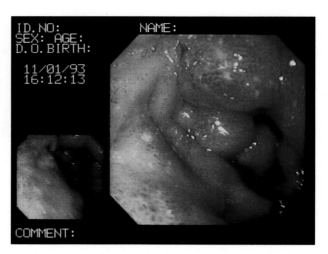

Fig. 10.3 Endoscopic appearance of duodenitis.

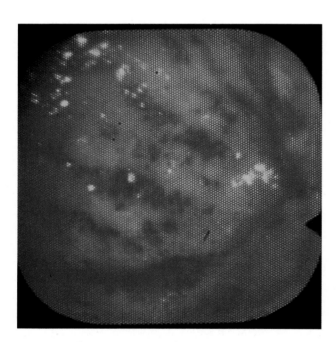

Fig. 10.2 Endoscopic appearance of gastritis. From *Atlas of Diseases of the Upper GI Tract.* © SmithKline Beecham, Welwyn Garden City.

the right shoulder well recognized. Colic is a misnomer, as in 80% of instances the pain is steady rather than colicky. There is no relief from antacids and the pain may last unabated for several hours. Whilst tenderness in the upper abdomen is not uncommon it is not accompanied by guarding. Where the stone impacts in the cystic duct as opposed to the common bile duct, derangement of liver function tests may be minimal or absent. There may or may not be accompanying pyrexia.

Acute cholecystitis

Acute cholecystitis presents with pain in the right upper quadrant perhaps radiating to the right shoulder tip and accompanied by a febrile illness. There is tenderness which may be accompanied by guarding in the right upper quadrant and Murphy's sign may be present. Murphy's sign is elicited by pressing the fingers gently but firmly into the right upper quadrant and asking the patient to take a slow deep breath. As the diaphragm contracts so the liver and gall bladder descend and the inflamed gall bladder descending onto the examiner's fingers produces pain. The accompanying systemic illness varies from mild pyrexia to severe sepsis with rigors, a leucocytosis and deranged liver function tests.

Acute pancreatitis

Acute pancreatitis is characterized by epigastric pain radiating to the back, occasionally improved by the patient leaning forward. By the time of presentation some 80% of patients have vomited and anorexia and nausea are the norm. Abdominal tenderness is present in the epigastrium and may extend to the upper abdomen whilst the lower abdomen is usually soft and non tender. Both Grey Turner's sign of ecchymosis in the flank and Cullen's peri-umbilical ecchymosis are uncommon (Fig. 10.4). The accompanying systemic disease may range from a trivial one in the early stages to a life-threatening illness with tachycardia, tachypnoea, hypoxia, circulatory collapse and shock.

Perforated peptic ulcer

Perforated peptic ulcer classically presents with epigastric pain spreading to the entire abdomen. Where the perforation walls off the pain may remain confined to the epigastric

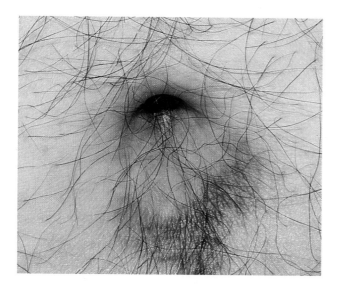

Fig. 10.4 Grey Turner's sign.

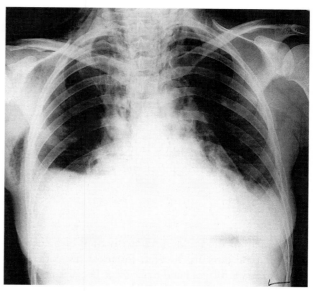

Fig. 10.5 Chest X-ray of ruptured oesophagus.

region or upper half of the abdomen. The onset is classically sudden, but a gradual onset is not uncommon. Pain in the shoulder tip is well recognized resulting from diaphragmatic irritation from gastric contents. While nausea is frequent, vomiting is unusual. Abdominal examination typically reveals a rigidity which may be confined to the epigastrium if the perforation is sealed but where there has been perforation into the peritoneal cavity board-like rigidity affects the entire abdomen. Generalized rebound tenderness is also present. After the initial stages bowel sounds are absent.

Mesenteric vascular occlusion

This gives rise to severe pain which typically has an onset of dramatic suddenness. In the early stages the pain is characteristically severe yet associated with minimal or no abdominal signs. This contrast between minimal signs, quite out of proportion to the severity of the pain, is said to be diagnostic of the condition. The pain is initially colicky and then progresses to a dull generalized abdominal pain. At this stage the abdomen can distend, become tender and as gut necrosis progresses the patient develops peripheral circulatory failure and shock. By the stage that infarction has involved the full thickness of the bowel wall, the features of peritonitis are present with anxiety, cyanosis, shock, oliguria and a profound metabolic acidosis.

Ruptured abdominal aortic aneurysm

Ruptured abdominal aortic aneurysm presents with devastatingly severe pain which may be generalized in the abdomen, confined to the central abdomen but commonly felt to radiate to the back. The condition is uncommon

below the age of 60. The patient will appear unwell, hypotension is common and the pulses in the lower limb may be diminished and are absent in about 20%. Abdominal examination may reveal abdominal swelling in a thin patient with a small aneurysm. The ruptured aneurysm may be palpable in some instances as a pulsatile swelling in the upper abdomen.

Spontaneous rupture of the oesophagus

Spontaneous rupture of the oesophagus is uncommon. Upper abdominal pain is usual and severe. It may radiate to the back particularly to the inter scapular region and retrosternally. The patient rapidly becomes unwell with tachypnoea, cyanosis and hypotension. Surgical emphysema in the supraclavicular fossae is a pathognomic sign (Fig. 10.5).

Peptic ulcer

The emergency presentation of peptic ulcer may be either as an acute ulcer or an acute manifestation of chronic peptic ulcer disease. It may be difficult or impossible to differentiate clinically between these.

The clinical features of acute peptic ulcer may begin with prodromal dyspeptic symptoms, often in the form of minor epigastric pain progressing to severe pain over several hours. The pain may be severe enough to suggest a diagnosis of perforated peptic ulcer. Characteristically the pain:
1 Is highly localized in the epigastrium (finger pointing sign);

2 May radiate through to the back (in the case of a posterior penetrating duodenal ulcer); and

3 Is improved or abolished by antacids, H₂ receptor antagonists or proton pump inhibitors (usually within a matter of minutes).

Acute ulcers may be associated with precipitating factors, commonly irritants like spices or alcohol. They are now being seen increasingly in association with aspirin, non-steroidal anti-inflammatory drugs (NSAIDs) or corticosteroids. A drug history, asking specifically about these, is essential in all patients presenting with suspected acute peptic ulcer.

Diagnosis

Differentiation from a localized perforation of a duodenal ulcer may be difficult. In both instances the patient has localized epigastric pain and tenderness. Localized guarding may be present. There may be no subdiaphragmatic gas on chest X-ray and no leakage of water-soluble contrast medium demonstrated on abdominal X-ray (Fig. 10.6). In the absence of other discriminating features a trial of intravenous H₂ receptor antagonist is appropriate. If the balance of evidence suggests a localized perforation then conservative treatment for this should include in addition: nasogastric aspiration, intravenous fluids and broad-spectrum antibiotics.

In such situations upper gastrointestinal endoscopy is contra-indicated. Normally, however, the diagnosis of acute peptic ulcer should be confirmed by early upper gastrointestinal endoscopy (Fig. 10.7). This allows assessment of the ulcer, its position, size and depth, providing a baseline for assessing healing at any subsequent examination. If the ulcer lies in the stomach multiple biopsies and brushings should be taken to ensure that the ulcer is not malignant.

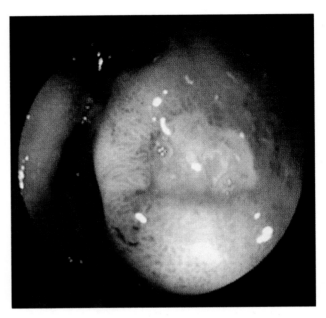

Fig. 10.7 Endoscopic appearance of duodenal ulcer. From *Atlas of Diseases of the Upper GI Tract.* © SmithKline Beecham, Welwyn Garden City.

Upper endoscopy also allows any associated pathology to be excluded. Most importantly it now allows assessment of *Helicobacter pylori* infection. This should be done routinely by taking antral biopsies for histology and for urease testing. Commercial preparations such as the CLO test enable a diagnosis of *H. pylori* infection to be made within minutes of sampling to allow treatment, where appropriate, to begin immediately. *H. pylori* infection is present in some 95% of patients with chronic duodenal ulcer and 80% of patients with chronic gastric ulcer. In NSAID-associated acute ulcers the incidence of *H. pylori* infection is the same as that in the general population (about 50% of adults in the UK).

Medical treatment

Treatment of peptic ulceration depends upon the position, size and depth of the ulcer and whether it is acute or chronic. Associated *H. pylori* infection should always be treated where present.

For all ulcers any provoking agents should be stopped and the patient advised to avoid these in future. Where NSAIDs cannot be avoided, patients should be prescribed Misoprostil, a synthetic prostaglandin, which protects gastric and duodenal mucosa against the ulcerogenic effects of these agents.

Treatment of *H. pylori* infection is determined by local policies which are in turn determined by local resistance patterns and cost of the drugs. Because resistance to *H. pylori*

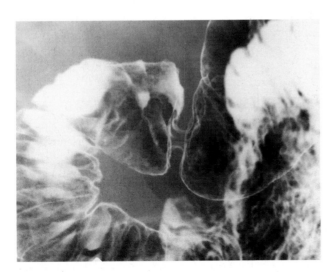

Fig. 10.6 Barium meal showing an acute duodenal ulcer.

develops readily, monotherapy is not advised. Dual therapy is based on a proton pump antagonist combined with an antibiotic. Triple therapy usually consists of a proton pump antagonist combined with two antibiotics, one of which is usually metronidazole. Other antibiotics commonly used include amoxycillin, clarithromycin and tetracycline. Currently there is no consensus about the ideal drug regimen.

Surgical treatment

Surgical treatment for uncomplicated peptic ulcer has now become an uncommon operation in developed countries.

Gastric ulcer

The gastric ulcer which fails to heal despite appropriate treatment with acid suppressing agents and *H. pylori* eradication therapy may require surgical treatment where symptoms persist. The choice of surgical procedure will depend upon the site of the ulcer within the stomach. The most common site is on the lesser curve straddling the incisura (Type I ulcers in Johnson's classification). For these ulcers the surgeon has the option of local excision. For Type II gastric ulcers (which are associated with duodenal ulcer) and Type III gastric ulcers (which occur in the prepyloric region) the only appropriate surgical option for an ulcer which has failed to heal is gastric resection. Billroth I gastrectomy and re-anastomosis is the traditional operation in this situation and remains the operation of choice. The extent of the resection will vary according to surgical preference but in general should include about one-third of the stomach so that the entire antrum is resected.

The Type IV gastric ulcer (situated within 2 cm of the cardia) is fortunately rare. Each of these must be judged on its merits according to the age, fitness and build of the patient.

Perforated duodenal ulcer

Perforated duodenal ulcer has undergone a remarkable demographic change over the past 50 years. Until the middle years of this century it was essentially a disease of young men. As the century draws to a close it has become a disease of elderly females. Throughout the world the age of the population affected by the problem has consistently increased, the increase being most marked in females over the age of 65. European studies have suggested that only some 50% of perforated peptic ulcers are associated with *H. pylori* infection, a proportion similar to that in the general population. This suggests that many of these ulcers are due to other factors. NSAIDs and corticosteroids have been increasingly recognized as precipitating factors.

Clinical features

The classic clinical features of perforated peptic ulcer are well recognized with sudden-onset epigastric pain which is severe and unrelenting and spreads to involve the entire abdomen. The patient quickly realizes that any movement aggravates the pain and characteristically lies still. The typical appearance from the end of the bed is of an immobile patient, in severe pain with pale, drawn facies. The abdomen is tender throughout with characteristic board-like rigidity on palpation. Bowel sounds may be heard for several hours after the perforation but in the majority of patients the abdomen is silent at the time of presentation.

Clinical variants include a presentation suggesting acute appendicitis where gastric contents track down the right paracolic gutter, presenting with features of peritoneal irritation in the right lower quadrant of the abdomen.

Another variation is of the walled off perforation where the perforation seals rapidly with fibrin or omentum and spillage of gastric contents into the general peritoneal cavity is limited. In such cases the pain and physical findings remain confined to the epigastrium.

Diagnosis

The clinical diagnosis may be confirmed by the presence of free intraperitoneal gas below one or both diaphragms on an erect chest X-ray (Fig. 10.8). Absence of this radiological sign does not exclude a perforation but the diagnosis may be enhanced by giving the patient water-soluble contrast medium and taking an abdominal X-ray 20 min later, after the patient has been lying on the right side (Fig. 10.9). Any contrast material lying outside the gastrointestinal tract is diagnostic of a perforation. Where the diagnosis remains in doubt and the radiological features are not clear, abdominal ultrasound may be useful in demonstrating free intraperitoneal fluid. The serum amylase test can be useful where diagnostic doubt remains. It is never elevated into the range diagnostic for acute pancreatitis but may be raised to levels below this value.

Management

Laparotomy with peritoneal toilet and primary closure of the perforation remains the most widely practised method of treatment. In some circumstances conservative treatment is appropriate and there is increasing interest in laparoscopic treatment.

Active fluid resuscitation is the initial part of any treatment regimen. Intravenous fluid, appropriate (usually opiate) analgesia and nasogastric aspiration and in most cases a urinary catheter to measure urine output is appropriate. Fluid replacement will depend upon the degree of

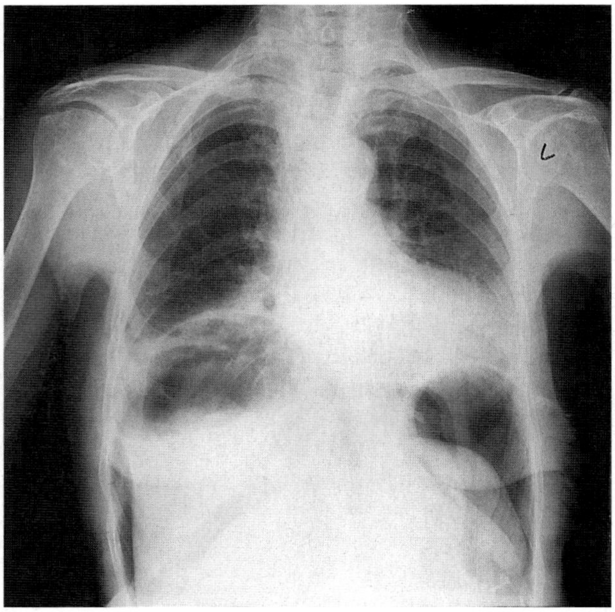

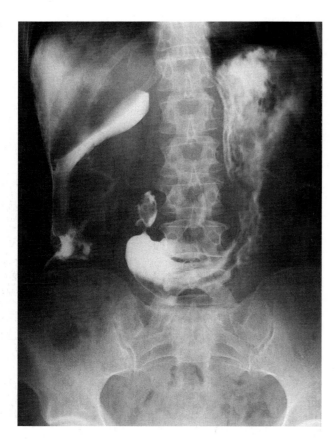

Fig. 10.8 Chest X-ray showing free subdiaphragmatic gas.

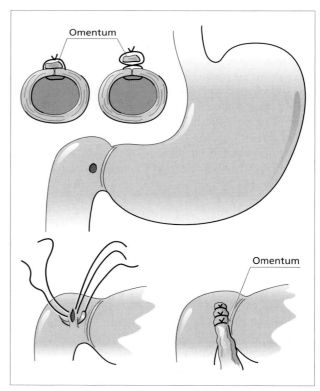

Fig. 10.9 Gastrografin for perforated duodenal ulcer showing contrast lying free in the peritoneal cavity.

hypotension and circulatory shutdown and crystalloid may have to be supplemented by colloid.

Operative treatment

Laparotomy should be performed through an upper midline incision. The diagnosis of perforated duodenal ulcer is usually apparent with a rounded punched out perforation freely leaking gastric or duodenal contents. The perforation may be plugged by fibrin or omentum.

Perforated duodenal ulcers should be closed by two or three absorbable (polyglycolic/polylactic acid (Vicryl), Ethicon UK; polydioxanone (PDS), Ethicon UK) sutures (Fig. 10.10). Perforated peptic ulcers are traditionally closed if the defect is small, using two or three absorbable sutures. Most surgeons would tie over a patch of omentum onto this repair. If the defect is too large to close primarily, or the surrounding tissues are so indurated that they fail to hold sutures satisfactorily, the greater omentum may be incorporated into the closure as a so-called omental patch as the primary procedure (Fig. 10.11).

Thereafter, thorough peritoneal toilet is important. This includes careful removal of all gastroduodenal contents and fibrin clot, followed by thorough lavage with either

Fig. 10.10 Diagram to show closure of a perforated duodenal ulcer. From Zinner, M.J. (1992) *Atlas of Gastric Surgery.* Churchill Livingstone, New York.

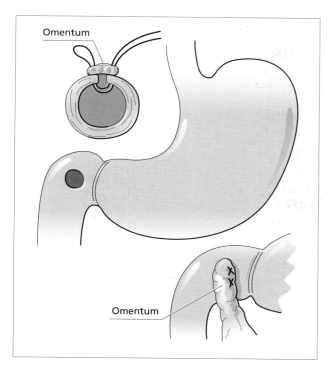

Fig. 10.11 Diagram to show Graham omental patch. From Zinner, M.J. (1992) *Atlas of Gastric Surgery*. Churchill Livingstone, New York.

normal saline or saline impregnated with an appropriate antibiotic.

In past years there has been considerable controversy about the place of a definite procedure such as truncal vagotomy as part of the treatment of perforated duodenal ulcer. In modern surgical practice, truncal vagotomy and closure of the perforation as a pyloroplasty is not recommended. Truncal vagotomy and drainage has become obsolete in the elective management of duodenal ulcer disease. Truncal vagotomy could, at best, only reduce acid output by 60% and H$_2$ receptor antagonists and particularly proton pump inhibitors are much more effective in this regard. Furthermore, in a small proportion of patients, truncal vagotomy resulted in an explosive diarrhoea. At its worst this can be incapacitating for the patient and even at best can be very difficult to manage. Modern acid-suppressing agents achieve more effective acid reduction without such side effects. Drainage procedures such as pyloroplasty, are associated with early dumping and with reactive hypoglycaemia in a small proportion of patients. The risk of these side-effects does not, in most cases, justify truncal vagotomy and drainage when more effective acid suppression is now available without the risk of such side effects.

A laparoscopic technique to treat perforated duodenal ulcers has been advocated and is practised in some centres. It has the appeal of avoiding the sequelae of an upper abdomi-nal wound. The suggestion that it is the initial insult to the peritoneal cavity and its sequelae which determines the patient's progress and rate of recovery has moderated enthu-siasm and the results of controlled trials are awaited before this treatment method can be recommended.

Non-operative treatment

Planned non-operative treatment was reported in the 1950s to have a similar mortality to that of operative treatment. Improvements in resuscitation techniques and the advent of powerful acid-suppressing agents have re-awakened interest in the technique. Using water-soluble contrast to define those patients who do not have a free perforation into the peritoneal cavity allows selection of patients in whom this treatment may be appropriate. In some studies mortality rates of 5% have been reported but conversion to operative treatment is required in up to a third. The technique has several problems:
1 Perforated gastric cancer is difficult to diagnose and will usually not respond.
2 Gastric ulcer is less likely to respond to conservative therapy.
3 Colonic perforation is difficult to exclude and a free per-foration will do badly with conservative treatment.
Conservative treatment is appropriate as the primary treat-ment in patients with severe accompanying medical illness, such as an acute myocardial infarction sustained a few days before, or overwhelming pneumonia.

Perforated gastric ulcer

Perforated gastric ulcer is much less common than perfo-rated duodenal ulcer and the diagnosis is usually only made at the time of laparotomy.

Initial resuscitation is as for perforated duodenal ulcer. The choice of operative technique will depend on the posi-tion and size of the ulcer and the age and fitness of the patient.

Where gastric resection is not felt to be appropriate the ulcer should always be biopsied before primary closure or, if amenable to excision, should be excised with primary closure.

Where the size and position of the ulcer suggests that resection would be more appropriate this may be carried out, provided the patient is sufficiently fit and the surgeon sufficiently experienced. Emergency radical gastric resection in an unfit elderly patient is rarely advisable.

Pyloric stenosis

Pyloric stenosis in infants is a true stenosis at the pylorus. The term in adults is used to describe gastric outlet obstruc-tion. Peptic ulcer causing gastric outlet obstruction may be in the pyloric channel or in the first part of the duodenum. Peptic ulcers in this situation may cause obstruction either by interstitial oedema and mucosal swelling caused by acute ulceration or by cicatrization and scarring as a result of repeated episodes of ulceration and healing. Whilst the former will usually respond to medical therapy, the latter will not.

Diagnosis

The diagnosis of gastric outlet obstruction is usually suggesed clinically. Characteristically the vomiting is projectile, and the vomitus contains recognizable food from earlier in the day or the previous day. Up to a litre may be vomited at any one time. The vomitus characteristically does not contain bile. On abdominal examination, gross distension of the stomach may be visible or palpable and the succussion splash 3 or 4 h after a meal is clinically diagnostic. The diagnosis is usually confirmed by barium meal. While this can readily diagnose gastric outlet obstruction it may on occasions fail to define the cause. Endoscopy may be made difficult by the residue within the stomach. An obstructing gastric carcinoma is usually readily recognizable. Outlet obstruction caused by peptic ulceration may be more difficult to diagnose as the pyloric channel may end blindly in oedema and the pylorus may not be recognizable, let alone negotiable.

Other causes of gastric outlet obstruction include: malignant infiltration from carcinoma of the head of the pancreas, or malignant infiltration of the prepyloric region by lymphoma or leukaemia. Benign tumours causing gastric outlet obstruction are excessively rare.

Medical treatment

The characteristic metabolic abnormality in pyloric stenosis is hyponatraemic hypokalaemic alkalosis as a result of a loss of sodium, chloride, potassium and hydrogen ions from the stomach (Fig. 10.12). This abnormality should be treated by intravenous infusion of normal saline with potassium. The rate of infusion will depend on the degree of dehydration and the ability of the patient to withstand an intravenous fluid load. In the presence of normally functioning kidneys the replacement of volume and sodium will allow the kidneys to correct the alkalosis. After fluid and electrolyte resuscitation the patient's haemoglobin should be reassessed lest an anaemia has been masked by haemoconcentration. In patients whose gastric outlet obstruction is the result of oedema from active ulceration (as opposed to fibrosis) treatment with nasogastric aspiration and intravenous H_2 receptor antagonists and parenteral nutrition, where appropriate, will result in resolution of the problem in the majority. Where the outlet obstruction is caused by scarring operative treatment will be necessary (Fig. 10.13).

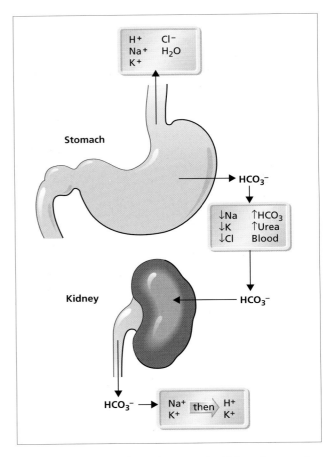

Fig. 10.12 Diagram to show pyloric stenosis with loss of water and electrolytes.

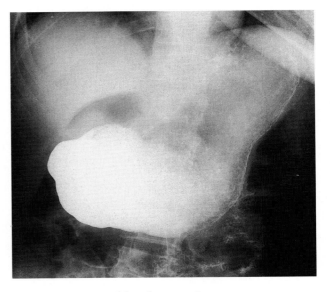

Fig. 10.13 Barium meal for pyloric stenosis.

Surgical treatment

Several options are available to treat gastric outlet obstruction caused by cicatrization from chronic prepyloric or duodenal ulcer.

Endoscopic balloon dilatation is only possible where there is a visible channel through which the balloon may be placed. In these circumstances balloon dilatation may have to be repeated on more than one occasion, and should be accompanied by appropriate acid suppression. The options for surgical treatment are truncal vagotomy with gastrojejunostomy or pyloroplasty, highly selective vagotomy with pyloric dilatation or Polya gastrectomy. In elderly, particularly female, patients, gastric resection should be avoided wherever possible. The sequelae of gastric surgery are more common in women and more common after an extensive gastric resection with Polya reconstruction. The sequelae include:

- Early dumping;
- Late dumping (reactive hypoglycaemia);
- Bile vomiting;
- Explosive diarrhoea;
- Nutritional sequelae/weight loss, iron deficiency anaemia, megaloblastic anaemia, osteomalacia;
- Afferent or efferent loop obstruction (Stammers' hernia);
- Retrograde jejunogastric intussusception.

Truncal vagotomy and drainage and highly selective vagotomy with pyloric dilatation both have their advocates. As highly selective vagotomy is performed so rarely for elective duodenal ulcer disease, the technically less challenging option of truncal vagotomy and drainage, although itself rarely required, is preferable.

Further reading

Wastell, C., Nyhus, L.M. & Donoghue, P.V. (1995) *Surgery of the Oesophagus, Stomach and Small Intestine* 5th edn. Little Brown & Co., Boston.

Cuschieri, A., Giles, G.R. & Moussa, A.R. (1992) *Essential Surgical Practice* 2nd edn. Butterworth Heinemann, Oxford.

CHAPTER 11

Acute biliary emergencies

Stephen J. Wigmore & O. James Garden

General introduction

Acute biliary disease accounts for a substantial proportion of the workload of the general surgeon. In the 1980s the development of endoscopic biliary diagnosis and intervention had a major impact on the surgical management of cholelithiasis, and was matched in the 1990s by the arrival of laparoscopic biliary surgery which resulted in a further re-evaluation of the conventional approach to the management of gallstones.

A clear understanding of the patterns of presentation and pathophysiology of biliary disease will facilitate diagnosis and management of patients. This chapter describes the most common acute biliary emergencies, their pathophysiology and current management strategies. Although variations in clinical practice do exist, this chapter attempts to address the fundamental principles of safe management of acute biliary emergencies. Effective management of acute biliary disease requires a co-ordinated and integrated approach involving specialities other than surgery such as radiology and gastro-enterology. Indeed in the management of certain diseases considerable cross-over exists and the responsibility for management may not always be clear. Close relations with such departments will optimize care of these patients, some of whom should only be managed in units with a full range of specialist expertise available.

Biliary colic

Biliary colic is the most common symptomatic manifestation of gallstones in the absence of infection. Gallstones may become impacted in the neck of the gall bladder or cystic duct and cause pain. In the absence of sepsis it is unusual for biliary colic to progress to ischaemia or perforation. The situation may resolve spontaneously with the stone falling back into the gall bladder.

Biliary colic typically presents as sudden onset of severe intermittent griping pain initially felt in the epigastrium but becoming localized to the right hypochondrium and which may also radiate to the back. Pain is not relieved by sitting or lying in any position and may be associated with nausea and, less commonly, with vomiting. The patient is apyrexial and

is not systemically unwell, although tachycardia related to pain is not uncommon. Patients with biliary colic recover quickly; however, recurrence of symptoms is common.

These symptoms should be differentiated from those which are associated with acute cholecystitis, acute pancreatitis, peptic ulcer disease and renal colic. Many patients have a history of similar episodes of pain. A family history of gallstone disease, obesity, hyperlipidaemia, cirrhosis or haemolytic anaemia are all predisposing factors to gallstone formation.

Clinical findings

The patient will be apyrexial and the blood pressure will be normal or elevated. A tachycardia may be present. There may be tenderness on deep palpation in the right upper quadrant, however the absence of tenderness does not exclude the diagnosis of biliary colic.

Investigations

Ultrasound examination is the investigation of choice to image the gall bladder. The presence of gallstones or biliary sludge combined with a typical history of symptomatic gallstones is often enough to confirm the diagnosis, but the presence of a thickened gall bladder wall or of a shrunken gall bladder in the fasted patient is indicative of gall bladder disease. By the time of investigation it is often not possible to demonstrate a stone in the neck of the gall bladder or cystic duct but the common hepatic duct should be assessed to exclude common bile duct stones or dilatation. The patient should have liver function tests performed. Mild elevation of serum alkaline phosphatase is common; however, gross derangement of liver function tests is uncommon unless common bile duct stones are present or there is some other co-existing pathology.

Management

Immediate management essentially involves providing adequate analgesia and preventing contraction of the gall bladder. The former may be achieved initially using pethi-

Table 11.1 Factors indicating choledocholithiasis and the requirement for intra-operative cholangiography.

Abnormal common bile duct
Wide cystic duct
*Elevated alkaline phosphatase
*Elevated bilirubin

*Within preceeding 6 months.
From: Wilson *et al.* (1986) Is operative cholangiography always necessary? *British Journal of Surgery* 73(8) 637–640.

dine or morphine, although in some patients the administration of intramuscular diclofenac may be as effective as opiate analgesia. Preventing further contraction of the gall bladder necessitates resting the gut and particularly avoiding fat which stimulates cholecystokinin release and gall bladder contraction. Centres differ in their approach to this problem, with some allowing continued drinking of clear fluids thereby avoiding the requirement for an intravenous infusion. More often, however, the gut is completely rested by placing the patient nil by mouth and starting an intravenous fluid regimen.

Early surgery

In a confirmed case of biliary colic there is no contra-indication to early cholecystectomy by either the laparoscopic or open approach. Ultrasound scanning preoperatively may demonstrate whether there is evidence of choledocholithiasis. Regardless of the approach used an operative cholangiogram should be performed to exclude the presence of bile duct calculi. Operative cholangiography is desirable in the majority of patients but in those with risk factors for choledocholithiasis it should be mandatory (Table 11.1). These may then be removed either by laparoscopic or open exploration of the common bile duct or by subsequent endoscopic retrograde cholangiopancreatography (ERCP).

Elective interval surgery

In many centres early surgery may not be feasible because of pressure on operating lists and beds. In this case, the patient should be discharged with advice to avoid high-fat foods and early elective surgery should be planned. Although a change in eating habits may ameliorate symptoms, the onset of further gall bladder symptoms will ensure these patients will eventually come to urgent or emergency surgical intervention. Patients with asymptomatic gallstones should not be considered for surgical intervention.

Acute cholecystitis

Acute cholecystitis is one of the major clinical presentations

of cholelithiasis and one of the most common surgical emergencies. It is three times more common in women than in men and this concurs with the demographic pattern of gallstones. The peak incidence of acute cholecystitis occurs in the middle aged to elderly population.

Pathophysiology

Gallstones are present in over 90% of cases of acute cholecystitis. The acute episode of cholecystitis is typically caused by impaction of a gallstone in Hartmann's pouch or in the cystic duct. However, the subsequent events leading to infection and inflammation are controversial. It is generally agreed that the underlying pathophysiology involves injury to the gall bladder mucosa and infection or inflammation. It has been suggested that mucosal injury might occur mechanically through abrasion or pressure from the stone or might arise as a consequence of chemical injury from concentrated bile acids. Infection is common and approximately three-quarters of patients have infected bile when operation is performed early. The incidence of positive bile cultures decreases with time from the initial presentation. The most common groups of organisms are those found in the gut including *Streptococcus faecalis*, staphylococci, *Escherichia coli*, enterococci, *Klebsiella*, *Bacteroides* and *Proteus*. Biliary stasis undoubtedly contributes to infection and it is rare for acute cholecystitis to occur in the presence of a patent cystic duct. The observation that a quarter of patients with acute cholecystitis have sterile bile lends weight to the hypothesis that bile infection is a secondary phenomenon. Macroscopically the gall bladder is typically tense and distended and may be two to three times larger than normal. The wall may be red and oedematous with transmural inflammation. Microscopic examination reveals a non-specific inflammatory change with oedema, neutrophil-rich leucocyte infiltrate and vascular congestion. In more severe cases focal abscess formation and areas of necrosis may be apparent.

When intraluminal infection occurs with the formation of pus the condition is termed **empyema**. The majority of cases of acute cholecystitis will resolve following conservative management using hydration and antibiotic therapy. In a minority of cases, compression of the arterial supply to the

> **Biliary colic and acute cholecystitis**
>
> • Approximately 90% of cases resolve without acute surgical intervention.
> • Recurrence of symptoms is extremely common unless the gall bladder is removed.
> • Acute cholecystitis is not a bar to early laparoscopic surgery.
> • Acalculous cholecystitis is rare but is associated with a high mortality.

gall bladder at its neck may lead to **ischaemia** and **necrosis**. Perforation may follow and this usually occurs either at the fundus, which is thin and also has the most tenuous blood supply or at the neck of the gall bladder, due to erosion by the calculus. Perforation may lead to local abscess formation with the formation of subhepatic or subphrenic abscesses. Diffuse peritonitis or the formation of a fistula into an adjacent structure, such as the duodenum, may also occur.

Presentation

The patient may feel generally unwell, with relatively rapid onset of epigastric and right hypochondrial pain. A prior history of biliary colic is found in approximately two-thirds of patients but in a third, acute cholecystitis is the first clinical manifestation of cholelithiasis. These symptoms should be differentiated from those of biliary colic, acute pancreatitis, perforated duodenal ulcer, renal colic and pyelonehritis/pyonephrosis. The patient may be pyrexial and tender on palpation of the right upper quadrant with involuntary guarding and rebound tenderness over the gall bladder. A further clinical sign indicating localized peritonitis is catching of the breath as a result of pain caused by palpation of the gall bladder on deep inspiration (Murphy's sign), is frequently present. The distended gall bladder may be palpable, particularly if omentum has become adherent to it.

Empyema

The patient may be extremely unwell with evidence of circulatory insufficiency, severe pyrexia, dehydration and severe pain, although the diagnosis may only become apparent at the time of early cholecystectomy in the patient with suspected acute cholecystitis. The risk of gangrenous cholecystitis, perforation and generalized peritonitis is high. The aetiology of empyema is uncertain. It is most common among the elderly and is usually associated with calculous obstruction of the cystic duct or Hartmann's pouch. It can occur in the absence of gallstones. It is thought that a number of cases develop in a similar fashion to acute cholecystitis with suppurative infection of bile, but in others empyema may represent infection of a mucocele.

High-risk patients

The incidence of gallstone disease is high in-patients with haemolytic anaemia. Sickle cell anaemia, auto-immune haemolytic anaemia and leukaemia can all result in the formation of pigment stones. Such patients are more prone to sepsis and, in the case of sickle cell anaemia, to hypoxic stress and therefore need careful management. Patients with sickle cell disease require aggressive fluid resuscitation and may require oxygen to reduce the likelihood of sickle cell crisis.

Antibiotic therapy should be instituted early and cognizance should be taken of the fact that antibiotic flora in these patients may be different with a higher incidence of *Salmonella* and staphylococci species. The sickle cell status of the patient should be ascertained prior to surgery (i.e. homozygotic or heterozygotic) and the anaesthetist informed early prior to surgery. Elective surgery is always safer in these high-risk patients.

Investigation

The patient will require hospital admission. A full blood count should be undertaken since the presence of a neutrophil leucocytosis supports the diagnosis. Gross derangement of urea and electrolytes is rare in a patient with uncomplicated acute cholecystitis and a serum amylase is required to exclude the diagnosis of concurrent acute pancreatitis. Slight elevation of alkaline phosphatase is not unusual, but if the serum bilirubin is abnormal, this may indicate the presence of a ductal stone. Ultrasound scanning of the abdomen will confirm the presence of gallstones, but the diagnosis of acute cholecystitis is confirmed if there is obvious oedema or thickening of the gall bladder wall or an associated fluid collection around the gall bladder. The diameter of the bile duct should be assessed to exclude the presence of choledocholithiasis.

Management

The patient is commenced on an intravenous hydration regimen and analgesia is given. Since three-quarters of patients have infected bile and modern antibiotics are capable of achieving effective concentrations in the bile, it is standard practice to commence intravenous antibiotics. Controlled trials have demonstrated questionable benefit of using antibiotics for acute cholecystitis; however, there is some evidence to suggest that their use may reduce the incidence of infective complications such as suppurative cholangitis and empyema. Broad-spectrum antibiotics, such as the cephalosporins, cover the majority of infecting organisms; piperacillin also has a broad spectrum of activity, but is specifically effective against *Streptococcus faecalis*, a not uncommon infecting organism. Failure of standard antibiotic therapy to reduce clinical signs of infection may indicate anaerobic infection in which case metronidazole is the antibiotic of choice. However, it should be remembered that persisting clinical signs are indicative of an increased risk of perforation in which case early surgery should be considered. In the unfit patient in whom aggressive conservative management fails percutaneous cholecystostomy under ultrasound guidance may be considered as a life-saving procedure and to avoid subsequent perforation and peritonitis. Usually, a more definitive procedure is required at a later date and the percutaneous procedure is not without problems. Common complications of cholecystostomy include the extrusion of the tube, formation of a permanent fistula, retained gallstones and recurrent cholecystitis.

Timing of cholecystectomy

With modern anaesthetic techniques and the advent of minimal access surgery the number of patients who are unfit or unsuitable for surgery is extremely limited. The number of patients undergoing laparoscopic cholecystectomy has increased in recent years although more than 10% of gall-bladder surgery is undertaken using an open technique (Fig. 11.1). Timing of the operation has been the subject of much debate. Traditionally urgent surgery was only advocated for patients with symptoms which did not resolve rapidly on supportive management, for patients in whom perforation seemed likely or if empyema was suspected. The indication for early surgery has since been extended. Clearly, hospital stay is greatly shortened if surgery is undertaken during the same admission and postoperative morbidity appears to be no greater (Table 11.2). Furthermore, approximately one-half of patients admitted with acute cholecystitis which settles on conservative therapy will develop complications or recurrence of symptoms whilst waiting for elective surgery. Pressure on elective operating lists, lack of adequately trained staff or laparoscopic facilities, or local practice ultimately dictate the timing of surgery in the group not requiring emergency surgery in many centres.

Laparoscopic cholecystectomy

Laparoscopic cholecystectomy can be undertaken safely in the majority of patients within 5 days of the onset of symptoms and indeed oedema of the gall bladder wall and surrounding tissues may actually facilitate dissection by making the plane between gall bladder and liver more clear. Nonetheless, an experienced surgeon should undertake the laparoscopic procedure, as there may be an increased risk for cholecystectomy in this clinical setting. Decompression of the gall bladder using needle aspiration may enable the gall bladder to be grasped more readily. In this way, exposure of Calot's triangle is facilitated and the cystic duct and artery

Table 11.2 Complication rates in patients undergoing early and delayed cholecystectomy.

	Early surgery	Delayed surgery
Number	80	75
Mortality	0	1
Complications	11 (14%)	13 (17%)
Wound infection	3	0
Hospital stay (days)	10.7 ± 4.9	18.2 ± 8.6
Loss of working capacity (days)	40.4 ± 4.4	54.4 ± 8.8

From: Jarvinen *et al.* (1980) Early cholecystectomy for acute cholecystitis. *Annals of Surgery* **191**(4) 501–505.

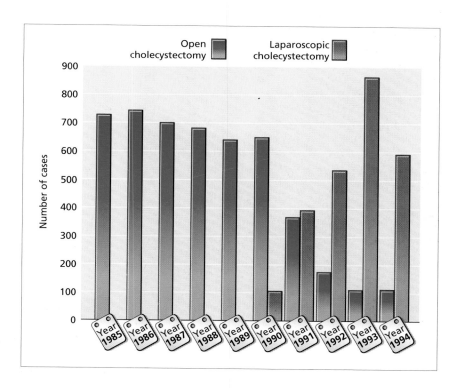

Fig. 11.1 Changing trends in cholecystectomy between 1985 and 1994 in the Lothian region.

are clearly identified prior to division. Operative cholangiography should be performed in all cases to confirm anatomy and to exclude choledocholithiasis which is thought to be more common in acute gall bladder disease (Fig. 11.2). Empyema of the gall bladder can similarly be managed by laparoscopic cholecystectomy. Prior aspiration of pus from the gall bladder may facilitate its manipulation and minimize the risk of peritoneal contamination. Care must be exercised due to the friability of tissues, particularly the gall bladder itself which may require to be delivered from the abdomen, along with any spilled stones in a retrieval bag. If dissection cannot be safely undertaken and the anatomy be clearly defined, conversion to open cholecystectomy should be considered. Although conversion constitutes a failure of laparoscopic surgery, it should not be seen as a failure of good surgical technique.

Emergency laparoscopic or open cholecystectomy

- Oedema may initially obscure anatomy but facilitate dissection.
- Friable tissues demand a more cautious approach.
- Decompression of the gall bladder may facilitate its manipulation.
- Spillage of bile and stones is more frequent than during elective operation.

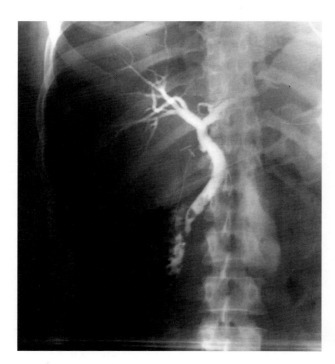

Fig. 11.2 An operative cholangiogram performed during laparoscopic cholecystectomy. A stone can clearly be seen at the lower end of the common bile duct.

Open cholecystectomy

The principles of cholecystectomy in the emergency setting are the same as those for elective operation. As for the laparoscopic procedure, decompression of the gall bladder makes manipulation of the gall bladder easier. In the presence of florid inflammation a 'fundus first' approach may be adopted and may be a safer option. Oedema and bleeding can make identification of the anatomy of the cystic duct and artery difficult and an operative cholangiogram should be performed to confirm the anatomy and exclude common bile duct calculi. Subtotal cholecystectomy should be considered for the grossly oedematous and friable gall bladder when the risk of damaging the biliary tree is considered too great to permit safe dissection of the cystic duct. In such cases the gall bladder should be opened and its contents removed. The gall bladder may be dissected free of the liver bed and transected at its neck. If it is not possible to develop a plane of dissection between the gall bladder and liver, the posterior wall may be left adherent to the liver. When this procedure is performed, the mucosa may be ablated using diathermy and the neck of the gall bladder closed by oversewing with a non-absorbable suture. If there is any concern regarding the definition of the anatomy at the free edge of the lesser omentum, no attempt should be made to close the cystic duct which should be drained, leaving the patient with a controlled biliary fistula.

Torsion of the gall bladder

This extremely rare condition can be difficult to differentiate from acute cholecystitis; however, it does not normally resolve with conservative management. In some instances it may only be diagnosed at laparotomy in the patient with an acute abdomen. Torsion can occur for one of two reasons. Firstly, the gall bladder may have a long mesentery and therefore float free with no close contact to the liver. In this instance torsion may occur about the transverse axis. Secondly, the gall bladder may have no mesentery at all, in which case its only attachments are the cystic duct and artery. In this instance torsion usually occurs about the longitudinal axis of the gall bladder. Torsion of part of the gall bladder has been described but is extremely rare. The clinical presentation is not dissimilar to a severe attack of acute cholecystitis which has a progressive rather than resolving course because of the associated gall bladder ischaemia. The patient may have a tender palpable subcostal mass, systemic

---

Routine operative cholangiography

- May identify unsuspected common bile duct stones.
- Delineates the biliary anatomy in all cases.
- Will establish proficiency.

upset may be marked as gangrene develops and perforation is likely if early surgery is not undertaken.

Acalculous cholecystitis

Less than 5% of cases of acute cholecystitis occur in the absence of gallstones. The precise mechanisms for acalculous cholecystitis are unclear; however there are a number of associations which allow some speculation as to the cause. The majority of cases of acalculous cholecystitis occur in very sick patients following recent major surgery, multiple trauma or severe burns, or in patients with severe sepsis. There is also an increased risk of this condition in women who have recently delivered, in diabetics and in patients with polyarteritis nodosa and other systemic arteritides. The association with the seriously ill may implicate hypoperfusion and infection of bile although in one third of cases bile cultures are sterile.

The substantial morbidity and mortality associated with this condition is accounted for by the serious concomitant illness and the diagnosis is often made late when sepsis or perforation and peritonitis may have developed.

Gallstone ileus

This is a rare complication of biliary disease. The patient presents with symptoms of intestinal obstruction: central colicky abdominal pain and vomiting. There is frequently a previous history of biliary colic. Abdominal X-ray demonstrates a typical small bowel obstruction with distended central loops of bowel and fluid levels on an erect film. Occasionally the opacified gallstone can be visualized typically at the ileocaecal junction where the gut is narrowest typically 1.5 cm in diameter.

Closer examination of the radiograph will frequently reveal air within the biliary tree from erosion of a solitary large calculus through the gall bladder wall into the duodenum. Stones which are large enough to obstruct the ileum are usually too large to pass through the sphincter of Oddi.

Initial management includes hydration and correction of electrolyte imbalance which may result from the obstruction and vomiting. Nasogastric aspiration will alleviate vomiting. A laparotomy is performed and the stone is milked through this proximally from its site of obstruction and delivered through an enterotomy. The gall bladder is generally densely adherent to the duodenum, and the safest strategy is to leave it *in situ* and avoid dangerous dissection at the porta hepatis.

Mirrizzi syndrome

Mirrizzi syndrome is an uncommon cause of obstructive jaundice. It occurs when a gallbladder calculus, normally impacted in Hartmann's pouch, impinges on the common hepatic or common bile duct resulting in partial biliary obstruction. Frequently, in these circumstances the gall bladder and bile duct are in extremely close apposition because of adhesions from previous inflammation. A variant of the classic Mirrizzi syndrome is described where a fistula has developed between the gall bladder and bile duct (Mirrizzi type II). This fistula probably arises as a result of pressure necrosis and erosion of the gall bladder and bile duct walls or as a consequence of infection adjacent to the calculus. If Mirrizzi syndrome is suspected a pre-operative ERCP is mandatory to establish whether a cholecystocholedochal fistula exists. In the frail or elderly patient a stent can be inserted to relieve the biliary obstruction. This can be undertaken as a definitive treatment if the patient is not then fit for elective surgery.

In the classic or type I Mirrizzi syndrome, in which the stone is prolapsing through the cystic duct and occluding the common hepatic duct, cholecystectomy may be undertaken. Although a laparoscopic approach has been described, this will require a skilled surgeon since drainage or closure of the defect may be required. The type II Mirrizzi syndrome is more challenging to manage due to the presence of the cholecystocholedochal fistula. If this fistula is simply taken down there is a high risk of subsequent biliary stricture. Some authorities have advised the fashioning of a viable rotation flap derived from the gall bladder wall to attempt to prevent this complication. The safest option however is to resect the fistula and perform a hepaticojejunostomy Roux-en-Y.

Ascending cholangitis

The triad of obstructive jaundice, fever and rigors may not always be present when infection of the biliary tree exists. Cholangitis may occur in the presence of biliary stasis due to any reason. The condition has commonly been associated with choledocholithiasis, but the presence of an obstructed biliary stent in the patient with malignant jaundice and endoscopic or percutaneous biliary intervention has been a more frequent cause in recent years. Rarer causes include primary sclerosing cholangitis, choledochal cyst, benign biliary stricture, peri-ampullary carcinoma and parasitic infestation by *Clonorchis sinensis* or *Opisthorcis viverinni*.

Ascending cholangitis

- Aggressive rehydration may be required.
- Intravenous antibiotics may reduce septic complications.
- Resolution of symptoms demands decompression of the biliary tree.
- Endoscopic or percutaneous decompression have a lower morbidity and mortality than open surgical decompression.
- An expectant approach to renal failure should be adopted.

The high incidence of septicaemia associated with cholangitis has been attributed in part to the unique arrangement of the portal triad within the liver parenchyma. It has been proposed that increased pressure in the intrahepatic bile ducts consequent upon biliary obstruction and infection may result in reflux of infected bile into the hepatic sinusoids and septicaemia. When the bile duct contains frank pus the condition is termed suppurative cholangitis. Prolonged and unrelieved obstruction of the bile duct may lead to the development of liver abscesses.

Presentation and investigation

Patients are frequently unwell. The onset of symptoms may be very sudden, although some patients describe an antecedent general malaise with flu-like symptoms. There is a high incidence of Gram-negative septicaemia in-patients with cholangitis which accounts for the high fever and rigors frequently associated with this condition. In addition, a number of patients will develop frank septic shock and urgent and aggressive management is therefore required.

Management

The diagnosis may be obvious from the clinical presentation (e.g. patient with malignant biliary obstruction having undergone biliary intervention), but is based on the presence of cholestatic liver function tests, positive blood cultures and on the presence of a dilated biliary system on ultrasound scanning. The main priority of management is to effect drainage of the obstructed biliary tree but initial resuscitation will include hydration by intravenous infusion. Serum levels of urea and creatinine should be measured to assess hydration and renal function. In the presence of shock, urinary catheterization will permit more accurate measurement of urine output and central venous pressure monitoring may be required. Intravenous antibiotic therapy using piperacillin or a cephalosporin should be commenced

Table 11.3 Outcome of therapeutic intervention by early surgery and endoscopic sphincterotomy in patients with acute cholangitis.

	Early surgery (n = 28)	Endoscopic sphincterotomy (n = 43)
Mean age	67	75
Medical risk factors	1	2
Positive blood cultures (%)	47	57
Complication rate (%)	36	23
Mortality (%)	21	5
Hospital stay (days)	23	20

From: Leese *et al.* (1986) Management of acute cholecystits and the impact of endoscopic sphinterotomy. *British Journal of Surgery* 73(12) 988–992.

following sampling of blood for culture. Non-invasive assessment of the biliary tree will include ultrasound scanning but early ERCP is indicated in the presence of choledocholithiasis. Similarly, a blocked stent should be replaced at the earliest opportunity once the patient is resuscitated. At ERCP, relief of the obstruction is often met with a flood of purulent bile. If satisfactory endoscopic drainage cannot be achieved, percutaneous transhepatic cholangiography should be considered in order to decompress the biliary tree. Surgery may be hazardous in the frail, elderly patient and is associated with increased morbidity and mortality when compared to non-surgical intervention (Table 11.3).

Obstructive jaundice

Jaundice caused by obstruction of the bile duct rarely occurs rapidly, but may present as an emergency when it becomes apparent to the patient or their family or because secondary cholangitis supervenes. The most common cause of obstructive jaundice is choledocholithiasis. Such patients frequently have an antecedent history of biliary colic or flatulent dyspepsia, may have epigastric colicky pain, may have a history of fluctuating jaundice and do not usually have associated weight loss. In addition, on examination, the gall bladder is rarely palpable but palpation is often tender in the right hypochondrium. By contrast, patients with malignant obstructive jaundice do not usually have an antecedent history suggestive of biliary disease, may be pain free, have progressive unremitting jaundice and may have marked weight loss. Malignant obstructive jaundice is most common in the elderly, although is being seen more frequently in the younger patient. It may arise as a consequence of a peri-ampullary carcinoma, cholangiocarcinoma, carcinoma of the head of the pancreas or by a tumour producing extrinsic compression of the biliary tree.

A detailed history must be taken to exclude viral hepatitis, particularly documenting the above features but also recent drug history, foreign travel, and details of social habits such as drinking or intravenous drug use. Patients with obstructive jaundice of whatever cause have dark urine and pale stools. Baseline investigations include liver function tests, serum urea and creatinine and abdominal ultrasound scanning. If gallstones are suspected or a low obstruction is demonstrated, ERCP may be of value, since stones may be removed by sphincterotomy or strictures dealt with by endoscopic insertion of a stent. If the ultrasound scan demonstrates a high bile duct obstruction, percutaneous transhepatic cholangiography should be considered.

Management of calculous obstructive jaundice

In the patient with obstructive jaundice the kidney is particularly sensitive to insult. It is thought that the excretion of conjugated bilirubin has a direct toxic effect on the kidney

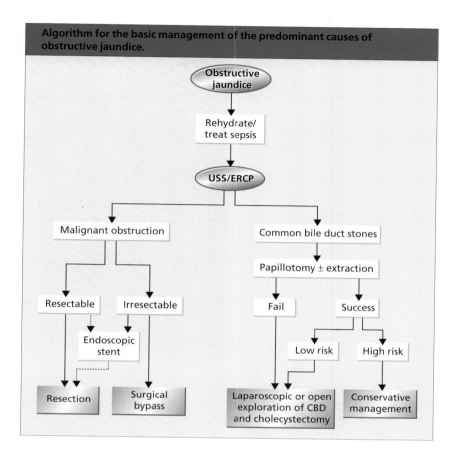

Algorithm for the basic management of the predominant causes of obstructive jaundice.

and that the development of hepatorenal syndrome may be compounded by dehydration and endotoxaemia. If acute tubular necrosis and renal failure are to be avoided patients should always be adequately hydrated and have broad-spectrum antibiotic cover prior to instrumentation of the obstructed biliary tree.

The majority of cases of calculous obstruction of the common bile duct can be managed by ERCP and sphincterotomy. Frequently the stone or stones will pass following papillotomy alone. Further stones may be removed using either a Fogarty catheter or a Dormier basket (Fig. 11.3). If large or multiple stones are present at endoscopic cholangiography but cannot be removed following sphincterotomy surgical exploration of the common bile duct may be indicated. However, in the frail, elderly patient, placement of a biliary stent may provide adequate decompression of the biliary tree. It is of interest to note that in patients presenting with severe acute pancreatitis secondary to gallstones, early endoscopic intervention on the biliary tree has been shown to be associated with an improved morbidity and mortality (Table 11.4). It has been suggested that this improvement has been due to the elimination of acute cholangitis as a contributing factor to the patient's deterioration.

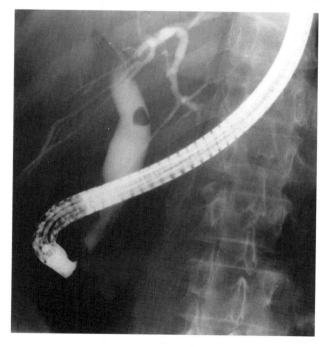

Fig. 11.3 A dilated common bile duct containing a solitary calculus seen at ERCP. A papillotomy has been performed and an endoscopic snare has been passed around the stone to facilitate its removal.

Table 11.4 Complications in patients with acute biliary pancreatitis undergoing ERCP and sphincterotomy and no procedure (control).

	ERCP+ sphincterotomy (n = 97)	Control (n = 98)
Mild		
Biliary sepsis	0	4
Phlegmon	6	1
Severe		
Biliary sepsis	0	8
Pancreatic abscess	0	3
Phlegmon	4	7
Renal failure	4	6
Death	5	9

From: Fan *et al.* (1993) Early treatment of acute biliary pancreatitis by endoscopic papillotomy. *New England Journal of Medicine* **328**(4) 228–232.

Management of malignant obstructive jaundice

The main priorities in malignant obstructive jaundice are to define the level and cause of the obstruction and to decompress the biliary tree. Although these may be achieved at operation, it is now established practice to undertake this by endoscopic or percutaneous means. The patient can subsequently be more fully investigated to determine whether surgical intervention is appropriate. If endoscopic decompression of the biliary tree cannot be achieved, a radiologist may be successful in percutaneously accessing the intrahepatic biliary tree (Fig. 11.4). Improvements in technique now allow the radiologist to insert either a biliary drain or stent without recourse to combined endoscopic and percutaneous technique. It is unusual for the interventional radiologist or endoscopist not to be able to achieve biliary decompression, but it should be borne in mind that it may be inappropriate to attempt any form of biliary decompression in the otherwise asymptomatic, elderly patient. Furthermore the

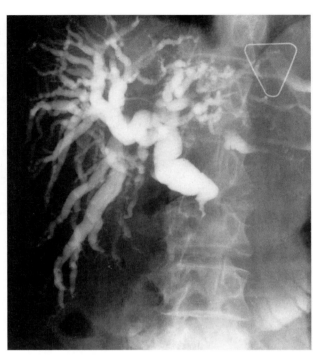

Fig. 11.4 Percutaneous transhepatic cholangiogram demonstrating a dilated intrahepatic biliary tree. A classical rat tail stricture can be seen leading to a complete occlusion of the common bile duct caused by a malignant tumour in the head of the pancreas. ERCP had failed and the immediate problem of obstructed bile flow was achieved by percutaneous transhepatic stent insertion.

likelihood of persistence or recurrence of symptoms is considerable in the patient with an unresectable tumour (Table 11.5).

Definitive management of malignant stricture is beyond the scope of this chapter but it should be borne in mind that inappropriate radiological or surgical intervention can compromise the subsequent management of the patient with apparently curable disease. The precise risks of disseminating malignancy by biliary stenting have not been adequately

Table 11.5 Incidence of cholangitis, jaundice and pain after treatment of cholangiocarcinoma in patients surviving beyond 30 days. Figures in parentheses indicate percentage.

	Number	Cholangitis	Jaundice	Pain
Extrahepatic bypass	16	3 (19)	6 (38)	3 (19)
Operative stent insertion	8	6 (75)	1 (12)	1 (12)
Segment III cholangiojejunostomy	16	3 (19)	3 (19)	2 (12)
Resection	15	1 (7)	1 (7)	4 (27)
Endoscopic and/or percutaneous stent	20	11 (55)	7 (35)	9 (45)

From: Guthrie *et al.* (1993) Changing trends in the management of extrahepatic cholangiocarcinoma. *British Journal of Surgery* **80**(11) 1434–1439.

quantified, although the risks of seeding of tumour with percutaneous intervention are not inconsiderable. For patients with irresectable high bile duct malignancy, attempts at percutaneous cholangiography or drainage may infect right-sided ducts which will not be decompressed by segment III cholangiojejunostomy. This operation has been proposed as a satisfactory means of achieving long-term drainage of the biliary tree, but in the patient with tumour involvement at the confluence of the hepatic ducts, prior manipulation of the right duct system may result in long-term biliary sepsis in the undrained right hemiliver.

Bile duct injury

The most common cause of bile duct injury is iatrogenic following elective cholecystectomy. The incidence of injury has increased with the advent of laparoscopic cholecystectomy and there is gathering evidence to suggest that such bile duct injuries which occur during this procedure may be more severe than those that occur during open cholecystectomy. The increased incidence of bile duct injuries and failure to recognize these injuries associated with laparoscopic cholecystectomy may be accounted for by changes in surgical practice. It has been suggested that the use of laser and more extensive use of diathermy in the laparoscopic procedure has accounted for some of the injuries to the duct. Such injuries may not declare themselves for several days following cholecystectomy because of the late necrosis of the damaged duct. Traction on the gall bladder and failure to clearly identify the anatomical relations in the region of the porta hepatis account for the severe injuries which result from excision of the tented hepatic duct. Extensive diathermy dissection may account for some of the devascularizing injuries which produce stricturing of the duct system. Imprecise placement of metal clips may result in bile leakage from the cystic duct or occlusion of the duct system (Fig. 11.5).

In addition to these potential factors, the reluctance of some surgeons to undertake routine operative cholangiography has resulted in failure to diagnose injuries at the time of surgery. It is generally agreed that the injury may arise before cholangiography has been performed, but early recognition and repair undoubtedly produces an improved outcome in the longer term.

The presentation of bile duct injuries is extremely variable. Transection of the duct may be apparent at the time of operation, either from leakage of bile or following examination of the excised gall bladder. Such injuries should be dealt with immediately, although it is accepted that the failure rate is high for the inexperienced biliary surgeon. Urgent and immediate referral to a specialist surgeon is more likely to produce a satisfactory long-term outcome.

When the duct has been transected, its blood supply is also likely to have been compromised and end-to-end anastomosis of the common bile duct or common hepatic duct

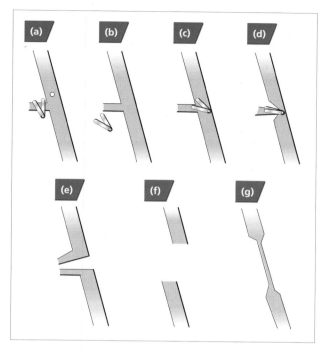

Fig. 11.5 Patterns of iatrogenic bile duct injury. The injuries (a–d) may be suitable for simple drainage procedures using either a T-tube or an endobiliary stent. The injuries listed (e–g) are more extensive and will probably require hepaticojejunostomy. (a) Pinhole injury caused by diathermy or laser injury; (b) cystic duct clip dislodged; (c) occlusion of the common hepatic duct; (d) occlusion of the common bile duct caused by application of the clip too close to the principal duct; (e) division of the common duct; (f) complete division and excision of the common duct; (g) stricture formation following devascularization of the common duct.

Avoiding bile duct injury

- Clear demonstration of the anatomy of Callot's triangle is essential.
- Operative cholangiography may assist identification of anatomy.
- Conversion to open operation if in difficulty represents good surgical practice not failure.
- Early recognition of bile duct injury and repair offers better prognosis than delayed diagnosis.
- Seek specialist advice early in the event of bile duct injury.

will often heal with subsequent stricture formation. It is for this reason that the operation of choice is hepaticojejunostomy Roux-en-Y. When the common hepatic duct has been transected close to the porta hepatis, effective biliary drainage can be obtained either by extending the opening into the left hepatic duct which pursues an extrahepatic course beneath segment IV.

Duct injuries from pinhole perforation or dislodgement of the clips from the cystic duct usually present either by persisting drainage of bile through a drain in the peritoneal cavity, if this has been used, or by collection of bile in the peritoneal cavity. On occasion, the right hepatic duct or an isolated sectoral branch may have been divided during cholecystectomy (Fig. 11.6). Bile in the peritoneal cavity frequently becomes infected, giving rise to subhepatic or subphrenic abscesses or diffuse peritonitis. Provided that there is no obstruction to the egress of bile at the level of the common bile duct, many of these lesions will close spontaneously. The key to their successful management, however, should consist of drainage of biliary peritonitis and control of the bile leak. Antibiotics should be continued to attempt to treat established infection and endoscopic retrograde cholangiography is used to define the level and size of the bile leak. Endoscopic sphincterotomy or stent placement may improve biliary drainage and expedite the healing of the biliary fistula. The surgeon should have a low threshold to surgical intervention for management of biliary peritonitis or for the subsequent development of subphrenic or subhepatic abscesses.

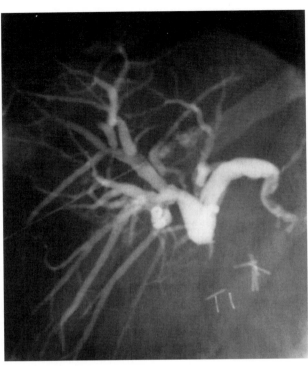

Fig. 11.7 Percutaneous transhepatic cholangiogram demonstrating a dilated intrahepatic biliary tree due to complete occlusion of the common hepatic duct by a metal clip placed at laparoscopic cholecystectomy. The remainder of the clips appear to be on the wrong side of the expected course of the common bile duct and indeed at laparotomy the right hepatic artery had been ligated and excised.

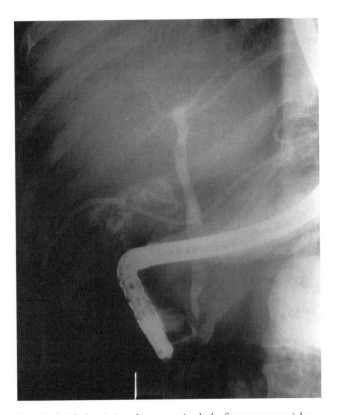

Fig. 11.6 Bile duct injury demonstrating leak of contrast material at the level of the cystic duct. Of greater concern is the complete failure of filling of the right intrahepatic duct system. Opacities within the common bile duct are air bubbles. A percutaneous tube drain can be seen crossing the collection.

For the jaundiced patient who may have sustained an injury to the bile duct from an inappropriately placed clip, an ultrasound scan is used to detect the presence of a dilated duct system and to exclude biliary peritonitis. Percutaneous transhepatic cholangiography will be required to demonstrate the level of the obstruction (Fig. 11.7), although it is more frequent for the endoscopic approach to be used in the first instance since the surgeon may (inappropriately) hope that the underlying pathology is that of retained common bile duct stones, rather than that of an injury to the ductal system. Endoscopic intervention may dislodge clips if these have been applied to the otherwise intact duct.

Late duct injuries usually present also with obstructive jaundice and/or cholangitis and may present many weeks or months after primary operation. The cause of these duct injuries is often over-enthusiastic dissection of the common bile duct rendering it avascular. Healing inevitably results in stricture formation. Management requires careful evaluation either by endoscopic or percutaneous transhepatic cholangiography. Although decompression of the biliary tree may be achieved by either of these approaches, it is preferable for the surgeon to be left with a dilated duct system which can be more easily anastomosed to a 70 cm Roux-en-Y limb of jejunum (Fig. 11.7). Higher bile duct injuries may also involve injury to the right hepatic artery. Such injuries require careful evaluation and on occasions right hepatectomy may be indicated.

Traumatic bile duct injury

Traumatic injury to the bile duct is extremely rare and usually occurs in association with major vascular injury or liver injury. The priority should always be to control haemorrhage and repair vessels if this is possible. Bile duct repair should only be contemplated after vascular injury has been dealt with. In the unstable patient, bile duct repair may be preformed most safely at a second operation when the immediate threat to life has subsided. In this instance simple drainage of the duct system by means of a stent or external drain should be used. In the stable patient, minor bile duct laceration can be repaired by insertion of a stent and direct suture of the tear. More complex injury is repaired most effectively by hepaticojejunostomy using a Roux-en-Y configuration.

Penetrating injuries caused by a sharp implement such as a knife are essentially similar to iatrogenic bile duct injuries and should be managed in the same way. Bullet wounds affecting the common bile duct are often fatal because they frequently involve the vena cava or other vital structures.

Blunt injury may result in obstruction of the bile duct because of oedema of the duct itself or of the pancreas. If the duct is intact, effective drainage can be achieved by endoscopic stenting and, provided the blood supply to the duct is intact, these injuries heal with minimal stricturing.

CHAPTER 12

Acute pancreatitis

Geoffrey Glazer & Darren Mann

Introduction

Acute pancreatitis is a common condition, accounting for 2% of all cases of abdominal pain admitted to hospital in Europe. Despite the frequency with which the disease is encountered there remains much controversy regarding its diagnosis, investigation and treatment. The true incidence of acute pancreatitis is contentious, with reports from the UK ranging from 21 to 283 cases per million population. This wide range results from variations in diagnostic criteria, threshold for investigation and use of autopsy data, although there is evidence that the true incidence is increasing. Until recently, the lack of consensus on the definition of the disease and its complications has contributed to the confusion. In this chapter we will use the Atlanta clinically based definitions, produced by consensus agreement by a group of internationally acknowledged experts and published in 1993.

Despite apparent improvements in the management of patients with acute pancreatitis, including the availability of computed tomography (CT) scanning, advances in intensive therapy unit (ITU) care of the critically ill and operative strategy for septic complications, the overall mortality has remained unaltered around 10–15% for the last 20 years. Multicentre audits have demonstrated deficiencies at every step in the management of the disease, with variation in management both within and between institutions. It is evident that potentially beneficial treatments are not being aimed at the appropriate patients, because the severity of the condition often goes unrecognized.

The term acute pancreatitis encompasses a spectrum of pathological changes from glandular oedema at one end to frank pancreatic necrosis at the other. The clinical course is dependent on a balance between the extent of disease in the gland and the physiological response of the patient. This complex clinicopathological process will be very variable, and thus a flexible approach to management is necessary. Nevertheless, it is clear that there are patterns to the illness and that management can be organized in some formal way in this disease. Figure 12.1 demonstrates an idealized pathway for the phases of management of acute pancreatitis, and the chapter will follow this outline.

Central to the clinical strategy in acute pancreatitis is the need to stratify patients into mild and severe disease, because such distinction guides the degree of subsequent investigation, monitoring and treatment. In the first instance, however, the diagnosis of acute pancreatitis must be made in a reliable and accurate fashion as other severe intra-abdominal catastrophes may mimic the condition.

Diagnosis

Clinical definition

Acute pancreatitis is an acute inflammatory process of the pancreas, with variable involvement of other regional tissues or remote organ systems. The range of diagnostic tests available for a patient with suspected acute pancreatitis is shown in Table 12.1. Few patients will require all these steps.

Clinical features

Acute pancreatitis is principally (and occasionally purely) a clinical diagnosis. The disease may affect patients of any age or sex, and the clinical presentation is usually one of sudden onset of upper abdominal pain (which often radiates through to the back) and vomiting. The physical findings are variable but frequently the patient is unable to lie still because of the pain, preferring to lean forwards and move about in an attempt to find some relief. General features may include fever and dehydration; jaundice should be specifically sought. The cardiovascular examination may reveal tachycardia and even hypotension, and in severe cases respiratory distress and pleural effusions may be present. The abdominal findings are characteristically of distension with epigastric tenderness and guarding and on occasion an ill-defined mass or 'fullness' may be appreciated. In severe forms of the disease the classically described body wall ecchymoses around the umbilicus (Cullen's sign) and in the flanks (Grey Turner's sign) may be visible, indicating retroperitoneal haemorrhage.

In a small proportion of cases acute pancreatitis may present atypically such as unexplained circulatory

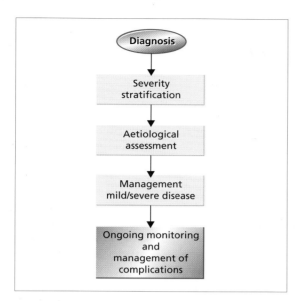

Fig. 12.1 Phases of management of acute pancreatitis.

Table 12.1 Diagnostic sequence for acute pancreatitis.

Clinical features
Serum amylase (× 4)/lipase (× 2)
Urinary amylase
Plain chest and abdominal X-rays
Ultrasound
Dynamic CT scan
Peritoneal aspiration
Laparoscopy
Laparotomy

Table 12.2 Other abdominal causes of hyperamylasaemia.

Penetrating/perforated duodenal ulcer
Penetrating/perforated gastric ulcer
Gangrenous cholecystitis
Generalized peritonitis
Intestinal obstruction
Mesenteric infarction
Ruptured abdominal aortic aneurysm
Ruptured ectopic pregnancy

the disease. Although the diagnostic confidence increases with the magnitude of amylase elevation (levels > 2000 IU are highly suggestive), hyperamylasaemia below this level is found in a number of common abdominal conditions, as summarized in Table 12.2. Furthermore, the release of amylase from the salivary glands in parotitis or mumps may cause confusion (easily resolved by measurement of serum lipase) as may incidental macroamylasaemia (indicated by a low urinary level). Conversely, a level of serum amylase within the normal range may be found in patients with severe pancreatitis presenting late, or in those with a mild attack. In these instances, confirmation may be achieved by the measurement of urinary amylase. If diagnostic doubt persists, then radiological studies will be required.

Radiology

Radiological investigation is used to exclude other possible causes of an acute abdomen as well as to confirm the presence of pancreatitis. An erect chest X-ray may detect air under the diaphragm, indicating a perforated viscus. Pleural effusions are sometimes seen in severe acute pancreatitis. A plain abdominal film is of most value in excluding alternative diagnoses such as intestinal obstruction, rather than in confirming the diagnosis of pancreatitis. In the presence of acute pancreatitis a number of non-specific features may be evident, including a sentinel loop (an isolated, paralytic segment of small intestine), absence of psoas shadows, and pancreatic calcification from chronic pancreatitis. Rarely, gas in the retroperitoneum is seen, indicating pancreatic infection with gas-forming organisms. As a diagnostic test, however, a plain abdominal X-ray is unreliable.

Ultrasound scanning is of greatest value in demonstrating cholelithiasis, cholecystitis or the presence of free intra-abdominal fluid. Clear views of the pancreas are unobtainable in over one third of cases and so this test is of limited use in confirming the diagnosis. When the gland is seen, however, pancreatic swelling and acute fluid collections are relevant to the diagnosis. The state of the common bile duct should be assessed whenever possible.

shock, coma or postoperative intra-abdominal crisis, and the diagnosis must therefore be borne in mind in such patients.

Laboratory investigations

The standard diagnostic test is an elevated serum amylase greater than four times the upper limit of the laboratory normal range. Lipase, which is less readily available, is of similar diagnostic value when the level is above twice the normal limit. These tests must be evaluated in the appropriate clinical context since they are not specific to pancreatitis. The amylase liberated by an inflamed pancreas and absorbed into the circulation is rapidly cleared by the kidneys (and reticulo-endothelial system), and so the serum level changes dynamically with time. The peak level usually occurs within the first 48 h of an attack, and thereafter declines (a process that is reflected in an increase in urinary amylase content). A normal serum amylase estimation therefore does not exclude

The most important means of confirming acute pancreatitis in cases of diagnostic uncertainty is contrast enhanced (dynamic) CT scanning, although this is not recommended routinely. This imaging technique not only provides the most accurate means of assessing the pancreas and the retroperitoneum but also provides information of prognostic import as will be discussed later. In obscure abdominal pain the dynamic CT scan may confirm the presence of pancreatitis. It should be appreciated, however, that in clinically proven cases with an elevated serum amylase the CT scan appearances may be normal in up to 20% of patients (representing the milder end of the disease spectrum) and so an unremarkable CT scan does not exclude pancreatitis.

Peritoneal aspiration and diagnostic lavage

If access to a CT scanner is not available, or when doubt persists as to the diagnosis, more invasive investigation is recommended, initially by the sampling of peritoneal fluid. This technique is usually warranted in the severely ill patient in whom the concern for a visceral perforation is high. Aspiration of fluid may be achieved under ultrasound guidance, or alternatively a flexible peritoneal dialysis catheter can be inserted into the abdominal cavity. If no free fluid is withdrawn, lavage may be performed with a few hundred mls of normal saline. The free fluid in cases of acute pancreatitis ranges from pale yellow to 'prune' juice, and characteristically has a high amylase content. Microscopy is essential, and the presence of bacteria on Gram staining, or of vegetable fibres or faecal matter indicates perforation which must be managed accordingly.

Laparoscopy and laparotomy

If all else fails and the diagnosis of a severe abdominal problem is unresolved, surgery may be necessary. Laparoscopy is an alternative to full laparotomy and can be used to exclude intestinal perforation, mesenteric infarction and cholecystitis. The pancreas and retroperitoneum will not be seen easily and the evidence for pancreatitis may be indirect, e.g. the presence of fat necrosis. On occasion, a formal laparotomy may be required to resolve the issue and it should be remembered that sometimes pancreatitis may coexist with some other intra-abdominal catastrophe (such as gangrenous intestine). Overall, with the clinical, biochemical, and radiological steps outlined above, diagnostic surgery should rarely be needed.

Severity stratification

It is necessary to stratify patients with acute pancreatitis as this has important implications for management, prognostication and use of resources. Failure to accurately stratify patients into predicted mild and severe forms of disease can be identified as the starting point for deficiencies in management and can be implicated in potentially avoidable deaths.

Clinical definitions

By the Atlanta criteria, mild acute pancreatitis is associated with minimal organ dysfunction and an uneventful recovery, the predominant pathological feature being interstitial oedema of the gland. Severe acute pancreatitis is associated with organ failure and/or local complications such as necrosis (with infection), pseudocyst or abscess; most often this is an expression of the development of pancreatic necrosis, although patients with oedematous pancreatitis may manifest clinical features of a severe attack.

A clinical assessment alone is inaccurate in the identification of patients who are likely to develop complications. In prospective studies purely clinical evaluation has been shown to miss nearly two-thirds of cases that went on to develop complications. For this reason, and some alternative objective laboratory or other measurements must be made early in the attack to assess severity.

Ranson/Imrie objective criteria

Apart from the patient's age, a number of routine haematological and biochemical variables have been shown to predict the eventual clinical outcome. These 'objective criteria' have been grouped to provide a multiple factor scoring system that can be used to predict the likelihood of complications for a given patient. Table 12.3 shows the prognostic criteria proposed by Imrie—the system most often used in the UK (these are based on the original, and similar, Ranson criteria often used in the USA). A combination of three or more positive criteria within 48 hours of admission indicates a severe attack, and the sensitivity of these scoring systems exceeds that of clinical assessment alone, being of the order

Table 12.3 Imrie prognostic scoring system. Three positive within 48 h = severe attack.

Age > 55 years
WBC > 15 000/mm³
Glucose > 10 mmol/L
Urea > 16 mmol/L
Po_2 < 60 mmHg
Calcium < 2 mmol/L
LDH > 600 UI/L
AST/ALT > 200 U/L
Albumin < 32 g/dL

LDH = lactate dehydrogenase; ALT = alanine amino transferase; AST = aspartate amino transferase.

of 80%. The risk of complications and death increases with the number of positive scoring criteria.

Acute physiology and chronic health evaluation (APACHE)

Criticisms of multifactorial scoring systems include the delay in obtaining results (up to 48 h) and the fact that they provide a 'one shot' prediction, and as such cannot be used for continued evaluation over the course of an attack. The APACHE II system (which uses not only measurements of the physiological response of the patient to an attack, but also includes in the assessment some contribution relating to the premorbid medical condition of the individual) has been used in the setting of acute pancreatitis (see Table 12.4). An APACHE II score of 8 or more is indicative of a severe attack. With predictive accuracy matching that of the objective scoring systems, the advantage of the APACHE II measurement is that it can be repeated serially on a daily basis to indicate changes in the course of the illness and may herald the development of local and systemic complications.

C-reactive protein (CRP)

An additional means of assessing the severity of an attack in the early phase is by measurement of serum markers of systemic inflammation, the most readily available of which is C-reactive protein (CRP). Initial trials have shown that levels of this acute phase reactant exceeding 210 mg/L in the

Table 12.4 APACHE II scoring system.

Acute physiology score	High abnormal range					Low abnormal range			
Variable	+4	+3	+2	+1	0	+1	+2	+3	+4
Temp (°C)	>41	39–40.9		38.5–38.9	36–38.4	34–35.9	32–33.9	30–31.9	<29.9
Mean arterial pressure (mmHg)	>160	130–159	110–129		70–109		50–69		<49
Heart rate (ventricular)	>180	140–179	110–139		70–109		55–69	40–54	<39
Respiratory rate	>50	35–49		25–34	12–24	10–11	6–9		<5
Oxygenation (mmHg)									
A_aDO_2 when $F_iO_2 > 0.5$	>500	350–499	200–349		<200				
P_aO_2 when $F_iO_2 < 0.5$					$P_O_2 > 70$	$P_O_2 61–70$		$P_O_2 55–60$	$P_O_2 < 55$
Arterial pH	>7.7	7.6–7.69		7.5–7.59	7.33–7.49		7.25–7.32	7.15–7.24	<7.15
Serum Na (mmol/L)	>180	160–179	155–159	150–154	130–149		120–129	11–119	<110
Serum K (mmol/L)	>7	6–6.9		5.5–5.9	3.5–5.4	3–3.4	2.5–2.9		<2.5
Serum creatinine (mg/100 ml) Double score for ARF	>3.5	2–3.4	1.5–1.9		0.6–1.4		<0.6		
Haematocrit (%)	>60		50–59.9	46–49.9	30–45.9		20–29.9		<20
White blood count (×10³/mm³)	>40		20–39.9	15–19.9	3–14.9		1–2.9		<1
Glasgow coma scale (GCS): Score = 15-actual GCS									

APACHE II score is given by the sum of the acute physiology score, the age points and the chronic health points. Age points are assigned: age < 44, zero; 45–54, 2 points; 55–64, 3 points; 65–74, 5 points and > 75, 6 points. Chronic health points are assigned if the patient has a history of severe organ system insufficiency or is immunocompromised as follows: for non-operative or emergency post-operative patients, 5 points; and for elective postoperative patients, 2 points. Organ insufficiency or an immunocompromised state must have been evident before hospital admission and must conform to the following criteria: *liver*, biopsy proven cirrhosis and documented portal hypertension, episodes of past upper gastro-intestinal bleeding attributed to portal hypertension, or prior episodes of hepatic failure/encephalopathy/coma; *cardiovascular*, New York Heart Association Class IV (i.e. symptoms of angina or cardiac insufficiency at rest or during minimal exertion); *respiratory*, chronic restrictive, obstructive, or vascular disease resulting in severe exercise restriction i.e. unable to climb stairs or perform household duties, or documented chronic hypoxia, hypercapnia, secondary polycythaemia, severe pulmonary hypertension (> 40 mmHg), or respirator dependency; *renal*, receiving chronic dialysis; and *immunocompromised*, the patient has received therapy that suppresses resistance to infection, e.g. immunosuppression, chemotherapy, radiation, long-term or recent high-dose steroids, or has a disease that is sufficiently advanced to suppress resistance to infection e.g. leukaemia, lymphoma, AIDS.
A_aDO_2, alveolar-arterial oxygen difference; P_aO_2, arterial partial pressure of oxygen; F_iO_2, fraction of inspired oxygen; ARF, acute renal failure

first 48 h (and >120 mg/L at 7 days) perform as well as objective scoring systems in prognostication. When used in combination with multifactor scoring systems the overall accuracy may be improved, each method providing a means of correcting the cases misclassified by the other.

The stratification of patients into predicted mild and severe disease early in the course of an attack provides the basis for subsequent investigation and management.

CT scanning in severe disease

It is recommended that all patients judged to have a severe attack should have a contrast enhanced (dynamic) CT scan performed within the first week of the disease. Dynamic CT scanning not only refines the process of disease prognostication, but sets a baseline for the subsequent monitoring of disease progression. The investigation is indicated when an attack is judged severe by the methods outlined above, but should not be withheld in the face of clinical deterioration even if objective criteria are negative. The CT scan will not only give an indication of the extent of the disease process but may be used as a prognosticating test in its own right. In the context of prognostication, it is essential that intravenous contrast enhanced (dynamic) scanning is performed. Before requesting this examination it is important to appreciate that intravenous contrast may exacerbate renal failure, and so should be used with caution in patients with an elevated creatinine as well as those with documented allergy. Non-iodinated compounds should be used in these circumstances. The initial CT scan in severe acute pancreatitis is best performed some 3–10 days after the onset of the attack. However, because scanning in this context is principally used for planning later management of complications (as distinct from the urgent scanning required in cases of diagnostic difficulty) the timing should be optimal for the patient. It may be dangerous to move a patient with fulminant acute pancreatitis and cardiovascular/respiratory failure to the radiology department with the attached ventilators and inotrope infusions when the diagnosis is not in doubt, for an investigation that is non-essential.

The prognostic information is derived from the extent of the locoregional changes in the pancreas and surrounding tissue and on the degree of pancreatic necrosis. The scan may reveal a spectrum of changes from normal appearances, through swelling confined to the pancreas (see Fig. 12.2), to pancreatic swelling and extension of inflammatory changes into the peripancreatic tissues, often with the presence of one or more acute fluid collections. The dynamic phase is required to demonstrate areas of the pancreas that fail to enhance, which is taken to indicate pancreatic necrosis; this may be interpreted in quartiles of 0, 25, 50, 75% or total necrosis (see Fig. 12.3). When the plain and dynamic appearances are combined, a 'CT severity grade' is produced (see Table 12.5). The extent of the local inflammatory

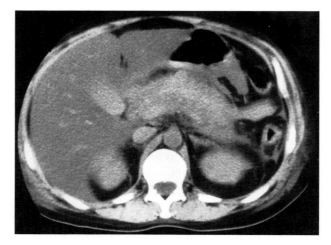

Fig. 12.2 CT scan demonstrating pancreatic swelling.

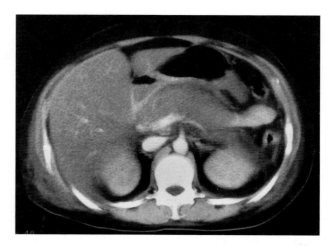

Fig. 12.3 Enhanced phase scan from patient in Fig. 12.2 showing small area of perfusion in head and >75% necrosis.

changes and the proportion of the gland that is necrosed correlates with the likelihood that the patient will develop infection in the dead tissue (infected necrosis). Over three quarters of patients with the combination of inflammatory pancreatic changes, multiple acute fluid collection and 50% or greater necrosis (grade E) will develop infected necrosis, and in these patients the mortality is much higher.

Dynamic CT scanning thus provides a reliable means of identifying that subset of all patients judged to have severe disease by objective criteria who are likely to develop life-threatening complications. Appreciation that the extent of pancreatic necrosis is a major determinant of the course of the disease has important implications for management of these patients, and there is an argument for concentrating such patients in specialist centres.

Table 12.5 Contrast enhanced CT grading system.

Grade	CT Morphology
A	Normal
B	Focal or diffuse gland enlargement Small, intrapancreatic fluid collection
C	Any of above plus Peripancreatic inflammatory changes <25% gland necrosis
D	Any of the above plus Single extrapancreatic fluid collection 25–50% gland necrosis
E	Any of the above plus Extensive extrapancreatic fluid collections Pancreatic abscess 50%+ gland necrosis

Magnetic resonance imaging (MRI)

The value of dynamic (gadolinium enhanced) MRI in the setting of acute pancreatitis is currently under evaluation. Early indications suggest that this modality can reliably detect necrosis, and improve the ability to distinguish solid matter from fluid and debris. The technique is limited by the requirement of the patient to remain still for longer periods of time than that required by CT, and is not universally available at present. However, the reduction in radiation exposure is an important consideration.

Assessment of aetiology

The aetiology of an attack influences therapeutic decision making and so early assessment should be made. The principal causes of acute pancreatitis are shown in Table 12.6. The patient's alcohol consumption should be accurately recorded in units/week (although it is appreciated that this information may not always be reliable). Previous drug consumption is important, as is the presence of any prodromal illness

Table 12.6 Causes of acute pancreatitis.

Gallstones
Alcohol
Idiopathic
ERCP
Postoperative
Drug induced
Hypercalcaemia
Tumour
Hyperlipidaemia
Viral

which may suggest a viral aetiology. A previous attack of dyspepsia (or jaundice) will suggest gallstones, whilst the development of clinical jaundice raises the possibility of gallstones or tumour.

Hyperparathyroidism is a rare cause of pancreatitis and calcium changes during the early stage of an attack may mask an underlying hypercalcaemia.

An early ultrasound scan is essential for the demonstration of gallstones. The investigation should be repeated if negative in the first instance because stones may be missed in severe disease when gas-filled loops of bowel and free fluid obscure the view.

In the convalescent stage, if no aetiology has been established, blood should be taken for calcium level and lipid profiles. If all tests are negative, then consideration should be given to a dynamic CT scan (to look for pancreatic tumours or other retroperitoneal pathology) and endoscopic retrograde cholangiopancreatography (ERCP) (to look for common bile duct stones, ampullary lesions and anatomical variants).

Management of acute pancreatitis

Phases of illness

The clinical course of patients with acute pancreatitis is variable and comprises a series of different phases. The timing of these phases will, likewise, be variable. The pathology which ranges from oedema and inflammation through to necrosis of the gland and subsequent infection will be reflected in different clinical syndromes. These may not marry up precisely as the clinical manifestations are a resultant of the pathological process in the gland and the physiological response of the patient. The older patient with comorbid conditions may have an unfavourable outcome with a high mortality in apparently mild pancreatitis.

The initial phase of the attack lasts for a week or so during which time a varying degree of multisystem failure can occur. In the subsequent phase lasting up to several weeks, most mild patients will recover, but others with underlying necrosis in the gland may be manifest as 'failure to thrive' with ongoing abdominal signs and periodic bouts of multisystem instability. The onset of infection in areas of necrosis can occur at any stage and may be suspected clinically by a systemic septic response and severe illness or by a progressive decline which can be difficult to distinguish from sterile necrosis. Later complications such as pseudocyst, biliary or duodenal obstruction, abscess or rarely haemorrhage can occur at any stage, even many weeks after onset.

Principles of management of acute pancreatitis

The principles of management of acute pancreatitis include:

1 Multisystem support for the patient during the initial phases of the attack.

2 Attempts to limit extension of the disease process by promoting pancreatic blood flow, suppressing secretions and preventing secondary infection.

3 The close monitoring of patients to detect and treat complications.

4 The eradication where possible of the underlying cause of the attack, in particular gallstones.

The degree of monitoring and intensity of treatment will be commensurate with the severity of the attack.

Management of mild disease

Pancreatitis predicted to be mild by objective criteria usually runs an uneventful self-limiting course and this form of disease constitutes 80% of all attacks. These patients can be managed on the general ward with basic monitoring of temperature, pulse, blood pressure and urine output. Although all will require a peripheral intravenous line for fluids and possibly a nasogastric tube, few will warrant an indwelling urinary catheter.

Antibiotics should not be used routinely, and a CT scan is unnecessary. The vast majority of these patients will make a full recovery. Occasionally an initially predicted mild case may transform into a more aggressive clinical picture, suggestive of the development of complications. These patients should be re-evaluated by APACHE II scores and CRP measurement and a dynamic CT scan, and should be managed along the lines of those with severe disease.

Initially predicted mild disease accounts for less than 5% of mortality from acute pancreatitis, and on those occasions when such an attack proves fatal, this is often related to comorbid diseases (ischaemic heart disease, long-standing obstructive airways disease, diabetes).

An important component of the management of mild pancreatitis caused by cholelithiasis is the eradication of the gallstones, preferably on the same admission (within 2 weeks of the attack). Failure to do so will result in at least half of the patients that are discharged being admitted with a further attack of biliary pancreatitis within 6 months. Definitive treatment of gallstones will consist of some form of common bile duct evaluation (either ERCP or intra-operative cholangiogram) and cholecystectomy (usually by the laparoscopic route). ERCP and sphincterotomy with pre-operative duct clearance should be aimed at those in whom there is a higher degree of suspicion of common bile duct (CBD) stones (e.g. persistent jaundice, deranged liver function tests (LFTs), dilated duct on ultrasound). Other cases should have peroperative cholangiography.

Management of severe disease

Severe acute pancreatitis is associated with organ failure and/or local complications, and is further characterised by three or more Imrie criteria or eight or more APACHE II points. Organ failure is defined as shock (systolic blood pressure less than 90 mmHg), pulmonary insufficiency (P_aO_2 60 mmHg or less), renal failure (creatinine level greater than 177 μmol/L after rehydration) or gastrointestinal bleeding (more than 500 ml/24 hours). Systemic complications, such as disseminated intravascular coagulation (platelets 100 000/mm³ or less, fibrinogen less than 1 g/L and fibrin degradation products greater than 80 μg/ml) or severe metabolic disturbances (calcium level less than 1.8 mmol/L) may be seen. Severe acute pancreatitis accounts for 20% of cases of the disease, but is responsible for the vast majority of deaths. Mortality from acute pancreatitis can be divided into four main groups: (1) early deaths from fulminant disease and MOSF (multiple organ system failure); (2) late deaths caused by infection related to complications, principally infected necrosis; (3) deaths related to other complications of acute pancreatitis, such as haemorrhage; and (4) death principally related to comorbid medical conditions. The principles of management of severe acute pancreatitis are aimed at counteracting to these causes of death.

Monitoring

The initial management in severe acute pancreatitis requires a degree of invasive monitoring and active resuscitation. In this way, the proportion of early deaths caused by circulatory and renal failure can be reduced. The patient must be managed in an intensive care unit (ITU) or high dependency unit (HDU). All of these patients require peripheral vascular access, a central venous line (for fluid administration and central venous pressure (CVP) monitoring), a urinary catheter and nasogastric tube. A pulse oximeter is an important adjunct. Nursing assessment must include regular hourly pulse, blood pressure, CVP, respiratory rate, oxygen saturation, urine output, and temperature. These recordings must be charted accurately, along with cumulative calculations of fluid balance. More aggressive monitoring with arterial lines and Swan–Ganz catheterization is required in a proportion of cases.

System support

Fluid replacement is provided with normal saline in the first instance, with plasma expanders (e.g. gelatins) and blood transfusion as necessary, guided by the circulatory haemodynamics. Oxygen is provided by face mask or nasal cannulae as required. Potent analgesia in the form of titrated opiates in adequate amounts is essential, accompanied by the appropriate antiemetic.

A fall in haematocrit usually reflects the large volume of infused fluid required to resuscitate the patient, although some blood may be lost into the retroperitoneal space, and transfusion may be required. Persistent elevation of blood glucose will necessitate insulin on a sliding scale. The onset of renal failure as indicated by a rising plasma urea and creatinine, worsening circulatory instability and/or respiratory failure evidenced by deterioration in arterial gas tensions with acidosis, indicate the need for a pulmonary arterial flotation catheter (Swan–Ganz catheter) to determine the optimal volume state (especially in the presence of non-cardiogenic pulmonary oedema adult respiratory distress syndrome (ARDS). Thereafter, renal failure will require treatment with frusemide infusion and renal dose dopamine. Persistent hypotension despite adequate filling pressure is managed by pressor agents (dopamine, dobutamine, adrenaline, noradrenaline). Respiratory failure (caused by non-cardiogenic pulmonary oedema) will necessitate endotracheal intubation and ventilation. Close liaison with the ITU anaesthetic staff and intensivists is essential.

Hypocalcaemia can rarely be demonstrable clinically by twitching, tetany and neuromuscular excitability and can be treated by intravenous injection of calcium gluconate. Asymptomatic albumin-corrected hypocalcaemia < 1.8 mmol/L should be corrected empirically. Derangement of clotting is common and should be reversed by administration of fresh frozen plasma if severe.

Antibiotics in the form of parenteral second- or third-generation cephalosporins (cefuroxime, cefotaxime) are indicated in severe disease, as some evidence is emerging that they reduce the overall infection rate in this group of patients. More potent broad-spectrum antibiotics such as imipenem have also been suggested to be efficacious, but the clinical data are relatively weak and coupled with their high expense this class of compounds cannot be recommended routinely. Specific infections in blood, urine or sputum will require appropriate therapy.

After 3 or 4 days, in the absence of improvement, parenteral nutrition should be commenced via a dedicated feeding line inserted with strict attention to asepsis. There are good data that indicate that indwelling vascular cannulae can serve as the source of organisms that ultimately colonize the necrotic pancreatic bed to produce infected necrosis. There is no evidence to suggest that low-lipid formulations have any benefit to offer over the conventional preparations. As soon as the patient can tolerate it, enteral nutrition should be used as emerging clinical data show this to be associated with a more rapid recovery with fewer complications. The place for selective decontamination of the gut and early enteral feeding is currently under review.

Ongoing assessment

Once the patient has been stratified and stabilized following admission it is important that regular reassessment is performed to detect and manage any complications. In the setting of acute pancreatitis, complications can be divided

Table 12.7 Complications of acute pancreatitis.

Local	General
Acute fluid collection	Circulation
Necrosis	Cardiovascular collapse
Infection	Coagulopathy
Pseudocyst	Respiratory
Pancreatic abscess	ARDS
	Pleural effusions
	Abdominal
	Ileus
	Intestinal ischaemia
	Fistulae
	Haemorrhage
	Renal tract
	Acute renal failure
	Metabolic
	Hypocalcaemia
	Hyperglycaemia
	Nutritional failure

into local and systemic types. Both forms are more likely to occur in severe disease (see Table 12.7). The systemic complications chiefly consist of individual or combinations of organ system dysfunction which may culminate in MOSF. The management of these critically ill patients requires organ system support in an ITU setting, as described above.

Detection of local complications of acute pancreatitis requires monitoring of the clinical status for signs of sepsis, together with judicious use of radiology. The commonest local complications are acute fluid collections, pancreatic necrosis sterile or infected, pseudocyst formation and true pancreatic abscess, and are discussed below.

The most accurate means of assessing the response of the patient to treatment during the course of an attack is by regular clinical evaluation with daily recording of the APACHE II score and measurement of CRP level in blood. Clinical signs of sepsis (high fever, tachycardia, circulatory instability), an increasing APACHE II score and/or laboratory signs suggestive of infection (leucocytosis, elevated CRP) demand active investigation. Peripheral sources of infection including chest, urinary tract and indwelling vascular cannulae must be considered and managed accordingly. Local retroperitoneal complications must be evaluated by radiological means — chiefly dynamic CT scanning, with fine needle aspiration and bacteriological culture of any collections suspected of being infected.

Some patients run an unremitting severe course, whilst others seem to improve and then deteriorate at a later stage with new symptoms or signs of sepsis. There is no clear pattern for the course of the disease.

Severe gallstone pancreatitis

It is important to recognize when gallstones are the cause of a severe attack. This may be evident if the patient has had gallstones previously documented, if ultrasound has shown gallstones within the gall bladder on this admission or if the clinical suspicion is high for example in the presence of jaundice and particularly if the transaminases are raised. In this instance, failure of the patient's condition to improve rapidly (within 48 h) following initial resuscitation is an indication for urgent ERCP and sphincterotomy. This measure should be covered by antibiotics and is not without risk of complications which include haemorrhage, sepsis or flare-up of the pancreatitis.

Available evidence from clinical trials suggests that this intervention may reduce overall mortality from severe attacks in this subset of patients. Similarly, an ERCP and duct drainage is essential in the presence of cholangitis which occurs in around 10% of patients in combination with acute pancreatitis.

Management of local complications

Acute fluid collections

Acute fluid collections occur early in the course of acute pancreatitis, are located in or near the pancreas, and always lack a wall of granulation or fibrous tissue. Acute fluid collections are common in patients with severe pancreatitis, occurring in 30 to 50% of cases (see Fig. 12.4). More than one half of these will resolve spontaneously and in an otherwise stable patient they do not require treatment. Thus in the absence

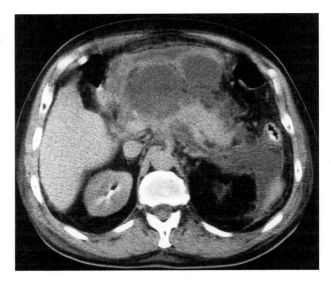

Fig. 12.4 CT scan showing acute fluid collection anterior to pancreas with further collection in the region of the tail.

of signs of sepsis, it is not recommended that percutaneous drains be inserted into these fluid collections. Such unnecessary attention merely increases the risk of introducing infection. Some acute fluid collections represent an earlier point in the development of a pseudocyst which will result if the collection persists and develops a defined wall.

Clinical features of sepsis demand assessment for the possibility of local infection. The development of infection in areas of necrosis or an acute fluid collection must be actively pursued by the use of CT (or ultrasound) guided fine needle aspiration. The aspirate should be examined by urgent Gram stain and culture. Subsequent management is determined by the extent of necrosis, as will be discussed below. Occasionally, however, an acute fluid collection (or an established pseudocyst) may become infected in the absence of large areas of pancreatic necrosis, and this may give rise over a period of weeks to a true pancreatic abscess. In such instances, percutaneous aspiration for diagnosis, and subsequent percutaneous drainage may suffice for treatment.

Pancreatic necrosis and infected pancreatic necrosis

Pancreatic necrosis is a diffuse or focal area(s) of non-viable pancreatic parenchyma, which is typically associated with peripancreatic fat necrosis. The diagnosis and extent of pancreatic necrosis is established on the basis of dynamic CT scanning as discussed above (see Fig. 12.3). In general, the degree of pancreatic necrosis determines the severity of an attack of acute pancreatitis and the subsequent risk of local or systemic complications and death. Extensive sterile pancreatic necrosis may produce a fulminating clinical picture with rapid onset of multisystem failure, circulatory collapse and death. The essential distinction to make, however, is between sterile and infected necrosis, since the onset of infection results in a trebling of the mortality rate. This discrimination can be made by the technique of CT-guided fine needle aspiration of the necrotic tissue and bacteriological culture. A negative aspirate does not completely exclude infection because of the chance of sampling error, and ultimately decisions regarding management must be made on the basis of the overall clinical picture.

Selected patients with sterile pancreatic necrosis can usually be managed non-operatively with full systems support. In a small number of cases, however, the clinical condition may continue to deteriorate, and there is some evidence that these patients may benefit from operation and debridement of necrotic tissue even in the absence of documented infection.

The majority of patients who run a persistently severe course, or who develop signs of sepsis will be found to have infected pancreatic necrosis and this complication now accounts for the majority of all deaths from acute pancreatitis. Infected necrosis is usually fatal if treated conservatively, and its diagnosis or high index of suspicion of infection is an absolute indication for operation. The risk of developing infection increases with the extent of parenchymal necrosis and the number of acute fluid collections. Those patients demonstrated radiologically to have a poor prognosis should therefore be monitored more closely. Although the onset of infected necrosis is often regarded as a relatively late occurrence usually declaring itself some weeks into an attack (the incidence increasing with time) it is important to note that up to 20% of infected cases will occur within the first week.

The surgical treatment of infected pancreatic necrosis is subject to debate, but the central principles of debridement and drainage are agreed. Individual units vary in the use of open packing ('laparostomy') and through irrigation (continuous retroperitoneal lavage) via bilateral flank drains placed in the retroperitoneum, with a sway towards the latter at the current time. It is wise to fashion a gastrostomy in anticipation of the requirement for prolonged gastric aspiration and a jejunostomy to establish early enteral feeding. Repeated operations and debridement may be required, as the process of peripancreatic necrosis and slough formation seems to continue, and these may lead to several complications. The commonest problems relate to small and large bowel fistulae, haemorrhage from the necrotic bed and into the gastrointestinal tract, colonic necrosis and mesenteric infarction. Although mortality still remains of the order of 30% in most units, in selected series of patients from specialized centres aggressive surgical intervention has resulted in improved outcome (mortality 6–11%). This may add to the argument in favour of managing these patients in specialist centres.

Acute pseudocyst

An acute pseudocyst is a collection of pancreatic juice enclosed in a wall of fibrous or granulation tissue that arises following an attack of acute pancreatitis. The formation of a pseudocyst requires 4 or more weeks from the onset of acute pancreatitis. The pseudocyst arises as a function of persistence and maturation of an acute fluid collection, which can be followed by serial ultrasounds and less frequently CT or MRI scans (see Fig. 12.5). The clinical features are usually of abdominal pain, fullness and vomiting, and a palpable mass in the upper abdomen. The serum amylase often remains persistently elevated during recovery from the attack, or becomes elevated after an initial fall. Some 50% of acute fluid collections resolve spontaneously, but fewer established pseudocysts resolve without surgery. Furthermore, established pseudocysts are at risk of developing complications, including haemorrhage, rupture, infection and mechanical obstruction to the stomach and duodenum. For these reasons, operation is recommended for pseudocysts greater

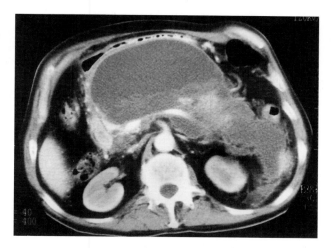

Fig. 12.5 CT scan from patient in Fig. 12.4 after 4 weeks, demonstrating mature acute pseudocyst.

than 6 cm in size and 6 weeks old. The procedure of choice is operative internal drainage into the stomach or small bowel. Internal stent drainage can now be accomplished by endoscopic and radiological means, and these techniques require long term evaluation.

Pancreatic abscess

A pancreatic abscess is a circumscribed intra-abdominal collection of pus, usually in proximity to the pancreas, containing little or no pancreatic necrosis, which arises as a consequence of acute pancreatitis. The clinical picture is variable, but the usual presentation is with signs of sepsis. Pancreatic abscesses tend to occur late in the course of an attack of severe acute pancreatitis, often after 4 or more weeks. Pancreatic abscesses probably arise in the context of limited pancreatic necrosis with subsequent liquefaction and infection, or as a result of infection of an acute fluid collection or pseudocyst. As such, the clinical expression differs from that of infected necrosis which typically displays a fulminant course from the outset with progressive systemic features. Rather, a pancreatic abscess runs a more indolent course, with initial recovery from the attack and subsequent late features of infection. The diagnosis is confirmed by dynamic CT scanning, which details the anatomical location and presence of associated necrosis. The distinction is important, as treatment and outcomes differ. A pancreatic abscess has less than half the mortality risk of infected necrosis, and may in the first instance be managed by percutaneous drainage techniques (although open operation may be required, particularly if necrosis is evident).

Summary

Acute pancreatitis represents a spectrum of disease ranging from a mild attack with rapid recovery to a fulminating illness with multisystem failure and death. Early stratification is central to the treatment of these patients, using objective criteria to identify those with a severe attack. These patients can then be targeted for more invasive monitoring and aggressive therapy, which should include a dynamic CT scan and management in an HDU/ITU setting. Subsequent ongoing assessment is required for the early detection and treatment of complications. Such measures may improve outcome from this disease which still has a mortality rate of 10%.

CHAPTER 13

Upper gastrointestinal haemorrhage

Robert J. C. Steele

Introduction

Currently, as in almost all areas of surgery, the management of upper gastrointestinal bleeding is undergoing a revolution. Of all forms of treatment, endoscopic therapy is perhaps having the greatest impact, but new interventional techniques and novel drug strategies are also evolving. The role of surgical intervention has been modified accordingly, and it is important for all surgeons who operate on the gastrointestinal tract to be aware of these developments even if they do not employ them directly. In this chapter, we shall start with sections on initial management and diagnosis and then consider the medical, endoscopic and surgical managements of variceal and peptic ulcer bleeding in turn.

Initial management of upper gastrointestinal bleeding

Patients bleeding from the oesophagus, stomach or duodenum will normally present with a history of haematemesis, melaena or rectal bleeding. It is important to bear the last of these in mind, as the patient with profuse fresh rectal haemorrhage, especially when accompanied by haemodynamic instability, may well be bleeding from the upper gastrointestinal tract. In assessing a patient with possible upper gastrointestinal bleeding there are three crucial questions to answer in the first few minutes:

1 *Is the airway clear?* It may be necessary to evacuate blood and clot from the upper airway.
2 *Is there evidence of active bleeding?* Although this may be difficult to ascertain, the patient who is losing fresh blood must be at high risk.
3 *Is there evidence of hypovolaemia?* Pulse rate and blood pressure must be measured at the first opportunity whether or not there are clinical signs of shock.
Management should then continue as follows:
1 Establish vascular access with a wide bore (14 gauge) cannula, and cross-match blood.
2 If haemodynamically stable, obtain a full history, carry out a thorough examination and arrange for an upper gastrointestinal endoscopy on the next available list, preferably within 24 hours.

3 If haemodynamically unstable, resuscitation must take priority. A reasonable rule of thumb is to institute and continue with aggressive fluid replacement therapy as long as the systolic blood pressure is less than 100 mmHg and the pulse rate greater than 100/min. In elderly patients or in those with cardiac disease, the central venous pressure (CVP) should also be monitored. It should be stressed, however, that a CVP catheter should only be inserted by an experienced operator, and that monitoring should be carried out in an adequate environment such as a high dependency unit. Severely ill or compromised patients should also have a urinary catheter inserted, and the urine volume maintained at not less than 30 ml/h.

Fluid replacement can start with 500 ml of normal saline over the first 15 min, followed by 500 ml of colloid (e.g. gelatin) over the next 15 min. Resuscitation should then continue with blood at one unit every 15 min. If the blood pressure fails to come up or falls, this infusion rate must be increased accordingly, but when the patient becomes stable (BP > 100 mmHg and pulse < 100/min) rapid infusion must be stopped, and maintenance fluids only given. If the CVP is being measured, then rapid infusion should proceed until it is more than 5 cm H_2O.

If the CVP remains greater than 12 cm H_2O and the BP greater than 100 mmHg, then overload has occurred and 40 mg of frusemide should be given. Frusemide should not be given solely to increase urine output, as this will exacerbate hypovolaemia. If the CVP remains greater than 12 cm H_2O, and BP less than 100 mmHg, then there is a degree of pump failure, and intensive care is necessary. It may be advisable to start an infusion of dopamine at 5 µg/kg/min while this is being arranged.

If stabilization is difficult to achieve by these measures, urgent investigation to locate the bleeding point and decide on further management is then necessary.

> **1** Adequate resuscitation is the first priority in upper gastrointestinal bleeding.
> **2** Endoscopy must be carried out in optimal circumstances by an experienced endoscopist.
> **3** Surgeons who operate for gastrointestinal bleeding should be familiar with endoscopic appearances.

Diagnostic endoscopy

For upper gastrointestinal bleeding, flexible endoscopy of the oesophagus, stomach and duodenum is the investigation of choice, and although techniques for this procedure are well established, special considerations have to be taken into account in bleeding.

Firstly, the patient must be prepared for the endoscopy, and the first priority is to ensure adequate resuscitation, as described above. In the patient who is bleeding rapidly, resuscitation should continue during the endoscopy, and in the unstable patient who is actively vomiting blood there should be no hesitation in contacting an anaesthetist so that general anaesthesia and cuffed endotracheal intubation can be established. This latter precaution has two advantages; firstly, it allows safer endoscopy with minimal risk of aspiration and secondly, it permits rapid progression to surgery if the bleeding cannot be controlled by endoscopic therapy.

Under most circumstances it is feasible to carry out the endoscopy under sedation in an endoscopy unit, but even then it is important that the patient is properly monitored. Pulse and blood pressure should be measured regularly, preferably by means of an automatic device incorporating an alarm system, and the use of a pulse oximeter is similarly mandatory. This latter device detects arterial desaturation, and it is a wise precaution to administer 40–60% oxygen via nasal prongs as this has been shown to prevent hypoxia during prolonged endoscopic procedures.

The endoscopy should be performed on a trolley which can be tilted in both directions, the head-down position may be required for the shocked patient, and the head up position can be useful to prevent blood from refluxing into the oesophagus from the stomach and obscuring the view. Initially the patient should be in the left-lateral position, as this will allow blood to pool in the fundus where bleeding lesions are uncommon (Fig. 13.1).

Most currently available endoscopes are suitable for the bleeding patient, but although video endoscopes now produce very high quality images under normal circumstances, the presence of large amounts of blood can degrade the video image to such as extent as to hamper the procedure. For this reason the ideal instrument is still a fibreoptic endoscope, and as a therapeutic manoeuvre may be required, this should have a wide working channel and a forward washing channel or two working channels (Fig. 13.2). Other equipment which should be available includes a wide bore (40 Fr) stomach lavage tube which should have an open end to allow aspiration of clots, and a pharyngeal overtube which facilitates repeated changes between the endoscope and the lavage tube, and protects the airway.

During the endoscopy, the air/water channel is at risk of becoming blocked by clot, and it should therefore be flushed at frequent intervals by fully depressing the

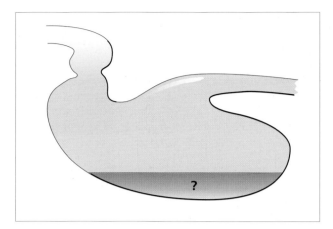

Fig. 13.1 In the left lateral position blood tends to pool in the fundus. Thus the view is obscured in the least likely site for a bleeding lesion.

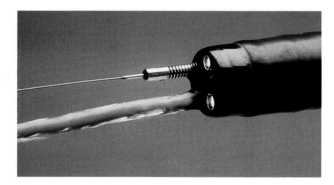

Fig. 13.2 Twin channel endoscope in action.

appropriate button. If clot adheres to the tip of the endoscope, obscuring the view, it can be cleared by a jet of water generated by injecting the entire contents of a 20 ml syringe through the working channel. This procedure is also useful for clearing clot in order to obtain a clear view of the bleeding lesion.

If blood is seen on entering the oesophagus, it can be difficult to decide whether it is originating from the oesophagus or whether it is refluxing back from the stomach. If aspiration of blood through the endoscope is insufficient, then tipping the patient head up will encourage the blood to fall back into the stomach, and the situation will usually become clear. Attention must be paid to identifying varices, and if too much insufflation pressure is used, small varices may be compressed and difficult to see. Mallory–Weiss tears and lesions within a hiatus hernia are often overlooked, and it should always be part of the routine to examine the lower end of the oesophagus by obtaining a retroflex view when the endoscope is in the stomach.

When the stomach appears to be full of blood clot, it is important to give the air insufflation time to distend the stomach fully. If the patient is correctly positioned, the clot will then lie in the fundus leaving the lesser curve, antrum and duodenum clear for inspection. However, if it is still impossible to obtain a good view, the endoscope is removed and, preferably with an overtube in position, a lavage tube is inserted and direct suction applied. This may remove enough blood and clot, but if it does not, it becomes necessary to carry out lavage by attaching a funnel to the tube and rapidly pouring in a litre of water. This will tend to break up the clot, which can then be siphoned out by placing the tube in a dependent position.

Loose clot lying in the duodenum can be washed out by a jet of water as described above, but active bleeding can be a problem. If this is massive, then fruitless struggling to obtain haemostasis can be dangerous, and surgery should proceed forthwith. If a definite lesion is seen in the first part of the duodenum, then the second part should not be entered for fear of traumatizing the lesion and initiating or exacerbating active bleeding.

Endoscopic appearances

For the gastrointestinal surgeon who may be called upon to operate for upper gastrointestinal bleeding, familiarity with the endoscopic appearances of the common pathologies is vital. Ideally, the surgeon should carry out the procedure, but if this is not possible, then every effort should be made to attend the endoscopy when there is a possibility of surgical intervention. The most likely causes are shown in Table 13.1, and these will now be dealt with in turn.

Oesophagitis

Peptic oesophagitis can be graded, as shown in Fig. 13.3, and with severe ulceration moderate sized vessels can become

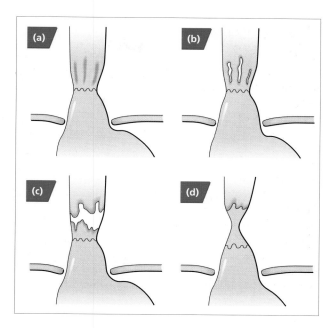

Fig. 13.3 Grades of peptic oesophagitis: (a) Linear streaks (I); (b) linear erosions (II); (c) confluent erosions (III); and (d) stricture (IV).

exposed. If these bleed, it can be difficult to distinguish from variceal bleeding although the clearly pulsatile nature of the haemorrhage should provide the diagnosis. Very occasionally, a peptic ulcer within a Barrett's oesophagus may be the culprit, and this 'Barrett's ulcer' must be distinguished from a carcinoma.

Varices

Oesophageal varices appear as bluish, longitudinal columns, with a wavy configuration (Fig. 13.4). There are usually four or more columns, and the extent to which they bulge into the lumen of the oesophagus can be used as a classification system (Fig. 13.5). Active bleeding is seen as a non-pulsatile jet of blood from a varix, and a 'cherry red' spot on a varix can be taken as a sign of recent haemorrhage.

Carcinoma

A carcinoma is usually exophytic and ulcerated.

Mallory–Weiss tear

This lesion, which inevitably follows a vomiting bout, tends to involve the gastric mucosa more than the oesophagus, and is therefore best seen in retroflexion. It is usually associated with oozing although active arterial bleeding can occur.

Table 13.1 Common causes of upper gastrointestinal bleeding.

Oesophagus	Oesophagitis
	Varices
	Carcinoma
	Mallory–Weiss tear
Stomach	Peptic ulcer
	Gastritis
	Dieulafoy lesion
	Varices
	Vascular malformations
	Tumours
Duodenum	Peptic Ulcer
	Aortoduodenal Fistula

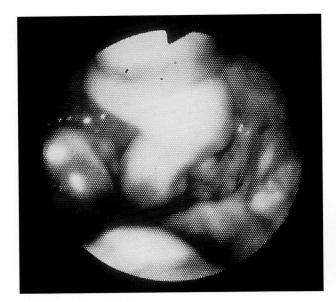

Fig. 13.4 Oesophageal varices.

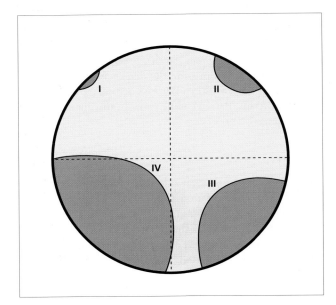

Fig. 13.5 Grading of varices according to protrusion into the lumen.

Peptic ulcer

In the stomach, the peptic ulcer is a round defect in the mucosa of highly variable size, usually situated in the antrum or along the lesser curve. In the duodenum, ulcers normally lie in the first part, but although anterior lesions are usually obvious on passing the pylorus, posterior ulcers

can be difficult to see. When an ulcer is identified, special attention must be paid to any stigmata of recent haemorrhage. These appearances can be classified as (a) active pulsatile bleeding (Fig. 13.6); (b) active non-pulsatile bleeding; (c) visible vessel (Fig. 13.7); (d) adherent blood clot (Fig. 13.8); and (e) flat red or black spots.

Although active pulsatile bleeding carries the highest risk, the non-bleeding visible vessel or adherent clot imply a 30–50% chance of rebleeding. Unfortunately, there is a large degree of interobserver variation in the interpretation

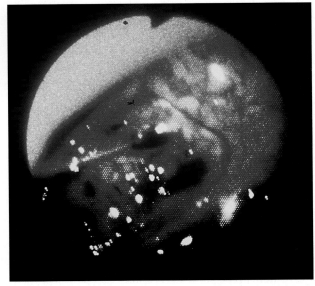

Fig. 13.6 Arterial bleeding from a peptic ulcer.

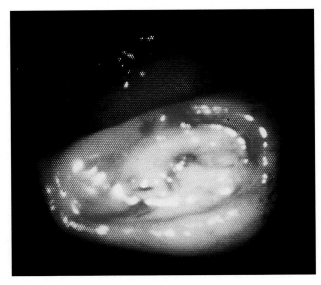

Fig. 13.7 Visible vessel in a peptic ulcer.

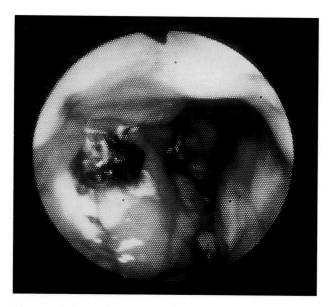

Fig. 13.8 Adherent clot in a peptic ulcer.

of these appearances and their usefulness is thereby limited.

Gastritis

Erosive gastritis is usually seen in the antrum, and consists of multiple shallow ulcers. The precise site of bleeding can be very difficult to ascertain in this condition.

Dieulafoy lesion

This consists of a tiny ulcer exposing a large vessel which sticks out of the mucosa anywhere in the stomach. Unless it is actively bleeding it can be very difficult to see.

Gastric varices

Situated in the fundus, these can be very difficult to distinguish from the normal gastric rugae, and full gastric distension is necessary for a confident diagnosis.

Vascular malformations

Haemangiomas may occur in the stomach, either singly or as part of the Osler–Weber–Rendu syndrome.

Gastric tumours

Bleeding gastric cancers are inevitably ulcerated, and they can be distinguished from benign ulcers by their typical, heaped-up mucosal rim. The commonest benign tumour is the leiomyoma, and this may bleed from a central, apical ulcer.

Aortoduodenal fistula

Usually the result of an aortic graft, the commonest site is in the third part of the duodenum. While there may be nothing to see, there may be a pulsatile mass or even visible graft material.

Medical therapy of acute variceal bleeding

The patient with variceal bleeding should be assessed and resuscitated as above, but there are some special considerations which have to be taken into account. Because the bleeding is often torrential, and because clotting abnormalities are common, it is advisable to send blood for a clotting screen and arrange fresh frozen plasma and platelet concentrate well in advance. It is also important to avoid large volumes of crystalloid, as this will exacerbate the ascites and peripheral oedema associated with portal hypertension and liver failure. The patient is also at risk of hepatic coma, and appropriate preventative measures should be taken. The use of opiates should be avoided, and blood glucose levels should be monitored with a 10% glucose infusion used to correct hypoglycaemia. In order to reduce the amount of protein in the gut, oral lactulose should be given at 10 ml q.i.d., and neomycin 1 g q.i.d. should be given to reduce the production of toxic metabolites by bacterial flora.

The main pharmacological agents which have been used to control acute variceal bleeding are vasopressin and somatostatin or its analogues. Vasopressin is a splanchnic vasoconstrictor, and infusion at 0.5–0.6 U/min will reduce portal pressure sufficiently to control acute variceal bleeding in 50–70% of cases. Unfortunately the side effects of vasoconstriction, notably angina and cardiac arrhythmias, can be a problem, and its use has been all but abandoned in many centres. Somatostatin, and its longer acting analogue octreotide, are much more selective in terms of their action on mesenteric smooth muscle, and there is evidence that a 50 μg bolus of octreotide followed by an infusion at 50 μg/h may be as effective at controlling acute haemorrhage as sclerotherapy (see below).

The risk of rebleeding from varices may be reduced by the long-term administration of β-blockers such as propranolol, but this has no place in the treatment of the acute bleed. Their negative inotropic and chronotropic effects may indeed compromise the hypovolaemic patient.

Endoscopic therapy for variceal bleeding

For many years, the mainstay of treatment for bleeding oesophageal varices has been endoscopic sclerotherapy, but endoscopic banding has gained favour recently. These techniques will be considered separately.

Sclerotherapy

It is now accepted that acute variceal bleeding can be treated by endoscopic treatment in the majority of cases. For sclerotherapy, a twin-channelled endoscope is ideal for three reasons. First, suction and irrigation are still available with the injector needle in place. Second, the size of the instrument is useful in obtaining a degree of tamponade, and third, the two channels provide flexibility in obtaining the correct position for the needle.

> 1 Active variceal bleeding can usually be controlled by endoscopic therapy.
> 2 Variceal banding is at least as effective as sclerotherapy and may be preferable.
> 3 Oesophageal transection using a staple gun is the procedure of choice when surgical intervention is necessary.
> 4 Transjugular intrahepatic portosystemic shunting may be of value in recurrent haemorrhage.

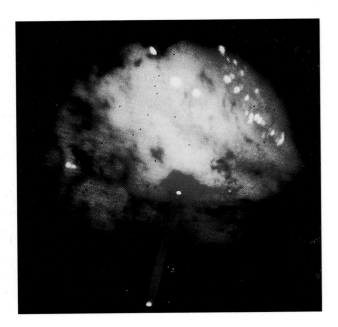

Fig. 13.9 Active variceal bleeding.

The most commonly used sclerosants are 3% sodium tetradecyl sulphate (STD), 5% ethanolamine, 1% polidocanol and absolute alcohol. Injection needles are available in many different designs and sizes, but it is generally agreed that the disposable type should be used in all cases to obviate any risk of disease transmission. When an oil-based sclerosant such as ethanolamine is used, it is necessary to employ a needle of at least 23 gauge, whereas the less viscous sclerosants can be injected by means of a thinner needle.

Under most circumstances, it is possible to inject varices using topical anaesthesia and sedation, and the flexible endoscope has now almost completely supplanted the rigid oesophagoscope for this purpose. There has been some debate as to whether injection should be performed directly into the varices or around them, but it is now generally agreed that the intravariceal technique leads to more rapid obliteration of the varices.

If varices are seen at endoscopy, it is still important to carry out a full examination of the stomach and duodenum if possible, as a significant proportion of varices patients may be bleeding from some other lesion. Active bleeding from a varix is usually seen as a jet of blood (Fig. 13.9), but if no active bleeding is seen, varices can be assumed to be the site of bleeding if no other lesions are found in the upper gastrointestinal tract. If one of the varices is bleeding actively, this should be injected first by puncturing it just proximal to the bleeding point and depositing 1–2 ml of sclerosant. Further injections should then proceed from the oesophagogastric junction upwards at 2-cm intervals in all the variceal columns until 15 ml of sclerosant have been used.

If massive bleeding obscures the view, the endoscope should be inserted into the stomach, and as much blood as possible should be aspirated. The shaft of the instrument will compress the varices, and should be left in position for at least 5 min. The endoscope should then be withdrawn slowly, with the patient in a head-up position if possible, and it is then usually feasible to obtain a view which is clear enough to place the injection precisely. Occasionally, of course, the bleeding is just too profuse, and under these circumstances the insertion of a Sengstaken–Blakemore tube becomes necessary (see below), and the endoscopy can be repeated at 24–48 h.

If the sclerotherapy is successful in controlling the haemorrhage, repeat sclerotherapy should be carried out at weekly intervals until the varices have been obliterated, and check endoscopy with repeat injections as necessary at 6-monthly intervals thereafter. Serious complications are relatively rare, but ulceration does occur in about 50% of cases. Stricture formation occurs after multiple injections in about 5% of cases, but can usually be managed by endoscopic dilatation. Perforation of the oesophagus is rare, but may occur if large amounts of sclerosant are used over a short period of time.

Banding

The technique of endoscopic banding has recently attracted a lot of interest, and a recent randomized trial has suggested that it may obliterate varices more quickly and with less rebleeding than sclerotherapy. It is also being used increas-

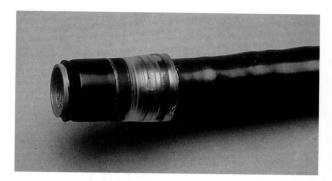

Fig. 13.10 Endoscopic band ligator.

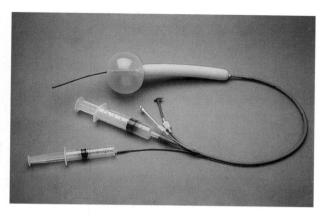

Fig. 13.11 Modified Sengstaken–Blakemore tube.

ingly for acute haemorrhage, and may in time supplant the use of sclerotherapy.

The equipment required for band ligation (the Stiegmann–Goff ligator) is made up of an outer cylindrical adaptor which fits onto the tip of the endoscope, an inner cylinder preloaded with an elastic 'O' ring and a trip wire for pulling the inner cylinder into the outer adaptor to release the ring (Fig. 13.10). When the use of banding is anticipated, it is necessary to use an overtube to allow easy passage of the device, and facilitate multiple loadings and re-insertions.

The steps for device assembly and application can be summarized as follows:

1 The outer cylinder is attached to the tip of the endoscope.
2 The trip wire is passed through the working channel of the endoscope.
3 The inner cylinder with its preloaded 'O' ring is attached to the end of the trip wire by means of a double groove system located inside the cylinder. It is important that the end of the cylinder with the 'O' ring closest to the edge faces away from the endoscope.
4 The inner cylinder is then fitted inside the adapter so that the 'O' ring is close to the edge of the adapter.
5 The endoscope is passed, and a portion of the varix to be treated is selected. In the non-bleeding case, this should be close to the gastro-oesophageal junction; if there is active bleeding, the actual bleeding point should be targeted.
6 Direct contact is then made with the varix, and suction applied to draw the tissue into the inner cylinder.
7 Keeping the suction button depressed, the trip wire is pulled to fire the 'O' ring. Suction can then be released to allow inspection. The process is repeated as often as deemed necessary.

Balloon tamponade

Balloon tamponade of varices is necessary when endoscopic therapy and octreotide infusion prove ineffective in controlling acute haemorrhage. The most commonly used device is the Sengstaken–Blakemore tube, or one of its variations.

This comprises a gastric balloon of about 400 ml capacity, an oesophageal balloon, and the best devices have aspiration lumens both distal and proximal to the balloons (Fig. 13.11).

The first step is to check the balloons for leaks. After thorough lubrication, the tube can then be inserted through the mouth or the nose; the latter may seem traumatic, but is in fact much more comfortable for the patient once it is in place. Once the tube has been passed, the gastric balloon must be inflated to about 350 ml using either water or air. If water is used, contrast medium such as Conray 280 should be added so that the position of the balloon can be checked on X-ray; if air is used, the balloon will be seen on a sufficiently penetrated chest X-ray. Of course, it is very important that the balloon is in the stomach when it is inflated, and this can be checked by insufflating air down the gastric lumen and auscultating over the stomach. Alternatively, if air is being used, this should be insufflated in series with a sphygmomanometer to ensure that the pressures that are being developed are not too high.

Once the balloon is inflated, it is important to apply traction in order to interrupt the blood flow into the varices at the gastro-oesophageal junction. The traction can then be maintained by taping the tube to the bridge of the nose if the nasal insertion route has been used. If the oral route has been used this is more difficult; it may then be necessary to develop traction using pulleys and weights which add another layer of complexity to the procedure. It is not usually necessary to deploy the oesophageal balloon, but if active bleeding continues, this should be connected to a sphygmomanometer and inflated to a pressure of 20–40 mmHg.

Balloon tamponade is very much a temporary measure, and traction should be released after a maximum period of 24 h to avoid necrosis of the gastro-oesophageal junction. This should be done in the endoscopy room, and if the bleeding has stopped, the tube can be removed, and immediate endoscopic therapy delivered.

Oesophageal surgery for variceal bleeding

Very occasionally all the above measures will fail, and direct oesophageal surgery will be necessary. Direct under-running of oesophageal varices has been supplanted by the use of the circular end-to-end anastomosis stapling gun, and the best approach is through an upper midline abdominal incision. The oesophagus is carefully mobilized with ligature of the surrounding high-pressure venous collaterals. Avoiding the vagus nerves, a strong silk suture is passed around the oesophagus, and a small gastrotomy is made in the upper aspect of the anterior gastric wall. A 30-mm circular stapler in the 'open' position is then inserted through the gastrotomy and into the lower oesophagus so that the silk suture can be tied firmly around the shaft of the stapling head (Fig. 13.12). The device is then closed and fired, simultaneously transecting and rejoining the oesophagus so that the portosystemic flow through the lower oesophageal veins is interrupted.

When gastric varices are bleeding, this is more difficult to control surgically, and when this becomes necessary, the stomach has to be opened via a high gastrotomy and the variceal columns under-run with a continuous suture. For any direct surgery to varices, the patient should come to the theatre with a Sengstaken tube in place, and the balloon

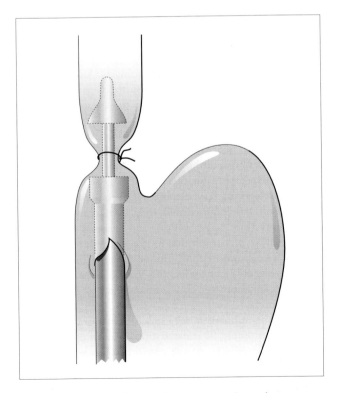

Fig. 13.12 Oesophageal transection using a circular stapler.

should only be let down at the last moment so that the stomach is not full of blood.

Portosystemic shunting

The rationale behind portosystemic shunting is to lower portal pressure by diverting portal blood into systemic circulation. The most common surgical procedures which have been employed to achieve this have been the direct portocaval shunt or the selective 'Warren' shunt in which the splenic vein is anastomosed to the left renal vein so that the short gastric veins are decompressed into the systemic system. Although good results have been reported from specialist centres for these operations, they are widely associated with a high operative mortality, and with increasingly good results from endoscopic therapy they have tended to lose favour.

However, the advent of a new technique has brought shunting back into the arena as a viable option for variceal bleeding. The transjugular intrahepatic portosystemic stent-shunt (TIPSS) is inserted by interventional radiological techniques which involve passing a sheath over a guidewire via the internal jugular vein into the right or middle hepatic veins. A stylet is then passed through the sheath to puncture a branch of the portal vein within the liver, the tract between the hepatic vein and portal vein is dilated with an angioplasty balloon, and an expanding metal stent (Wallstent) is inserted to keep the tract open.

The preliminary results of this procedure indicate that it may be useful in the control of refractory variceal bleeding, but in common with the open procedures, it is associated with the development of encephalopathy in patients with severe liver disease. In addition, shunt dysfunction may occur over a 6–12 month period in 15–60% of cases.

With the introduction of TIPSS, the indications for portosystemic shunting may change, and there are current trials comparing TIPSS with endoscopic treatment for the first episode of bleeding. The jury is still out on shunting, but it should certainly be considered in good-risk patients (Child's grade A and B) when there is recurrent haemorrhage despite vigorous endoscopic therapy.

Medical therapy of acute peptic ulcer bleeding

Most patients with bleeding from a peptic ulcer will recover spontaneously, and drug therapy can only be considered to be of value if it can reduce the need for surgery and, if possible, mortality rates.

The two main approaches which have been tried are, first, reduction of gastric acid secretion and, second, inhibition of fibrinolysis. The rationale behind acid inhibition is based on the observation that acid impairs platelet function and haemostasis, so that a high intragastric pH might be expected to reduce the rate of rebleeding or continued bleeding from peptic ulcers. Twenty-seven trials of H_2 receptor antagonists have been reviewed in a meta-analysis, but although this suggested that such drugs might reduce surgery and mortality rates, meta-analysis is subject to various types of bias which are impossible to eliminate completely. More important information is available from two large independent placebo-controlled trials, one which studied the H_2 receptor antagonist famotidine and the other the proton pump inhibitor omeprazole. Unfortunately, neither of these studies was able to demonstrate an effect, and it must be concluded that acid inhibition has no clinically useful influence on acute gastrointestinal bleeding.

Fibrinolysis inhibition would seem a reasonable approach, and the plasminogen inhibitor tranexamic acid has been tested in at least six randomized, double-blind controlled trials. A meta-analysis of the various trials has suggested that treated patients do benefit in terms of rebleeding, need for surgery and mortality, but as this was greatly influenced by a single study it cannot be taken as conclusive evidence.

Somatostatin and its analogues have been tried in peptic ulcer bleeding owing to their abilities to inhibit acid secretion and reduce splanchnic blood flow, but trials have proved disappointing. Somatostatin infusion may, however, ameliorate torrential bleeding from multiple erosions. The prostaglandin misoprostol has also been tried, and has been found to reduce the need for surgery in a small trial, but its role has not been fully established.

In summary, therefore, pharmacological therapy still has a long way to go before it can make an impact on peptic ulcer bleeding in terms of emergency surgery and mortality rates, but future studies are awaited with interest.

Endoscopic haemostasis

At present, there are five main endoscopic methods of controlling non-variceal bleeding: laser photocoagulation, bipolar diathermy, heater probe treatment, injection sclerotherapy and adrenaline injection. Other methods have been tried (Table 13.2), but none have proved particularly satisfactory. As the majority of patients with peptic ulcer bleeding will settle without intervention, it is very important that all new techniques are subjected to controlled trials before they are accepted.

In these trials, it is important that the end points are clearly defined. Mortality is the most important, but, given an average death rate of no more than 10%, it would take a very large trial to demonstrate a significant improvement attributable to any specific treatment. The next most useful end-point is the need for urgent operation; this can be associated with a mortality of around 20% and it is therefore likely that a reduction in emergency surgery would translate into a lowering of mortality and morbidity rates. In this

Table 13.2 Different methods which have been employed in endoscopic haemostasis for non-variceal bleeding. Commonly used techniques are marked with an asterix.

Thermal methods	Laser photocoagulation
	Argon
	Nd–YAG*
	Diathermy
	Monopolar
	Bipolar (BICAP)*
	Heater probe*
	Microwave
Injection methods	Adrenaline*
	Alcohol*
	Sclerosant
	STD
	Ethanolamine
	Polidocanol*
	Clotting factors
Topical applications	Collagen
	Clotting factors
	Cyanoacrylate glue
	Ferromagnetic tamponade
Mechanical methods	Balloon tamponade
	Clips
	Staples
	Sutures

---

1 There is no good evidence that pharmacological intervention alters the outcome in upper gastrointestinal bleeding.
2 Adrenaline injection is the most effective endoscopic treatment for active bleeding.
3 Heat probe and injection sclerotherapy are also effective but laser treatment is no longer considered appropriate.
4 Rebleeding after endoscopic treatment should be regarded as a major indication for surgery.
5 The main aim of surgery is to obtain secure haemostasis and the role of the vagotomy is controversial.

---

section each of the widely used methods are discussed, emphasizing the results of randomized trials comparing endoscopic treatment with conventional therapy. In addition, more recent studies which have set out to compare different techniques are considered.

Laser photocoagulation

Laser light transmits energy which is converted into heat on contact with tissue, and the resultant coagulation can produce haemostasis. The two types of laser which have been used with fibreoptic endoscopes to treat bleeding are the argon ion and the neodymium–yttrium aluminium garnet (Nd–YAG). The argon laser has a wavelength of 440–520 nm, and the coagulation effect is superficial. The Nd–YAG, on the other hand, has a wavelength of over 1000 nm, and the greater depth of tissue penetration means that it is more effective in treating haemorrhage from large vessels. As it is difficult to estimate the direction in which a vessel is running in the base of an ulcer (Fig. 13.13), the bleeding point or visible vessel should be surrounded by a ring of laser pulses in order to maximize the chances of coagulating the main vessel trunk (Fig. 13.14). Care must be taken as it is possible to precipitate bleeding by vaporizing protective clot overlying a hole in an artery.

There have been three randomized studies of the argon laser, and although the first was unable to demonstrate any significant benefit, two subsequent trials did suggest a reduction in the need for emergency surgery. The Nd–YAG laser has been subjected to nine trials, but four of these were poorly designed and do not merit consideration. Of the remainder, four produced favourable results in terms of rebleeding of need for surgery, and one was unable to demonstrate any effect.

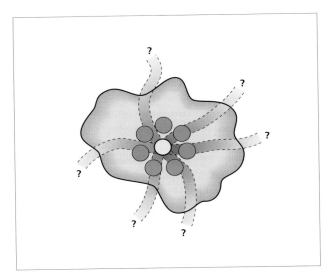

Fig. 13.14 Vessel surrounded by a tight ring of coagulation points in order to obliterate the feeding vessel.

Bipolar diathermy

Bipolar diathermy has been adapted for use in gastrointestinal bleeding by means of the BICAP® probe which consists of three pairs of longitudinal electrodes separated by ceramic insulators and arranged in a radial pattern around the tip. The current delivered to the tissue is dependent on the electrical resistance of that tissue, and this in turn increases with desiccation. Thus, as the treated tissue dries out, the current is automatically reduced so that the degree of damage is limited, and sticking of the probe to the tissue is less likely to occur than with a monopolar electrode.

To achieve haemostasis, this device relies on the principle of 'coaptive coagulation' in which external pressure of the probe is used to tamponade the vessel to be treated before the current is applied (Fig. 13.15). By this means, dissipation of heat by the blood flow in the vessel (the 'heat-sink' effect) is minimized, and in active bleeding, effective tamponade will confirm that the heat is being delivered to the correct spot. If there is no active bleeding it is more difficult to know where the probe should be positioned, and it is necessary to produce a ring of coagulation around the vessel by multiple applications of the probe, just as in laser therapy.

Three controlled trials of bipolar diathermy have demonstrated no benefit in ulcer bleeding, and although one did show a reduction in clinical rebleeding, it was unable to demonstrate any differences in the need for emergency surgery between the treated patients and the controls. However, in two other randomized studies, both carried out by a single operator, much better results were obtained.

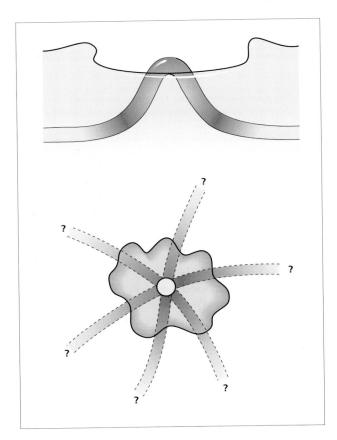

Fig. 13.13 The visible vessel loops up to the ulcer base (top), but the endoscopic view cannot indicate the direction in which the vessel is running (bottom).

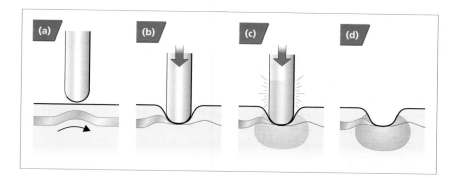

Fig. 13.15 Coaptive coagulation.

Heat probe

The heat probe is operated in much the same way as bipolar diathermy, using the same basic principle of coaptive coagulation. It consists of a hollow metal tip containing a heating coil which can rapidly raise the temperature of the probe to 150 °C, and because no electrical current has to pass into the tissue, the metal can be coated with insulating 'non-stick' material which helps to prevent adherence to coagulated tissue.

The heat probe has two theoretical advantages over bipolar diathermy. First, because the temperature produced is independent of desiccation of the treated tissue, there is no interruption to the flow of energy as coagulation proceeds, and tissue bonding may be stronger. It is possible, however, that this same property may increase the risk of perforation. The second advantage of the heat probe is that the power settings allow delivery of a pre-set amount of energy, and the duration of the pulse is governed by a silicon chip sensor built into the probe tip. Thus, unlike diathermy, the energy used can be very precisely controlled, although whether this represents a real advantage is open to debate.

To date, there have been four randomized studies comparing heat probe therapy with no active intervention; two of these reported no measurable benefit from the endoscopic therapy, but two showed a significant reduction in rebleeding when active treatment was compared with sham treatment.

Injection treatment

Ulcer bleeding can be treated by the endoscopic injection of either adrenaline or sclerosant. Some work has also been done on the injection of clotting factors, but this is still at an early stage. Adrenaline (1 : 10 000) can bring about permanent haemostasis by a combination of tissue pressure from the injected fluid and active vasospasm producing initial haemostasis and hence allowing the formation of platelet and fibrin thrombus within the vessel lumen. Adrenaline

also has a role in the activation of platelets, and this may aid the process. Sclerosants act in a quite different way; the detergent sclerosants such as polidocanol or STD cause thrombosis by damaging the endothelium, and absolute alcohol produces rapid dehydration and fixation of tissue with the same result.

The technique of injection is essentially the same regardless of the agent used, although it must be stressed that excessive use of sclerosant, especially alcohol, will cause extension of the ulcer and may lead to perforation. A standard endoscopic injection needle of the type used for variceal bleeding is used, and if the ulcer base is fibrotic it is better to rely on the metal, type as firm pressure will be required. Even if sclerosant is to be used, it is now standard practice to start with adrenaline to provide initial haemostasis if there is active bleeding. The needle is advanced into the base of the bleeding point, and 0.5–1.0 ml of the adrenaline solution is injected. This will usually stop the bleeding, but if it does not, the position of the needle should be changed, and further injection carried out. When the bleeding has been controlled, sclerosant or extra adrenaline should be injected around the vessel. In the case of a non-bleeding visible vessel, the sclerosant can be injected in 0.5 ml aliquots around the vessel from the outset.

Adrenaline injection has been widely used in conjunction with both sclerotherapy and laser, and the results of laser treatment have been shown to be improved by the initial adrenaline. With such combined therapy, it is impossible to know which component has exerted the major therapeutic effect, but in a randomized controlled trial of patients with actively bleeding ulcers, adrenaline injection alone significantly reduced transfusion rates, the need for emergency surgery and the duration of hospital stay.

No true randomized study of alcohol injection has been reported, but extremely good results have been achieved by Japanese workers using this technique. The sclerosant polidocanol has been examined in two randomized trials, both of which also utilized pre-injection with adrenaline. In both, reductions in rebleeding were seen.

Comparative studies and conclusions

Recently, a number of randomized comparisons of different methods of endoscopic haemostasis have been reported. The Nd–YAG laser has been compared with bipolar diathermy, heat probe and injection treatment. Bipolar diathermy has been compared with heat probe, alcohol injection and adrenaline injection. The heat probe has been compared with alcohol injection, and studies have looked for differences between adrenaline injection alone and combinations of adrenaline and sclerosant or heat probe.

These studies have produced conflicting results, and are not very useful in establishing the ideal method of endoscopic haemostasis. There is little doubt, however, that in the right hands endoscopic haemostasis for non-variceal bleeding can be effective in producing initial haemostasis, reducing the rate of rebleeding and diminishing the need for urgent or emergency surgical intervention. It is also possible that it may have an effect on mortality in certain high risk groups, and in a recent comprehensive meta-analysis of the available trials comparing the various techniques with untreated controls, it was found that, overall, endoscopic therapy did significantly reduce mortality (odds ratio 0.55; 95% confidence interval 0.40–0.76). This is open to all the criticisms of meta-analysis, however, and convincing evidence on mortality from a single study has yet to be provided.

A major problem in this field is deciding on which of the various methods to use. In practice, the decision comes down to personal preference, individual expertise and the availability of equipment. It should be pointed out, however, that laser therapy does not appear to have any advantages over the other simpler and cheaper techniques, and it must be stressed that in some of the trials which have demonstrated its efficacy cases were excluded if the bleeding point was not accessible to the laser beam.

Injection methods are simple and relatively inexpensive, and adrenaline injection has the attraction of being the most 'physiological' and least traumatic of all the available techniques. However, its efficacy has only been proven in active bleeding, and its effect on the non-bleeding visible vessel is less certain. At present, therefore, it would seem sensible to opt for sclerosant or one of the thermal techniques in the high-risk non-bleeding lesion, and to await further developments and the results of larger comparative trials.

Surgery for acute gastrointestinal bleeding

The two main problems when considering surgery for acute peptic ulcer bleeding are the timing of the operation and deciding on which procedure to perform.

Timing of surgery

Before endoscopic haemostasis, the decision to operate for upper gastrointestinal bleeding was arguably simpler to make. Obviously, when continuing massive fresh bleeding is evident, surgery should not be delayed, but when the patient has stopped bleeding by the time endoscopy takes place the surgeon has to decide between an expectant policy and early 'prophylactic' surgery.

The most important factors in predicting the likelihood of rebleeding appear to be age over 60 years, shock and/or anaemia on admission and the presence of endoscopic stigmata of recent haemorrhage (active bleeding or visible vessel in an ulcer base). There has been a randomized trial comparing early with delayed surgery, and the results indicated that for patients over the age of 60, early surgery was associated with a lower mortality. Despite doubts as to whether the endoscopic criteria in this trial were entirely appropriate, it did serve to emphasize the need for prompt surgical intervention in high-risk elderly patients.

When endoscopic haemostasis is introduced, the situation can be more complicated. If endoscopic attempts to stop active bleeding fail, there is little argument about the need for surgery. However, the problem of rebleeding after initially successful endoscopic haemostasis has not been fully addressed, and there is a temptation to persist with non-operative interventions, especially in the older patient. This can be dangerous, and personal experience would strongly suggest that a single rebleed after endoscopic treatment should warrant surgery. It would therefore be very useful to have some means of predicting rebleeding after endoscopic haemostasis, and although very little work has been done in this area, it does seem that a visible vessel on the posterior wall of the duodenum or on the lesser curve of the stomach has a high risk of rebleeding after injection treatment.

Choice of procedure

Conventionally, the bleeding duodenal ulcer is treated by under-running followed by truncal vagotomy with pyloroplasty (or gastrojejunostomy if a pyloroplasty cannot be performed safely), although a giant ulcer will occasionally necessitate a partial gastrectomy. The bleeding gastric ulcer has for many years been taken as an indication for partial gastrectomy.

Two developments have led to a partial change of attitude towards these operations: highly selective vagotomy (HSV) and the advent of effective medication for peptic ulcer in the form of H_2 receptor antagonists, proton pump inhibitors and regimes to eradicate *Helicobacter pylori*. Because of the reduced incidence of side effects following HSV as compared with truncal vagotomy, it has been suggested that after local control of the bleeding, HSV should be performed as the definitive procedure. Unfortunately, the results of HSV are highly operator dependent, and as elective surgery for peptic ulcer disease has all but disappeared, there is little opportunity for most surgeons to become proficient at this procedure.

Acid-reducing drugs are now so effective that some authorities believe that surgery for bleeding peptic ulcer should be restricted to simple control of haemorrhage, and developments in *Helicobacter pylori* eradication, which have radically improved the long-term medical treatment of the disease, reinforce this view.

Clearly, the ideal operation for the bleeding peptic ulcer is still a subject for debate and the only sensible course to follow is to ensure that haemostasis is secure. For the duodenal ulcer, simple oversewing is usually adequate, but for the chronic gastric ulcer this approach is associated with a high rate of rebleeding. Thus it may be necessary to carry out a gastrectomy, although many gastric ulcers are amenable to formal local excision. In any event, despite advances in other areas, we can be sure that surgery will retain an important role in gastrointestinal haemorrhage for many years to come. For the future, therefore, it is important that interested surgeons work together with like-minded endoscopists and radiologists in order to provide a service aimed at minimizing mortality and morbidity from gastrointestinal bleeding.

Further reading

Cook, D.J., Guyart, G.H., Salena, B.J. *et al.* (1992) Endoscopic therapy for acute non-variceal upper gastrointestinal haemorrhage: a meta-analysis. *Gastroenterology* **102** 139–148.

Dronfield, M.W. (1987) Special units for acute upper gastrointestinal bleeding. *British Medical Journal* **294** 1308–1309.

Fleischer, D. (1986) Endoscopic therapy of upper gastrointestinal bleeding in humans. *Gastroenterology* **90** 217–234.

Gimson, A.E.S., Ramage, J.K., Panos, M.Z. *et al.* (1993) Randomised trial of variceal banding ligation versus injection sclerotherapy for bleeding oesophageal varices. *Lancet* **324** 391–394.

Jalan, R., Redhead, D.N. & Hayes, P.C. (1995) Transjugular intrahepatic portosystemic stent-shunt in the treatment of variceal haemorrhage. *British Journal of Surgery* **82** 1158–1164.

Moss, S. & Calam, J. (1992) *Helicobacter pylori* and peptic ulcers: the present position. *Gut* **33** 289–292.

Steele, R.J.C. (1989) Endoscopic haemostasis for non-variceal upper gastrointestinal haemorrhage. *British Journal of Surgery* **76** 219–225.

Steele, R.J.C., Chung, S.C.S. & Leung, J.W.C. (1993) *Practical Management of Acute Gastrointestinal Bleeding.* Butterworth Heinemann, Oxford.

Sung, J.J.Y., Chung, S.C.S., Lai, C.W. *et al.* (1993) Octreotide infusion or emergency sclerotherapy for variceal haemorrhage. *Lancet* **342** 637–641.

CHAPTER 14

Lower gastrointestinal bleeding

Akhtar Qureshi, James Gunn & Graeme S. Duthie

Introduction

Acute lower gastrointestinal bleeding is usually defined as bleeding distal to the ligament of Trietz; however, massive haemorrhage from the upper gastrointestinal tract can also present with rectal bleeding. Massive blood loss results in a haemodynamically unstable patient and therefore the primary concern is to resuscitate the patient. In the majority of these patients, the bleeding will stop spontaneously following adequate resuscitation. Once the patient has been adequately resuscitated, identify the source of bleeding.

The commonest source of the bleeding is the colon, accounting for 85% of the cases. The upper gastrointestinal tract accounts for 10% and the small intestine 5%.

Causes of lower gastrointestinal tract bleeding

The commonest causes of massive lower gastrointestinal bleeding are, diverticular disease and angiodysplasia. However, there are a wide variety of gastrointestinal lesions that can cause rectal bleeding, including upper gastrointestinal lesions (Table 14.1).

Clinical features

While the patient is being resuscitated, obtain a thorough history and physical examination. The age of the patient can be a helpful guide in determining the cause. The elderly patient is more likely to have diverticular disease and angiodysplasia compared to the younger patient in whom inflammatory bowel disease is more common. A history of haematemesis suggests an upper gastrointestinal source of bleeding. Other symptoms suggesting possible diagnoses are shown in Table 14.2.

General examination usually reveals a shocked patient with tachycardia and hypotension. A rough guide to the amount of blood loss is detailed in Table 14.3.

Abdominal examination is usually unremarkable, apart from scars resulting from previous surgery for peptic ulcer disease or colonic pathology. Digital rectal examination, proctoscopy and sigmoidoscopy is mandatory, and should be performed as soon as the patient is resuscitated.

A nasogastric tube should be inserted and the aspirate checked for bile and fresh/altered blood (coffee grounds). Testing the aspirate for occult blood is unhelpful as the trauma of insertion of the nasogastric tube can give a positive result. The presence of bile alone without any blood suggests that the bleeding is unlikely to be from the upper gastrointestinal tract.

Investigations

Proctoscopy and rigid sigmoidoscopy

Proctoscopy and rigid sigmoidoscopy should be performed as part of the initial investigations. Proctoscopy inspects the anal canal and identifies any bleeding haemorrhoids or anal fissures. Sigmoidoscopy allows the visualization of the rectal mucosa for any obvious inflammation, tumour masses or bleeding polyps.

Colonoscopy

The role of colonoscopy in the acute lower gastrointestinal bleed remains controversial. In experienced hands, diagnostic accuracy of colonoscopy varies from 70 to 90%. In the majority of these patients the bleeding will stop spontaneously and therefore colonic preparation is possible. Colonoscopy is useful to identify and arrest bleeding from tumours (Fig. 14.1) or angiodysplasia. In the patient with active bleeding, however, as a result of blood within the colonic lumen, visibility is impaired and the risk of perforation is increased. Thus the diagnostic accuracy of the procedure is diminished. Despite the drawbacks of colonoscopy in the active bleeder, the only contra-indication to colonoscopy is shock. If blood clots are seen coming from the ileocaecal valve, the colon is unlikely to be the source of bleeding.

Technetium sulphur colloid scintigraphy

This technique involves the use of technetium sulphur colloid which is injected intravenously. The accumulation of

Table 14.1 Gastrointestinal lesions that cause rectal bleeding.

Site	Cause
Upper gastrointestinal tract	Peptic ulcer disease
	Angiodysplasia
Small bowel	Jejunal diverticulosis
	Aortoenteric fistula
	Meckels diverticulum
	Lymphoma
	Trauma
Colonic	Diverticular disease
	Angiodysplasia
	Colonic carcinoma
	Colonic polyps
	Ulcerative colitis
	Ischaemic colitis
	Juvenile polyps
	Trauma
Rectal	Carcinoma
	Rectal prolapse
	Juvenile polyps
	Trauma
Anal	Haemorrhoids
Miscellaneous	Mucosal telangiectasia
	(Osler–Weber–Rendu syndrome)
	Anticoagulants
	Coagulopathy

Table 14.2 Clinical features and diagnoses.

Symptom	Possible diagnoses
Abdominal pain	Inflammatory bowel disease
	Ischaemic bowel
Painless bleeding	Diverticular disease
	Angiodysplasia
	Haemorrhoids
Constipation	Malignancy
	Haemorrhoids

the radiopharmaceutical into the bowel lumen is detected even with slow bleeding rates (0.5 ml/min). The disadvantage of this technique is the rapid clearance by the reticuloendothelial system resulting in a very short half-life ($t_{1/2} = 3$ min); this requires the patient to be actively bleeding during the few minutes the agent is in the blood.

Technetium-labelled red blood cells

The patient's red blood cells are labelled with the technetium *in vitro* and then injected intravenously into the patient. Abdominal images are then obtained at 5-min intervals for the first 30 min followed by images every few hours for up to 24 h (Fig. 14.2). The longer intravascular duration of the technetium-labelled red blood cells offers a clear advantage over the sulphur colloid technique. Pitfalls in the interpretation of the scintiscans include misinterpretation of abnormalities such as abscesses and fibroids.

Angiography

Selective arteriography has become an important diagnostic and therapeutic tool in the management of acute lower gastrointestinal bleeding. This technique involves the cannulation of superior mesenteric artery and is usually performed

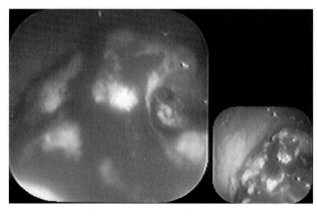

Fig. 14.1 Colonoscopic appearance of bleeding tumour.

Table 14.3 Blood loss and its effects.

Blood loss	< 750 ml	750–1500 ml	1500–2000 ml	> 2000 ml
Heart rate (per min)	<100	>100	>120	>140
Blood pressure	Normal	Normal	Decreased	Decreased
Urine output (ml/h)	>30	20–30	5–15	Negligible

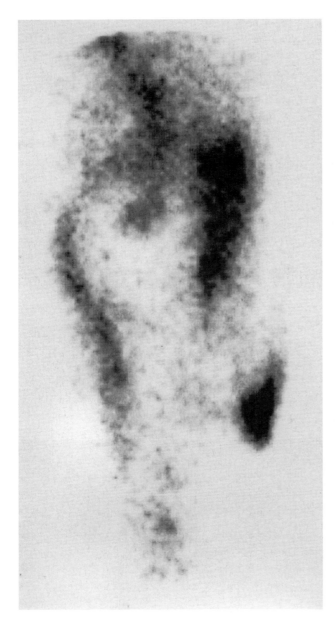

Fig. 14.2 Red cell scan.

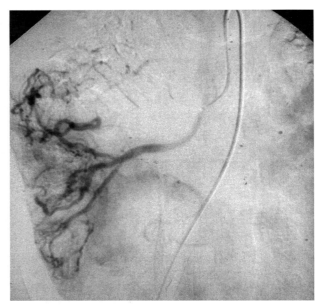

Fig. 14.3 Angiogram of angiodysplasia.

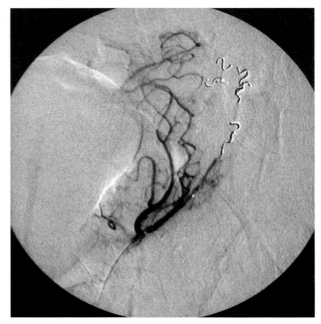

Fig. 14.4 Angiogram of embolization.

through a common femoral artery stab, and if negative, is followed by selective angiography of the inferior mesenteric artery and coeliac trunk separately. As the patient may continue to bleed during the procedure which can be prolonged, the patient has to be carefully monitored. Extravasation of contrast material is seen if the bleeding is at least 1 ml/min (Fig. 14.3). The advantages of angiography include precise localization of the bleeding point, and not requiring any bowel preparation. In addition, therapeutic options available include injection of vasopressin and embolization of gelfoam or cyanoacrylate (Fig. 14.4). The

disadvantages of selective arteriography include timing of the procedure, the need for active bleeding, a skilled interventional radiologist, arterial thrombosis, haematoma, bleeding from puncture site, and complications as a result of embolization such as bowel infarction and renal failure.

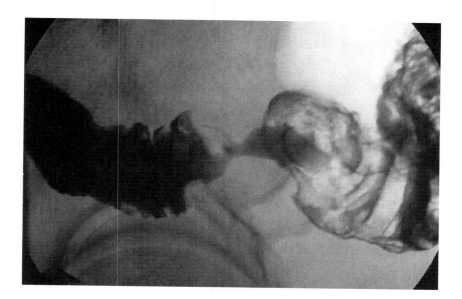

Fig. 14.5 Barium enema of colonic carcinoma.

Barium enema

Air contrast barium studies are largely discouraged in the early phase of acute lower gastrointestinal bleed, as the barium may obscure selective angiography interpretation. There have however been anecdotal reports on cessation of diverticular bleeding following barium studies. Barium enema or water-soluble studies are useful in cases of suspected carcinoma for operative planning (Fig. 14.5).

Enteroscopy

The small bowel distal to the ligament of Trietz is usually difficult to visualize directly. Until relatively recently, apart from intra-operative enteroscopy using a colonoscope introduced orally, a small bowel enema was the only method of assessing the small intestine. At present there are three types of enteroscopes. The push enteroscope utilizes a stiffening overtube to enable the enteroscope up to 150 cm beyond the ligament of Trietz. The sonde enteroscope is passed nasally and guided to the distal duodenum by an orally introduced gastroscope and depends on peristalsis to guide it to the distal ileum. Once in position, it is pulled back and the small bowel visualized. The sonde type of enteroscopy may take up to 6 h to perform. Enteroscopy is indicated in patients in whom both upper gastrointestinal and colonoscopy have been shown to be negative.

A common cause of small bowel bleeding is a Meckel's diverticulum. If enteroscopy is not readily available a Meckel's scan may be performed (Fig. 14.6).

Diagnostic approach

The diagnostic approach to the patient with acute lower gas-

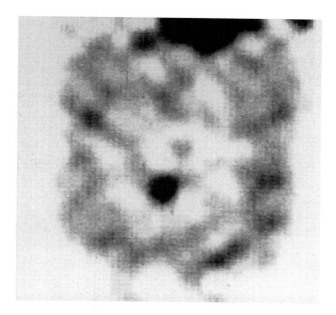

Fig. 14.6 Meckel's scan.

trointestinal bleeding depends on the rate of bleeding and whether or not the bleeding has stopped. In the patient in whom the bleeding appears to have stopped, once resuscitation has been achieved, an initial nasogastric lavage/aspirate is performed. Unless the nasogastric lavage/aspirate is unequivocally negative (the presence of bile alone with no blood), an upper gastrointestinal endoscopy must be performed. If the nasogastric lavage/aspirate or upper gastrointestinal endoscopy are negative, proceed to lower gastrointestinal investigations. These include proctoscopy and rigid sigmoidoscopy to begin with followed by semi-elective colonoscopy in a prepared colon, according to the algorithm shown in Fig. 14.7.

In the patient with active bleeding, follow the same protocol as above. However, if the nasogastric lavage/aspirate or upper gastrointestinal endoscopy are negative, proceed to lower gastrointestinal investigations beginning with proctoscopy and rigid sigmoidoscopy, to be followed by either colonoscopy in an unprepared colon, selective angiography or radionuclide scanning, depending on what is available. If an experienced colonoscopist is available proceed to colonoscopy. Should the colonoscopy be unsuccessful or an experienced colonoscopist is unavailable then proceed to selective angiography, as shown in Fig. 14.8.

Management of common causes of acute lower gastrointestinal bleeding

Diverticular disease

Although diverticular disease is more common on the left side of the colon, bleeding from diverticular disease tends to be more common on the right side of the colon (Fig. 14.9). Diverticular bleeding tends to be severe as it is arterial in nature. Overall, the bleeding will stop spontaneously in 80% of cases; however up to 25% will rebleed. Colonoscopic management of diverticular bleeding has been described in a small number of patients with the use of a heater probe. These reports are still largely experimental and require further assessment and long-term follow-up. Surgery for bleeding diverticular disease is necessary only if it does not stop on conservative treatment.

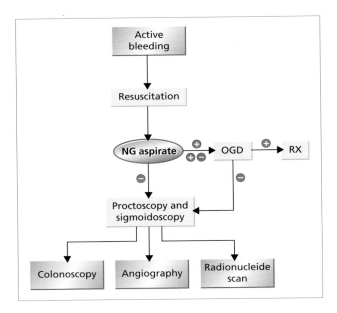

Fig. 14.8 Algorithm for diagnosis when bleeding is still active.

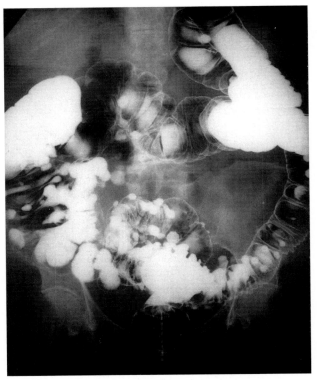

Fig. 14.9 Barium enema of diverticular disease.

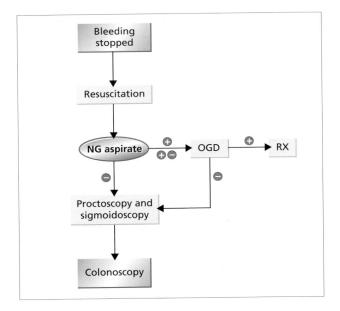

Fig. 14.7 Algorithm for proctoscopy and sigmoidoscopy when lower gastrointestinal bleeding has stopped.

Angiodysplasias

Angiodysplasias are specific mucosal vascular ectasia that develop as a degenerative process of ageing. These lesions are most commonly seen in the caecum and the ascending colon. There is some controversy as to the treatment of choice for these lesions. Colonoscopy with heat (hot biopsy forceps) or laser (YAG laser) coagulation is effective in up to 80% of patients but with higher rebleeding rates. Twenty percent of these patients require more than one colonoscopic treatment. The main risks of coagulation of these angiodysplasia lesions are perforation, delayed bleeding and postcoagulation syndrome. The postcoagulation syndrome is defined by the features of abdominal pain, localized rebound tenderness, raised white cell count but without any evidence of colonic perforation. Surgical resection is more effective but with obvious greater risks.

Ischaemic colitis

Massive bleeding from an infarcted colon usually requires surgical resection. Ischaemic colon should always be suspected in cases of bloody diarrhoea following abdominal aortic aneurysm repair.

Inflammatory bowel disease

Massive rectal bleeding occurs in extensive ulcerative colitis as well as localized Crohn's disease. In these patients surgery is the treatment of choice.

Meckel's diverticulum

Bleeding from Meckel's diverticulum usually occurs in children and adolescents. It occurs in 2% of the population and although of equal incidence between the sexes, it is twice as symptomatic in males. It is estimated that 10–20% of these Meckel's diverticulae are complicated by bleeding. The diverticulum lies about 30–90 cm from the ileocaecal valve and is often lined with heterotropic gastric epithelium. The presence of the diverticula may be diagnosed by a small bowel enema or sodium pertechnetate isotope scan. Treatment is by surgical resection.

Treatment

Endoscopic techniques

When the bleeding source is the colon, therapeutic options available at endoscopy include the use of snare polypectomy to excise bleeding polyps, Nd–YAG laser ablation of tumour mass within the rectum and occasionally when the bleeding is not as a result of a polyp, injection with adrenaline may be useful. Although the relatively thin wall of the colon may be more susceptible to perforation. Angiodysplastic lesions can be treated using laser or heat ablation.

Angiographic techniques

Following the identification of the bleeding lesion at angiography, localized infusion of vasopressin can result in cessation of the bleeding point, particularly in diverticular disease. An alternative technique is the use of embolization techniques to stop the bleeding. This is used with great caution as irreversible ischaemia leading to infarction and perforation may occur. Materials used in therapeutic embolization include, gelfoam, oxycel and cyanoacrylate.

Surgery

Surgery should be considered in the following patients.
- Estimated blood loss greater than 4 units.
- Recurrent bleeding following therapeutic angiography or colonoscopy.
- Extensive angiodysplasia.

It is ideal to have localized the site of bleeding before laparotomy; however, this is not the case in every situation. When the site of the bleeding is known the appropriate resection is performed. If the site of bleeding is not known, on-table colonoscopy can be carried out. In addition an on-table colonic lavage can be helpful. This is achieved by performing an appendicectomy and passing a large bore Foley catheter through the stump of the appendix, through which the irrigation is carried out.

In patients with recurrent bleeding without a localized bleeding site, a subtotal colectomy with or without a primary anastomosis is performed, blind segmental resections should never be carried out. Rarely, with severe bleeding from the rectum, an abdominoperineal resection may be required. The overall mortality for emergency surgery in patients with acute lower gastrointestinal bleeding is 2–10%.

Further reading

Goligher, J. (1984) *Surgery of the Anus, Colon and Rectum.* Baillière Tindall, Eastbourne.

CHAPTER 15

Small bowel obstruction

Gerard P. McEntee

Introduction

Some bowel obstruction is a common surgical emergency accounting for approximately 5% of all acute general surgical admissions. There are several possible causes and the epidemiology varies considerably from region to region. Adhesions, strangulated hernias and metastatic malignancy account for the vast majority of cases of adult small bowel obstruction in western Europe whereas in other regions strangulated hernias and volvulus obstruction predominate (Table 15.1).

Pathophysiology

Obstruction of the bowel results in proximal distension with accumulation of gas and upper gastrointestinal tract secretions. The normal process of small bowel reabsorption of intestinal fluid is impaired resulting in a nett loss of extracellular fluid and electrolyte imbalance. As the bowel distension increases oedema of the bowel wall occurs. This oedema inhibits venous return causing further swelling and eventual compromise of arterial circulation with ischaemia and subsequent infarction and perforation (Fig. 15.1). Bowel ischaemia is associated with increased translocation of enteric bacteria which proliferate in the stagnant fluid of the obstructed bowel lumen. The consequences of bowel obstruction therefore are progressive dehydration, electrolyte imbalance and systemic toxicity associated with bacteraemia and toxin production.

Clinical features

Symptoms

The predominant symptoms of small bowel obstruction are abdominal pain and vomiting. The pain is typically central and colicky in nature, occurring every 3–5 min but where strangulation of the bowel has occurred the pain may become constant. Vomiting is typically bilious in nature and rarely faeculent — the frequency and volume are related to the level of the obstruction, occurring earlier and in greater volumes with high jejunal obstruction. Small bowel obstruction is also associated with central abdominal distension, the degree of distension related to the level of the lesion; high small bowel obstruction close to the ligament of Treitz may be associated with minimal or no distension whereas obstruction close to the ileocaecal valve typically produces gross abdominal distension which is maximal centrally. Constipation is rarely a feature except in patients who present late.

Signs

Signs depend on the degree of dehydration, the cause and level of the obstruction and the presence or absence of underlying bowel strangulation. In addition to the unreliable clinical signs of dehydration such as reduced skin turgor, dry tongue and sunken eyeballs, significant dehydration is indicated by hypotension, tachycardia and oliguria. The abdomen is typically distended and a previous history of abdominal surgery raising the possibility of adhesive obstruction may be confirmed on inspection. A careful check of the hernial orifices may reveal an irreducible inguinal, femoral or para-umbilical hernia, all of which may be missed in obese patients. Raising the foot of the bed to the Trendelenberg position may facilitate groin examination in such obese patients. The presence of a hernia may be unrelated to the obstruction but if the hernia is tense, tender or irreducible with no cough impulse, it not only implicates the hernia but suggests that strangulation is present. Palpation of the abdomen may detect tenderness, guarding and rebound tenderness, the latter in particular suggesting peritonism and possible bowel strangulation. Previous surgery for malignancy, abdominal or otherwise, raises the possibility of metastatic disease and in advanced cases, tumour mass or masses may be palpable in the abdomen or liver. Auscultation typically reveals increased high pitched 'tinkling' bowel sounds which may be heard without the aid of the stethoscope (borborygmi). Obstruction with strangulation may result in reduced or absent bowel sounds.

Investigations and management

The majority of patients with intestinal obstruction are dehydrated and management priority is to establish ade-

Table 15.1 Causes of small bowel obstruction.

	Europe (%)	Africa (%)
Adhesions	60	10
Strangulated hernias	20	50
Malignancy	10	5
Volvulus	5	30
Others	5	5

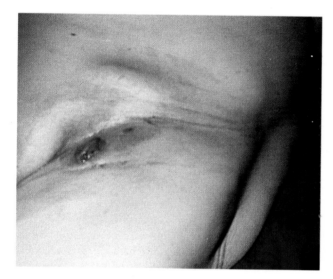

Fig. 15.1 Enterocutaneous fistula secondary to perforated strangulated femoral hernia.

Symptoms and signs of small bowel obstruction	
• Pain	• Tender +/– rebound
• Vomiting	• Increased bowel sounds
• +/– Constipation	• +/– Abdominal distension

quate venous access and commence resuscitation with intravenous fluids. A large bore cannula (14–16 French gauge) is inserted into a large peripheral vein such as the ante-cubital vein or a major central vein such as the internal jugular or subclavian. At the same time as venous access is established, blood is taken for laboratory estimation of serum urea and electrolytes, haemoglobin, full blood count, blood glucose and a serum amylase which may be moderately elevated in intestinal obstruction. The volume and nature of fluid resuscitation required is determined by the degree of dehydration and the extent of electrolyte imbalance. Evaluation of the degree of dehydration usually requires more invasive means than simple monitoring of pulse, blood pressure and skin turgidity. A urinary catheter should be inserted and if urinary output does not respond promptly to a moderate fluid challenge (e.g. 1 L of Hartmanns over 2 h) a central

Intravenous fluids	Central venous line
Urinary catheter	? Swan–Ganz line
Nasogastric tube	

venous line should be inserted. Patients with a previous history of cardiac failure or pulmonary hypertension may require insertion of a central venous line or preferably a Swan–Ganz catheter at the outset. It has been demonstrated convincingly by the CEPOD (Confidential enquiry into perioperative deaths) Report that patients with intestinal obstruction who are hypovolemic have a much higher morbidity and mortality if not adequately resuscitated prior to surgery. The nature of intravenous fluid used depends on the degree of electrolyte imbalance; compound sodium lactate (Ringer's solution) is used most frequently because of its balanced electrolyte content which can be adjusted by appropriate additions based on serum electrolyte levels. Once intravenous access has been established, a nasogastric tube is inserted which reduces the tendency to vomit by decompressing the upper abdomen of both fluid and gas. Resuscitation is continued until the central venous pressure is restored and a consistent adequate urinary output (> 0.5 ml/kg/h) obtained.

Once resuscitated, radiological confirmation of small bowel obstruction is then obtained by erect and supine films of the abdomen. The former may identify multiple fluid levels, a feature which may be absent in high level obstruction and in long-standing obstruction where bowel loops are filled with fluid and gas is minimal. A supine abdominal film may demonstrate dilated loops of bowel and the degree of dilated loops might give some indication as to the site of the obstruction—obstruction close to the duodenojejunal flexure is associated with minimal or absent dilated loops whereas lesions of the terminal ileum may be associated with multiple distended central loops. Jejunal obstruction is indicated by the presence of dilated central loops with its valvulae coniventes producing a regularly spaced 'coin stacking' appearance running from antimesenteric to mesenteric border (Fig. 15.2) whereas ileal obstruction typically produces distended but featureless loops. Only rarely is the cause of the obstruction detectable on plain films of the abdomen (e.g. gallstone ileus) but small bowel barium contrast studies may help identify the cause (e.g. intussusception).

Further management

Having commenced appropriate resuscitation a decision is then made regarding the need for and timing of surgical intervention. The presence of strangulated bowel is an absolute indication for surgical intervention but the difficulty lies in accurately identifying strangulation. Constant pain, marked abdominal tenderness together with rebound tenderness, a silent abdomen, fever and raised white cell

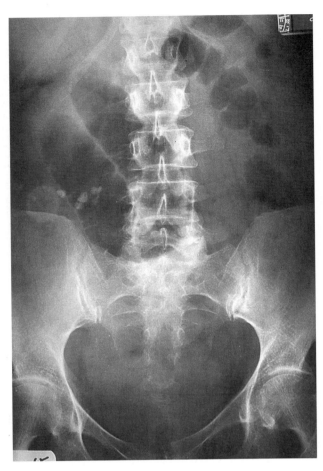

Fig. 15.2 Small bowel obstruction with dilated central loop.

count have all been considered useful indicators of underlying bowel ischaemia but several studies have shown that none of these findings alone are sensitive enough to accurately predict strangulation. The old American adage that 'the sun should never set on an intestinal obstruction' ensures that no patient with underlying strangulation will suffer as a result of delayed surgery but it also means that a significant proportion of patients particularly those with adhesive obstruction may undergo unnecessary surgery. In general patients with marked abdominal tenderness and rebound tenderness together with signs of systemic toxicity such as tachycardia, fever, hypotension or raised white cell count should undergo surgery once adequate resuscitation has been carried out. Patients with minimal tenderness and no systemic signs may settle on conservative management alone thereby avoiding surgery. It is important, however, that such patients be reviewed on a regular basis and a decision regarding conservative management be revised if necessary.

Adhesions

A significant proportion of patients with adhesive obstruc-

tion may settle in response to conservative management. If, however, surgery is indicated, it is best performed through a mid line abdominal incision. The peritoneal cavity is carefully entered avoiding, if at all possible, enterotomies of the underlying adherent bowel. The site of adhesive obstruction is identified by tracing the distended proximal bowel distally and the offending adhesion is divided. In general, and where possible, all adhesions should be divided from the duodeno-jejunal flexure to the caecum. Bowel that is clearly ischaemic should be resected. If bowel is of questionable viability, it is worth wrapping it in hot moist packs for 10–15 min then re-examining. Return of regular bowel colour, the presence of visible pulsations in the mesentery and active peristalsis all indicate bowel viability. In the event of recurrent extensive adhesive obstruction one may consider insertion of an extra long small intestinal tube (e.g. Miller–Abbott tube) via the nose or just below the duodenojejunal flexure at laparotomy which is then passed distally to the ileocaecal junction. This is used to establish and maintain an ordered alignment of small bowel and reduce the likelihood of bowel angulation and subsequent re-obstruction. Such tubes are typically left in situ for 2–3 weeks.

Obstructed hernias

The operative approach for an obstructed hernia varies depending on the site and the likelihood of underlying bowel strangulation (see Chapter 9). Obstructed femoral hernias may be approached directly by a transverse incision approximately 1 cm below the inguinal ligament and 3–4 cm in width. The sac is identified and mobilized completely down to and around the boundaries of the femoral canal. The neck of the hernia sac may be so constricted that one has to divide the lacunar ligament medially recognizing that in a significant proportion of cases there is an overlying small artery which may be transected in the process and subsequently require suturing. The sac which may be very thickened by overlying fat, is then opened and the contents examined. If the bowel is obviously not ischaemic, it is returned to the abdomen, the sac is transfixed at the neck, the distal portion excised and the femoral canal closed by two or possibly three interrupted non-absorbable sutures, which are all laid in initially and subsequently tied approximating the inguinal ligament anteriorly to the pectineal ligament posteriorly. The lateral suture should be tied first ensuring that the adjacent femoral vein is not compromised.

If the bowel is ischaemic, it should be resected. It may be difficult to withdraw sufficient bowel through the femoral canal to safely perform an anastomosis and subsequently return the bowel to the abdomen (Fig. 15.3). It is advisable if strangulation has occurred therefore to make a separate incision through a lower paramedian extraperitoneal approach or alternatively through the posterior wall of the inguinal canal using a standard inguinal hernia repair incision is made, the spermatic cord is then mobilized and retracted

Obstructed hernia	
• Relieve constriction	• Transfix sac
• ? Resect bowel	• Repair defect

and the transversalis fascia divided from the deep ring to the pubic tubercle, exposing extraperitoneal fat but taking care not to damage the inferior epigastric vessels. The femoral canal is then approached extraperitoneally from above the inguinal ligament. The contents are reduced if necessary by dividing the lacunar ligament medially with the obvious advantage that any overlying vessels can be identified and secured beforehand. Bowel resection if required can be performed safely through this incision and the femoral canal closed using interrupted sutures inserted into the same tissues as described above but tied on the superior rather than the inferior aspect of the canal. The transversalis fascia is then repaired using a fine non-absorbable suture (3/0 nylon or prolene) and the anterior wall of the inguinal canal closed in standard fashion. A similar approach may be used for obstructed inguinal hernias and once the bowel has been safely returned to the abdomen the sac is transfixed at the neck and the distal portion excised. The posterior wall is then repaired as in a standard elective inguinal hernia repair. The transversalis fascia which is attenuated by the obstructed hernia and has been divided from the deep ring to the pubic tubercle is repaired in two overlapping layers using a continuous 3/0 non-absorbable suture as in the Shouldice hernia repair. The conjoint tendon is then approximated to the inguinal ligament using a continuous 2/0 non-absorbable suture and the external oblique closed anterior to the cord.

An obstructed para-umbilical hernia is approached by a directly overlying transverse incision down to the fascia of the linea alba and the adjoining anterior rectus sheath. The sac is mobilized down to and around the neck if necessary dividing the tight constricting fascia laterally on either side. The sac is then opened and the bowel inspected. If viable, the bowel is returned to the abdomen, the sac emptied, transfixed at the neck and reduced. The defect is closed using two layers of interrupted non-absorbable sutures (e.g. 0 or 2/0 prolene or nylon), the first layer approximating the edge of the lower leaf of fascia to the under surface of the upper leaf. The edge of the upper leaf is then approximated as a flap to the fascia beneath.

Volvulus obstruction

Small bowel obstruction caused by volvulus is again approached through a midline abdominal incision and extended superiorly or inferiorly depending on the site and exposure. The offending segment is identified and the underlying cause which usually consists of an adhesive

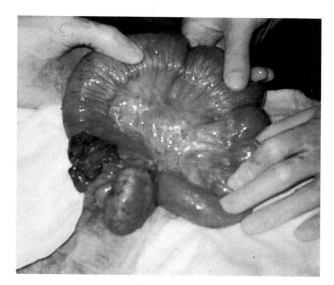

Fig. 15.3 Perforated small bowel with proximal dilatation secondary to an obstructed hernia.

band from the apex of the obstructed loop to the abdominal wall is divided, the bowel untwisted and, if necessary, any ischaemic bowel resected. Occasionally volvulus occurs because of malrotation of the small intestine. In this case, it may be necessary to relieve the volvulus and prevent recurrence by transfixing the offending portion of the small bowel to the posterior abdominal wall with a seromuscular non-absorbable suture.

Intusussception

Intusussception in the western world is usually seen in young children, the offending agent typically being an enlarged node or nodes intussuscepting into the distal bowel. The majority of intussusceptions in childhood can now be reduced radiologically and do not warrant surgery. Intussusception in the adult however is more commonly due to benign (e.g. lipoma) or malignant tumours and radiological reduction is not therefore an option. The abdomen is opened through a midline abdominal incision. If possible, the intussusceptum is reduced by traction on the proximal small bowel combined with retrograde compression of the apex of the intussusceptum. If reduction is not possible or if the bowel is obviously ischaemic when reduced then the diseased segment is resected together with the offending area.

Malignancy

A history of previous gastro-intestinal surgery for malignancy raises the possibility of recurrent malignant disease and small bowel obstruction has also been reported secondary to spread from extra-abdominal malignancies (e.g. melanoma, breast). Less commonly, small bowel obstruction may be due to a primary tumour of the small bowel either adenocarcinoma or lymphoma. If the obstruction is localized the involved segment is resected. If on the other hand, there is extensive tumour and many of the loops of bowel are fixed, it may only be possible to perform a palliative bypass from an appropriate mobile dilated proximal loop to a mobile distal collapsed loop using a side-to-side anastomosis with a similar technique to that described below.

Gallstone ileus

Rarely obstruction may be due to a large gallstone which has eroded from the gall bladder or common bile duct into the intestine, typically the duodenum, and has passed distally until it obstructs the lumen. The radiological combination of air in the biliary tree together with small bowel obstruction is strongly suggestive while a large calcified intra-abdominal calculus clinches the diagnosis (Fig. 15.4). The abdomen is opened through a midline abdominal incision. An enterotomy is performed at the site of the impacted stone taking care to avoid gross spillage of intestinal contents, and the offending stone removed. If the bowel is of questionable viability at the site of impaction, a small segment may be resected. The exact nature of the underlying cholecyst- or choledocho-enteric fistula may be difficult to determine at the time of laparotomy without detailed cholangiography and is best left alone for later elective investigation and subsequent repair.

Technique of small bowel resection

Once a decision has been made to resect small bowel the appropriate loops are mobilized and taken on to the anterior abdominal wall. The wound edges are protected from contamination by moist saline packs and the proposed segment emptied of fluid by milking proximally and distally and applying non-crushing clamps only to the bowel wall, well removed from the proposed resection margins. The proposed resection margins are then identified and the plane of mesentery resection incised superficially with a scissors from the bowel edge to the root of the mesentery (Fig. 15.5). The mesenteric vessels crossing the proposed resection site are divided between haemostats and ligated. Crushing clamps are then applied to the small bowel which is divided on the viable sides of the clamps. Cut edges are inspected for brisk bleeding which is controlled and the lumen is cleaned with antiseptic solution. The bowel edges are then approximated ensuring correct alignment of mesenteric and antimesenteric borders. If there is a gross discrepancy between the proximal dilated segment and the distal collapsed segment, the distal bowel circumference may be enlarged by an appropriate incision along the antimesenteric border. Alternatively in this situation, the diseased bowel may be resected using an appropriately sized stapling device and a

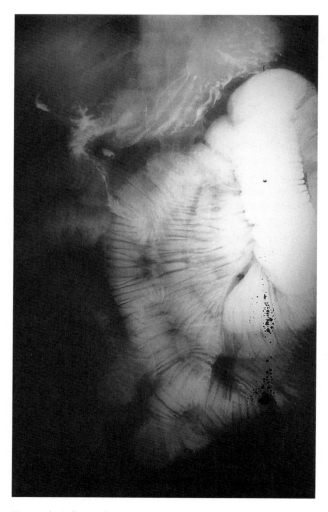

Fig. 15.4 Gallstone ileus. Barium study confirming obstruction from gallstone with contrast in gall bladder.

side-to-side anastomosis performed using the following technique.

A suture (2/0 Polydioxone, 30-mm needle) is inserted incorporating all layers of both proximal and distal bowel commencing in the central portion of the posterior wall (Fig. 15.6). The suture is then ligated and held. A continuous all layer suture is then inserted along the posterior wall towards the mesenteric border. One or two inverting Connell sutures may be inserted at the corner to invert the mucosa and the suture continued anteriorly for approximately one third of the anterior wall. A second suture is then inserted again centrally in the posterior wall and tied to the first suture and again an all layer suture incorporating the posterior layer towards the antimesenteric border and continued anteriorly to meet the initial suture (Fig. 15.6). Interrupted seromuscular sutures are then inserted (2/0 Polydioxone, 20-mm needle) commencing at the mesenteric border and continued on both anterior and posterior rows of the anastomosis (Fig.

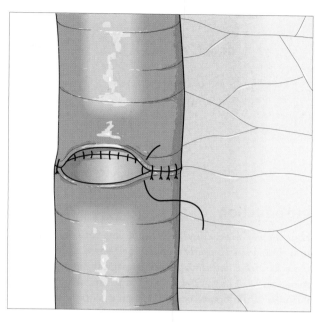

Fig. 15.7 Interrupted inverting seromuscular sutures.

15.7). The anastomosis is then checked for an adequate bowel lumen and the mesenteric defect closed by carefully approximating the mesenteric edges with a number of interrupted sutures avoiding the important mesenteric vessels running in the free edge of the mesentery. If peritoneal contamination has occurred, the abdomen is irrigated with warm saline. Intraperitoneal drainage is not required and the wound is closed in standard fashion.

Minimally invasive surgery

If the provisional diagnosis is one of adhesive obstruction, thought to be caused by a single band adhesion and surgery is indicated, it may be worth considering the laparoscopic approach. Obviously the pneumoperitoneum and the laparoscopic port should be carefully introduced under direct vision using the 'open' Hassaan technique. If a single band adhesion is identified as the cause it can be safely divided, thus avoiding a major laparotomy incision.

Summary

In conclusion, small bowel obstruction is a common surgical emergency. The overall mortality is approximately 10% and is greatest in patients with ischaemic bowel which may or may not have perforated prior to surgery. The most common causes of death are intra-abdominal sepsis, myocardial infarction and pulmonary embolism. The initial CEPOD report highlighted the importance of adequate pre-operative resuscitation of those patients who require operative intervention.

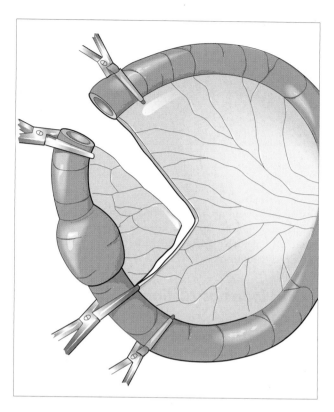

Fig. 15.5 Transection of bowel on 'remaining side' of crushing clamps.

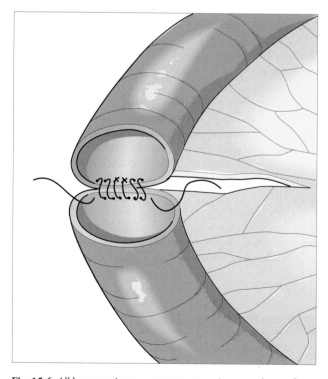

Fig. 15.6 All layer continuous suture commencing central part of posterior row.

CHAPTER 16

Large bowel obstruction

Simon P. L. Dexter & John R. T. Monson

Introduction

Large bowel obstruction (LBO) presents between three and four times less frequently than its small bowel counterpart. It remains, nonetheless, a common surgical emergency. The main causes of large bowel obstruction are malignancy, and volvulus of the sigmoid colon, the prevalence of both being subject to wide geographical variability. Colorectal cancer is particularly prevalent in the West, accounting for three-quarters of cases of large bowel obstruction. This proportion alters in Africa and Eastern Europe where sigmoid volvulus is the cause of obstruction in up to 40% of cases. Less common causes of large bowel obstruction are diverticular disease, either as a result of stricture or acute inflammation with oedema, and obstructed groin hernia. Inflammatory bowel disease is a very unusual cause of obstruction but strictures from any cause may precipitate obstruction by proximal faecal impaction. Faecal impaction alone rarely causes obstruction.

Causes of large bowel obstruction
• Cancer (primary or recurrent)
• Volvulus
• Diverticular disease
• Hernia
• Faecal impaction
• Inflammatory bowel disease
• Ischaemic stricture
• Anastomotic stricture

Classification of LBO

Mechanical large bowel obstruction is classically divided into chronic or acute-on-chronic obstruction depending on the clinical presentation. Chronic obstruction implies the presence of progressive symptoms over a period of time. If intervention is not forthcoming acute-on-chronic obstruction may supervene.

In fact there is a complete spectrum of clinical presentation and patients may present with acute large bowel obstruction without a pre-existing history of obstructive symptoms. Non-mechanical large bowel obstruction does occur and is dealt with under the separate heading of pseudo-obstruction.

Closed loop obstruction

The clinical features of large bowel obstruction are largely dependent on the function of the ileocaecal valve. Patency of the ileocaecal valve implies that the valve functions correctly and only allows antegrade passage of gas and faeces. When there is distal obstruction the valve often becomes incompetent and both small and large bowel become distended. If left untreated, the patient will start to vomit, but ischaemia or peforation of the bowel is unlikely. When the valve functions correctly, distal obstruction results in a *closed loop obstruction* of the segment of colon between the valve and the obstructing lesion. Failure to decompress this allows intracolonic pressure to build up rapidly. Intramural ischaemia causes patchy necrosis and may lead to perforation, which is a disastrous complication of obstruction.

In cases where the ileocaecal valve forms one end of a closed loop obstruction, the caecum is a common site of perforation. Perforation occurs here as it is the widest point of the colon. According to the Law of Laplace, tension (in this case in the wall of the colon) is proportional to the radius*, and is therefore higher in the caecum than elsewhere (Fig. 16.1).

$$*2T = PR$$

where P is the transmural pressure, T is the wall tension and R is the radius of a sphere.

Large bowel obstruction
• Chronic obstruction
• Acute-on-chronic obstruction
• Acute obstruction
• Pseudo-obstruction (Ogilvie's syndrome)

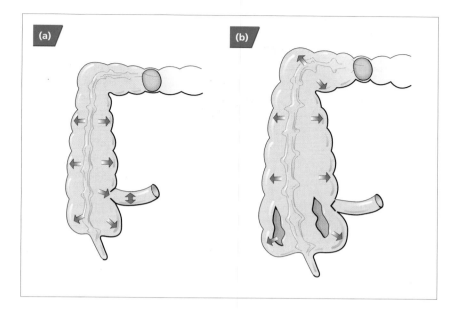

Fig. 16.1 Obstruction from a transverse colon carcinoma. In (a) ileocaecal valve remains open, but in (b) the valve is stopping reflux into the ileum resulting in closed loop obstruction.

Clinical presentation

Symptoms

The cardinal symptoms of intestinal obstruction are constipation, vomiting, abdominal pain and abdominal distention. In large bowel obstruction, the lesion is very distal within the intestine and constipation and distension are the earliest and most predominant symptoms. Vomiting of intestinal contents occurs late. In addition to these symptoms, the clinical history may establish other features indicative of the likely aetiology of the obstruction. A past history of colorectal or other intra-abdominal malignancy, recent alteration in bowel habit or the passage of blood is suggestive of neoplasm. Patients who are institutionalized and have cognitive impairment have a high incidence of sigmoid volvulus and severe constipation, and pseudo-obstruction tends to occur in patients with a history of recent non-gastrointestinal surgery or severe concurrent medical illness.

In relation to bowel obstruction, *constipation* implies that the patient has difficulty evacuating their bowels, and has reduced frequency of bowel action. Absolute constipation occurs when there is complete lumenal obstruction and the patient is unable to pass either faeces or flatus.

Paradoxically, partial obstruction may result in the frequent passage of liquid or soft stools. This occurs as the pressure in the proximal obstructed colon forces liquid faeces through the stricture. Episodes of such spurious diarrhoea are met with a sensation of incomplete evacuation and often alternate with episodes of constipation.

Abdominal distension is a prominent feature of large bowel obstruction and is commonly noticed by the patient. *Vomiting* of obstructed intestinal content (faeculant vomiting) is a late symptom of large bowel obstruction and implies a state of severe volume depletion. *Pain* is derived from a number of sources. Abdominal distention, colic from the bowel proximal to the obstruction and peritoneal irritation where ischaemia or perforation supervenes, all cause pain. Colicky pain is typical of small bowel obstruction and acute large bowel obstruction, but may be absent in chronic large bowel obstruction. The pain of intestinal colic is usually referred towards the midline rather than being localized. Pain derived from the embryological midgut is appreciated in the central abdomen, whereas hindgut pain (beyond the distal third of the transverse colon) is felt in the lower abdomen. Pain is most marked with closed loop obstruction.

Clinical examination (Fig. 16.2)

Examination findings will depend on the stage at which the patient presents. The patient with chronic obstruction may appear generally quite well with normal vital signs. On the

Symptoms of LBO

• Constipation
  — usually progressive
  — may alternate with diarrhoea
• Distension
• Pain
  caused by distension, gut colic, peritoneal irritation
• Vomiting
  — occurs late

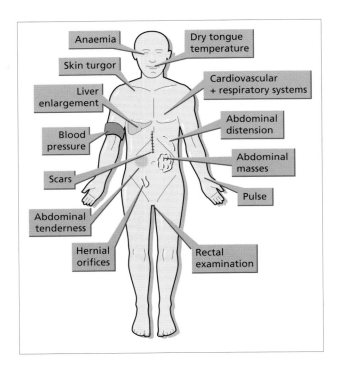

Fig. 16.2 Clinical examination for suspected large bowel obstruction.

other hand the patient who has an acute large bowel volvulus or an acute closed loop obstruction may be profoundly ill at the time of presentation.

Dehydration is assessed by asking the patient whether he or she feels dry, and by examination of the mucous membranes and skin turgor. The pulse, blood pressure and temperature may be altered as a result of pain, hypovolaemia or sepsis.

The clinical examination should include an assessment of the cardiovascular and respiratory systems as most of these patients will require surgery. Clinical examination is supplemented by an electrocardiogram (ECG) and chest X-ray.

Abdominal examination usually reveals marked distension, often to such an extent that further assessment of the intra-abdominal contents is impossible. Rarely a mass may be felt, or an irregular enlarged liver may suggest a malignant lesion as the cause of obstruction. Hernias are an unusual cause of large bowel obstruction but the hernial orifices must be examined as with all cases of intestinal obstruction.

Bowel sounds are frequent and high pitched often with audible borborygmi. Rectal examination will rarely provide a diagnosis. However, as a true rectal lesion rarely causes large bowel obstruction, the presence of blood and mucus on the glove is suggestive of a distal neoplasm.

Pain on movement or reluctance to move with shallow respiration is an indicator of peritonitis. Localized abdom-

inal tenderness in the presence of gross distension is a worrying feature suggesting strangulation or imminent perforation and indicates the need for urgent decompression. Localized peritonitis at the site of the obstruction may occur when there is a perforation at, or just above, a cancer or where acute diverticulitis has precipitated obstruction. Peritonitis rapidly becomes generalized following perforation, as the obstructed colon decompresses itself into the peritoneal cavity.

Rarely, acute appendicitis occurs in association with an obstructing lesion of the right colon. Appendicitis in the elderly should be approached with this in mind and the appendicectomy incision should be sufficient to allow inspection or palpation of the right colon and hepatic flexure.

Resuscitation and initial management

The majority of patients with large bowel obstruction present with chronic progressive symptoms, have incomplete obstruction and are not critically ill. The patient with acute large bowel obstruction on the other hand requires urgent assessment and resuscitation. A baseline full blood count and biochemical profile are taken on arrival, and serum is grouped and saved. Blood will require crossmatching for surgery (usually four units). Dehydration should be assessed and corrected as a fluid deficit of several litres may occur with complete obstruction, especially if the patient is vomiting. In extreme cases hypovolaemic shock may ensue. Fluid resuscitation should be aimed at restoring the circulating blood volume with colloid in the first instance, and the overall fluid and electrolyte deficit with appropriate crystalloid. Much of the fluid deficit is accrued by the loss of iso-osmolar body fluids and should be replaced by saline or Hartmann's solution. Potassium should not be added until the serum potassium is known and renal function is adequate. A low or normal haematocrit in the presence of dehydration is suggestive of underlying anaemia and volume replacement should include whole blood. Fluid balance must be carefully monitored and where active resuscitation is required a urinary catheter is essential. The urine output is monitored hourly and maintained above 0.5 ml/kg/h. Measurement of the central venous pressure (CVP) greatly aids the assessment of fluid balance both pre- and postoperatively.

Localized abdominal tenderness or peritonitis, fever, tachycardia, and leucocytosis are all indicators of actual or impending ischaemia or perforation. Shock, hypothermia, generalized peritonitis, leucopenia and acidosis indicate a particularly poor prognosis. In this situation aggressive resuscitation should be initiated, ideally within the intensive therapy unit (ITU) environment, but surgery should not be unduly delayed when there is a risk of impending perforation.

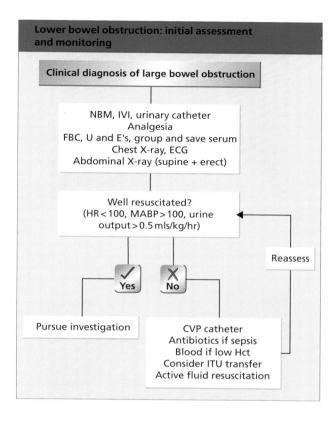

Lower bowel obstruction: initial assessment and monitoring

Clinical diagnosis of large bowel obstruction

NBM, IVI, urinary catheter
Analgesia
FBC, U and E's, group and save serum
Chest X-ray, ECG
Abdominal X-ray (supine + erect)

Well resuscitated?
(HR < 100, MABP > 100, urine output > 0.5 mls/kg/hr)

Reassess

Yes / No

Pursue investigation

CVP catheter
Antibiotics if sepsis
Blood if low Hct
Consider ITU transfer
Active fluid resuscitation

Plain radiography

A good quality plain abdominal radiograph and erect chest X-ray are mandatory baseline investigations. The colon may be identified on the abdominal radiograph by its peripheral distribution and the presence of haustrations, which are only lost with massive dilatation. Small bowel dilatation occurs when the ileocaecal valve becomes incompetent. Erect abdominal X-ray will demonstrate small bowel fluid levels in this situation and may help to clarify the distribution of gas shadows when the supine film is inconclusive. An erect chest X-ray is essential in the diagnosis of perforation. (Fig. 16.3)

In mechanical large bowel obstruction, colonic distension occurs proximal to the obstructing lesion with little or no gas beyond. The level of the obstructing lesion is often estimated by the point of distal cut-off of the gas shadow. This is subject to inaccuracy as the presence of impacted faeces proximal to the lesion can displace the cut-off to a more proximal level.

Volvulus of the colon results in a number of specific radiological features. Sigmoid volvulus produces a characteristic double loop shadow extending up towards the right upper quadrant. The coffee bean sign is produced by three lines converging towards the pelvis on the apex of the volvulus. The two outer lines are produced by the edges of the bowel and the central line by the two loops of bowel pressed together (Fig. 16.4). These features may be more difficult to interpret if there is significant proximal colonic dilatation.

In caecal volvulus there is only one distended loop which is directed up towards the left upper quadrant. Erect abdominal radiography shows the single fluid level within the hugely distended caecum (Fig. 16.5). Caecal volvulus is usually accompanied by some degree of small bowel distention.

Colonic pseudo-obstruction may appear radiologically indistinguishable from mechanical obstruction. In some case gaseous distension may extend as far as the anal canal, implying the absence of an intrinsic lesion, but there is commonly a more proximal gaseous cut-off.

Contrast studies

There may be considerable difficulty in differentiation between mechanical large bowel obstruction and pseudo-obstruction on plain abdominal X-ray alone. The penalty of misdiagnosis in pseudo-obstruction is an unnecessary laparotomy in a poor risk patient Contrast radiology is therefore indicated in all cases of apparent large bowel obstruction although it is contra-indicated in the presence of peritonitis and in toxic megacolon. Incomplete contrast examination is insufficient to exclude an obstructing lesion, and pseudo-obstruction can only be confidently diagnosed if contrast passes freely around to the caecum. A positive

Opiate analgesia is prescribed where indicated, but repeated doses should not be given without reassessment of the patient, unless surgery is imminent.

Broad-spectrum antibiotics are indicated for prophylaxis when surgery is undertaken, and to cover all intervention (e.g. sigmoidoscopy) in the case of cardiac valvular disease or when synthetic prostheses are present. The choice of prophylactic agents vary, but typical regimes include three perioperative doses of cefuroxime (1.5 g pre-operatively, 750 mg at 8 and 16 h postoperatively) and metronidazole (500 mg) i.v., or a single dose of cefotaxime 1 g plus metronidazole (500 mg).

Established peritonitis or gross faecal contamination during surgery requires a treatment regime of antibiotics for at least 5 days. The antibiotics used in this situation are usually the same as those used prophylactically, but may be altered according to the patient's response and local microbiological guidelines.

Investigations

Sigmoidoscopy

Rigid sigmoidoscopy is indicated in all patients with suspected large bowel obstruction. Distal obstructing cancers may be seen directly, and sigmoidoscopy may be therapeutic in patients with sigmoid volvulus or pseudo-obstruction.

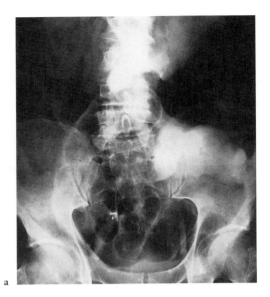

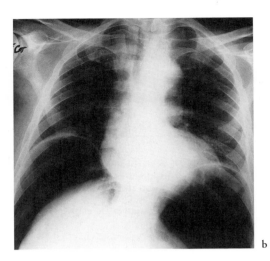

Fig. 16.3 Perforated large bowel obstruction. (a) Supine abdominal radiograph; (b) Erect chest radiograph.

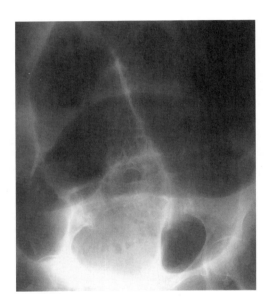

Fig. 16.4 The coffee bean sign.

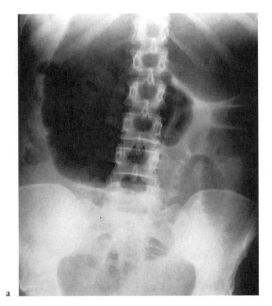

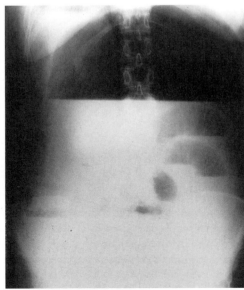

Fig. 16.5 Caecal volvulus: (a) supine film; (b) erect film.

finding on the contrast study may demonstrate a sharp shouldered cut-off in the case of malignancy, the beak sign at the apex of a volvulus or a long tapered stricture with mucosal oedema in the case of a diverticular stricture. However, the main role of the acute contrast examination is to establish that mechanical obstruction exists, the specific diagnosis being less critical.

The contrast media of choice for acute contrast studies are water soluble media such as Gastrografin or Urografin. Gastrografin in particular is very hyperosmolar and draws fluid into the colon. In some cases, where there is faecal impaction above a narrow lesion Gastrografin can be therapeutic as well as diagnostic by softening the inspissated faeces and allowing it to pass through the obstruction. Pseudo-obstruction also responds frequently to the hyperosmolar contrast enema with good result. Barium is contraindicated as it adds to any inspissation and is difficult to

evacuate completely from the peritoneal cavity in the case of perforation during the examination.

Ultrasound

Ultrasonography is not good at imaging bowel, especially when distended, and offers little in the routine evaluation of large bowel obstruction. However, an ultrasound may offer helpful information on the presence of liver metastases when the decision to operate on an elderly or debilitated patient is otherwise borderline.

Computerized tomography (CT)

CT can be used to evaluate large bowel obstruction but is usually not superior to conventional plain X-rays and contrast imaging. CT is indicated when there is a palpable mass

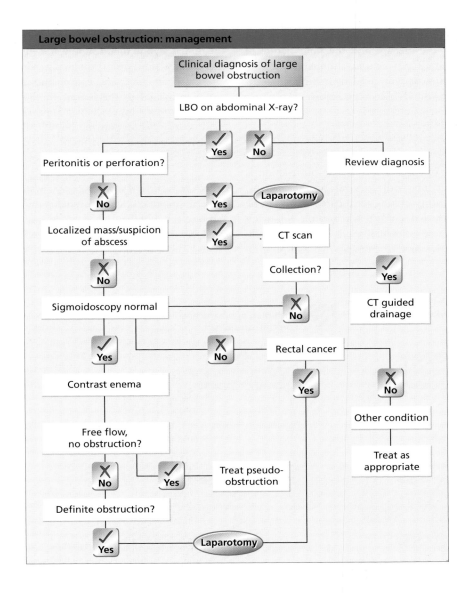

with low grade obstruction as can occur with a diverticular abscess. Percutaneous drainage of an abscess may relieve the obstruction and allow surgery to be deferred until the patient is fit.

Surgical management of large bowel obstruction

Malignant large bowel obstruction

Malignancy is the commonest cause of large bowel obstruction in the UK. The likelihood of a carcinoma of the colon causing obstruction is dependent on the nature of the cancer and the consistency of faeces proximal to the lesion.

Obstruction is the most likely outcome for cicatrizing tumours which involve the narrower parts of the colon (Fig. 16.6). Left-sided lesions precipitate obstructive symptoms at an earlier stage because the content of the left colon is more solid than the right side. Carcinomas of the caecum may become quite large before obstruction ensues, because of the large volume of the caecum and the fluid nature of the intestinal content. Rectal cancer, although common, rarely causes obstruction as symptoms such as rectal bleeding and tenesmus herald its discovery before obstruction ensues.

Surgical principles

The short term aim of surgery for colonic obstruction is relief of the obstruction with survival of the patient. However, the opportunity of long-term cure should not be overlooked. The corrected survival for patients following emergency resection of colorectal cancers is universally worse than after elective surgery. In order that compromise in surgical technique does not contribute to this statistic, surgery for obstructing colorectal carcinoma should be performed with the same surgical and oncological principles in mind as for elective colorectal cancer surgery. These principles include high ligation of the appropriate vessels, full excision of the adjacent mesentery and *en-bloc* resection when abdominal wall or adjacent organs are involved by tumour. Anastomoses should be well vascularized and without tension, and faecal spillage during the operation should be minimized.

Where possible, primary resection of the cancer is indicated. Local resections and other non-curative procedures should only be employed if there is non-remediable metastatic spread or the patient's life would be placed at risk by a resectional procedure.

Carcinoma of the right and transverse colon

Obstruction from carcinoma of the right side of the colon is usually amenable to resection and primary anastomosis. The ileum has a good blood supply and there is rarely a need to defunction the bowel proximally. Moreover a right-sided colectomy removes the cancer and all of the obstructed colon proximal to the lesion. In the rare event that the tumour proves unresectable, a proximal loop ileostomy will usually defunction the bowel, but a side-to-side ileotransverse anastomosis is more preferable. This avoids the necessity for a stoma and provides a very satisfactory bypass.

Right hemicolectomy and extended right hemicolectomy
The abdomen is opened through a midline incision centred around the umbilicus. The site of obstruction is confirmed and any metastases noted. The distended caecum and small bowel can be decompressed with a sucker via an enterotomy

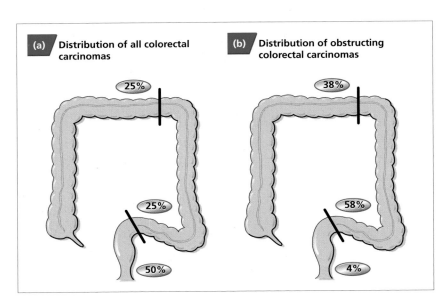

Fig. 16.6 Comparative distribution of elective and obstructing colorectal cancers.

in the terminal ileum. Decompression collapses the tense caecum, and reduces the risk of mesenteric tears caused by traction from heavy fluid filled loops of small bowel. The enterotomy is closed with a pursestring suture and is resected with the specimen.

The right colon, including the hepatic flexure and right transverse colon, is mobilized, taking care not to damage the underlying duodenum. If the lesion is large or adherent posteriorly, the right ureter should be clearly identified and protected during the mobilization. The ileocolic and right colic pedicles are divided and the consequent mesenteric defects are extended to the points of division of terminal ileum and transverse colon. The transverse colon is divided close to the middle colic pedicle to ensure a good blood supply (Fig. 16.7). For lesions of the transverse colon, the middle colic pedicle is also divided and an extended right hemicolectomy performed, in which case the splenic flexure needs to be taken down. The anastomosis is fashioned between ileum and the upper descending colon with the distal limb of the anastomosis dependent on the left colic blood supply.

Intestinal continuity may be restored by end-to-end, end-to-side or side-to-side ileocolic anastomosis, depending on the preference of the surgeon and the relative discrepancy in width of the bowel ends.

Carcinoma of the splenic flexure

Obstruction is a common complication of cancers around the splenic flexure. Elective surgery for these lesions usually involves left hemicolectomy or extended right hemicolectomy with ileo-descending anastomosis, depending on the preference of the surgeon. When the colon is obstructed by a carcinoma of the splenic flexure, the most logical procedure is an extended right hemicolectomy. This removes the cancer and the obstructed right colon and results in a well vascularized ileocolic anastomosis. Postoperative diarrhoea is rarely problematic, as the sigmoid and rectum are preserved.

> Obstructing carcinomas of right colon are treated by right hemicolectomy and of splenic flexure by extended right hemicolectomy.

Carcinoma of the left colon

The commonest sites of malignant large bowel obstruction are the sigmoid and rectosigmoid junction. The surgical treatment of such lesions will depend on the general status of the patient, the findings at operation and the preference of the operating surgeon.

Traditionally, left-sided large bowel obstruction was treated by a three-stage procedure, involving a primary proximal colostomy, subsequent definitive resection, and finally reversal of the stoma. More recently surgical practice has moved towards two-stage and, increasingly commonly, one-stage procedures for large bowel obstruction. The procedures and their relative merits and demerits are discussed below.

Left sided segmental resection without primary anastomosis
Perhaps the commonest procedure performed for acutely obstructed left sided colonic cancer is Hartmann's operation. In this operation the lesion is resected, the rectum is stapled or oversewn and the proximal colon brought out as an end colostomy. This is appropriate for sigmoid and rectosigmoid lesions, and rarely for obstructed rectal cancers. The advantages of Hartmann's operation are that the potential for anastomotic failure following acute resection is completely avoided, and the operation is less complicated than a restorative resection. In particular, although the resection may still be technically difficult in some cases, it is usually unnecessary to take down the splenic flexure, and there is no anastomosis.

The major disadvantage of Hartmann's operation is the difficulty in reversal once the patient has recovered from the initial resection. Reversal requires a full laparotomy, and in many cases a tedious dissection in the presence of dense adhesions in order to take down the stoma and find the rectal stump. The mortality of Hartmann's reversal is around 5%, and the morbidity somewhat higher. A significant proportion of patients never come to reversal because they are not considered fit enough, or are not prepared to undergo further major surgery.

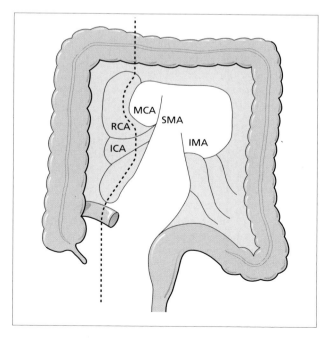

Fig. 16.7 Extent of resection for right hemicolectomy.

Hartmann's operation for malignant obstruction

Advantages
- No anastomosis
- Limited mobilization required
- Obstructing lesion resected
- Proximal colon preserved

Disadvantages
- Stoma
- High morbidity of reversal
- Up to 50% not reversed

Left-sided segmental resection with primary anastomosis
Primary left sided anastomosis on an unprepared obstructed colon is not generally regarded as appropriate, although some surgeons have achieved good results in selected cases. However, intra-operative decompression and preparation of the colon can be achieved by *on-table colonic lavage* (Fig. 16.8). The proximal colon is washed out via a catheter introduced through the appendix stump (or a caecotomy). The effluent is diverted into a sealed bag via a length of anaesthetic tubing, the proximal end of which is tied into the open distal end of the proximal colon. Once the effluent is clear the tubing is removed and primary anastomosis performed with the decompressed, 'prepared' bowel.

Results from on-table lavage with primary anastomosis vary considerably, but in experienced hands anastomotic leakage remains infrequent. A recent multicentre trial of lavage and anastomosis versus subtotal colectomy had a respectable leak rate of 5% with in-hospital mortality of 11% (The SCOTIA study group, 1995).

The technique is most appropriate for obstructing rectal lesions amenable to primary resection, where preservation of colon above a low anastomosis is desirable.

Primary resection with anastomosis

Advantages
- No stoma
- Lesion resected
- Proximal colon preserved

Disadvantages
- Potential for leakage
- Possibility of synchronous proximal lesion

Subtotal colectomy with ileosigmoid or ileorectal anastomosis
In the obstructed colon, the quality of the proximal bowel can be poor with respect to anastomosis because of oedema, distension, faecal loading, shutdown of the splanchnic blood supply and an inconsistent marginal vessel. Use of the proximal colon for anastomosis can be avoided by resection of the whole of the obstructed segment followed by primary ileorectal or ileosigmoid anastomosis. The anastomosis has a good blood supply from the ileum and proximal diversion is

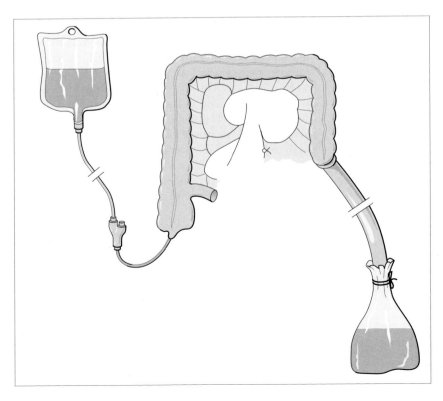

Fig. 16.8 On-table colonic lavage. Lavage fluid is poured through a catheter in the caecum, and the effluent drained into a bag from the distal end of the colon.

unnecessary. As the whole of the proximal colon is removed, undetected synchronous lesions, which may be missed in the absence of pre-operative imaging are removed and subsequent colonoscopic surveillance can be avoided.

The main perceived disadvantage to subtotal resection is postoperative bowel frequency. In most patients this is overstated as the median frequency after ileosigmoid anastomosis is in the region of two bowel actions per day, increasing to three per day after ileorectal anastomoses. Subtotal colectomy would of course be inadvisable in patients with known sphincter dysfunction or faecal incontinence.

Technically the operation is more demanding and takes longer than a segmental resection. With anastomotic leakage occurring in 9% of patients with a mortality of 13% in the SCOTIA trial.

Surgical technique for left-sided resection

For all left-sided colonic resections the Lloyd–Davis position is used. A generous midline incision is made taking great

Subtotal colectomy with ileorectal anastomosis
Advantages
• No stoma
• No need for lavage
• Lesion resected
• Obstructed colon resected
• Healthy bowel for anastomosis
• Proximal synchronous lesions resected
Disadvantages
• Extensive procedure
• Potentially normal colon removed
• Postoperative bowel frequency

care not to damage the distended bowel. If the colon is hugely distended and at risk of rupture during mobilization it should be decompressed before it is mobilized. When the caecum is likely to be resected or used to perform colonic

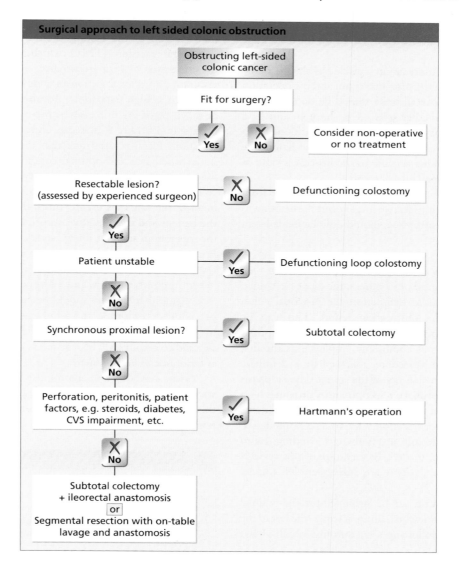

lavage, the colon can be decompressed by a lavage sucker introduced through the centre of a purse-string in the caecal wall. If a Hartmann's operation is anticipated, limited mobilization is required and decompression is rarely indicated before the stoma is exteriorized.

The left colon is mobilized taking care to identify and protect the left ureter. Once the colon has been mobilized, the inferior mesenteric vessels can be divided. The inferior mesenteric artery may be followed up and divided at its origin, but it is acceptable to leave the ascending left colic branch intact when the lesion is at or distal to the sigmoid. The inferior mesenteric vein is ligated separately from the artery. For restorative segmental and subtotal resections the splenic flexure is mobilized.

The distal margin of excision should lie at or close to the pelvic brim, provided that the resection margin is at least 5 cm distal to the tumour. Unnecessary dissection of the mesorectum for sigmoid lesions places the presacral nerves at risk of injury and opens up the presacral space, producing a cavity which could potentially harbour sepsis. For lesions of the upper rectum, however, the mesorectum should be dissected and cleanly divided at least 5 cm below the distal edge of the cancer.

The proximal resection margin is guided by the site of the cancer, the viability of the proximal colon and the operation being performed. Above all there should be no tension on the residual colon whether it is to be brought out as a colostomy, or a primary anastomosis is to be fashioned. If a subtotal colectomy is performed for a left sided lesion, the terminal ileum is divided as close to the ileocaecal valve as possible to preserve small bowel length.

The technique for anastomosis should not differ from that which is used during elective surgery, but the decision to perform a primary anastomosis should only be made by an experienced operator.

Decompression without resection for left-sided obstruction

The least invasive surgical procedure in the case of left-sided colonic obstruction is to defunction the proximal colon without resecting the obstructing lesion. This can be achieved by a loop transverse colostomy. At one time, proximal loop colostomy was commonly employed as the first stage of a three-stage procedure, followed by a definitive resection and finally by closure of the stoma. The emphasis has now changed to primary resection and a proximal loop colostomy is only used as a temporizing measure for patients considered too unfit for resection. The stoma is fashioned to the right of the middle colic artery thereby avoiding risk to the marginal artery on the left. Preservation of this vessel is important for the vascularity of any subsequent left colonic anastomoses.

A transverse colostomy can be fashioned through a small right transverse incision, which limits access to the rest of the peritoneal cavity, or following a laparotomy, which allows accurate assessment of the cause of obstruction at the expense of greater surgical trauma. However, whilst the unfit patient may survive the initial assault, they are still committed to a resectional procedure to rid them of their obstructing lesion. Clearly, a significant number of such patients will never actually have a resection because of their comorbidity. In those who do end up having a resection and then a reversal of the loop, the cumulative mortality from all three procedures approximates to the mortality from an emergent primary resection.

Obstruction from rectal cancer

Cancer of the sigmoid and rectosigmoid junction commonly obstruct, but acute large bowel obstruction from a lesion below the peritoneal reflexion is rare. This is because other symptoms such as rectal bleeding, tenesmus and altered bowel habit usually lead to the diagnosis before obstruction occurs. When rectal cancer does present with obstruction, the diagnosis should be made either by digital rectal examination or by sigmoidoscopy.

Current thinking in elective rectal cancer surgery is that excision of the rectum should include *en-bloc* total mesorectal excision (TME) which dramatically reduces the incidence of local recurrence, and that the ratio of restorative anterior resection to abdominoperineal excision should be as high as possible. Advanced rectal cancers may be downstaged in some cases by pre-operative neo-adjuvant chemoradiotherapy which can be followed by restorative resection. Elective rectal resection therefore requires planning, experience and optimal conditions to achieve good long term results. In the emergency situation, when the colon is obstructed by a rectal cancer, imaging and assessment of the cancer is usually incomplete, the condition of the patient and the operative exposure are suboptimal, and the operating surgeon may be relatively inexperienced. Primary resection, whilst appropriate for tumours of the rest of the colon, is therefore best avoided for middle or lower third rectal lesions, and a defunctioning left iliac fossa loop sigmoid colostomy should be fashioned instead. This procedure decompresses the colon and allows for the patient to be fully worked up before their definitive resection. The sigmoid colostomy will be resected as part of the subsequent anterior resection specimen.

Primary resection and anastomosis may in some circumstances be undertaken after on-table colonic lavage. Whilst this empties the bowel, the risk of anastomotic failure still remains high and there should be a low threshold for proxi-

Rectal cancer
• Rarely obstructs
• Diagnosis by PR examination/sigmoidoscopy
• Defunction with LIF colostomy
• Definitive treatment should involve colorectal surgeon

mal diversion. The diverting stoma should be, by preference, a loop ileostomy which will defunction the enterotomy used for the lavage, and does not endanger the marginal blood supply to the colon.

The use of Hartmann's operation for middle or low rectal cancers carries all the disadvantages of an acute primary resection and creates a difficult short rectal stump when it comes to reversal. For these reasons it is not recommended.

Non-surgical options in left-sided obstruction

Radiological techniques for decompressions of the obstructed colon are currently being developed. Self-expanding metal stents, similar to those used for the palliation of oesophageal carcinoma, can be placed transanally across the obstructing cancer over a guidewire. In the few cases reported to date the colon has been successfully decompressed, allowing for standard bowel preparation and operation on an elective basis. Details on the limitations and complications of the technique are awaited.

Non-malignant obstruction

Diverticular disease

Diverticular disease may unusually precipitate large bowel obstruction as a consequence either of an acute inflammatory mass or collection, or a chronic diverticular stricture. In the absence of local tenderness, a contrast enema is appropriate. This will demonstrate obstruction but will rarely exclude malignancy with any confidence as a cause of the obstruction. The presence of local peritonitis in the presence of colonic obstruction is a contraindication to contrast studies and should prompt urgent laparotomy.

At laparotomy it may still be impossible to differentiate between a diverticular mass and a locally invasive or perforated cancer. If doubt exists, resection should take the form of a radical en bloc cancer resection when resection would be considered potentially curative. Where the diagnosis is clearly benign, local excision is appropriate.

Immediate reconstruction is unwise in the presence of both obstruction and an inflammatory mass, or where locally invasive malignancy cannot be excluded. Hartmann's operation is therefore the operation of choice in this situation.

Hernia

The sigmoid colon is often drawn into left-sided sliding groin herniae. Obstruction of such herniae is uncommon, as there is usually a broad neck to the sac. However, as with all cases of obstruction, the groins should be carefully examined, and the reducibility of any hernia assessed.

Large bowel volvulus

Volvulus, or twisting of the colon occurs at sites where the colon has a free mesentery, either naturally, as a result of congenital failure of peritonealization or in some instances following surgical mobilization. The commonest site of large bowel volvulus is the sigmoid colon, which accounts for some 80% of volvulus in UK practice, followed by the caecum and much more rarely the transverse colon or splenic flexure. An unusual form of volvulus almost exclusive to Africa is ileosigmoid knotting, in which a complex twist occurs between a loop of ileum and a hypermobile sigmoid. It has a particularly rapid onset and course which progresses speedily towards ischaemia, usually of the ileum.

Factors which predispose to volvulus are excessive mobility of a segment of bowel and a narrow mesentery. Increased mobility is important in caecal volvulus, where the usual peritoneal fusion of the right colon is absent. Sigmoid volvulus, on the other hand often occurs when there is a long redundant sigmoid loop based on a narrow mesentery. The narrow mesentery allows a twist to occur.

Sigmoid volvulus

In the UK sigmoid volvulus is a condition predominantly of the elderly and the mentally handicapped. There may be a history of chronic constipation, and a number of patients have had previous episodes of volvulus treated conservatively. In other parts of the world, particularly parts of Asia and Africa a younger population is affected. In these cases high fibre diet may be a contributary factor in the pathogenesis of the condition.

Clinical presentation

Most cases of sigmoid volvulus are of a subacute progressive form in which abdominal distension and constipation are the predominant symptoms. Pain may be surprisingly mild for the degree of abdominal distension. A smaller group of often younger patients present with an acute fulminating picture of severe pain, distension, vomiting and early progression to gangrene of the affected loop.

Abdominal X-ray is usually diagnostic, showing the characteristic appearance of the hugely distended sigmoid extending towards the right upper quadrant. In most cases, however, an acute contrast enema may be required to differentiate between volvulus and other causes of obstruction or pseudo-obstruction. Contrast studies may show complete obstruction to flow with a typical beak appearance at the base of the torsion. If some contrast does pass through the apex of the twist, the distended sigmoid loop will be demonstrated. In some cases the contrast enema may be therapeutic by untwisting the volvulus (Fig. 16.9), or facilitating decom-

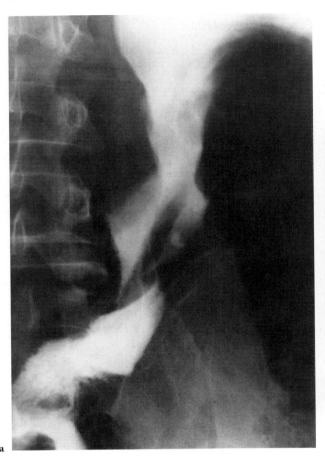

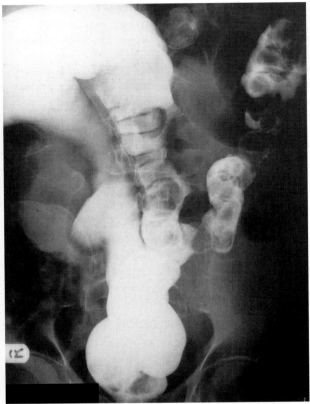

Fig. 16.9 Gastrografin enema for sigmoid volvulus. (a) The initial beak of contrast continues through the apex of the volvulus, in this case causing it to untwist. (b) Following decompression, the contrast-filled sigmoid loop fills the right upper quadrant. Proximal faecal loading can also be seen.

pression of the volvulus by manipulation of a flatus tube under radiological guidance to a position above the colonic twist.

Treatment

Decompression of uncomplicated sigmoid volvulus is usually achieved by the passage of a rigid sigmoidoscope up to the apex of the torsion, with the patient in the knee–chest position where possible. Decompression is met by a flood of gas and liquid faeces down the sigmoidoscope. A flatus tube can be passed down the sigmoidoscope under direct vision and the scope withdrawn around it. Flexible sigmoidoscopy may be used if the apex of the volvulus cannot be reached or negotiated with the rigid sigmoidoscope.

Failure to untwist the sigmoid endoscopically, or the presence of peritonitis or perforation should prompt urgent laparotomy.

In the acute situation, surgical resection carries a mortality upwards of 25%, which reflects the fact that surgery is

Volvulus of the colon
• Sigmoid—80%
• Caecum
• Transverse colon
• Splenic flexure
• Ileosigmoid knot

only performed acutely in the sickest of these frail patients. Ideally endoscopic detorsion should be followed by elective surgery after several days. The risks of elective surgery, although still substantial, should be balanced against the risks of recurrent volvulus without surgery (about 40%) and its complications. Surgery usually involves resection of the redundant sigmoid colon (Fig. 16.10).

Non-resectional procedures such as mesosigmoidopexy have had variable degrees of success, advocates claiming low morbidity and a low recurrence rates. Despite these claims, mesosigmoidopexy is rarely employed in the UK.

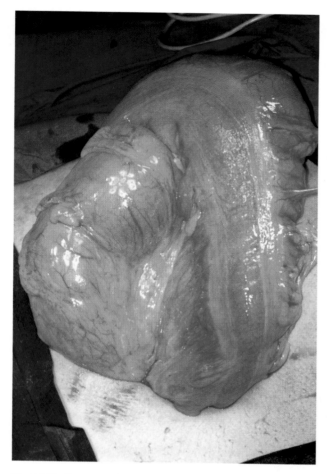

Fig. 16.10 Operative photograph prior to elective sigmoid resection for recurrent volvulus. Note the thickened mesentery at the base of the sigmoid.

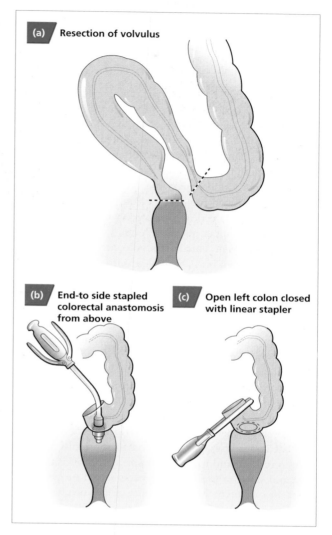

Fig. 16.11 Technique for stapled anastomosis after resection for sigmoid volvulus.

In the acute situation, care must be taken not to perforate the hugely distended colon during the abdominal incision. Resection of the sigmoid loop, including the points of torsion may be followed by primary anastomosis or by the creation of an end colostomy (Hartmann's operation). Where endoscopic detorsion has been successful, a primary anastomosis is usually possible. A colostomy is advisable in the presence of gangrene of the loop, perforation or gross proximal obstruction. Some of these patients, however, would have major difficulties managing a colostomy and the chance of surviving a second major procedure to close the stoma is limited. In such circumstances primary anastomosis may be the best overall option despite the grave outlook in the event of anastomotic failure.

Surgical technique (Fig. 16.11)

One of the problems of primary anastomosis after sigmoid resection for volvulus, particularly when chronic or recur-rent, is the size discrepancy between the proximal and distal bowel lumen. Moreover, the wall of the proximal bowel may be much thicker than that of the distal loop. This can be taken into account with a hand-sutured end-to-end anasto-mosis by taking wider bites of the proximal bowel, but stapling may be difficult because of the bulk of tissue pro-duced within the purse-string of thickened proximal bowel. An alternative is to suture or staple an end-to-side anastomo-sis. This requires a little extra length of proximal bowel but avoids the problems of discrepancy. A stapled end to side anastomosis is fashioned by placing the anvil into the rectal stump, using a purse-string, and passing the gun into the open end of the proximal bowel. The spike is advanced to pass through the antimesenteric aspect of the bowel, taking care to leave enough length beyond the staple line to close the open end of the proximal bowel after the gun is fired and removed. The open end may be closed with a linear stapler.

Caecal volvulus

Non-fixation of the right colon permits excessive mobility of the caecum. Caecal volvulus is primarily a consequence of the mobility of the non-fixed caecum, although other factors such as high fibre diet and a history of previous surgery may also be important. The symptoms of caecal volvulus are of crampy abdominal pain and distension. The distended caecum may be visible or palpable.

The diagnosis may be apparent from the plain abdominal film, which shows the distended caecum extending upwards towards the left upper quadrant, often with several dilated small bowel loops proximal to the volvulus. Contrast studies may demonstrate a bird's beak deformity at the apex of the volvulus, as with sigmoid volvulus.

Treatment is usually surgical although occasional cases of successful decompression by colonoscopy are described. The caecum is untwisted and if viability is doubtful, should be resected by right hemicolectomy. There is some debate as to the best procedure when the bowel is viable. The options are simple detorsion alone, caecopexy, caecostomy or resection. Retrospective data from the literature suggest that resection is safe and has the best long-term results. However, simple detorsion and caecopexy carry the lowest morbidity with little to choose between them in recurrence rates (around 13%). Caecostomy appears to add to morbidity and has little to recommend it. Whilst simple detorsion is the simplest and safest procedure, most experienced surgeons will resect the caecum to avoid recurrence of the volvulus.

Acute colonic pseudo-obstruction (Ogilvie's syndrome)

Colonic pseudo-obstruction is a condition of reduced motility, and dilatation of the colon. Patients present with many of the signs of large bowel obstruction, although there is no mechanical obstruction. Pseudo-obstruction usually occurs in patients who are ill from non-colonic conditions and in patients who have had surgery, often for non-gastrointestinal disease. The exact aetiology of the condition is unknown, but many of the factors which predispose to its development affect autonomic activity or colonic motility.

Presentation

Patients with pseudo-obstruction are commonly encountered by way of an in-hospital referral to the on-call general surgical team from a medical, gynaecology, neurosurgery or orthopaedic ward. The patient, who may be recovering from an operation, or suffering from multiple medical problems usually presents with abdominal distension, which is often painless. Constipation is a common feature although some leakage of liquid faeces may occur. Vomiting may or may not occur. On occasions, pseudo-obstruction presents without any obvious predisposing cause.

Examination reveals a hugely distended abdomen which is very resonant to percussion. The rectum is usually empty, although rectal examination may be met by a gush of flatus and liquid faeces on removal of the examining finger. The presence of tenderness over the caecum requires urgent intervention.

Plain abdominal X-rays reveal marked distension of the colon as far as the splenic flexure. Less commonly the gaseous cut-off occurs either at the hepatic flexure or in the left colon. A water-soluble contrast enema should be performed in all cases to confirm the diagnosis and exclude a mechanical cause for obstruction. In a number of cases the enema may prove therapeutic.

Treatment

The treatment of pseudo-obstruction involves the removal, where possible of precipitating factors and decompression of the distended colon. Surgical resection is rarely appropriate except following a colonic perforation.

A nasogastric tube is placed and oral intake discontinued. Opiates and drugs with anticholinergic or sympathomimetic actions should be stopped and any electrolyte imbalance, particularly hypokalaemia, corrected. Decompression may be achieved by the passage of a sigmoidoscope which, if successful, should be replaced by a flatus tube which is taped in place for 24 hours. Gentle enemas may also be used to encourage motility and decompression distally.

In the event of progressive distension or failure of the above measures to decompress the distended colon, a colonoscope can be used to enter and decompress the distended proximal colon. Insufflation should be kept to a minimum to avoid perforating the caecum, although in experienced hands perforation is an infrequent event.

Recurrence is a common problem but should be treated in the same fashion as the initial episode of pseudo-obstruction. Treatment of any predisposing acute condition will be more effective at reducing the chance of recurrence.

Surgery is indicated when there is actual or impending rupture of the caecum. Progressive distension of the caecum beyond 10–12 cm diameter usually heralds perforation, as does the development of peritoneal irritation over the caecum.

The most common method of surgical decompression of the caecum is by tube caecostomy. This can be performed under local anaesthesia if the patient is too unwell to tolerate a general anaesthetic. A transverse incision is made over the caecum, which may be decompressed partially by needle puncture and aspiration of some gas. A wide-bore rubber

Conditions associated with acute colonic pseudo-obstruction in 378 patients	
Surgical patients	
• Trauma (non-operative)	11%
• Pelvic surgery	15%
• Caesarian section	4%
• Orthopaedic surgery	7%
• Cardiothoracic surgery	4%
Medical patients	
• Infection	10%
• Cardiac disease	10%
• Neurological disease	9%
• Pulmonary disease	6%
• Metabolic disturbance	5%
• Renal failure	4%
Source: Vanek & Salti (1986)	

catheter or a cuffed endotracheal tube is introduced into the caecum via a caecotomy and held in place by a double purse-string suture. The caecum is hitched up by sutures to the abdominal wall around the caecotomy and the wound closed around the tube. Continued decompression is ensured by daily irrigation of the catheter with saline to avoid blockage of the lumen. If the pseudo-obstruction resolves, the catheter can be removed after 10 days and the caecostomy will usually close spontaneously.

If there is perforation, or the viability of the caecum is in doubt, resection is indicated. In contaminated cases it is safest to bring out both ends of the resection as an ileostomy and mucus fistula. Primary anastomosis without decompression can be followed by prolonged post-operative ileus and the same principles of avoiding precipitant drugs and maintaining the electrolyte balance should apply after surgery as before.

Further reading

Deans, G.T., Krukowski, Z.H. & Irwin, S.T. (1994) Malignant obstruction of the left colon. *British Journal of Surgery* **81** 1270–1276.

Rabinovici, R., Simanski, D.A., Kaplan, O., Mavor, E. & Manny, J. (1990) Caecal volvulus. *Diseases of the Colon & Rectum* **33** 765–769.

Vanek, V.W. & Al Salti, M. (1986) Acute pseudo-obstruction of the colon (Ogilvie's syndrome). An analysis of 400 cases. *Diseases of the Colon & Rectum* **29** 203–210.

Reference

The SCOTIA study group (1995). Single stage treatment for malignant left sided colonic obstruction: a prospective randomised clinical trial comparing subtotal colectomy with segmental resection following intra-operative irrigation. The SCOTIA study group. Subtotal colectomy versus on-table irrigation and anastomosis. *British Journal of Surgery* **82** 1622–1627.

CHAPTER 17

Abdominal hernias

Brendan McIlroy & Andrew N. Kingsnorth

Introduction

With refinements in the organization and delivery of health care in the developed world, including particular emphasis on the provision of day care surgical services, the emergency presentation of abdominal hernias has changed to occupy a smaller proportion of the acute surgical workload. However, the emergency management of abdominal hernias demands a familiarity with the basic principles of resuscitation and surgical technique if the best outcomes are to be achieved in this group of patients who are often frail, elderly and with intercurrent medical problems.

Various presentations of abdominal hernias will be described followed by a discussion of general principles of management. Specific hernias are then discussed along with alternative operative strategies.

Presentation and pathophysiology

The vast majority of emergency presentations of abdominal hernias occur along the spectrum of incarceration, with or without obstruction, leading to strangulation, again, with or without obstruction. Incarceration is defined as an external hernia which cannot be reduced into the abdomen. Although in itself not life threatening, it is an important finding as it implies that there is an increased risk of obstruction and strangulation. Incarceration is usually caused by a tight neck of the hernia sac. However, the examining surgeon should be alert to other causes of incarceration caused by pathology within the hernia's contents, such as diverticulitis or carcinoma. Strangulation implies that the blood supply of the hernia's contents is compromised or cut off entirely with the danger of tissue death. The ischaemia of a strangulated hernia may be reversible, i.e. the contents are viable, or irreversible with necrotic or gangrenous contents. The possibility of an abdominal hernia as the cause of obstruction should be entertained in all such cases (Fig. 17.1). At least a quarter of all cases of obstruction result from hernias and, in patients without previous abdominal surgery, hernias are the leading cause of obstruction. The source of the problem may be obvious in certain situations, such as inguinal or incisional hernia but it is easy to overlook

a small femoral hernia in an obese patient. Indeed, there may be no external manifestation in cases of obturator hernia. In patients with scars from previous abdominal surgery, all hernial orifices should still be carefully examined.

Bowel obstruction occurs frequently in cases of strangulated hernia but if the hernia sac contains omentum, mesentery or even a solid organ, strangulation is less common. The examining surgeon should, however, be aware that, in certain situations, obstruction may not occur even when bowel is contained in the sac of a strangulating hernia, including cases where only the appendix is involved, a Meckel's diverticulum (Littre hernia; Fig. 17.2), or only part of the circumference of the bowel (Richter's hernia).

Although strangulation may be due to occlusion of a mesenteric blood vessel, it is much more commonly a local phenomenon. The process begins with bowel becoming distorted because of angulation at the neck of the hernial sac. Lymphatic and venous outflow from the sac is impeded with resultant oedema of the contents. Capillary blood flow next becomes compromised. The arterial supply is eventually occluded by this course of events leading to ischaemic changes within the bowel wall. The demarcation of this process is clearly seen at the edge of the fascial defect. Although usually involving only a short segment of small intestine, a strangulated hernia may contain several contiguous or non-contiguous loops of small or large bowel.

In untreated cases of strangulation, gangrene of the bowel will ensue. The gut mucosal defences break down and Gram-negative aerobic and anaerobic bacteria invade the bowel wall and multiply. If the bowel were returned to the peritoneal cavity in this condition, it would almost certainly perforate, or, less likely, heal by fibrosis resulting in a stricture.

Bowel in a strangulated hernia eventually perforates, releasing bowel content with multiplying bacteria into the surrounding tissues. Thus decompressed, the hernia contents may reduce into the abdomen followed by diffuse peritonitis. Perforation can also result in abscess formation which, if it discharges through the skin, can cause a bowel fistula.

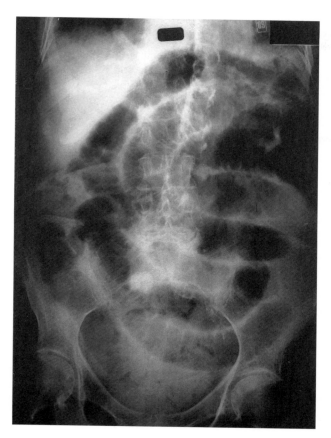

Fig. 17.1 A plain supine abdominal X-ray showing small bowel obstruction.

Initial management

A case of strangulating hernia causing small bowel obstruction will, in the majority of cases, be apparent from the history and examination of the patient. Most patients will be aware of a previously reducible lump which has become enlarged, hard, tender and irreducible. A full abdominal examination is required and it is essential not to overlook all

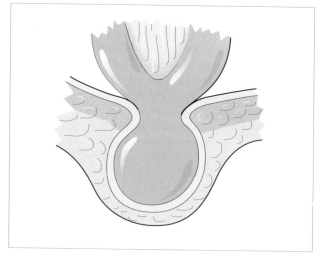

Fig. 17.2 A Meckel's diverticulum may form the content of a hernia sac.

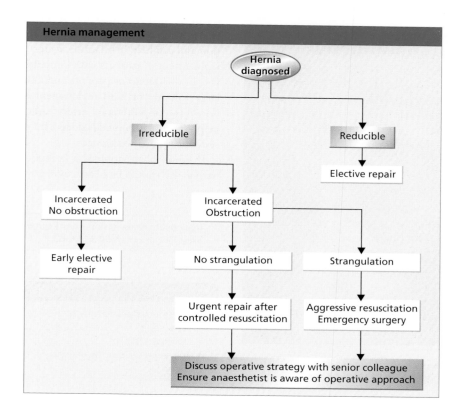

Hernia management

Hernia diagnosed

Irreducible — Reducible

Reducible → Elective repair

Irreducible → Incarcerated No obstruction → Early elective repair

Irreducible → Incarcerated Obstruction

Incarcerated Obstruction → No strangulation → Urgent repair after controlled resuscitation

Incarcerated Obstruction → Strangulation → Aggressive resuscitation Emergency surgery

Discuss operative strategy with senior colleague
Ensure anaesthetist is aware of operative approach

potential hernia sites in cases of obstruction. The patient's general condition and the presence of intercurrent medical problems will guide the surgeon towards the amount and speed of resuscitation required. Investigations will confirm the clinical impression and can help to establish the degree of physiological derangements. A full blood count with blood urea and electrolytes are, at the very least, needed. Arterial blood gas analysis may also be required in patients who have been vomiting, diabetics, and in co-existing respiratory disease. A plain, supine abdominal X-ray may demonstrate a gas-filled structure in the area of a palpable mass and will confirm the diagnosis of obstruction (Fig. 17.3). In the elderly, especially, the X-ray may show dual or alternative pathology. Patients over the age of 50 years require a pre-operative electrocardiograph (ECG). A chest X-ray should be taken in the presence of any cardiorespiratory disease and where there is a history of vomiting to determine whether aspiration pneumonia is present.

A patient with a strangulated hernia may need a significant period of resuscitation before surgery is undertaken. Dehydration is compounded by bowel obstruction which

> Check all potential hernia sites in all cases of obstruction even when the cause appears to be adhesions.

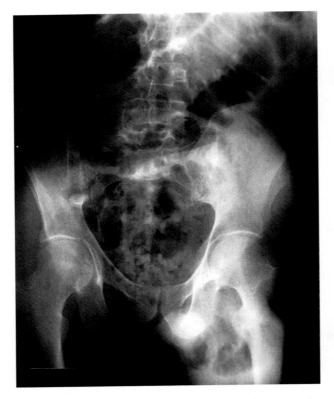

Fig. 17.3 Small bowel obstruction with a loop of bowel incarcerated in a left inguinal hernia.

causes vomiting and fluid sequestration within the bowel. Bacterial translocation from necrotic tissue or infarcted bowel will lead to endotoxaemia with systemic sepsis or frank septic shock. Cardiovascular collapse is almost inevitable if general anaesthesia is induced under these conditions. A period of resuscitation prior to surgery virtually always improves the patient's physiological variables which, in the majority of cases, will translate to better surgical outcomes. Despite the fact that these patients are often ill and elderly, inadequate resuscitation and hasty surgery is still seen not infrequently with disastrous consequences. It must be remembered, however, that in the presence of dead gut or established peritonitis, there is nothing to be gained by continuing aggressive resuscitation, where deterioration will continue despite this. In these cases, resuscitation and emergency surgery go hand in hand. It should be noted, particularly by junior surgeons, that in gravely ill, elderly patients, non-operative management may be a more humane course of action. This decision should be made at a senior level.

In assessing the amount and speed of resuscitation required, signs of shock must be sought even if the patient appears well with a normal blood pressure. Tachycardia is an important sign and, if present, should prompt intravenous fluid replacement with regular monitoring of pulse, blood pressure and urine output. An initial fluid challenge with crystalloid may be all that is required in a young, previously fit patient. In all other cases, and where the response is not as expected, additional information is needed. Invasive monitoring may be necessary and, at the very least, a urinary catheter should be inserted. Central venous pressure monitoring via a right subclavian or internal jugular catheter is valuable in confirming the clinical impression of dehydration and can help in guarding against overenthusiastic fluid replacement in patients with limited cardiovascular reserve. It is in this group of patients and also in the elderly where large volumes of fluid replacement are anticipated that a flow-directed pulmonary artery catheter (Swan–Ganz) can be positioned to provide added data on cardiac output and systemic vascular resistance.

If bowel obstruction is a complication of strangulated hernia, this should be treated as in any complete mechanical

> Inadequate resuscitation + hasty surgery – surgical experience = potential disaster.

> **A question of resuscitation**
>
> - How much fluid do I give?
> - What sort?
> - How quickly?
> - The answer: assess the degree of shock and closely monitor.

obstruction. Fluid replacement and gastric decompression via a nasogastric tube are mandatory. In all cases, once adequate resuscitation has been carried out, operative exploration and hernia repair must proceed forthwith. Any delay could mean the difference between dead and viable bowel, or between perforated and intact bowel.

Attempts at reduction

It has been argued by some that reducing an acutely incarcerated hernia converts a surgical emergency into an elective operation, thereby reducing the mortality risk. There is no evidence to support this argument and, in addition, there is the attendant risk of reducing dead bowel into the abdomen. Another complication of forced attempts at reduction is reduction-en-masse. This refers to a reduction of the external hernial mass but the contents of the hernia are still incarcerated or strangulated within the hernial sac most commonly caused by a narrow, fibrosed neck.

No attempt should be made to reduce a hernia if it has been incarcerated for more than 24 hours, remembering that strangulation can cause gangrene in a hernia in under 5 h. Other contra-indications to attempts at reduction include, skin discoloration over the hernia, diffuse abdominal tenderness, signs of systemic sepsis, and in the presence of extraluminal gas on abdominal X-ray.

Principles of operative management and anaesthesia

Once adequate resuscitation has taken place, any further delay for operation for strangulating hernia is unacceptable. In the emergency setting, it is easy to overlook the provision of prophylaxis against deep vein thrombosis. At the very least, all patients require subcutaneous heparin and graduated compression stockings. Patients who are at an increased risk of thrombo-embolism should be considered for additional prophylaxis with intravenous Dextran or intra-operative pneumatic leggings.

All strangulating hernias must be presumed to contain gangrenous or perforated bowel and, for this reason, pre-operative broad-spectrum antibiotics must be administered, preferably at least 15 min before anaesthetic induction. Unless gross peritoneal contamination has occurred, antibiotics need not be continued beyond the first postoperative day, except in certain circumstances (see below).

The experience of not only the operating surgeon but also the attending anaesthetist should be a match for the condition of the patient undergoing emergency hernia surgery. Surgical and patient factors determine the chosen anaesthetic technique for a given operation. The primary concerns are for the patient's safety and the provision of optimum operating conditions. Although the repair of many abdominal wall hernias can be performed safely and

with little difficulty under local anaesthesia in the elective setting, a strangulated hernia will often require an alternative anatomical approach and, coupled with the possibility of bowel resection and anastomosis, local anaesthesia alone can be inadequate. In terms of patient safety, local anaesthesia may not be superior when faced with a poorly patient 'not fit for a general anaesthetic.' Such patients' anxieties will be increased by pain caused by inadequate local anaesthesia with deleterious effects on their physiological status. Increasing the dose of local anaesthesia and providing intravenous sedation can often amount to a virtual general anaesthetic with the added risk of cardiovascular side effects from local anaesthetic toxicity.

Regional anaesthesia can be an attractive proposition in the management of strangulated hernia. Spinal and epidural anaesthesia require a skilled anaesthetist but appear to have advantages in terms of speed and quality of patient recovery. Either technique can produce anaesthesia below a dermatomal level of T9 to T10 which is adequate for groin hernia surgery. In cases of strangulated groin hernias, anaesthesia can be extended up to the level of T5 which will produce a block of the abdominal viscera. Surgeon and anaesthetist alike must be aware of producing a more extensive sympathetic blockade as the effect of the anaesthetic extends up the neuroaxis. Peripheral vasodilatation occurs with less compensatory vasoconstriction above the block. The resultant tendency to hypotension can be disastrous especially in the emergency setting and again the importance of preoperative resuscitation cannot be over-stressed. A further advantage of epidural anaesthesia is that incremental doses of anaesthetic can be given via an indwelling catheter in the epidural space with enhanced patient safety. Postoperative analgesia can also be given in this way.

Despite the alternatives, modern general anaesthesia can provide smooth, controlled induction and recovery for even the most sick patients while offering the surgeon muscle relaxation for what may be a lengthy and technically demanding procedure.

In planning an operative strategy in a case of strangulating hernia, the surgeon must remember that the aim to repair the hernia defect is his least consideration. More important is the removal of gangrenous tissue and the prevention of further sepsis as well as the relief of obstruction. This may mean employing an alternative operative approach from the one that would be used in a case of non-strangulating hernia. The requirements of any such approach are that the bowel must first be controlled to avoid gangrenous or perforated

> - An unfamiliar approach to a strangulated hernia may have the same potential for disaster as a poorly judged familiar approach.
> - Tailor the operation to suit the patient, not the surgeon!
> - If in doubt, get help.

bowel slipping back into the peritoneal cavity, spreading sepsis. Any approach used for strangulating hernia must include access to the peritoneal cavity.

The advantages of prosthetic material for hernia repair are that the techniques for its use are easily learnt and recurrences are reduced. Mesh should not be used in cases of strangulating hernia in the presence of gangrenous or perforated bowel. However, provided certain precautions are taken, it can be used in cases of ischaemic but viable bowel when the surgeon assesses the risk of bacterial contamination to be negligible. The most widespread prosthetic mesh in use is polypropylene, e.g. Marlex, which is more tolerant to infection than other material. The mesh must be placed in an uncontaminated position. Although prophylactic antibiotics are not required for the placement of Marlex mesh in elective hernia repair, where there is even the slightest risk of contamination of the operative field from ischaemic bowel, a 5-day course of antibiotics is mandatory. Mesh should not be placed in a position of established infection. It is safer in such situations to resect bowel and control infection and to leave the repair of the hernia defect for another day.

Operative technique

Dealing with a strangulated or incarcerated hernia as an emergency is not the time for the surgical trainee to attempt an alternative operative approach with which he or she is not familiar. Although a junior surgeon will be aware of various techniques, detailed descriptions of which will be found in operative textbooks, an easily applicable approach to all the common emergency hernia conditions should be learnt.

A midline laparotomy incision, which could be considered excessive in many cases, nevertheless permits a thorough inspection of the contents of the abdominal cavity. All abdominal hernias can be repaired via this route and additional hernias can be found and dealt with. Also, early control of bowel which may be entering the hernia sac can be gained. Alternative or dual pathologies may be found. A laparotomy incision is strongly recommended in the presence of bowel obstruction where an incarcerated/strangulating hernia co-exists with previous abdominal surgery. In this situation, adhesions may be the cause of obstruction. Laparotomy is mandatory when generalized peritonitis follows a strangulated hernia.

Inguinal hernia

Most strangulating hernias encountered will be inguinal, about half of all cases. This is not because of any special propensity for inguinal hernias to strangulate but is because inguinal hernia is by far the commonest abdominal wall hernia. The risk of strangulation seems to lie at between 0.3 and 2.9% per year. However, this risk is probably at its greatest in the first several months after the hernia is first noticed.

Indirect hernias are ten times more likely to strangulate than direct.

The easiest approach to a strangulated inguinal hernia is the same as that used for an elective repair (Fig. 17.4). Certain points should be borne in mind. As in the standard approach to inguinal hernia, the external oblique aponeurosis is split along the line of its fibres. It should be remembered that the constricting neck of the hernia sac is often at the external ring. Once this constriction is released, the contents of the hernia could easily slip back into the abdomen. Sufficient mobilization of the cord and sac deep to external oblique in order to hold the contents in place should be attempted before the incision in external oblique is carried to its medial limit (Fig. 17.5) More often than not, the internal ring is dilated. If gangrenous bowel is resected and anastomosis performed, easy reduction back into the abdomen is possible. If the internal ring is not dilated, anastomosis may be awkward, if not impossible. Division of the inferior epigastric vessels allows the internal ring to be incised medially, through attenuated transversalis fascia, any extraperitoneal fat and peritoneum (Fig. 17.6).

Repair of the defect should follow the same principles as those that govern elective inguinal hernia repair. Except in situations of sepsis or suspected contamination, as described above, a tension-free repair with polypropylene mesh is recommended for its ease of use and low recurrence potential.

Preperitoneal repair of a strangulating inguinal hernia is an alternative approach and has particular value where the hernia is recurrent. A grid-iron, or preferably a Pfannensteil, incision allows the preperitoneal space to be entered. This serves the dual purpose of allowing control of bowel entering the sac, eliminating the danger of spreading sepsis into the peritoneal cavity, and carrying out the repair utilizing

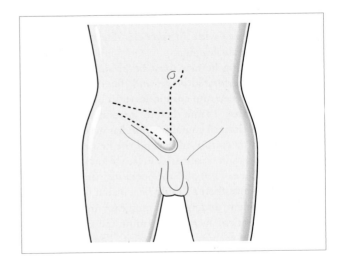

Fig. 17.4 Alternative approaches to a strangulated right inguinal hernia.

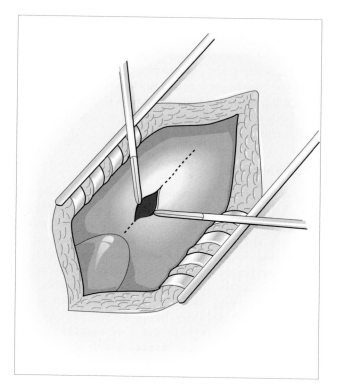

Fig. 17.5 The external oblique aponeurosis should not be split to its medial extent until the hernia contents can be prevented from reduction.

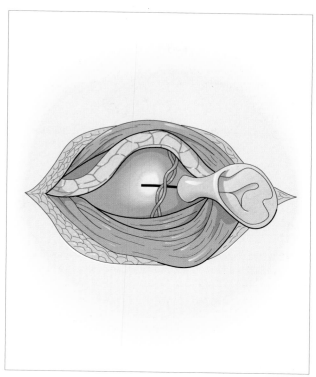

Fig. 17.6 A constricting internal ring can be extended medially.

healthy, unscarred tissue. The defect is closed by placing several interrupted non-absorbable sutures between the transverse aponeurotic arch and the inguinal ligament. The decision to reinforce with mesh will result from the same considerations as in the anterior approach.

Femoral hernia

Although less common than inguinal hernia, femoral hernias are at greater risk of strangulation, a much higher proportion initially presenting in this way. Bowel resection is about twice as likely to be needed in strangulated femoral hernias compared to strangulated inguinal hernias. The low approach to a strangulated femoral hernia is, therefore, to be condemned. A preperitoneal approach is advised (Fig. 17.7).

Of all the eponyms associated with femoral hernia repair, the approach associated with the British surgeon, Henry, should be remembered. Henry 'discovered' the preperitoneal approach to groin hernias in his surgery on the lower ureter, treating the complications of schistosomiasis. His initial description included a lower midline incision but he was to later recommend a Pfannensteil incision. In utilizing this route, the surgeon is afforded a clear view of the anatomy surrounding a strangulated femoral hernia. Any bowel entering the hernia sac can be visualized. If any

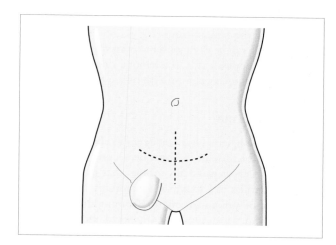

Fig. 17.7 Incisions for a preperitoneal approach to a strangulating femoral hernia.

ischaemia is thought to be irreversible, initial control can be secured. In this situation, it is advisable to divide the bowel as it enters the hernia sac which is most easily done with a surgical stapling device. The bowel is anastomosed and

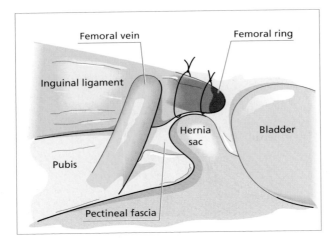

Fig. 17.8 The femoral canal is closed with interrupted monofilament sutures with a clear view of the surrounding anatomy.

returned to the peritoneal cavity which can then be closed. At this point the hernia can be reduced without the risk of spreading sepsis into the peritoneal cavity. If reduction is difficult, it can be better achieved by incising the insertion of the posterior inguinal wall into Cooper's ligament on the medial side of the hernia. The excellent view obtained with a preperitoneal approach has several further advantages. An aberrant obturator artery may be clearly seen as it passes over the medial margin of the femoral ring. The femoral vein is seen and protected as interrupted monofilament sutures are used to close the femoral ring (Fig. 17.8). A contralateral femoral hernia can be dealt with but even when no hernia is found on the opposite side, the femoral ring is often found to be dilated, requiring closure with two or three sutures.

Obturator hernia

This uncommon hernia has a tendency to effect frail, elderly females. It is because of its infrequent occurrence and the fact that it is never externally visible, that the majority of obturator hernias are found at laparotomy for intestinal obstruction of unknown origin. Commonly a Richter's hernia is found. Most cases of strangulated obturator hernia will need bowel resection. A clue to the presence of a strangulating obturator hernia can be the Howship–Romberg sign, which may only be present in around half of cases when specifically sought. This is pain down the medial aspect of the thigh which can usually be relieved by flexion at the hip joint and is exacerbated by extension, adduction or internal rotation. A tender mass felt through the lateral fornix of the vagina may also be due to a strangulated obturator hernia.

If a strangulated obturator hernia could be reliably diagnosed pre-operatively, then a preperitoneal approach would be most suitable. Otherwise, a lower midline laparotomy is

recommended. If a strangulation cannot be reduced, the constricting ring must be incised. Because of the varying relationships between the hernia sac and obturator nerves and vessels, the safest place to incise is at the lower edge. Difficulty may be encountered in closing the defect as the obturator foramen is a rigid structure. A plug of polypropylene mesh secured to the margins of the defect provides a reliable repair.

Umbilical hernia

Frequently encountered in obese and multiparous women, umbilical hernias have a high incidence of strangulation (Fig. 17.9). Another group at risk are cirrhotics with ascites. Although, electively, small hernias may be repaired with a subumbilical incision, in the presence of strangulation, a large elliptical incision is needed. This allows for ease of dissection down to the neck of the hernia sac on all sides. The umbilicus, skin and underlying fat can be excised at this point. The sac should always be opened at its neck as adhesions are more likely at the fundus. Care must be taken not to overlook a small Richter's hernia in a multiloculated sac. All the contents of the sac are carefully evaluated. If nonviable transverse colon is present, it is resected and an end colostomy either with or without a separate mucous fistula created. Repair is carried out with interrupted monofilament sutures using Mayo's overlapping repair, which has stood the test of time for 100 years.

Epigastric hernia

A large, strangulated epigastric hernia should be relatively simple to diagnose. However, caution is advised in ascribing vague or atypical epigastric symptoms to a small epigastric

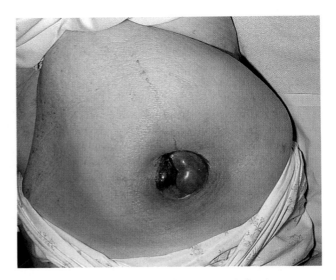

Fig. 17.9 A strangulated umbilical hernia in a typical patient.

hernia—numerous alternative pathologies may be the cause. Having said that, incarceration is especially common in small hernias. Strangulation, on the other hand is uncommon and usually involves extraperitoneal fat or, at the most, a small portion of omentum, giving rise to localized pain and tenderness. Strangulation of intra-abdominal viscera is extremely rare. A small strangulation may not be palpable, particularly in the obese patient. Ultrasound or computerized tomography (CT) examination have been shown to be useful adjuncts to diagnosis.

A vertical incision over the hernia should be of sufficient length so as not to overlook multiple defects in the linea alba which may co-exist with a strangulated epigastric hernia. The defect is closed with interrupted sutures without tension which usually requires a vertical closure.

Spigelian hernia

Also rare, Spigelian hernias because of their intramural position may not be diagnosed until strangulation of their contents occurs. However, the fundus of the sac may be visible along the semilunar line, most often below the umbilicus. Diagnosis even at this stage may remain elusive and may only come to light at an exploratory laparotomy for symptoms of strangulation or for undiagnosed bowel obstruction. If a strangulated Spigelian hernia is palpable, a grid-iron incision over the fundus is adequate to deal with the strangulation and close the defect.

Incisional hernia

With laparoscopic procedures increasing in frequency as well as variety, particular mention must be made of the increasingly numerous case reports of strangulation occurring in port site hernias. An awareness of this complication should prevent late diagnosis of a small, strangulating Richter's hernia, for example.

For most incisional hernias, what starts as a small defect, caused by tearing through of suture under tension, can soon become a large rupture. As well as incarceration and strangulation, an uncommon event in large incisional hernias is external rupture. The thin skin covering an incisional hernia can become necrotic and ulcerate. To prevent rupture, urgent repair is carried out.

The operation for strangulating incisional hernia begins by excising the previous abdominal scar with an extension at either end so that the sac and margin of the defect are approached through fresh tissue. Flaps of skin and subcutaneous fat are raised to well beyond the margins of the hernia defect. If possible, the peritoneum is mobilized at the margin of the defect and the extraperitoneal plane is developed. The sac is opened and the contents dealt with as required. Once excess sac is excised, the peritoneum is closed, provided the extraperitoneal plane has been dissected

widely enough to enable large bites of fascia to be taken with sutures. The defect is closed in the direction of least tension. In the majority of cases, primary closure is possible with a series of interrupted sutures. All are placed and then tied in turn. This is especially important if closure of the peritoneum has not been possible, to enable wide bites of fascia to be taken without risking trapping a loop of bowel between a loop of suture and the anterior abdominal wall. A 'Cardiff repair' of far–near–near–far sutures is advised (Fig. 17.10). If the fascia appears weak, it can be reinforced with an onlay polypropylene mesh.

When, on the infrequent occasion, it is impossible to close the defect without undue tension. A prosthetic mesh of polypropylene should be placed in the retromuscular preperitoneal space and the rectum sheath closed over it. Haematoma and seroma are complications due to the wide reflection of skin flaps. Closed-suction drains are placed prior to skin closure.

Parastomal hernia

A strangulating parastomal hernia may also compromise the blood supply to the stoma itself (Fig. 17.11). Ideally, for an effective repair, the stoma must be repositioned and if possible the new stoma should be brought through the mid portion of the rectus sheath well away from the hernia. A tissue defect is almost inevitable at the stomal hernia site and prosthetic mesh should be used to reinforce the repair in the absence of actual or potential sepsis.

Other abdominal wall hernias

Lumbar, supravesical and sciatic hernias are all rare and all

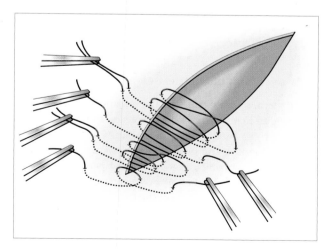

Fig. 17.10 Incisional hernia repair. Interrupted monofilament 'far–near–near–far' and 'far–near–near–far–near–near–far' sutures.

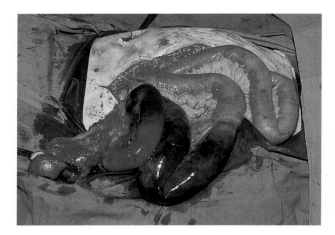

Fig. 17.11 Strangulated small bowel from a long-standing para-ileostomy hernia showing clear demarcation between viable and non-viable bowel.

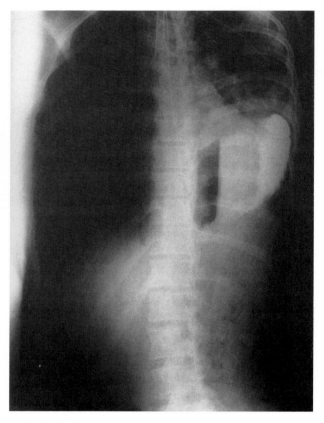

Fig. 17.12 Traumatic diaphragmatic hernia.

can be further subdivided depending on their relationships to surrounding neurovascular anatomy. Suffice it to say that strangulation in any of these hernias is a notable event indeed. As long as the surgeon is aware of their existence, then he may one day have the occasion to congratulate himself for his diagnostic abilities.

Intra-abdominal herniation

Internal herniation occurs when a loop of bowel protrudes through an opening in the visceral peritoneum. The commonest cause is a mesenteric defect either congenital or iatrogenic. As these hernias are intraperitoneal, they have no sac. An incarcerated internal hernia can lead rapidly to strangulation. Severe abdominal pain and vomiting, often with signs of bowel obstruction should lead to early laparotomy if the patient's condition is not to worsen. Previous bypass procedures and the formation of stomas can lead to the creation of a potential space for herniation.

Para-oesophageal hiatus hernia

These hernias occur through an enlarged defect at the oesophageal hiatus. The stomach rolls up in front of and to the left of the fixed gastro-oesophageal junction. Patients may be asymptomatic until they present as an emergency with bleeding, volvulus, strangulation or perforation where mortality can be as high as 50%. An erect chest X-ray often shows an air–fluid level behind the heart with contrast radiology confirming the diagnosis. Orientation at endoscopy can be confusing because of distortion of the stomach.

Through an upper midline laparotomy, the herniated stomach is reduced. The stomach must be decompressed pre-operatively for this to be achieved. Previous perforation

and ensuing sepsis may cause difficulty and a left lateral thoracotomy may be needed. The hernia sac should be excised to prevent a potential fluid collection. An incision at the margin of the hernia defect then allows the sac to be peeled off the mediastinal tissues. It is important not to mobilize the lower oesophagus as recurrence is more likely if the crural repair fails. The defect is closed with interrupted mattress sutures placed in the crura behind the oesophagus and, for large defects, the crura should also be brought together in front of the oesophagus. In the emergency setting, an antireflux procedure may not only be unnecessary but will also significantly increase the operating time. If, however, the stomach appears at risk of volvulus following reduction, a subtotal gastrectomy by an experienced surgeon may be required. Alternatively, with a redundant fundus but no true volvulus, a tube gastrostomy placed high on the anterior stomach wall is the best option. A nasogastric tube is then unnecessary and early feeding via the gastrostomy tube can be introduced.

Traumatic diaphragmatic hernia

Abdominal viscera can herniate through a previously

acquired traumatic defect in the diaphragm (Fig. 17.12). If early diagnosis is not achieved, the clinical presentation of incarceration or strangulation can be delayed for a considerable time. Strangulation with shock and respiratory distress can develop rapidly. Chest X-ray is diagnostic in the majority of cases but if difficulties in interpretation arise, oral contrast followed by CT scanning will usually delineate the offending loop of small bowel.

Late presenting diaphragmatic hernias are approached through a full lateral thoracotomy on the side of the herniation. There is no hernia sac and multiple adhesions are found between loops of bowel and the lung. The fibrosed margin of the diaphragmatic defect may need to be incised to allow the reduction of contents back into the abdomen. Often primary closure with interrupted mattress sutures cannot be achieved, any resulting gap should be bridged with prosthetic mesh. Bowel loops are much less likely to adhere to PTFE mesh, reducing the risk of subsequent adhesive obstruction.

Further reading

Nyhus, L.M. & Condon, R.E. (eds) (1995) *Hernia*, 4th edn. JB Lippincott, Philadelphia.

Devlin, H.B. & Kingsnorth, A.N. (1998) *Management of Abdominal Hernias*. Chapman and Hall, London.

CHAPTER 18

Acute right iliac fossa pain

Ridzuan Farouk, Graeme S. Duthie & Tonia Young-Fadok

Introduction

Acute abdominal pain is defined as a previously undiagnosed abdominal pain of recent (less than 72 h) duration. Within an acute general surgical ward, it represents the commonest presenting complaint, accounting for approximately 1% of all hospital admissions within the UK. Right iliac fossa pain usually accounts for between a third and a half of all such admissions with a considerable proportion of these patients undergoing surgery.

Appendicitis is the most common cause for such pain (Table 18.1) although this is somewhat dependent on the age and gender of the patient. At the Hull Royal Infirmary for example, there were 332 patients who underwent emergency surgery between January and March of 1997. Forty-eight of these patients underwent diagnostic laparoscopy or open appendicectomy. In Western countries, it is estimated that up to 16% of the population will undergo an appendicectomy. It is of interest to note that admissions for acute appendicitis are falling. In England and Wales for example, the number of admissions for acute appendicitis fell from 113 000 in 1966 to 69 000 in 1978. It is nevertheless still fair to say that acute appendicitis should be on the list of differential diagnosis of any patient who is admitted with abdominal pain, particularly in the right iliac fossa.

Pathophysiology

Intraperitoneal structures are poorly innervated and tend to exhibit visceral type pain when inflamed or distended by affecting the overlying visceral layer of the peritoneum. Embryologically derived foregut structures (stomach, first and proximal second part of duodenum, hepatobiliary tract including pancreas) primarily exhibit midline epigastric pain as a result of this pattern of innervation. The midgut (inclusive of the distal second part of duodenum to the level of the colonic splenic flexure) will refer pain to the midline in the peri-umbilical region. Hindgut structures (inclusive of the colon from splenic flexure to the transitional zone of the anal canal) when inflamed will refer to the midline but in the region of the hypogastrium. A shift in pain laterally signifies irritation of the somatic peritoneum which is innervated by the overlying dermatome. Thus an inflamed appendix will frequently first manifest itself by vague peri-umbilical pain, which as the inflammation progresses then shifts to a more constant, severe right iliac fossa pain (classically at McBurney's point). Inflamed foregut structures will first present with epigastric pain. In the event of a perforation which may complicate peptic ulcer disease or cholecystitis, fluid may track down into the right iliac fossa mimicking appendicitis or result in generalized peritonitis. An acutely distended, inflamed gall bladder may similarly attain sufficient size to extend into the right iliac fossa causing overlying peritoneal irritation, presenting with right iliac fossa pain.

History and physical examination

History

The ultimate diagnosis of cause for acute abdominal pain may only agree with the preliminary diagnosis in 45–65% of patients. This is particularly so for women, and patients at the extreme end of the age spectrum. The history and physical examination will nevertheless often provide crucial information in an attempt to achieve the correct diagnosis. When taking a history, the pertinent points to note are the age and gender of the patient, the duration of pain, the nature of onset of the pain (sudden versus gradual), the site of onset and any radiation of the pain, whether the pain is constant or colicky and whether there are any aggravating or relieving factors. In addition, concurrent gastrointestinal symptoms (e.g. vomiting, diarrhoea), genitourinary symptoms (last date of menses, whether sexually active, pain on intercourse, the presence of vaginal discharge, urinary frequency, dysuria or haematuria), current medication including alcohol intake and cigarettes, and previous medical history are usually relevant, even if negative.

The principal clinical features which will help distinguish acute appendicitis from other causes of abdominal pain are given in Table 18.2. Patient age will help further in coming to a diagnosis. While appendicitis can occur at any age, it is rare in patients below the age of 2 years and in those over 65

Table 18.1 Common causes of right iliac fossa pain.

Appendicitis
Urinary tract infection
Non-specific abdominal pain
Pelvic inflammatory disease
Renal colic
Ectopic pregnancy
Constipation

Table 18.2 Principal features of history and examination which indicate appendicitis.

Pain which has shifted to the right iliac fossa
Nausea, vomiting, anorexia
Low-grade temperature
Focal tenderness in right lower quadrant, aggravated by movement
    or coughing
Right iliac fossa guarding with/without rebound tenderness
Localized right-sided tenderness on rectal examination

Table 18.3 Causes of a right iliac fossa mass.

Common causes
Appendix mass
Crohn's disease
Caecal carcinoma

Less common causes
Empyema/mucocele of the gall bladder
Psoas abscess
Pelvic kidney
Ovarian cyst
Iliac vessel aneurysm
Intussusception
Spigelian hernia
Actinomycosis/tuberculosis

Table 18.4 Clinical features of a perforated viscus.

Raised temperature
Sudden onset of pain which is constant and severe
Pain aggravated by movement, deep inspiration, coughing
Silent, rigid abdomen
Diffuse tenderness

years of age. The peak incidence of developing appendicitis is age 10–20 years.

Examination

Unfortunately, only about half of patients with acute appendicitis give a typical history. About a third of patients will have a history that exceeds 24 hours, with similar proportions of patients never vomiting or having shifting abdominal pain. Physical examination and re-examination are therefore important. This should include pulse, temperature and blood pressure assessment with bedside urine analysis. The patient should be supine, and comfortable ensuring that they are sufficiently warm. A cold hand can make a difficult examination impossible and can be masked by use of an overlying blanket, particularly in children. Specific aspects to be considered in trying to establish a diagnosis are the point of maximal tenderness (ask the patient to point to this area before palpation), the presence or absence of muscular guarding/rigidity, rebound tenderness, and the presence of a mass. A mass may sometimes be palpated (Table 18.3). *A rectal examination should be routine*, specifically assessing the patient for areas of focal tenderness, and in women for the presence of cervical excitability or adnexal masses. A suspicious history in combination with urinary symptoms and pelvic tenderness usually suggests a pelvic appendicitis.

Frequent re-examination will usually confirm or refute the preliminary diagnosis. The examination should adhere to basic principles of abdominal examination including light followed by deeper palpation, quadrant by quadrant, with the most tender area being examined last. Palapation of the left iliac fossa may reproduce the pain in the right iliac fossa (Rovsing's sign). The patient may lie with their right hip partially flexed if there is psoas irritation. In patients with acute, severe abdominal pain, asking the patient to cough will often elicit peritonism (Table 18.4) and may be used to replace palpation. Similarly, gentle percussion of the abdomen may be used to elicit signs rather than palpation in these patients. The extent of peritoneal contamination is not always reflected by the physical findings. In particular, young muscular men, the morbidly obese, and those patients who take steroids may mask their signs until severe contamination from a perforated viscus has occurred. Important considerations should be given to including the loin, groin and genitalia as areas that must be examined. Rarely, the presence of flank or peri-umbilical bruising may be observed and should alert the examiner to causes of retroperitoneal bleeding (ruptured aortic aneurysm; ectopic pregnancy; warfarin overdose).

Judicious use of vaginal examination combined with a high vaginal swab in the presence of a suggestive history may establish a gynaecological cause for the pain. When this is contemplated, awaiting the result of a pregnancy test to exclude an ectopic pregnancy is advised. If an ectopic pregnancy is suspected, a vaginal examination should be deferred and early gynaecological opinion should be obtained.

In children, assessment of tonsils, and cervical lymph nodes are essential. The presence of foetor should be sought. Use of the child's hand to palpate the abdomen is frequently useful in gaining confidence while eliciting signs. Talking to the child about an unrelated matter (e.g. school, siblings, hobbies, etc.) can also be useful in drawing their attention from the ongoing examination. Younger children may be examined on the lap of a comforting relative.

Achieving a differential diagnosis

The main consideration after taking a careful history and performing an examination is whether the patient requires an urgent operation or whether there is time available for further observation with reassessment combined with supplementary tests. Virtually all patients fall into the latter category. The primary conditions that can present with acute right iliac fossa pain requiring emergency surgery are ruptured aortic aneurysm and ectopic pregnancy.

Acute appendicitis should never be lower than second on the differential diagnosis list of a patient presenting with acute right iliac fossa pain. Difficulty in achieving the correct diagnosis is most common in women within their reproductive age, and at the extremes of age.

Right iliac fossa pain in children

Up to 90% of all children who present to a surgical ward with abdominal pain will have non-specific abdominal pain or appendicitis (Table 18.5).

Important differential diagnoses for this age group include mesenteric adenitis (will often have concurrent signs of viral infection and lymphadenopathy elsewhere), constipation (pain tends to be left-sided), urinary tract infection (may have strong smelling urine, complain of urinary symptoms, have loin tenderness or have a previous history), and in younger children (<30 months old), intussusception. The latter should be considered when the child has severe, central abdominal pain associated with distress. A plain abdominal film may show evidence of small bowel obstruction or paucity of intestinal gas with a soft tissue mass. The diagnosis is confirmed by barium enema which may be therapeutic by means of hydrostatic pressure. Consideration for surgery should be given if this fails (Table 18.6). A palpable mass, altered bowel sounds and the presence of bloody stool are additional possible findings in this condition. Infective gastro-enteritis should also be considered, especially if other members of the family are affected. Occasionally, a chest infection or pleurisy may cause referred pain to the abdomen. Additional enquiries concerning the health of siblings as well as any problems that may be causing psychological disturbances, e.g. difficulties in school, or with the family should be sought wherever necessary.

Right iliac fossa pain in women of child-bearing age

In women, a careful history including the date of last menses, whether the patient is sexually active (and the presence of dyspareunia if so), their contraception history, the presence and nature of vaginal discharge combined with physical examination, and a pregnancy test are mandatory in trying to achieve an accurate diagnosis. Appendicitis must be actively excluded in every patient (Table 18.7).

Right iliac fossa pain in older patients

Patients over the age of 50 years also suffer appendicitis, but other pathology should also be considered. Acute cholecystitis, peptic ulceration with perforation, pancreatitis, mesenteric ischaemia, and cancer of the colon are the primary pathologies which may mimic appendicitis.

Suggested investigations

There can be a tendency to drift towards a 'biochemical bingo' in the assessment of a patient with acute right iliac fossa pain. Clearly, the extent of investigation should be tailored to the age of the patient, the physical findings and the clinical impression. Furthermore, the extent that each is investigated is based on one's own clinical training, experience, and the facilities that are available. Most patients can safely have a diagnosis achieved by physical examination in combination with the baseline investigations suggested in Table 18.8. Where the clinical condition of the patient allows and the diagnosis is not immediately clear, a 'second-line' of investigations that may be instituted is given in Table 18.8.

Table 18.5 Common causes of right iliac fossa pain in children.

Appendicitis
Mesenteric adenitis
Non-specific abdominal pain
Urinary tract infection

Table 18.6 Indications for surgery in intussusception.

Peforation
Failure of hydrostatic barium reduction
Suspected anatomical abnormality
Prolonged evidence of small bowel obstruction
Severe shock prior to resuscitation

Table 18.7 Common causes of right iliac fossa pain in women of child-bearing age.

Appendicitis
Urinary tract infection
Pelvic inflamatory disease
Pregnancy
Ectopic pregnancy
Ruptured ovarian cyst

Table 18.8 Suggested tests for patients with right iliac fossa pain.

Baseline tests Urine analysis Pregnancy test Full blood count *Additional tests* Electrolytes and glucose Serum amylase ECG and erect chest X-ray Ultrasound

Immediate tests

Specific recommended tests include bedside *urine analysis* (for blood, ketones, glucose, bilirubin and protein), a *midstream sample of urine* for immediate microscopy (note the presence of red cells, white cells, organisms and casts), Gram staining of organisms where relevant followed by culture, and urine for *pregnancy testing*. All patients with a history of hypertension or one suggestive of ischaemic heart disease should have an *electrocardiograph* (ECG) as should all patients over the age of 50 years. Serum amylase should be selectively tested for to help exclude pancreatitis but can also be nonspecifically abnormal in a number of other important conditions such as acute cholecystitis, perforated peptic ulcer, appendicitis, mesenteric ischaemia, and ruptured aortic aneurysm. A *full blood count* is often requested for assessment of white cell count but may show other abnormalities such as anaemia in the presence of a colon carcinoma. A normal white cell count does not specifically exclude appendicitis. In addition, a blood count is a test which is also frequently requested as a baseline test by the anaesthetist for medicolegal reasons. A high white cell count combined with an abnormal ECG should alert the clinician to the possible presence of a mesenteric thromboembolic event. Serum amylase (raised) and arterial blood gases (metabolic acidosis) are also commonly abnormal in such patients.

A plain supine abdominal film is often not justified in patients with acute right iliac fossa pain, particularly in patients aged below the age of 50 years. These patients usually have appendicitis, urinary tract infection, cholecystitis or non-specific abdominal pain. Older patients can justifiably have an abdominal film, particularly where an obstruction is suspected. Additional useful information that may be obtained in a small proportion of these patients include vascular, renal tract or biliary tract calcification. Erect abdominal films are rarely performed in the UK now. Patients suspected of having a perforated intra-abdominal viscus are likely to have an erect chest X-ray instead, irrespective of age.

Additional (optional) tests

Other blood tests that may be useful depending on the clinical impression include serum *urea and electrolyte* measurement (mandatory in the presence of prolonged vomiting and/or diarrhoea), 'liver function tests', coagulation profile, serum glucose, and cardiac enzyme profile. Additional radiological assessments are dependent on the patient's condition as well as the facilities and expertise available. *Ultrasonography* is increasingly playing an important role. Although accuracy is operator dependent, exclusion of acute cholecystitis, hepatic, renal tract and gynaecological pathology can easily be undertaken via the transabdominal and transvaginal routes. The aorta similarly can be quickly assessed if there is doubt about the diagnosis. In addition, the presence or absence of free intraperitoneal fluid can be sought. The development of higher-frequency transducers has resulted in an increasing experience in identifying the appendix and associated pathology.

Additional modes of radiology that can be used are dependent on the mode of presentation. An acutely ill, unstable patient who despite resuscitation continues to be unwell may well require emergency laparotomy without further assessment. This scenario is rare. Where the facilities are available, and baseline tests including ultrasound have failed to show a cause for on-going pain, there are two distinct choices. The first is to carry out a diagnostic laparoscopy in the absence of any contra-indications. Additional radiological assessment represents a second option. With very few exceptions, our own preference is the former. Additional radiological assessments that can be carried out include a radiolabelled white cell scan to rule out appendicitis, a HIDA scan for suspected cholecystitis, a Gastrografin swallow for suspected perforated peptic ulcer, a CT scan for possible subclinical obstruction, or a barium enema.

Treatment

Once a working diagnosis is achieved, treatment may be *conservative* (analgesia, bowel rest by intravenous fluids combined with observation), *medical* or *surgical*. Many patients, by default, undergo a period of conservative treatment during which time a diagnostic work-up is being carried out. After a period of 'active' observation, the patient will either get better or require treatment. Analgesia and fluid replacement during this phase are important considerations.

Medical

Medical treatment is usually reserved for patients with a urinary or gynaecological infection and takes the form of antibiotics. Such treatment is often commenced empirically after suitable culture material has been obtained and should

Table 18.9 Uncommon medical causes of right iliac fossa pain.

Diabetic ketoacidosis
Porphyria
Shingles

also take into account subsequent culture and sensitivity results. An ultrasound of the pelvis will usually corroborate or refute suspicions of a gynaecological cause for pain. Infective gastroenteritis is often self-limiting and the primary aim of treatment should be supportive (analgesia, fluid and electrolyte replacement). Stool culture is needed and affected patients should be isolated from other patients. Ureteric stones tend to pass spontaneously. Failure to pass a stone merits urological referral for consideration of lithotripsy or endoscopic retrieval. Occasional medical conditions that may mimic appendicitis are shown in Table 18.9.

Surgical

Virtually every child undergoing surgery for right iliac fossa pain will have a diagnosis of appendicitis. A Lanz incision is appropriate for these patients.

The advent of laparoscopy has altered standard surgical approaches to the diagnosis and treatment of adult patients with acute right iliac fossa pain. Most young adult males with right iliac fossa pain will have appendicitis and a Lanz incision is arguably the most appropriate for these patients. Randomized trials of open versus laparoscopic appendicectomy have failed to show any early benefit for the laparoscopic approach in these patients.

The primary advantage of laparoscopy lies with its ability to undertake a diagnostic process prior to performing a definitive surgical procedure such as appendicectomy. The recent development of 2-mm diameter cameras will reduce the invasiveness of this procedure even further. Between 70 and 90% of all appendicectomies undertaken are subsequently confirmed to be genuinely inflamed. Many of these 'negative appendicectomies' will be carried out in young women who will be found to have a gynaecological cause for their pain, or in older patients with unsuspected pathology.

Careful laparoscopy will occasionally diagnose a 'surgical astonishment'. Acute cholecystitis or perforated peptic ulcer are among these. Other rarer findings include Meckel's diverticulum, Crohn's disease, a solitary perforated/inflamed caecal diverticulum, lymphoma or carcinoma. The authors (R.F.) have experienced all of these on at least one occasion having embarked on a Lanz incision. Most of these pathologies can be managed by an extended incision—however, their discovery by laparoscopy may alter the surgical approach. For example, acute cholecystitis or peptic ulcer

disease may be managed laparoscopically or if the open approach is to be used, the choice of incision may be altered. The finding of a carcinoma or Crohn's disease, controversially may also be managed laparoscopically but again, a midline incision would be more appropriate depending on one's surgical experience than a Lanz incision if a laparotomy is to be undertaken. A minor but useful point to be made is that the initial peri-umbilical stab incision made for insertion of the laparoscopic port should be vertical rather than transverse if it is felt that a laparotomy may be subsequently undertaken. This will facilitate the subsequent incision and wound closure.

If laparoscopic facilities are not available or if the surgeon does not feel comfortable with the technology, a Lanz incision is recommended for children and for adults up to the age of 55 years where appendicitis is suspected (Fig. 18.1a–e). Where there is a suspicion of alternative pathology and in older patients, a midline laparotomy is recommended.

Special surgical situations

As in all unusual surgical situations, three courses of action should be considered when one encounters unexpected pathology or experiences an intra-operative complication: (1) Seek senior advice. (2) Inform the anaesthetist that there is a problem. (3) Decide whether the incision (size, site) is appropriate.

Crohn's disease

The finding of Crohn's disease frequently causes consternation to the basic surgical trainee but generally should be treated in one of two ways. If the base of the appendix is not macroscopically affected and there is no indication to resect the disease, performing an appendicectomy may be undertaken safely. The risk of fistula formation in these patients is less than 2%. If this does not appear to be a safe option, then doing no more and closing the wound or performing a limited right hemicolectomy should be considered in consultation with someone senior. In all patients, a peritoneal swab should be obtained and any free fluid cultured as infective cases of terminal ileitis may mimic Crohn's disease. An attempt should also be made to determine whether there are any other areas of bowel affected by Crohn's disease.

Meckel's diverticulum

This is usually an incidental finding and is found as an anatomical variant in about 1% of the population. Occasionally, however, it is the primary cause of the patient's pain. A pre-operative technetium scan may diagnose the condition in those patients who present with acute, recurrent pain. Resection of the diseased segment is definitive.

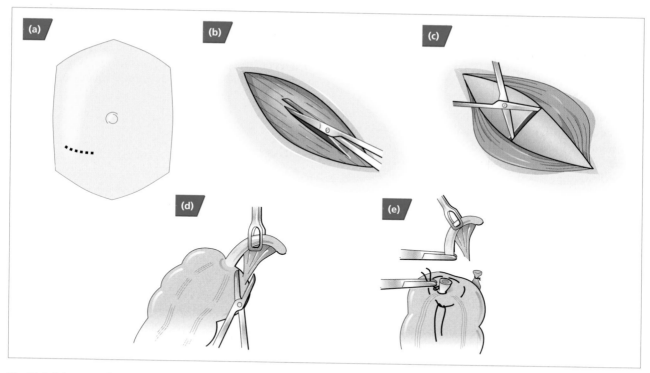

Fig. 18.1 Schematic of appendicectomy through a Lanz approach.

This may be performed by diverticulectomy or by wedge resection of the affected segment of bowel. Without becoming embroiled in the debate over hand-sewn versus stapled procedures, diverticulectomy can be judiciously performed where stapled instruments are available by the application of a cross-stapler (TA gun) across the base of the diverticulum.

The controversy that exists about a Meckel's diverticulum is what should be done about it in an asymptomatic patient. Resection has been variously reported to be free of complications by some and to be associated with anastomotic leakage by others. Diverticulae which are greater than 1 cm in length or with a base that is greater than 1 cm in width have previously been identified to be those which are at greatest risk of subsequently developing complications. My own approach (R.F.) in the absence of inflammation would be to note the finding but do no more.

Colon carcinoma

The incidental finding of a caecal carcinoma should be managed by alerting a senior colleague and the anaesthetist, ensuring adequate exposure by extending the incision or reverting to a midline incision, and performing a right hemicolectomy in the usual manner.

Appendicitis in pregnancy

Appendicitis does occur in pregnant women but should be differentiated from urinary tract infection, pyelitis, red degeneration of a fibroid and torsion of an ovarian cyst. Rarer causes of pain include a curious phenomenon related to 'over-stretching' of the round ligament, the pain of which may be reproduced by palpating the inguinal canal, and acute fatty degeneration of the liver. Later in the pregnancy (second trimester onwards), there is a chance that the associated tenderness of appendicitis is higher and more lateral than is usual because of displacement by the gravid uterus. Specific anaesthetic-related considerations are a higher risk of aspiration because of oestrogen-related relaxation of the gastro-oesopheal sphincter mechanism, as well as compromise of cardiac return because of compression of the inferior vena cava. There is a recognized risk of abortion and the patient should accordingly be counselled. Gentle handling of tissues intra-operatively and avoiding undue manipulation of the gravid uterus are advised. The author's own experience (R.F.) is small (11 patients) but abortion was not encountered.

The appendix mass

In the absence of peritonitis, the initial approach should be conservative by observing the size of the mass, the pulse, and temperature. Prolonged use of antibiotics may result in a honeycombed 'antibioticoma'. Percutaneous drainage may be employed in selected patients which may result in early resolution. Where resolution occurs, interval appendicectomy may be undertaken after 3 months. A minority of cases fail to resolve and may not be suitable for ultrasound drainage. Surgery is then required but this can be tedious.

Summary

A careful history combined with physical examination will allow an accurate impression of whether a period of observation followed by re-examination is warranted or whether urgent resuscitation followed by surgery is indicated. Appendicitis should be among the primary differential diagnosis of all patients who present with acute right iliac fossa pain. Supplementary diagnostic tests including urine analysis and pregnancy testing should be noted. Additional tests should be requested where indicated but should not completely influence one's clinical judgement. Where surgery is indicated, careful consideration should be given to the type of incision based on the likely pathology. Where there is doubt about the diagnosis, diagnostic laparoscopy can be invaluable.

Further reading

Jones, P.F. (1974) *Emergency Abdominal Surgery in Infancy, Childhood and Adult Life*. Blackwell Scientific Publications, Oxford.

Taylor *et al.* (1984) *Surgical Management*. Heinemann Medical Books, London.

CHAPTER 19

Acute anorectal conditions

Steven D. Wexner & Deborah DeMarta

Introduction and anorectal evaluation

Most patients who present with anorectal complaints attribute their symptoms to haemorrhoids. Usually, a careful history and physical examination will allow proper diagnosis within a few minutes. The history should include the patient's chief complaint, type and duration of symptoms, bowel frequency habits and their relation to presenting symptom and level of continence. Similar queries should address the presence and character of pain, bleeding, pruritis, and the relation of these symptoms to bowel activity. Similarly, a careful medical history should include any prior anorectal surgery, history of inflammatory bowel disease and personal or family history of neoplasia. If the history does not include significant acute pain then two disposable phosphate enemas are administered prior to examination. Time and labour can be saved if patients are instructed to self-administer the enemas prior to presentation to the clinic.

Important elements of the anorectal examination include optimal patient position, adequate lighting, and the appropriate anoscope. Under any circumstance, this examination is difficult for the patient who is anxious, frightened, embarrassed and possibly in pain. The ideal position is prone-jackknife as it affords excellent visualization and the enlistment of an assistant without the need for contortionary manoeuvres. However, this position requires a manual or electric tilt table which is clearly more expensive than is a stretcher or simple table. In the absence of such a table, the knee–chest position is best avoided because of its awkwardness. The second choice position is the Simm's or left lateral decubitus position. The lithotomy position should not be used in the awake patient. Regardless of position, good direct lighting and a choice of anoscopes should be available.

The examination should begin with careful inspection of the perineum and perianal skin. Special attention should be paid to the presence of any skin irregularities, scarring, inflammation, mucous or fecal soiling and approximation of the anal canal. Additionally, the patient should be asked to bear down to assess the presence of partial or complete rectal prolapse. By gently parting the buttocks and anus, one can visually inspect for an anal fissure (Fig. 19.1). Next, careful palpation of the perineum and perianal skin should be done to exclude any lesions. A gentle but thorough digital examination is then accomplished with a well lubricated examining finger by systematic palpation of the rectum in a circular manner, taking care to palpate to a level cephalad to the puborectalis muscle. The patient should be asked to squeeze to assess and compare resting and squeeze pressures and high pressure zone length. If a mass is palpated, one should note its consistency, size, location, mobility and distance from the dentate line. The size and consistency of the prostate gland or the cervix should also be evaluated and noted. Anoscopy should then be performed with a well-lubricated anoscope to visualize the mucosa and grade the hemorrhoids. If the diagnosis of anal fissure is obvious, one need not submit the patient to undue pain, and the digital and anoscopic examinations can be deferred. The least acceptable method of examination of the anal canal is by retroflexion of a flexible instrument as such a manoeuvre occludes the anus and physically prevents haemorrhoidal prolapse.

A proctosigmoidoscopy should be performed. We prefer to use the flexible endoscope, if clinically indicated, for better patient comfort and greater distance of insertion. However if this instrument is not readily available then rigid sigmoidoscopy should be performed. Colonoscopy, anal ultrasound, other physiological tests and radiographic investigations should be done, when indicated, based on history and physical findings.

For the purpose of simplicity, the various anorectal conditions discussed here in this chapter will be categorized under the broad symptom headings of pain only, and pain and bleeding.

Pain only

1 Anorectal sepsis: anorectal abscess, fistula in ano, necrotizing anorectal infection, hidradenitis suppurativa, pilonidal disease.
2 Strangulated internal haemorrhoids.
3 Thrombosed external haemorrhoids.

Anorectal evaluation

- Good lighting.
- Assortment of anoscopes.
- Prone-jackknife position.
- Assistance available.
- If too tender, proceed to examination under anaesthesia.

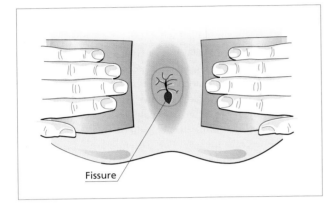

Fig. 19.1 Anorectal examination: parting the anus. Arrow demonstrates a posterior midline anal fissure.

Anorectal sepsis

Abscess and fistulous disease

Fistula in ano and anorectal abscess represent a continuum of anorectal sepsis; anorectal abscess representing the acute suppurative process and the more chronic stage of communication between two epithelial lined spaces in fistulous disease.

Pathogenesis

The majority of abscesses (90%) are of a cryptoglandular origin as a result of anal gland and/or duct obstruction. As an abscess expands, purulent material tracts to the perianal region where either spontaneous or surgical drainage can result in an external opening, thereby creating a fistula. The patient with an acute abscess usually presents with pain that gradually increases over a few days. Its character is usually throbbing and may be exacerbated by defecation. Pyrexia, a painful perianal swelling and possibly drainage of purulent material may be noted by the patient. Classification of anorectal abscesses depends on the relationship to both the external anal sphincter and the puborectalis muscle as depicted in Fig. 19.2. The origin of a perianal or intersphincteric abscess is from simple downward extension of pus into the intersphincteric space. Ischiorectal abscess and transphincteric fistulae form by penetration of the external sphincter caudad to the puborectalis muscle. The more

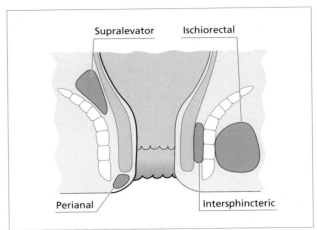

Fig. 19.2 Classification of anorectal abscess.

uncommon supralevator abscess is an upward extension of pus from the intersphincteric space cephalad to the puborectalis muscle.

Examination of the patient with a perianal or ischiorectal abscess typically reveals an erythematous tender swelling with fluctuance; localized or surrounding cellulitis may also be present. The diagnosis of intersphincteric or supralevator abscess may not be so obvious as external signs are lacking. A good rule of thumb is that any acute pain out of proportion to physical findings, or occurring in a patient too tender for clinic evaluation warrants an examination under general anaesthesia.

Treatment

The mainstay of treatment for acute anorectal abscess is prompt surgical incision and drainage. There is no role for antibiotic therapy unless used as an adjuvant in patients with immunosuppression, diabetes, with a valve or other prosthetic device, or with evidence of soft tissue cellulitis. Most small perianal and ischiorectal abscesses can be drained under local anaesthesia as a day case. The patient is best placed in the prone-jackknife position; next, the tissue circumferential to the area of maximal fluctuance is subcutaneously infiltrated with a solution of 0.5% lidocaine with 1 : 200 000 epinephrine. Injection directly into the abscess should be avoided because the acid environment of the abscess will bind the basic compound of the local anaesthetic rendering it of limited effect. Furthermore, the localized anaerobic environment is a poor one for diffusion of anaesthetic.

A cruciate or elliptical incision is made over the area of fluctuance to evacuate the pus and the skin edges are excised to allow adequate drainage. Growth of enteric microorganisms on culture confirms an anorectal rather than cutaneous source (as in a carbuncle or furuncle). In general

Abscess drainage

- Ischiorectal or perianal as outpatient.
- Intersphincteric or supralevator in theatre.
- Avoid primary fistulotomy unless an obvious low transsphincteric or intrasphincteric tract.
- Avoid packing wounds.

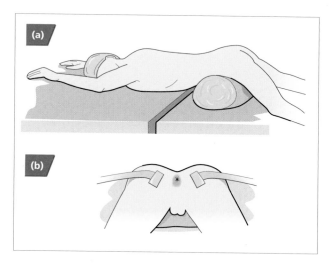

Fig. 19.3 The prone-jackknife position is utilized for most anorectal surgery. (a) In the operating room, the patient is positioned with the pelvis over the 'break' in the table. A Kraske roll is placed under the pelvis. (b) The buttocks are then taped apart and to the operating room table. This is best done using Benzoin spray and applying cloth tape.

however, Gram stain and culture have limited value. After satisfactory drainage and debridement, the cavity can be loosely packed. No effort is made to perform a primary fistulotomy. Most ischiorectal abscesses can be drained in the same manner unless large or horseshoe in nature, whereby operative drainage under general anaesthesia is required. In the operating room the patient is placed in the prone-jackknife position over a Kraske roll in the lithotomy position (Fig. 19.3). A careful examination under anaesthesia is performed. An attempt is made to identify the primary opening in the posterior midline. The postanal space is then drained by dividing the subcutaneous and superficial external anal sphincter and the distal most fibres of the internal anal sphincter. Counter incisions should then be made over each ischiorectal fossa to allow adequate drainage of a horseshoe abscess. Soft mushroom catheters can be left in the cavity to avoid packing. The patient with an intersphincteric abscess typically presents with pain out of proportion to physical findings, so again one should proceed with examination under anaesthesia. Surgical treatment involves division of the internal anal sphincter up to the most proximal extent of the abscess. The wound is best managed by marsu-

pialization of the edges with meticulous postoperative wound care. The treatment of supralevator abscess depends on its aetiology; whether from upward extension of an ischiorectal or intersphincteric abscess or from downward extension of a pelvic abscess or an intra-abdominal process. For supralevator abscesses that originate from an ischiorectal source, drainage should be through the ischiorectal fossa. When the sepsis originates from an intersphincteric source it should be drained through the rectum. A pelvic or intra-abdominal source of supralevator abscess can be drained either through the rectum or the ischiorectal fossa or percutaneously through the abdominal wall as determined by appropriate pre-operative radiographic studies. We prefer to delay definitive fistulotomy at this time to avoid unnecessary division of sphincter muscle.

Following surgical drainage of anorectal abscesses the patient should be instructed to keep the wounds clean, sitz baths or irrigation with a pulsatile water-pik device is particularly useful. We place our patients on bulk-forming psyllium agents, non-constipating analgesics, and a diet including 25–30 g/day of fibre. The patient should be seen in follow-up until all wounds have healed. It is essential to allow healing from the depths of the wound so as to avoid loculation and recurrent sepsis.

Fistula in ano

A fistula is an abnormal communication between any two epithelial lined surfaces. A fistula in ano consists of a single primary internal opening and one or more secondary external openings connected by a primary track, and possibly one or more secondary tracks. The internal opening is the point at which an anal gland duct enters the anal canal; the majority lie in the posterior midline location. One should always attempt to identify the internal opening; however, in about 10% of the cases attempts are unsuccessful, despite the aid of endoanal ultrasound. Classification of anorectal fistulae, like anorectal abscess, is anatomically based and depends on the relationship of the fistula to the external anal sphincter and the puborectalis muscle (Fig. 19.4).

The most common type of fistula in ano is the intersphincteric type (approximately 70%) caused by perianal abscess. Transsphincteric fistulae represent approximately 23% of all fistulas, and are usually secondary to an ischiorectal abscess. The rectovaginal fistula is an example of a transsphincteric fistula. Less common is the suprasphincteric fistula (5%) which originates from the supralevator abscess. The extrasphincteric fistula (2%), should prompt the clinician to search for aetiologies such as Crohn's disease, diverticulitis, appendicitis, and foreign body or penetrating injuries of the perineum.

The cardinal symptom on presentation of fistula in ano is that of purulent drainage that has been either continuous or intermittent in nature. Often the patient will relate a history

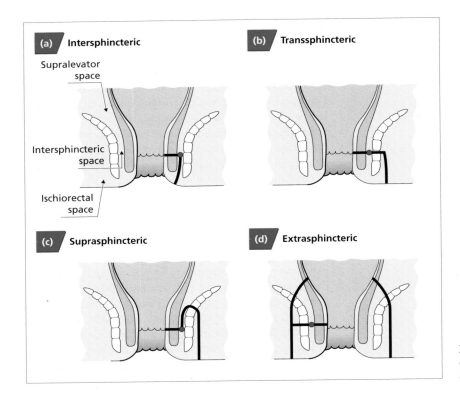

Fig. 19.4 Classification of fistula in ano:
(a) Intersphincteric; (b) Transsphincteric;
(c) Suprasphincteric; (d) Extrasphincteric.

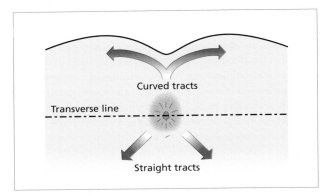

Fig. 19.5 Goodsall's Rule: if the anus is transected with an imaging transverse line, anterior fistulous tracts are straight and posterior tracts are typically curved entering into the posterior midline.

of pain which resolves with passage of purulent discharge. On physical examination, the external opening(s) may be seen on careful inspection of the perianal area. The surrounding skin is usually indurated but one may be able to palpate the primary tract. The internal opening may also be identified by careful digital rectal examination as an area of induration, similarly the tract is palpable as a firm 'cord like' structure. Goodsall's rule is useful when identifying the course of fistulous tracts (Fig. 19.5).

Treatment

Fistulotomy is the preferred procedure over fistulectomy for fistula in ano as the former procedure creates a smaller wound with less healing difficulties and less sphincter damage. The principle of 'laying open the fistula' serves to 'open up' and drain both the primary and secondary tracts, while simultaneously preserving continence. Pre-operatively it is important to assess sphincter tone and continence. The procedure should be done in the prone-jackknife position, local anaesthetic is infiltrated along the fistulous tract after its identification. Figure 19.3 demonstrates the patient positioning in the operating room. Next a probe is inserted into the tract taking care not to create any false passages. Using cautery, the tissue overlying the probe is incised. The tract should be curetted of all chronic granulation tissue and the wound left open to heal by secondary intention. If, however, the tract crosses the sphincters at a high level, only a small amount of muscle should be cut and a seton inserted.

A seton, whether cutting or non-cutting, is indicated in settings in which continence may be compromised. Such scenarios include high transsphincteric fistulas and fistulas in patients with Crohn's disease, advanced age, weak sphincters and previous/multiple fistula operations. Furthermore, the seton may be preferred in anterior fistulas in women. A drainage seton is essentially a drain which is left in place to prevent recurrent abscess or to temporize until a more definitive procedure can be undertaken. In patients with Crohn's disease, a seton may be left in place indefinitely. Alternatively, a cutting seton slowly cuts the sphincter muscle while at the same time stimulating fibrosis to prevent a gaping defect. Anorectal advancement flap is an alternative option in any setting in which consideration is given to either type of seton (Fig. 19.6).

Anorectal advancement flap is an attractive option for these high risk patients since no division of sphincter muscle is required. The procedure requires a full mechanical and antibiotic bowel preparation. Technically, the tract is identified as for a fistulotomy or seton placement. A full thickness

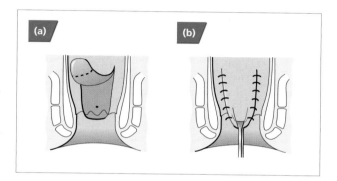

Fig. 19.6 Technique of anorectal advancement flap. (a) After 'coring out' the internal opening of the fistula and gently curetting the tract, the opening is sutured closed and a full thickness flap is raised. The distal most tip of the flap is excised. (b) The flap is then advanced beyond the external opening and sutured down to the anal canal in a tension free manner with interrupted absorbable sutures.

flap of mucosa, submucosa and internal anal sphincter is fashioned. The internal opening is sharply excised and the defect is then closed with absorbable suture material. The flap is mobilized in a cephalad direction several centimetres beyond the internal opening. Once adequate length is achieved to allow a tension free flap, the fistula at the proximal tip is excised. After closure of the internal opening, the flap is sutured in place with interrupted sutures. A mushroom-tipped drain can be left in the tract and sutured to the skin at the external opening. The drain is generally removed 4–6 weeks later after the flap has healed. Because the primary source of sepsis has been eradicated, the tract should promptly close.

Necrotizing infection

The importance of prompt surgical treatment of anorectal abscesses cannot be over emphasized as a delay in treatment can lead to disastrous complications such as a necrotizing anorectal infection. Such sepsis can result from delay in diagnosis, an immunocompromised host and/or a particularly virulent organism. Signs of systemic toxeamia, widespread cellulitis, crepitus in the tissues or necrosis that appears as 'black patches' should alarm the physician, that rapid and aggressive surgical intervention is mandatory (Fig. 19.7).

Prior to proceeding to the operating suite, the patient must be adequately resuscitated with large bore intravenous

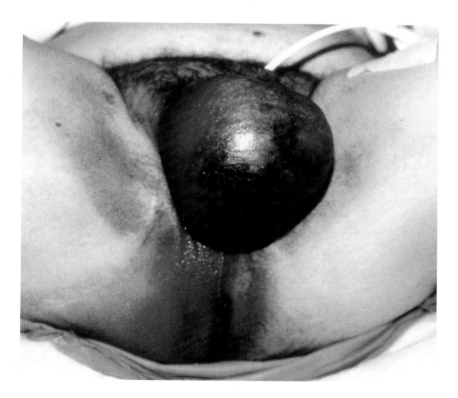

Fig. 19.7 Anorectal sepsis and necrotizing anorectal infection. Note the areas of necrosis on the scrotal skin (black tissue).

catheters, massive fluid replacement and a bladder catheter. The affected area can be aspirated and examined for microorganisms, but should not delay surgery. High doses of broad-spectrum antibiotics should be immediately administered. The surgical approach is one of wide radical debridement; all involved areas must be excised to healthy tissue, often to include fascia. Creation of a colostomy may also be advisable. All wounds are left open and burn-type dressings are applied. Postoperatively, the patient should be nursed in the intensive care unit. Repeat debridements and initial wound care is probably best done in the operating room. When available, hyperbaric oxygen may be used as added therapy, but should never delay surgical treatment. Its use is controversial and results are not uniformly convincing.

Hidradenitis suppurativa

Aetiology and pathogenesis

Like pilonidal disease, hidradenitis is a chronic inflammatory condition; however it predominantly affects the apocrine glands with their surrounding skin and soft tissue. The disease was first described in 1839 by Verlpeau and its association with the sweat glands is credited to Verneuil in 1854. Literally translated, hidradenitis suppurativa means sweat gland, from the Greek roots *hydros* and *adeno*, respectively. The perineum is affected in 30% of cases, with axillary and groin involvement as the most common presenting sites. Additionally, the areolar, perianal, inframammary and periumbilical areas may be affected.

If one remembers that apocrine sweat glands become active only after puberty, it is intuitive that age of presentation is commonly between 16–40 years. There seems to be a male predominance with hidradenitis suppurativa; however the literature is conflicting in this regard. The most agreed upon aetiological basis for this disease is obstruction of these apocrine sweat glands with keratinous plugs, resulting in glandular dilatation and ectasia, bacterial overgrowth, leukocyte infiltration and eventual ductal disruption. This disruption leads to extensive scarring and fibrosis of the surrounding tissues and finally, fistula formation to the skin. An endocrine or androgen aetiology has also been suggested. There is an association of hidradenitis with obesity, diabetes mellitus, hyperhidrosis, Cushing's disease, poor hygiene, acne, anaemia, and other cutaneous diseases that cause pore occlusion.

Clinical presentation

Initially, the patient may present with one or more areas of perianal abscess and cellulitis; however more commonly the patient presents with chronic recurrent subacute infection of the hair bearing areas of the perineum which may extend to the inner thighs, scrotum, labia and natal cleft. Although unusual, severe cases with fistulization to the anal canal have been reported. The early lesions typically fail to heal and instead go on to form fistulas and sinus tracts, albeit superficial.

Examination reveals marked induration of the involved hairbearing skin with multiple burrowing sinuses that express malodorous, thin, purulent drainage upon palpation. The lesions can be tender and erythematous; signs of low-grade systemic toxicity may also be present (low-grade fever, leukocytosis and adenopathy). Repeat bouts of cutaneous sepsis can lead to decreased range of motion of involved areas secondary to extensive fibrosis. Social stigmata may be secondary to offensive malodorous discharging lesions. Rarely, squamous carcinoma has been reported in longstanding cases (Figs 19.8 and 19.9).

Hidradenitis suppurativa
• Exclude Crohn's disease.
• Exclude fistula in ano.
• Unroof and debride.
• Do *not* perform incision and drainage only.

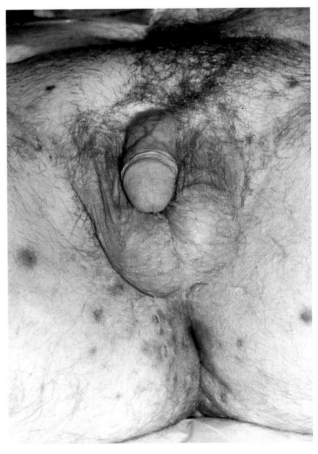

Fig. 19.8 Hidradenitis suppurativa of the perineum. Reprinted with permission.

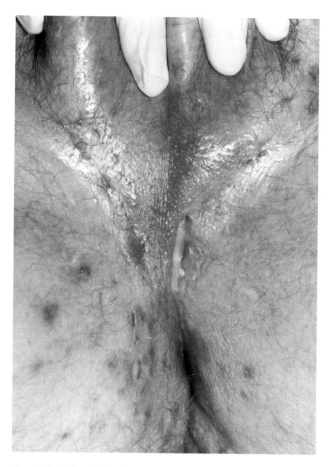

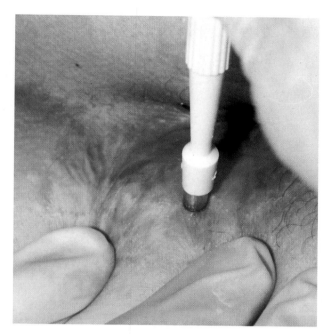

Fig. 19.10 Technique of obtaining a 'punch biopsy'; the area is first infiltrated with local anaesthesia.

Fig. 19.9 Perineal hidradenitis. Here the scrotum is held cephalad to demonstrate the extent of disease. Reprinted with permission.

Differential diagnosis

Hidradenitis suppurativa may mimic perianal Crohn's disease, fistula in ano and pilonidal disease, however several differentiating features will aid in the differential diagnosis.

Firstly, if the diagnosis is in question, a biopsy of the chronically inflamed and fibrotic area will reveal apocrine gland destruction, which is not found in Crohn's disease although the two disorders may co-exist. Figure 19.10 demonstrates the technique of punch biopsy. The presence of disease at extra perineal sites such as the axilla or groin is also highly suggestive. If the diagnosis at this point is still in doubt, it is advisable to obtain endoscopic colonic mucosal biopsy and radiographic gastrointestinal series. The differentiation between hidradenitis and fistulous disease may be easier to delineate as only the distal one-third of the rectum is involved in the former. Similarly, all reported cases of hidradenitis are located caudad to the dentate line and do not involve the internal anal sphincter or intersphincteric tissues. Conversely, fistula in ano usually arises from the dentate line and as previously described is classified based on relationship to the sphincters.

Treatment

Conservative medical management is only indicated for mild cases and includes short courses of broad-spectrum antibiotics, warm soaks, antiseptic solutions and improved hygiene. A number of bacteria have been isolated in hidradenitis suppurativa including: staphylococci, streptococci, *Escherichia coli*, *Proteus*, *Pseudomonas* and *Bacteroides*. There is no evidence that long-term antibiotic therapy changes the natural course of this disease and therefore should be avoided. Incision, drainage and deroofing of the infectious process is of course indicated in the acute or recurrent setting. The mainstay of treatment for hidradenitis is surgical ablation with radical excision of all involved areas. Simple incision and drainage alone does not remove the risk of recurrent sepsis and recurrence is as high as 83%. Similarly, local excision is useful in only localized disease and results in high recurrence rates.

In severe, chronic forms of hidradenitis, wide ablative excision of all diseased skin and soft tissue down to the fascia is recommended. Figures 19.11 and 19.12 demonstrate the extensive scarring and fibrosis. The wounds may be treated with a combination of primary closure, marsupialization, packing, rotation or pedicle flaps, or split thickness skin grafts. It should be cautioned that graft take is poor in this setting. Despite this aggressive approach, wound breakdown and recurrence is still a problem. Approximately 25% of recurrences are due to *de novo* disease developing at a new anatomical site. Diversion of the faecal stream is occasionally

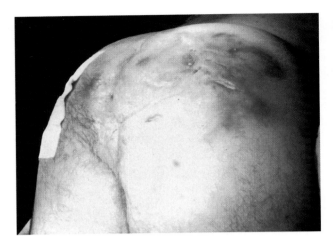

Fig. 19.11 Extensive involvement of the perineum with hidradenitis suppuratia (pre-operative). Note the extensive scarring and fibrosis.

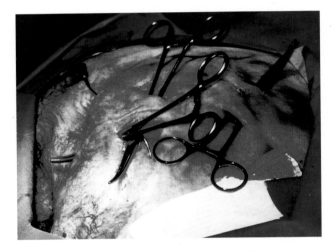

Fig. 19.12 The same patient in the operating room. The haemostat clamps are placed within the burrowing sinus tracts to demonstrate the extent of disease.

warranted although no data exist to support any improvement in healing.

Pilonidal disease

Pilonidal disease is an inflammatory condition of the natal cleft area that commonly presents in young adulthood. Pilonidal disease is rare after age 40, and a male predominance is noted at all ages. Some predisposing factors may include a deep hirsute natal cleft, buttock friction causing local trauma, obesity, increased sweating, prolonged sitting, and perhaps a hormonal influence. Pilonidal disease is usually a self-limiting condition; however, complications such as abscess and recurrent sepsis can occur.

> **Pilonidal disease**
>
> - Drain abscesses away from the midline.
> - Maintain depilatory status of surrounding skin during healing.
> - Aid wound healing with daily mechanical home debridement.
> - Lay open and curette sinuses *without* excision of the fibrous base.
> - Marsupialize wounds.

Aetiology and pathology

Understanding the aetiology and pathogenesis of pilonidal disease are fundamental prerequisites to the diagnosis and management. Pilonidal disease was originally described by Anderson in 1847, later Hodges in 1880 coined the term 'pilonidal', literally translated to be 'nest of hairs', as hair is often found within the pilonidal sinus. The aetiology of this disorder has been debated for years; originally thought to be congenital in origin, it is now thought to be more of an acquired problem. Although the pits through which the hair enters may be congenital, there is often an acquired chronic foreign body reaction involving the hair and hair follicles. Close examination of the hair reveals 'barbs' or scales on its surface, thereby providing the explanation for how a remote hair can burrow into the subcutaneous tissue and cause repeated local trauma to the area. This trauma promotes the inflammatory process of a foreign body giant cell reaction.

Generally, one or more midline pits are noted; each with its own hair follicle, lined by squamous epithelium within the natal crease. The direction of the pilonidal sinuses are characteristically cranial and lateral to the pits. The sinuses can be lined with either granulation tissue or squamous epithelium and often secondary pits and sinuses may form. Lord observed that lateral sinus openings were always cephalad to the pits. It should be noted that squamous cell carcinoma has been reported in the sinus tracts; but invariably involves chronic disease and is exceedingly rare.

Symptoms and diagnosis

The diagnosis of this condition is usually not difficult. When the patient presents with an acute pilonidal abscess, the signs and symptoms are the same as for an abscess of skin and subcutaneous tissue elsewhere on the body. Typically pain, swelling and a localized fluctuant mass are noted while pyrexia and leukocytosis are uncommon. However, cellulitis and induration may also be present (Fig. 19.13).

The chronic form of pilonidal disease often presents with chronic symptoms of discomfort while sitting and persistent drainage of seropurulent material. Alternatively, patients may relate repeated episodes of acute abscess that either drain spontaneously or have been previously incised. This cycle of repeated abscess formation and drainage leads to much patient frustration. Bascom estimated that approxi-

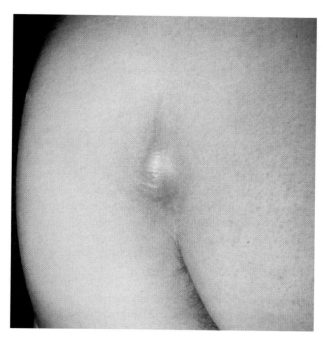

Fig. 19.13 A simple pilonidal abscess.

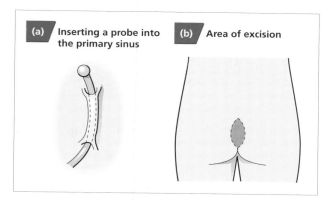

Fig. 19.14 Pilonidal disease. (a) Inserting a probe into the primary sinus. (b) The dotted line demonstrates the area of proposed excision.

mately 80% of patients present with this chronic form of disease.

Physical examination of chronic pilonidal disease may be almost unimpressive in comparison to the patient's symptoms. One or more pits or dimples are seen in the midline of the sacrococcygeal area, which may be absent if the patient had previous surgical therapy. Often, close inspection of the pit reveals hair protruding from this orifice, the hair should be removed with a small forceps. Often, without much patient discomfort, a probe can be gently inserted through this opening to assess the depth and course of the sinus (Fig. 19.14).

Treatment of acute pilonidal disease

The treatment of acute pilonidal abscess is always surgical, with immediate incision and drainage. This can usually be done with local anaesthesia in the clinic or emergency room setting. We recommend using a mixture of equal volumes of 1% lidocaine mixed with 0.5% bupivicaine with 1 : 200 000 epinephrine, yielding a final solution of 0.5% lidocaine, 0.25% bupivicaine with 1 : 400 000 epinephrine. To minimize pain, one should use a very small (30 gauge) needle and injection should be done slowly. Additionally, some authors recommend the addition of sodium bicarbonate to help lessen injection site discomfort. Again the local anaesthetic should be injected around the inflammatory process (and not into the area of fluctuance), as the anaesthetic will not function in an acid environment. Next the hair surrounding the natal cleft should be shaved. Corman recommends making a longitudinal incision slightly off the midline as

intergluteal wounds are known to heal poorly. Additionally, the edges of the wound should be removed to facilitate continued drainage and wound care. Meticulous hygiene and wound care is crucial to promote adequate healing. We recommend t.i.d. sitz baths or irrigations with a shower head attachment or portable dental water-pik device and a toothbrush for added mechanical debridement. During follow up, the intergluteal cleft should be shaved of all surrounding hair and exuberant granulation tissue should be debrided until complete healing occurs.

Jensen and Harling prospectively showed that incision, drainage and postoperative wound care relieves symptoms in all patients and leads to cure in 58%. Unfortunately, a 20–40% recurrence rate exists after simple incision and drainage procedures, requiring further therapy. Adjunctive antibiotics have little role in the treatment of either acute or chronic disease.

Treatment of chronic pilonidal disease

Unlike the treatment for acute pilonidal abscess, there is no general agreement about how chronic, nonhealing pilonidal disease should be managed. One must consider average healing time, time lost from work or school, treatment cost, and recurrence rates of the various procedures before choosing one over the other. Although up to 40% of acute pilonidal abscesses develop into chronic draining pilonidal sinuses, the majority resolve by the age of 40. For this reason some authors advocate a more minimally invasive surgical approach.

The laying open technique with cystotomy and curettage, aims to excise as little tissue as possible. Excision of only the midline pits or sinuses is advocated and curettage to remove debris and hair from the abscess bed. Advantages of this procedure include small wounds with quicker healing time (3–6 weeks), and no need for general anaesthesia as it can be done under local anaesthesia. This technique is best performed with the patient in prone-jackknife position. After infiltration of the area with local anaesthetic, a Lockhart–Mummary probe is inserted into the primary orifice and diathermy cautery is used to open the tissue of the tract and abscess cavity. All rectal secondary tracks are opened in a similar manner. One should also curette the cavity bed and all side sinuses as well as trim the wound edges to allow for a flat wound contour. No effort is made to excise the fibrous base of the cavity. Postoperative instructions include warm sitz baths and mechanical hydrodebridement two or three times per day. Reported recurrence rates using this technique range between 7–15% at one year follow-up.

A more conservative variation of the laying open technique is the closed technique, which involves simply coring out or debriding the epithelial pits. As with the lay open technique, the procedure can be done on an outpatient basis with local anaesthesia. Repeated brushings of the tract are done in follow up with a reported recurrence rate of 18%. Bascom reported a 15% recurrence rate after excision of the affected epithelial pits 5 days after initial incision and drainage of the acute suppurative process. Other authors have described the addition of phenol or cryotherapy to the closed technique but these are only isolated case reports and success is not clearly documented in the literature. In attempts to lower the recurrence rates of pilonidal disease, wider excisions have been advocated.

Wide excision of pilonidal disease differs from simpler techniques in that it requires a general anaesthetic and results in a larger wound. The procedure is done with the patient in the prone-jackknife position with the buttocks taped apart. Next, an elliptical incision is made to include all involved primary and secondary tracts, healthy intervening tissue and fat, down to the presacral fascia. The result is a large wound with prolonged healing up to several months with recurrence rates of 13% at 1 year follow-up. In an attempt to decrease healing time, variations to the wide excision method have been proposed.

Wide excision coupled with marsupialization of the wound edges both decreases healing time and recurrence rates to 4% at 1 year follow-up compared to the simple laying open technique.

Excision of pilonidal disease and primary wound closure appears to be an attractive option with healing within approximately 2 weeks; however healing is at the expense of a 15% recurrence rate at one year, and failure of primary healing in up to 30% of patients. This procedure also requires heavy retention sutures, restriction of activity, prolonged hospitalization and much time lost from work or school.

We believe that a more aggressive approach should be reserved for extensive or recurrent pilonidal disease. In such circumstances, wide excision is followed by reconstruction of the large primary tissue defect with one of a variety of different rotational flap procedures.

Presently, the most popular reconstructive procedures are the Z-plasty and the gluteus maximus rotation flaps. Other options include the modified Z-plasty, rhomboid fasciocutaneous flap and the U-flap. All of these procedures result in flattening of the natal cleft and transposition of the wound away from the midline. Most published series report primary healing within 14 days, with a flap complication rate of up to 50% including infection, decreased sensation, and flap tip necrosis. The recurrence rates for these procedures range between 0–8% in published series. Because they require general anaesthesia, prolonged hospitalization, antibiotics, suction drains and often bulky dressings and a period of immobilization, they should be reserved for use in complex or exceptionally recalcitrant disease.

In recent years some authorities have advocated complete avoidance of surgery by using the so-called 'buddy' system of skin care. This requires meticulous attention to hair removal under direct vision by a partner or friend. Although not universally accepted the early results are encouraging.

In summary, pilonidal disease can present as either acute suppuration with abscess, as a simple sinus or as a complex disease state. For the simple case of pilonidal sinus, we recommend the excision and marsupialization technique as it affords both low recurrence rates and short healing time. Incision and drainage is indicated for the acute suppurative process, with definitive treatment applied at a later date and only if symptoms persist. Finally, the use of reconstructive flap procedures should be reserved for complex cases of pilonidal disease associated with a large tissue defect.

Strangulated internal haemorrhoids

Anatomy

Symptomatic haemorrhoids are one of the most common afflictions of Western civilization. They can occur at any age and afflict both sexes equally. Haemorrhoids are highly specialized vascular cushions within the anal canal. They consist of a thickened submucosa containing blood vessels (arteriovenous connections), elastic connective tissue, and Treitz's muscle (smooth muscle derived from the conjoined longitudinal muscle and the internal anal sphincter). The submucosa, instead of forming a continuous ring of tissue in the anal canal, characteristically forms three discrete bundles. These vascular cushions are typically found in the left lateral, right anterior and right posterior positions dictated by the location of the middle rectal veins. These structures are believed to play a role in maintaining normal continence. The blood supply of these cushions is derived from the superior, middle and inferior rectal arteries. Bleeding from haemorrhoids is thus bright red and arterial in nature, and occurs when haemorrhoidal sinuses are disrupted.

This complex is important in maintaining adherence of the muscle and submucosa to the underlying internal anal

---

Strangulated internal haemorrhoids

- Appropriate anaesthesia.
- Reduce haemorrhoids to restore anatomy prior to excision.
- Maintain adequate anoderm and anal mucosal bridges to avoid stenosis.
- Avoid Whitehead procedure.

---

sphincter. These vascular cushions are normal anatomic structures; thus haemorrhoids are not pathological unless symptomatic. Repeated stretching of these complexes and Treitz's muscle is associated with chronic straining, irregular bowel habits and the natural aging process. Chronic stretching may lead to eventual detachment of the muscle from the submucosa thereby allowing prolapse to occur. Therefore, the goals of nonoperative and operative therapy are to cause fixation of these tissues to prevent prolapse from occurring.

Classification

External haemorrhoids (piles) comprise the vascular plexus that lies caudad to the dentate line and is covered by anoderm (squamous epithelium). They may swell with straining or evacuation, thus assuming a purplish discoloration. External skin tags may result as the residual of thrombosed external haemorrhoids. Because of their somatic nervous innervation and the presence of sharp pain fibres, any manipulation of external haemorrhoids requires adequate anaesthesia as they are exquisitely sensitive. For this reason, external piles are never ligated via the rubber band technique.

Internal haemorrhoids are located caudad to the dentate line and are covered with columnar epithelium. They therefore lack somatic innervation, making them amenable to treatment by rubber band ligation and other non-operative methods without anaesthesia.

Internal haemorrhoids are graded according to their symptoms. First-degree haemorrhoids may bleed but do not prolapse. Second-degree haemorrhoids prolapse during evacuation but spontaneously reduce. Manual reduction of the prolapsed mass is required in third-degree haemorrhoids, whereas fourth-degree haemorrhoids are irreducible and remain incarcerated in the prolapsed state (Fig. 19.15). Incarceration can lead to strangulation and eventual necrosis, the treatment of which will be discussed below.

'Mixed' haemorrhoids are those in which elements of both internal and external haemorrhoids are present in the same quadrant.

Symptomatology and diagnosis

Because patients invariably attribute any anorectal problem,

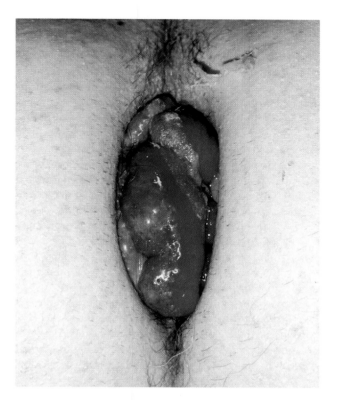

Fig. 19.15 Fourth degree haemorrhoids. The patient is placed in the prone-jackknife position.

whether pruritis, prolapse, a fissure, skin tags or the presence of a palpable mass to haemorrhoids, the task of the treating physician is to differentiate these various problems from symptomatic haemorrhoids. After taking a detailed history, the patient is examined as previously described. Careful inspection of the anal area with good illumination is combined with digital examination, anoscopy and sigmoidoscopy. With the anoscope in place, the patient should be asked to bear down as if evacuating to allow assessment of the degree of prolapse.

Description of haemorrhoidal position should include the relation to the dentate line (internal or external), the degree (1st through 4th) and the position (left lateral, right anterior, or right posterior). One should avoid descriptions based upon the hours on the clock (i.e. 3 o'clock) as the position of the clock is contingent upon the position in which the patient is examined. Attention should be made to any ulceration, tags, or visible bleeding. A picture drawn in the medical record will be invaluable in saving time writing such descriptions and allowing for rapid reassessment and comparison after therapy. A complete colonic evaluation to include either contrast enema or colonoscopy is indicated for any patient greater than 40 years of age who presents with bleeding or any patient with a recognized risk for colorectal neoplasia.

Bleeding is the most common presenting symptom with internal haemorrhoids. The Greek word *haemorrhoides* literally translates to 'flowing of blood'. Classically, the bleeding is bright red and painless, and it usually occurs at the end of evacuation. The patient usually complains of blood 'dripping' or 'squirting' into the toilet water. The bleeding is usually self-limiting but can be profuse at times and on rare occasions may even lead to anaemia. Blood may be noted by the patient in the toilet bowl or on the stool. Blood mixed in with the stool is not secondary to haemorrhoidal bleeding.

The next most common symptom of haemorrhoidal disease is protrusion or the presence of an 'anal mass'. Any protruding mass must be differentiated from other aetiologies such as mucosal prolapse, rectal polyps, a protruding hypertrophied anal papilla, procidentia and carcinoma. A comparison is made between the characteristic radial folds seen with procidentia (Figs 19.16 and 19.17) and their absence in fourth-degree haemorrhoids (Fig. 19.18).

Pain, as such, is not a primary symptom of uncomplicated haemorrhoidal disease and usually indicates either co-existing anal disease, such as an associated fissure or abscess, strangulated internal haemorrhoids or thrombosed external haemorrhoids. Strangulated, prolapsed haemor-

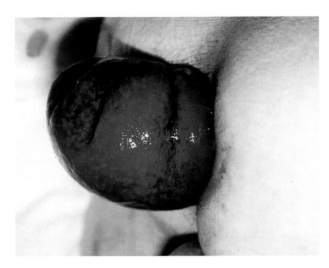

Fig. 19.17 Procidentia.

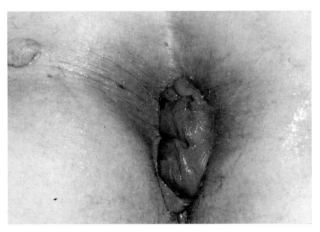

Fig. 19.18 Fourth-degree haemorrhoids. Note the presence of radial folds as seen with full thickness rectal prolapse. Reprinted with permission.

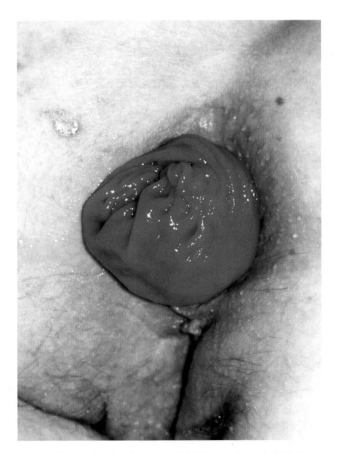

Fig. 19.16 Procidentia. Note the radial folds seen in the full thickness rectal prolapse. Reprinted with permission.

rhoids present with intense pain associated with oedematous, tender, irreducible haemorrhoids. If untreated, gangrene and rarely infectious complications may result; sloughing may lead to secondary bleeding.

External haemorrhoids may swell or cause itching and discomfort. However, unlike internal haemorrhoids, bleeding from external haemorrhoids is uncommon unless associated with the acute phase of thrombosis. Several days after the onset of an acute (usually painful) thrombosis of an external pile, the overlying skin may slough and the patient may relate the passage of blood. Typically the pain resolves much sooner than the swelling, which may persist for several weeks. A skin tag may result when the process resolves.

Most patients with symptomatic grade one or two haemorrhoidal disease are successfully treated with conservative medical management. It is estimated that only 5% of symptomatic haemorrhoids will require surgical intervention.

Treatment

Strangulated internal haemorrhoids occur in patients with fourth-degree haemorrhoids. This condition causes intense pain and can be accompanied by urinary retention. Examination reveals marked and unsightly oedema of both the internal and external haemorrhoids protruding from the anus, as well as an associated oedematous skin tag. If untreated, the oedema and venous congestion can progress to ulceration and necrosis.

Medical therapy is extremely painful, is associated with a high recurrence of symptoms and has no role in this acute emergency setting. In 1975, a study of 117 patients treated conservatively with bedrest, ice packs and elevation of the foot of the bed, 87% continued to have symptoms, 51 with bleeding, 58 with continued prolapse and 39 with both bleeding and prolapse.

Appropriate treatment of strangulated internal haemorrhoids requires urgent haemorrhoidectomy. The procedure is done in the operating room suite with an anaesthetized patient in the prone-jackknife position. It is helpful to tape the buttocks apart to aid in visualization. Once the patient is under general anaesthesia, the unsightly ring of almost circumferential oedema can be easily reduced manually. Injection of local anaesthetic and hyaluronidase may assist in reduction of the oedema and thereby the mass. After a few moments, much of the oedema will be noted to subside, as reduction of this mass of tissue enables venous return to occur. Next, a standard three-quadrant excisional haemorrhoidectomy is performed, taking extreme care not to excise excess anoderm as anal stenosis will ensue. Emergency haemorrhoidectomy in this setting gives immediate and maximal relief to the patient and surgeon. The patient is usually discharged to home as soon as oral analgesia is acceptable and the patient is able to void freely, generally on the first or second postoperative day.

The reported results of emergency haemorrhoidectomy for strangulated internal haemorrhoids are good with no more complications in the emergency haemorrhoidectomy group than in elective operations. One must keep in mind, however, that excision of minimal anoderm is of paramount importance, to avoid the complication of anal stenosis as in the elective setting.

Thrombosed external haemorrhoids

Thrombosed external haemorrhoids are a fairly common complication of haemorrhoidal disease. The patient usually presents with acute severe anal pain and a painful, tender

bluish nodule at the anal verge. The patient may report that the small mass appeared following heavy physical activity, straining during evacuation, after a bout of diarrhoea, or following long periods of sitting. Sometimes the patient cannot recall an eliciting event. The treatment depends on the time of patient presentation. If the patient presents during the acute painful episode, within the first 48 to 72 hours, the preferred treatment is ideally surgical excision, or simple incision and evacuation of clot. This condition is self-limiting, therefore the treatment is aimed at relief of pain and prevention of recurrent thrombosis and skin tags. For this reason, if the patient presents with pain that is already starting to improve, then the thrombus has already begun to involute and it is wise to employ conservative measures. Management should include warm sitz baths, non-constipating analgesics, and bulk-forming agents such as psyllium seed.

Once the diagnosis is made there is no need to place the patient in additional undue discomfort by anoscopic or sigmoidoscopic examinations. Excision of the thrombosed external haemorrhoid can easily be done under local anaesthesia (Fig. 19.19). The area should be slowly infiltrated with local anaesthetic using a very small (30 gauge) needle. We prefer a mixture of equal parts of 1% lidocaine and longer acting 0.5% bupivicaine with 1:400 000 epinephrine. Using forceps and a Metzenbaum scissors, the thrombosis and overlying anoderm and skin is excised in an ellipse. Care should be taken to excise all septations and any adjacent smaller clots.

Haemostasis can usually be achieved with simple pressure; however, cautery can be used if needed. The wound can be closed with absorbable loosely placed sutures. A dressing is applied for the first few hours. The patient will note immediate relief of pain with this simple procedure. Postoperative care involves keeping the area clean with sitz baths or washing. A mild non-constipating analgesic may

Thrombosed external haemorrhoid
• Excise under local anaesthesia.
• Role for incision only.

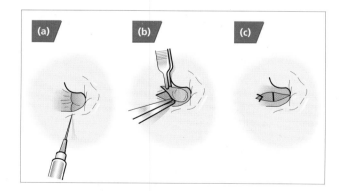

Fig. 19.19 Treatment of external haemorrhoids. (a) Local anaesthetic is infiltrated around the thrombosed varix. (b) The thrombosis is completely excised, including separations. (c) After obtaining adequate haemostasis, the wound is closed with simple absorbable sutures.

also be used. Although the treatment of both strangulated internal and thrombosed external haemorrhoids is initially surgical, most symptomatic haemorrhoids can be adequately managed conservatively.

General treatment principles

It is important to remember that asymptomatic haemorrhoids do not require treatment. Many patients with symptoms of bleeding and prolapse can be successfully treated with dietary regulation by a high fibre diet, with the addition of fibre supplements, liberalizing fluid intake and frequent sitz baths. One should aim for a goal of 25–30 g of fibre per day. The increase in fibre should be gradual to prevent poor patient compliance, as a rapid increase in fibre content can cause cramping and bloating. The clinician should also aim to correct co-existing constipation or diarrhoea as these altered bowel states lead to exacerbation of symptoms. Again, adding commercially available psyllium supplements is quite useful. The patients should also be instructed to drink 8 to 10, 250-ml glasses of water per day. This regimen should be continued even after symptomatic relief is achieved.

Commercially available haemorrhoidal preparations consisting of a myriad of topical creams, ointments or suppositories have never been shown to either shrink haemorrhoids or promote healing.

Many non-surgical techniques are available for the treatment of first, second-and third-degree symptomatic internal haemorrhoids that fail to respond to conservative medical therapy. Most of these patients are successfully treated in the clinic on an ambulatory basis. Treatments of these prolapsed or bleeding internal haemorrhoids include rubber band ligation, sclerosant injection and photocoagulation; surgical haemorrhoidectomy is reserved after failure of other treatments. The aim of treatment is to create scarring and fixation of the prolapsing mucosa to the underlying internal anal sphincter to prevent further prolapse and bleeding. These procedures are solely for the treatment of internal and not external haemorrhoids that fail to respond to initial dietary regulation.

Sclerotherapy involves the submucosal injection of sclerosing agents into the apex of the haemorrhoidal tissue to cause scarring and fixation of the tissues. Its use is limited to small first and second degree haemorrhoids with little or no prolapse. Various sclerosing agents have been used including 5% phenol in oil, quinine and urea hydrochloride. Possible complications with this technique include mucosal sloughing, ulceration, necrosis, abscess, stricture formation, and thrombosis of an adjacent external haemorrhoid. We do not routinely advocate the use of this procedure.

Infrared coagulation is a newer technique that employs administration of infrared radiation, generated by a tungsten–halogen lamp, directly to the haemorrhoidal bundle.

This electromagnetic radiation is converted to heat within the haemorrhoidal tissue which causes protein denaturation and coagulation, which leads to inflammation, scarring and fixation of the tissue. Thus far, reported success rates seem to approach that of rubber band ligation; however, each haemorrhoidal bundle usually requires three or four applications of heat in one setting to be effective, which can be uncomfortable for the patient and repeated applications may be required at a later date. This technique is best suited for first and second degree haemorrhoids that are difficult to band.

Rubber band ligation remains the mainstay of non-operative therapy for symptomatic grades one through three internal haemorrhoids. The procedure was first described by Blaisdell in 1958 and further refined by Barron in 1963. Rubber band ligation is easily done as an ambulatory procedure. With the patient in the prone-jackknife position, the haemorrhoid is grasped or suctioned up through a specially designed applicator device, and the instrument is fired, causing the placement of two tight rubber bands about the apex of the haemorrhoid (Fig. 19.20). Obviously, the rubber bands must be placed above the dentate line, where there is an absence of sharp pain fibres. For this reason the procedure does not require anaesthesia and indeed should not be performed under general anaesthesia. Placement more distally will require immediate removal of the bands. Ligation of several haemorrhoids using this technique can be done in one setting; however treatment may require more than one session of rubber band ligation. Rare but potential complications include possible delayed haemorrhage 7 to 10 days after band application, thrombosis of an external haemor-

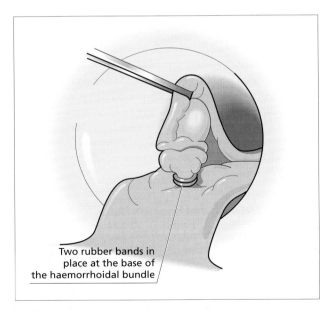

Fig. 19.20 Technique of rubber band ligation of internal haemorrhoids. Note the two bands in place at the base of the haemorrhoidal bundle.

Two rubber bands in place at the base of the haemorrhoidal bundle

rhoid after banding an internal pile, and perineal sepsis. Rubber band ligation is a fast, simple and effective treatment for symptomatic grade one, two and three internal haemorrhoids. Most large series demonstrate symptomatic relief in 80–90% of patients, and complications are rare. There are other non-operative interventional treatments for this condition, but rubber band ligation is the current gold standard of therapy.

Initially when cryotherapy was first introduced, it was advertised as a painless alternative treatment for both internal and external haemorrhoids. This technique rapid freezing and thawing of tissue using a nitrous oxide probe. This method should not be employed as subsequent studies have shown it to be an extremely painful procedure associated with long-standing foul-smelling drainage, and delayed wound healing often requiring greater than 6 weeks to heal.

Laser haemorrhoidectomy, despite the public attention it has received, has never been shown by any prospective randomized, controlled study to be more effective compared to traditional surgical haemorrhoidectomy. In fact, one study in 1992, prospectively comparing the laser to classic scalpel haemorrhoidectomy showed the only significant difference to be greater wound inflammation and dehiscence in the laser group.

When initial dietary regulation and other non-operative intervention fails to adequately treat the symptoms of haemorrhoidal disease, surgical therapy is indicated. It is also indicated in patients with fourth-degree haemorrhoids, those with combined haemorrhoids and a significant external component, for those with thrombosed gangrenous haemorrhoids, and when an associated anorectal condition requires operative intervention.

Operative haemorrhoidectomy can be performed under general, spinal or local anaesthesia with intravenous sedation. The basic principle of sugery is conservation of anoderm to prevent stricture formation. There are many techniques that can be employed but the closed haemorrhoidectomy, in which the anoderm is reapproximated after haemorrhoidal excision and mobilization of anoderm, has the added benefit of rapid wound healing (Figs 19.21–19.30).

Most patients are treated on a same day surgery basis, with admission to the ward postoperatively, for overnight observation. The most common problem encountered is

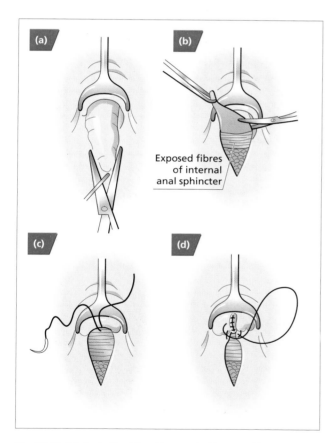

Fig. 19.21 Method of excisional haemorrhoidectomy (diagramatic representation). (a) Initial incision. The Metzenbaum scissors are placed with blades parallel to beneath the haemorrhoidal bundle. The jaw of the scissors should be open and pressed down against the external anal sphincter. (b) After sharply excising the haemorrhoidal complex, fibres of internal anal sphincter are clearly visible. The arrow points to the exposed fibres of internal anal sphincter. (c) Ligation of the haemorrhoidal pedicle. (d) After ligation of the haemorrhoidal pedicle, the anoderm is re-approximated with absorbable suture in a running fashion.

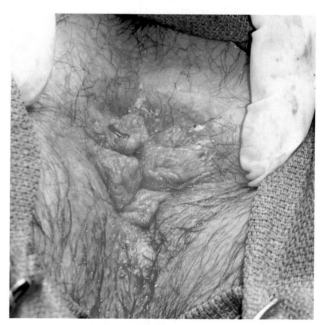

Fig. 19.22 Pre-operative view of fourth-degree haemorrhoids.

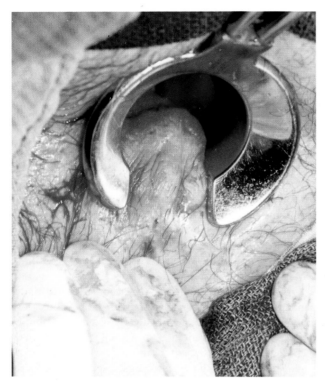

Fig. 19.23 The right posterior haemorrhoid is depicted within the anoscope.

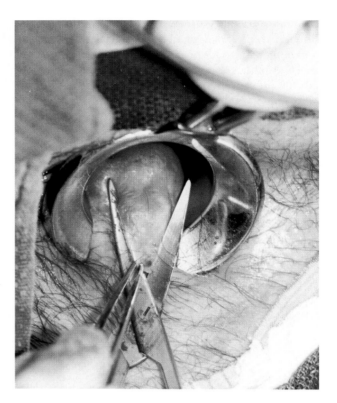

Fig. 19.24 Initial incision.

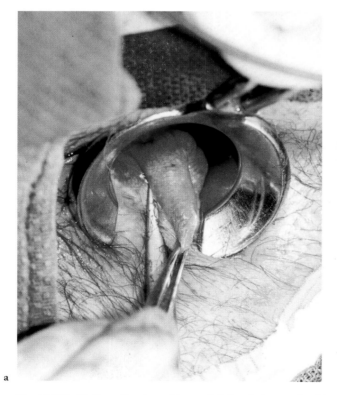

a

b

Fig. 19.25(a, b) Extending the excision cephalad to the haemorrhoidal pedicle.

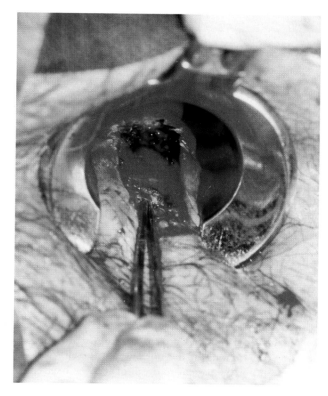

Fig. 19.26 The haemorrhoid has been excised. The forceps are pointing to the internal anal sphincter.

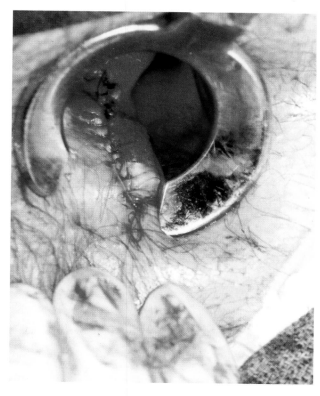

Fig. 19.28 The anoderm has been reapproximated using a running absorbable suture.

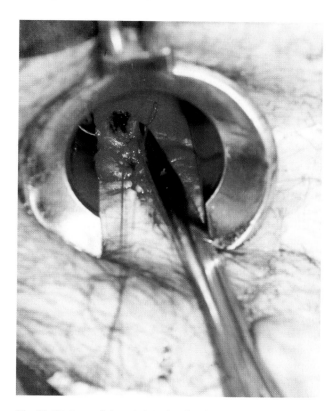

Fig. 19.27 A transfixing stitch is placed at the haemorrhoidal pedicle.

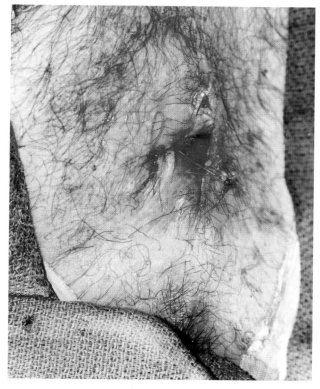

Fig. 19.29 Completion of a three-quadrant haemorrhoidectomy (right anterior, right posterior, and left lateral).

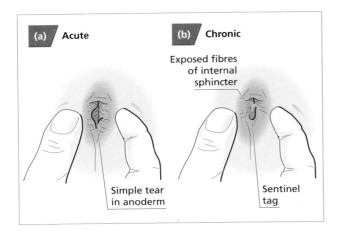

Fig. 19.30 Classification of anal fissure. (a) *Acute:* By gently parting the anus, a simple tear in the anoderm (arrow) can be visualized. (b) *Chronic:* Examination of the chronic fissure typically reveals exposed fibres of internal anal sphincter, a posterior 'sentinel tag' and a hypertrophied anal papilla.

postoperative urinary retention. For this reason, we limit peri-operative intravenous fluids by using a microdrip system and preoperatively a single 100 ml bag of intravenous fluid is hung to prevent inadvertant fluid overload. Bleeding complications are uncommon but may occur within the first 24 to 48 hours, suggesting a technical problem with inadequate haemostasis. Bleeding can also occur up to 7 to 10 days after the operation, indicating possible breakdown of the previously haemostatic suture line.

Pain and bleeding

Anal fissure

Aetiology and pathogenesis

An anal fissure, by definition, is simply a tear in the anoderm or lining of the anal canal that lies between the anal verge and dentate line. Fissures present in the posterior midline position in 99% of cases in males and in 90% of cases in females; therefore, when a fissure is located at an atypical position one should entertain the possibility of other aetiological or co-existing disease states. The condition may present at any age and both sexes are equally affected. The precise aetiology of anal fissure is unclear but thought to be related to an increased resting tone or mechanical trauma by the passage of either hard stool, diarrhoea, or foreign body as in an iatrogenic injury during endoscopy. Some authors have suggested that the observed increase in resting anal pressure, as noted by manometric studies with the 'overshoot' phenomenon, is a result of sphincter spasm induced by pain rather than a primary internal anal sphincter problem. Conversely, an ischaemic aetiology has been suggested from the studies done in cadavers where the course of

Anal fissure

- If eccentric location exclude other aetiologies.
- Do not pursue digital or any endoscopic exam if the patient is too tender.
- Sphincterotomy is preferable to the Lord's procedure.
- Maintain high-fibre diet with psyllium supplements after surgery.

the inferior rectal artery has been dissected revealing a less well vascularized pattern in the posterior anal wall than elsewhere in the anal canal. Regardless of the aetiology, the diagnosis of anal fissure is usually made by history alone, before actually examining the patient.

Diagnosis and treatment of acute anal fissure

The patient with an acute anal fissure usually presents with the acute onset of 'burning pain' at the onset of evacuation which usually lasts for several hours thereafter as a duller pain. Often the patient notes a small amount of blood on the toilet paper, but they can present with blood streaking on the stool or dripping in the toilet water as well. It is not uncommon for the patient to dread or fear the next bowel movement because of the severity of the pain. This classic history usually confirms the diagnosis of anal fissure so it is important to reassure the patient that the physical examination will be done in a gentle fashion.

Examination of the patient with an acute anal fissure is preferably done with the use of a topical anaesthetic lubricant. The fissure is easily visualized by simply and gently spreading the buttocks apart to view the anal verge. The typical appearance reveals a posterior based tear in the anoderm with sharply demarcated edges and granulation tissue within its base (Fig. 19.31). Once the fissure is seen, there is no need to proceed with an anoscopic or proctosigmoidoscopic examination—indeed the patient will not accept this. If further evaluation for bleeding is indicated, it should be done at a later date when the patient is not in significant pain. The patient should be placed on a high-fibre diet supplemented with additional bulking agents and reassured that most fissures respond to this regimen. They should be instructed to drink approximately 8–10 250-ml glasses of water per day. Sitz baths three times daily and after each bowel motion serve to ensure good hygiene as well as relax some of the sphincter spasm. A short course of topical glyceryl trinitrate GTN creams may also be helpful, although may be limited by headaches if applied too frequently. A bidet, detachable showerhead or water pik device can be used if preferred. One should avoid the use of mineral oil preparations and suppositories.

Chronic fissures typically present with less pain and less bleeding. Patients may complain more of pruritis ani, mucous drainage or 'haemorrhoids'. By definition, a fissure

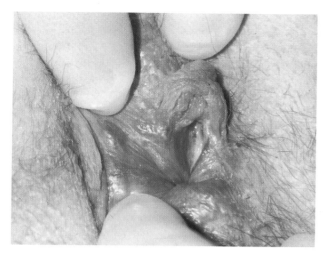

Fig. 19.31 Chronic posterior fissure.

is considered 'chronic' if present for greater than 2 weeks. We prefer to determine chronicity based on the appearance of the fissure. The chronic fissure has a classic appearance of undermined indurated edges surrounding visible transverse fibres of internal anal sphincter muscle, a hypertrophied anal papilla, and an external skin tag or 'sentinel tag'. See Fig. 19.30 for comparison of acute and chronic fissures and Fig. 19.31 for chronic posterior fissures.

The preferred surgical treatment of a chronic anal fissure is internal sphincterotomy whether open or closed; however, 40% of chronic fissures heal with conservative therapy using bran and topical anaesthetics. The first surgical sphincterotomy was described by Eisenhammer, but his initial description of the posterior midline approach led to an unacceptable anatomic malformation, namely, a 'keyhole' deformity and soiling. For this reason, the lateral internal sphincterotomy became widely practiced.

The open technique of lateral internal sphincterotomy is performed by first identifying the intersphincteric groove and hypertrophic internal anal sphincter. This is best done by inserting a bivalved anal speculum into the anal canal and opening it enough to slightly put the internal anal sphincter on stretch. The internal sphincter can then be easily palpated as a tight band or 'bow-string' between the speculum blades. Next, a small radial or circumanal incision is made distal to this groove. We prefer the right lateral side to avoid the left lateral haemorrhoidal complex. Either the tip of a curved haemostat or the Metzenbaum scissors can be used to delineate this plane. The distal one half of the internal anal sphincter is then divided. We prefer to loosely approximate the wound with absorbable sutures once haemostasis is achieved. Surgical treatment should result in 90–95% healing and various reported rates of mild soiling or incontinence of flatus, depending on the degree of muscle divided.

Alternatively, the closed technique of lateral external sphincterotomy as described by Notaras can be done. Here, the intersphincteric groove and internal anal sphincter is again identified with the bivalved anoscope in place. A narrow bladed scapula (number 11 blade or 'beaner' cataract knife) is inserted at the mid-lateral or 3 o'clock position with the flat of the blade beneath the anoderm but immediately above the internal anal sphincter (the flat of the blade should be sandwiched between the anoderm and internal anal sphincter). The blade is advanced to a point just cephalad to the dentate line. The scalpel is then rotated in a counter-clockwise direction, caudad to the dentate line towards the internal sphincter (which lies immediately beneath the blade). This is the 'out to in technique' as the internal anal sphincter fibres are outwardly incised, there is a characteristic 'gritty' sensation as the scalpel divides the fibres or hypertrophied internal anal sphincter muscle. The operating surgeon can also sense a 'sudden give' of the tissues upon completion of the sphincterotomy. Another variation of the closed sphincterotomy is the 'in to out technique'; here the scalpel blade is inserted into the intersphincteric groove, between the internal and external anal sphincter muscles. The sphincterotomy is then performed by rotating the blade inwards towards the mucocutaneous lining. Alternatively, an anal advancement may be employed to treat a chronic anal fissure. This has the advantage of requiring no sphincter division, thereby reducing the incidence of temporary or long-term incontinence.

Other procedures have been described and are used in certain centres for the treatment of chronic fissures but we discourage their use. The sphincter stretch, originally described by Lord does indeed result in sphincter stretch and adequate healing, but this technique is an uncontrolled fracturing of the internal anal sphincter which results in varying degrees of incontinence and faecal soiling as recently documented by anal ultrasonography.

Anorectal trauma and foreign bodies

Fortunately, trauma to the anorectal area is rare. In general, preservation of life in the trauma setting takes precedence over the intricacies of completing a perfect anatomic repair of the anal sphincters and restoring normal continence. Because the rectum is protected anatomically by the bony pelvis, it is not surprising that penetrating trauma is the most common aetiology. Gunshot wounds cause most rectal injuries, followed by stab and impalement injury. Blunt anorectal injury is seen less commonly and requires a significant force of impact to cause the same degree of injury.

Anatomical considerations

The relationship of the visceral peritoneum to the rectum is important as related to the treatment required. The upper

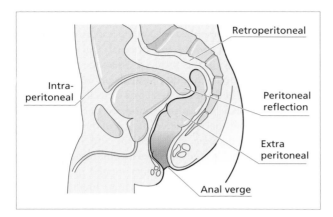

Fig. 19.32 Classification of rectal injuries: the rectum and its relationship to the peritoneal reflection.

rectum is completely intraperitoneal in location. The mid-rectum is covered by peritoneum only on its anterior surface, the posterior aspect is retroperitoneal. The distal rectum lies below the peritoneal reflection and is therefore extra-peritoneal. All of the sphincter muscles (puborectalis and levator ani muscles) lie below the peritoneal reflection. The total length of the rectum, from anal verge to sacral promontory is approximately 12–15 cm. Most anorectal wounds involve that portion that is intraperitoneal or extraperitoneal (Fig. 19.32).

Aetiology of penetrating and blunt anorectal trauma

Gunshot wounds to the perineum, buttock, thigh, and lower abdomen or torso cause most penetrating rectal injury. Missiles may cause injury by either direct penetration, blast effect or indirectly by injury from associated fragments of bone or missile. The degree of tissue damage caused by a missile depends both on the velocity (v) and the mass (m) of the projectile as depicted in the equation for kinetic energy ($E = 1/2 \, mv^2$) and because the velocity is squared, it is the factor that most determines the kinetic energy of the projectile. The degree of injury also depends on the trajectory of the missile. Multiple organ injury is common as the missile traverses the various structures within the pelvis. The tissue damage is not limited to that in direct contact with the offending bullet (as in other penetrating injuries), but also to blast effect. The kinetic energy of the missile creates a surrounding high-pressure zone around the trajectory which can result in extensive tissue damage some distance from the missile. Management of rectal injury has evolved from our military experience with rectal trauma. These wounds were typically high velocity in nature with extensive tissue loss and contamination. The principles learned during wartime combat are evident when one reviews the successive decline in morbidity and mortality over the last century as a result of

our broad application of these principles. During the American Civil War the mortality associated with penetrating anorectal injuries approached 90%. By World War I, the mortality declined to 67%. Ogilvie was able to demonstrate a decrease in mortality to 35% in the UK by employing the routine use of faecal diversion for all rectal injuries, which thereafter became standard of care. During this time surgeons also adopted the routine use of presacral drainage, antibiotics and blood transfusions as needed. The mortality was further reduced to 14% in the Vietnam era with improved antisepsis, antibiotic therapy, more rapid evacuation and resuscitation, and the addition of distal rectal washouts. Our current management of penetrating anorectal injuries is based on these principles outlined above.

Penetrating anorectal injury may also be caused by stab wounds to the buttocks or perineum, impalement injury, iatrogenic injury and foreign bodies inserted into the rectum. Both stab and impalement injuries are similar to gunshot wounds in that they are usually associated with concomitant injuries to other pelvic organs. Blunt rectal trauma is far less common than penetrating injury owing to its safe location within the sacral hollow of the pelvis and excellent blood supply. As a result a significant high-energy insult is often required to elicit such an injury.

Unlike penetrating trauma to the anorectum, the magnitude of blunt trauma required to cause significant anorectal injury is great and often results in multisystem injury. The mechanism of injury is related to either penetration of bony fragments, shear injury causing anorectal lacerations, direct or indirect trauma to the sphincter mechanism and rectal wall, or rarely devascularization with disruption of the blood supply to the rectum. Blunt injuries are most commonly seen in association with severe pelvic fractures, especially the open book type. Rectal injury from a pelvic fracture is almost always located below the peritoneal reflection. Associated genito-urinary injury and haemorrhage secondary to tearing of the presacral venous plexus from shear force with severe pelvic fractures are common. Causes of significant blunt injury include high-speed motor vehicle acci-

Table 19.1 Classification of rectal injuries.

*Grade	Description of injury
I	Contusion or haematoma without devascularization or partial thickness laceration
II	Laceration < 50% circumference
III	Laceration ≥ 50% circumference
IV	Full thickness laceration with intraperitoneal extension
V	Devascularized segment

* Multiple injuries to the same organ advances the grade by one.

dents, motorcycle accidents, pedestrian struck accidents, or fall and crush injuries. As a result, the rectal injury is often a small part of the multitrauma patient who often presents in shock. Blunt trauma can also cause disruption of the anorectum from the muscular sphincter apparatus, and also occurs below the peritoneal reflection.

Classification of rectal injury

A system for the classification of rectal injuries has been developed by the Committee of the American Association for the Surgery of Trauma (AAST). This Rectal Organ Injury Scale (OIS) grades rectal injuries based on the anatomic description of the rectal injury from 1 to 5, from the least severe to the most severe (Table 19.1).

Further reading

Fielding, L.P. & Goldberg, S.M. (eds) (1993) *Rob & Smith's Operative Surgery. Surgery of the Colon, Rectum and Anus*, 5th edn. Butterworth-Heinemann, London.

Barkin, J.S. & Rogers, A.I. (eds) (1994) *Difficult Decisions in Digestive Diseases*, 2nd edn. Mosby-Yearbook Inc, St. Louis.

Corman, M.L. (ed.) (1995) *Colon and Rectal Surgery*, 3rd edn. J.B. Lippincott, Philadelphia.

Falcone, R.E. Wanamaker, S.R. Santanello, S.A. & Carey, L.C. (1992) Colorectal trauma: primary repair of anastomosis with intracolonic bypass vs. ostomy. *Diseases of the Colon and Rectum* **35** 957–963.

Zudima, G. (ed.) (1996) *Shackleford's Surgery of the Alimentary Tract*, Vol IV. W.B. Saunders, Philadelphia.

Gordon, P.H. & Nivatvongs, S. (eds) (1992) *Principles and Practice of Surgery for the Colon, Rectum and Anus*. Quality Medical Publishing, St. Louis.

O'Connell, P.R. (1995) Hidradenitis suppurativa. In: *Clinical Decision-making in Colorectal Surgery*, (eds S.D. Wexner & A.M. Vernava III), pp. 169–172. Igaku-Shoin, New York.

Dent, T.L. Kukora, J.S. & Leibrandt, T.J. (eds) (1988) *Surgical Tips*. McGraw-Hill, New York.

Beck, D.E. & Welling, D.R. (eds) (1991) *Manual of Patient Care in Colorectal Surgery*. Little, Brown and Co, Boston.

Keighley, M.R.B. & Williams, N.S. (eds) (1993) *Surgery of the Colon, rectum and anus* Vol I. W.B. Saunders: London.

References

Anderson, A.W. (1847) Hair extracted from an ulcer. *Boston Med Surg* **36** 74.

Barron, J. (1963) Office ligation treatment of haemorrhoids. *Dis Colon Rectum* **6** 109–113.

Blaisdell, P.C. (1958) Prevention of massive haemorrhage secondary to haemorrhoidectomy. *Surg Gynecol Obstet* **106** 485–488.

Hodges, R.M. (1880) Pilo-nidal sinus. *Boston Med Surg* **103** 485–486.

Lord, M.R. & Thomson, J.P.S. (1977) Fissure in ano: the initial management and prognosis. *Br J Surg* **64** 355–358.

Lord, P.H. & Millar, D.M. (1965) Pilonidal sinus: a simple treatment. *Br J Surg* **52** 292–300.

Notaras, M.J. (1993) Lateral subcutaneous internal anal fissure. In: *Rob and Smith's Operative Surgery. Surgery of the Colon, Rectum and Anus* (eds L.P. Fielding & S.M. Goldberg), 5th edn, pp. 871–879. Butterworth-Heinemann, London.

Oglivie, W.H. (1944) Abdominal wounds in the Western Desert. *Surg Gynecol Obstet* **78** 225–239.

CHAPTER 20

Abdominal trauma

Alastair C. J. Windsor & Pierre J. Guillou

Introduction

Civilian trauma remains a significant cause of death in all age groups and the most frequent cause of death in the under 45s. Abdominal trauma accounts for a large fraction of this tragic loss of life and unrecognized abdominal injury remains a distressingly frequent cause of preventable death. Subtle physical signs, often overshadowed by pain from extra-abdominal injuries and masked by intoxication or significant head injury seem the principal reasons for these missed abdominal injuries. Additionally, up to one-third of patients with abdominal injury requiring urgent operative intervention will have an initial benign physical examination, misleading the unwary clinician into assuming no injury exists.

Clinical aims

The key to successful management of abdominal trauma and injury is a high index of suspicion. Any patient who has sustained significant blunt or penetrating trauma should be assumed to have suffered visceral injury until such time as this can be confidently ruled out. Furthermore, the primary clinical aim of the attending clinician should be to determine whether an intra-abdominal injury exists and that urgent operative intervention is or is not required, rather than an exhaustive attempt to diagnose or define specific organ damage. As a rule of thumb, some 75–90% of patients with abdominal gunshot wounds will require emergency laparotomy, 25–35% with abdominal stab wounds and only 15–20% with blunt abdominal trauma. With this in mind, and the acceptance that unnecessary laparotomies carry a definable operative risk, the less the potential need for operative intervention the greater the clinical difficulty in defining those who do and do not need surgery. In simple terms, faced with a gunshot wound to the anterior abdominal wall, a clinician can reasonably expect there to have been significant intra-abdominal injury and many accept this as a mandate for emergency surgery. However, faced with a patient involved in a road traffic accident, with fractured lower ribs, and semi-conscious following head injury, identification of intra-abdominal injury and the decision to proceed to laparotomy is significantly more complex. As blunt trauma is by far the commonest cause of abdominal injury in the UK it is critical that clinicians involved in trauma management follow an objective, systematic and thorough approach to these patients, so minimizing the likelihood of missed potentially fatal injury.

General considerations

Anatomical considerations

The abdominal cavity is, by convention, divided into three distinct regions: (1) the peritoneal cavity; (2) the retroperitoneum; and (3) the pelvis. The peritoneal cavity may be further divided into thoracic and abdominal segments. The thoracic portion lies between the costal margin and the diaphragm, and may rise to the fourth intercostal space on full expiration. This exposes critical organs such as the liver, spleen, stomach and transverse colon to injury following lower thoracic trauma.

The retroperitoneum contains the major vessels, pancreas, duodenum and colon in addition to the upper urinary tract. Often contained and hidden from all but advanced radiological procedures, injuries in this area are difficult to assess and treat. The pelvis though protected by a significant bony cage is still prone to injury particularly from blunt trauma. It contains rectum, bladder, iliac vessels, female genitalia and a rich plexus of veins all of which may be compromised in the event of pelvic injury.

Anatomical regions and contents	
Anatomical site	Visceral and vascular contents
Peritoneum	
Thoracic	Liver, spleen, stomach, colon
Abdominal	Small bowel, colon
Retroperitoneum	Major vessels, pancreas, duodenum, colon, urinary tract
Pelvis	Rectum, bladder, major vessels, female reproductive organs, rich venous plexus

Diagnostic aids and adjuncts
• History and physical examination
• Laboratory investigation
• Plain radiology
• Diagnostic peritoneal lavage
• Computerized tomography and ultrasound
• Laparoscopy

Diagnostic adjuncts

The diagnostic tools available to the clinician making decisions regarding the need for operative intervention include, history, physical examination, laboratory investigation, radiology, diagnostic peritoneal lavage and direct emergency laparotomy. The choice and application of these tools and the significance placed on their results will depend upon a number of factors including: (1) the mechanism of injury; (2) haemodynamic stability of the patient; (3) availability and expertise of surgical personnel; (4) presence of other life-threatening injury. The following section will discuss these diagnostic adjuncts with reference to generic abdominal trauma, their more defined roles in blunt and penetrating trauma and algorithms for their application in these settings will be discussed later in the chapter.

History

Information about the nature of the traumatic insult may be critical in deciding the extent of injury. Eye-witness accounts, notes from emergency personnel and acute admitting staff in hospital are all relevant to the final clinical decisions regarding management. In road traffic accidents for example, the speed and direction of impact, damage to vehicles, and the use of seat belts will determine the type of shearing, crushing or decelerating injuries suffered by the victim and thus potential underlying injuries. Ejection from a motor vehicle at the time of impact more than trebles the likelihood of major injury. In the case of a gunshot wound, the calibre and muzzle velocity of the weapon, number of shots and distance between gun and victim are all related to the nature and extent of intra-abdominal disruption. This information is therefore as important as much of the complex diagnostic tests available to the clinician in the final decision to operate or not.

Physical examination

Physical examination of the injured abdomen is less informative and potentially more misleading than in any other system involved in trauma. It has already been emphasized that in 30% of patients needing urgent operative intervention the initial physical examination may be benign. This figure rises to nearly 50% in patients with altered conscious level from head injury or intoxication. This is particularly evident in blunt trauma, and illustrated in a classic series by Davis *et al.* (1976) of 437 blunt abdominal trauma patients in whom 47% had no positive physical signs at initial evaluation. 44% of these patients were eventfully explored as a result of other diagnostic tests and significant intra-abdominal injury was found in 77% of them.

In stark contrast to the negative physical examination, a positive physical examination revealing signs of peritoneal irritation is possibly the most reliable sign of significant intra-abdominal injury requiring intervention. Indeed overt signs of peritonitis mandates urgent laparotomy without the need for further diagnostic delays. Therefore, meticulous, systematic abdominal examination in an ordered sequence is mandatory in all cases of abdominal trauma.

Inspection
A rapid but thorough examination should be performed, with the patient fully undressed and log-rolled to examine perineum, buttocks, back and posterior chest. Evidence of penetrating injury, bruising, abrasions and imprints from clothing should be noted. In particular the imprints and abrasions associated with the seat-belt sign dramatically increase the likelihood of injury even in the presence of an otherwise normal examination.

Auscultation
The presence or absence of bowel sounds in the abdomen is of little diagnostic use, their presence in the chest, however, may suggest significant diaphragmatic injury. Bruits may suggest major arterial/arteriovenous injury.

Palpation and percussion
Early visceral pain tends to be poorly localized and unhelpful. However, definitive signs of peritoneal irritation (localized pain, tenderness with guarding and rebound tenderness) should not be attributed to local body wall injury and further investigation of the peritoneal cavity is required. Acute gastric dilatation should be sought and treated with nasogastric decompression (beware of cribriform plate damage in patients with head injury). Rectal examination is essential to look for sphincter tone to assess spinal injury, blood suggesting rectal injury and the level of the prostate indicating posterior uretheral disruption. In addition, the penile meatus should be examined for blood, and the presence of scrotal haematoma further suggests the possibility of urethral injury. 'Springing' of the pelvis and the lower ribs will indicate potential bony injury, whose presence once again significantly increases the risk of underlying visceral injury such as bladder and urethra, and liver and spleen, respectively.

As with much of trauma management the initial examination should be treated as a baseline measure from which to judge further repeated examination. Undoubtedly regular returns to the patient watching for changing or developing physical signs are very much more valuable than an isolated finding. In addition, such repeated examinations should continue throughout other investigative procedures until such time as the need for operative intervention is ruled out.

Laboratory investigation

Initial blood and other laboratory tests are, on the whole, of little value except as baselines from which to monitor clinical progress such as serial haematocrit to monitor blood loss, or amylase to monitor evolving pancreatic injury. The exceptions are perhaps urinalysis for haematuria indicating urinary tract injury, blood gases in intubated patients and a coagulation screen following massive resuscitative transfusion. Nevertheless blood should be drawn for baseline measurement, cross match and to screen for anaesthetic risk (sickle cell) as with any other operative workup.

Plain radiology

Plain radiology is again of limited use in abdominal trauma, it is estimated that at least 800 ml of free peritoneal fluid is required to be evident on a plain abdominal film. However, an erect chest X-ray may demonstrate free intraperitoneal gas indicating hollow visceral perforation. Further, it may demonstrate a nasogastric tube in the chest cavity as a sign of diaphragmatic rupture. A careful radiological search for bony injury to the chest, pelvis and abdominal skeleton may direct attention to possible, associated, secondary visceral injury (Table 20.1).

Diagnostic peritoneal lavage

Introduced in 1965 by Root and colleagues, diagnostic peritoneal lavage (DPL) provides a rapid, inexpensive, accurate and for the most part safe method of assessing both blunt and penetrating abdominal trauma. Although criticized over the years for: (1) over sensitivity, leading to unnecessary laparotomies for minor self-limiting intra-abdominal injury; (2) lack of organ-specific detail; (3) failure to detect retroperitoneal injury, DPL consistently achieves a 95% accuracy rate and less than 1% morbidity.

Table 20.1 Associated visceral injuries following skeletal fractures.

Bony injury	Associated tissue injury
Lower left ribs	Spleen
Lower right ribs	Liver
Pelvis	Bladder, urethra
Lumbar transverse process	Renal

Indications

According to guidelines laid down by the Advanced Trauma and Life Support course, the indications for DPL fall into three main categories centred around the physical examination. DPL is indicated when the abdominal examination is considered:

1 *Equivocal*, i.e. when associated local soft tissue and bony injury obscure findings.
2 *Unreliable*, i.e. when the patient's conscious level is depressed following head injury or intoxication.
3 *Impractical*, i.e. when it is anticipated that the patient will require lengthy general anaesthesia for other injuries.

In addition, in patients who have sustained abdominal trauma, who have unexplained hypotension, DPL may be a reliable way of excluding intra-abdominal injury.

Absolute contra-indications

The only absolute contra-indication to DPL is considered to be the presence of an existing indication for laparotomy.

Relative contra-indications

Technical difficulty with the procedure increases the likelihood of complications and increases the false positive rate and thus unnecessary laparotomies. Conditions such as morbid obesity, previous abdominal surgery, and advanced pregnancy should be considered relative contra-indications to DPL. In addition, an established coagulopathy might significantly decrease the accuracy of DPL and an alternative assessment may be advisable.

Technique of DPL

There are a number of different approaches to DPL described as closed, semi-open and open. Most institutions now favour the semi-open technique as giving the most accurate approach, whilst minimizing complications. Following urinary catheterization and insertion of a nasogastric tube, the patient's anterior abdominal wall should be prepared and draped as if for an elective operative procedure. The peri-umbilical area should then be infiltrated with local anaesthetic and a 5-cm incision made infra-umbilically. This incision is deepened through subcutaneous fat and superficial fascia until the rectus sheath and linea alba are reached. A 5-mm incision is then made in the linear alba and the edges grasped with tissue forceps. It is essential that haemostasis is maintained to prevent iatrogenic bleeding soiling the lavage fluid. While elevating the anterior abdominal wall by traction on the tissue clips a peritoneal dialysis catheter with trocar are inserted through the preperitoneal fat into the peritoneal cavity. The catheter should be directed away from the major retroperitoneal vessels and aimed into the sacral hollow. Once in the peritoneal cavity the trocar should be withdrawn and the catheter advanced into the pelvis. At this stage an attempt is made to aspirate any peritoneal fluid. The tap should be considered positive if >10 ml of fresh blood can be aspirated at this stage. It should be noted that even in a normal peritoneal cavity it is often possible to aspirate 5 ml of serous fluid. If no fresh blood is encountered, 1 L of 0.9% saline (15 ml/kg in children) should be run into the peritoneal cavity. If possible, the patient should then be rolled gently to allow contact between the fluid and all the peritoneal structures. The empty bag of saline is then placed on the floor allowing the lavage fluid to be retrieved. A minimum of 75% return of fluid is required to validate the test. Aliquots of the fluid should then be sent to haematology for red cell count (RBC) and white cell count (WBC) and to chemistry for amylase (LAM) and alkaline phosphatase (LAP) analysis.

Interpretation of results (Table 20.2)

In blunt abdominal trauma, a RBC of greater than $100\,000/mm^3$ is considered a positive lavage. The figure was originally based on a gross tap of 20 ml fresh blood diluted in 1 L of saline giving an haematocrit of 1%. It is thus very sensitive and some clinicians have argued for a reduction in this positive limit. However, in patients with a positive lavage with a RBC of $>100\,000/mm^3$, significant visceral injury is found in some 90–95%. If this positive limit is lowered to $20\,000/mm^3$ the incidence of significant visceral injury falls to $<5\%$. Counts of between $20\,000/mm^3$ and $100\,000/mm^3$ reveal significant injury in between 15–25% of cases. Many clinicians thus consider a RBC count in lavage fluid of $>100\,000/mm^3$ to be positive, and counts of $<20\,000/mm^3$ to be negative. Counts between $20\,000/mm^3$ and $100\,000/mm^3$ are considered to be equivocal requiring further evaluation by an alternative diagnostic test or by repeated lavage at a later time. The migration of white cells into the peritoneal cavity following trauma may be delayed by a number of hours and thus the use of lavage WBC counts as a definitive diagnostic tool is to be avoided. Rather, the finding of WBC counts of $>500/mm^3$ should alert the clinician and initiate further investigation to rule out the possibility of occult injury. Many institutions do not rely on lavage enzyme levels to diagnose injury. However, the trauma team in Denver, Colorado, USA have reported in over 2000 DPLs that an isolated finding of LAP $>3\,IU/L$ and LAM $>20\,IU/L$ is 97% specific and 78% sensitive for

hollow visceral injury; this may assist the otherwise difficult diagnosis of this problem.

The role of DPL in penetrating abdominal trauma is less certain, although its use in conjunction with local wound exploration is considered to reduce the incidence of unnecessary laparotomy. The levels at which lavage is considered positive vary greatly from institution to institution. However, in two published series from Houston, Texas, USA, RBC counts of $>100\,000/mm^3$ diagnosed significant visceral injury with an accuracy of $>90\%$, which is comparable to DPL in blunt trauma.

Complications

Complications of the technique are infrequent (1%) and usually relate to the use of the closed technique or attempting DPL in patients with relative contra-indications. Injury to bladder and stomach can be limited by decompression. Other injuries include major vessel, mesenteric vessels, small bowel and colonic perforation. False positive lavage usually results from poor haemostasis at the time of DPL. However, fractured pelvis and self limiting intra-abdominal injury can also initiate unnecessary operation. False negative lavage is typically the result of an isolated perforation of a hollow viscus; however, retroperitoneal injuries to vessels, kidney, duodenum and colon also contribute to this.

Computerized tomography (CT)

In recent years accessibility to machines and specialized interpretation has allowed the widespread use of CT scanning in the assessment of trauma. A significant body of literature exists comparing and contrasting CT scan with DPL in the initial evaluation of abdominal trauma, with the result that champions of one technique or the other have emerged and the indications for, and the value of, each technique has become somewhat confused. Most clinicians would now agree, however, that the two techniques are far from mutually exclusive, rather they should be viewed as complementary. The principal advantage of CT over DPL lies in its ability to diagnose organ-specific injury, thus, in certain cases obviating the need for unnecessary laparotomy. Modern conservative management of non-life-threatening injuries to liver and spleen for instance has been facilitated by the ability to sequentially monitor the extent of organ damage by serial CT scans. In addition, CT is able to examine both intra- and retroperitoneal injury and is essentially non-invasive, and as such, has fewer side effects or complications. The principal disadvantages of CT scanning stems from the time required to organize, carry out and interpret the findings. Even in specialist trauma centres this may be upwards of 1 hour. This transgresses an abiding principle in trauma management that delay in diagnosis is potentially life threatening. In addition, CT requires specialist personnel and specialist equipment, thus the expense is

Table 20.2 Positive diagnostic peritoneal lavage criteria.

Parameter	Aspirate	Lavage
Blood	>10 mL	
Red cells		>100 000/mm³ (20 000–100 000 mm³ equivocal)
Enzymes		Amylase > 20 IU/L Alkaline Phosphatase > 3 IU/L

significantly greater than DPL. In terms of diagnostic accuracy CT's popular failing is in the diagnosis of isolated hollow viscus, in particular perforation. However, the use of contrast techniques has improved this failing though not without the hazards of aspiration and allergy to the contrast media. Despite these failings CT is widely reported to be able to achieve a diagnostic accuracy for significant abdominal injury of between 90–98%, and is therefore comparable to DPL.

Indications
Indications for CT scan in abdominal trauma include:
1 Delayed presentation—delay of more than 12 h.
2 An equivocal DPL.
3 A relative contra-indication to DPL.
4 Suspected retroperitoneal injury—such as haematuria without obvious uretheral or bladder injury.

Contra-indications
Absolute contra-indications include the presence of an indication for laparotomy and pregnancy. Relative contra-indications include allergy to the contrast media required for some of the more definitive scanning protocols and in many institutions paediatric trauma is now preferentially investigated by ultrasound because of the relatively high radiation doses required for CT.

Ultrasound

Ultrasound (U/S) has been used extensively in Europe in the evaluation of abdominal trauma in particular in the paediatric population; however it has yet to gain such acceptance in the USA. With improvements in ultrasound resolution, modern scanning provides quick, cheap and relatively organ specific evaluation of the abdominal cavity. In addition modern machines are eminently portable and can be used in the resuscitation room for instant evaluation.

Undoubtedly the accuracy of U/S is more operator dependent than other forms of evaluation. It readily demonstrates free intraperitoneal fluid and solid organ injury, and is capable of evaluating the retroperitoneum, though without the finesse of CT. However, its limitations lie in identification of hollow viscus perforation and with a paralytic ileus gas filled loops of bowel render U/S interpretation extremely difficult.

In 1993 Rothlin *et al.* from Switzerland studied 300 patients with blunt abdominal trauma and demonstrated 90% sensitivity and 99.5% specificity for intra-abdominal injury. In the same year Rozycki *et al.* from the USA evaluated both blunt and penetrating abdominal trauma and demonstrated a 79% sensitivity and 95.6% specificity. The key message in these and other publications however, is that U/S provides very rapid patient assessment, allowing prioritization of injury. Increasingly it is available in the trauma or resuscitation room and increasingly the surgeon as well as the radiologist has a role in scanning and interpretation.

Laparoscopy

With the advent of modern minimally invasive surgery, the rapid advancement of technology has allowed the application of diagnostic and therapeutic laparoscopy in a wide variety of pathologies. Abdominal trauma is included as one of these growing applications. Its indications are still to be clarified but it does have a role in both penetrating and blunt trauma. In particular the difficulty of establishing whether or not a tangential penetrating injury to the abdomen has breached the peritoneal cavity can, at times, easily be resolved with diagnostic laparoscopy. Two independent series by Fabian and Ivatury from the USA demonstrated some 60% of tangential abdominal injuries were not associated with violation of the peritoneum and so avoided laparotomy. Furthermore Ivatury *et al.* were able to show a significant decrease in hospital stay in the negative laparoscopy group compared to the negative laparotomy group.

The role of laparoscopy in blunt abdominal trauma is less clear. Fabian *et al.* found no advantage in laparoscopy compared to DPL in this setting. Laparoscopy is poor at evaluating the whole peritoneal cavity, and like DPL, does not evaluate the retroperitoneum. Its role, however, may lie in the diagnosis, evaluation and treatment of solid organ injury, such as liver and spleen. Although as yet very much experimental, several authors have demonstrated its potential to control haemorrhage from solid organs in animal models. Its other definitive role is in the evaluation of suspected diaphragmatic injury. Few would argue that laparoscopy gives possibly the most complete view of the diaphragm, even surpassing formal laparotomy.

Blunt abdominal trauma

Mechanisms of injury

Pathophysiology

Essential to the rapid and effective management of specific injury following blunt abdominal trauma is a clear understanding of the potential mechanisms of such injury. They include:
1 Sudden rise in intra-abdominal pressure, giving rise to burst injury of solid organs such as liver and spleen, or rupture of hollow organs such as bowel.
2 Shearing forces, classically initiated by rapid deceleration in a road traffic accident, can lead to tearing of vascular pedicle such as mesentery, porta hepatis and splenic hilum.
3 Compression injury of viscera trapped between a force

applied to the anterior abdominal wall and the thoracic or lumbar spine.

Identifying high risk injury

Appreciation of these mechanisms allows the clinician to target specific areas of the abdominal cavity as high risk for injury, thus reducing the incidence of missed injury. In addition certain features of the history subclassify patients as either potentially high or low risk of injury and should further alert and direct the clinician's therapeutic efforts. Motorcyclists, pedestrians struck by cars and victims ejected from a motor vehicle are considered to be at high risk of abdominal injury. Falls from greater than 4.5 m, episodes of hypotension in the field or upon admission and associated injuries to chest and/or pelvis also indicate high risk. The distinction between potentially high and potentially low risk of injury, although by no means absolute, has been included in many algorithms for trauma care. In addition it has been ratified by prospective studies and as such provides a further useful adjunct for the clinician.

Management of blunt abdominal trauma

Physical examination

Earlier in this chapter the potential for a negative physical examination to mislead the clinician has been stressed. However, it should be re-emphasized that a positive physical examination, demonstrating features of peritonism, such as: localized tenderness, guarding and rebound tenderness, is possibly the most helpful and definitive indication of intra-abdominal injury. Thus, a careful, thorough and ordered physical examination as outlined above should be carried out on all patients. Specific features such as: seat belt sign, bruising, Kehr's sign of diaphragmatic irritation and evidence of bony injury to ribs or pelvis should all alert the clinician to the possibility of intra-abdominal injury. Furthermore, revaluation by serial examination is an essential part of preventing missed injury.

Plain radiology

Plain X-rays of the abdomen tend to be much less revealing than a chest X-ray performed in chest trauma. One series by Strauch et al. suggesting that plain abdominal films only contributed to the decision to operate in 3.2% of patients with blunt abdominal trauma. However, radiological evidence of rib fractures, for instance, increases the risk of liver and spleen injury by 10% and 20%, respectively. In addition, free intraperitoneal gas mandates emergency laparotomy for ruptured hollow viscus.

Laboratory investigations

Once again the results of laboratory investigations should be seen as contributory rather than definitive. An abnormal result may indicate further investigation but a normal result should never dissuade from investigation or intervention. Most haematological results in isolation are non-contributory in blunt abdominal trauma. Even serial haematocrits, suggested by some workers to help monitor resuscitation, are often confounded by changes in the parameters they are monitoring, such as, blood loss, fluid replacement and compartmental fluid shifts. Despite this, Knottenbett et al. in a South African study demonstrated that an admission haemoglobin of 8 g/L or less was a strong indicator of ongoing haemorrhage.

Serum enzyme levels have been studied at length in an attempt to correlate raised levels with specific organ injury. In the case of amylase and the pancreas and of transaminases and the liver, at best, raised levels should alert the clinician to potential injury. Retrospective studies from units such as Nassau County Medical Center who directly correlated raised transaminases with degree of hepatic injury, have yet to be ratified by prospective analysis.

Management algorithm

Figure 20.1 sets out a proposed algorithm for patients with blunt abdominal trauma. As with all such management aids it is designed as a guide to assist, not to instruct, the clinician in decision making.

Patients admitted with overt signs of intra-abdominal injury, with or without massive haemoperitoneum should not be delayed by further investigation. Resuscitation and emergency laparotomy may be lifesaving. Likewise, patients who are delayed more than 12 h in presentation who have suffered low-risk trauma and have no abnormal physical findings should either simply be observed or should undergo an ultrasound as a screening investigation, looking for free fluid with or without signs of organ injury. Those patients with delayed presentation who are at high risk of significant injury and/or with positive physical findings should undergo CT scan and further management based on the findings at scan.

Management of the patient with an acute presentation provides the real diagnostic dilemma. This is where all contributory pieces of information should weigh either for or against emergency surgery. Patients considered by history and examination to be low risk, i.e. no positive findings on examination and low-risk mechanism of injury who are haemodynamically stable should undergo an ultrasound or may simply be observed. Those with low-risk injury and equivocal or positive physical findings who are haemodynamically stable should undergo CT scan. Those who are haemodynamically unstable should be subjected to emer-

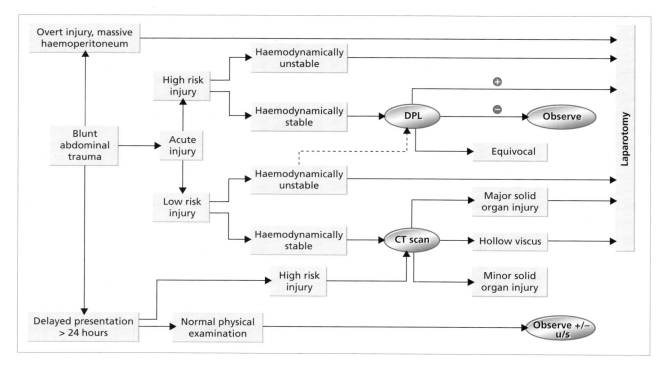

Fig. 20.1 Management algorithm for blunt abdominal trauma (Modified, with permission from A. Read & E. E. Moore, Abdominal trauma. In: *Current Practice Of Surgery* Levine *et al.* (eds). Churchill Livingstone, Edinburgh).

gency laparotomy, although some clinicians would undertake DPL as proof of an intra-abdominal source of bleeding in a multiply injured patient. High-risk injury in a haemodynamically unstable patient once again mandates emergency laparotomy. In a stable patient, the speed and accuracy of DPL makes it the safe diagnostic option; although once again some clinicians would be swayed by the more organ-specific CT scan if facilities for an expeditious investigation and expert interpretation were available. Positive DPL findings in high risk patients warrant emergency laparotomy, and negative findings further observation, whereas equivocal findings should initiate further investigation and CT scan is currently the investigation of choice.

CT scan findings of major solid organ injury or suspicion of hollow viscus injury mandates emergency laparotomy. Minor solid organ injury in a patient who remains haemodynamically stable may be observed and should undergo serial scans to re-assess the injury and to monitor healing or alert to the presence of complication which requires subsequent intervention.

Non-operative management of splenic injury

Up to this point the key message in this chapter has been identification of patients who have suffered abdominal trauma, have evidence of a significant intra-abdominal injury and who require emergency laparotomy. With our increased understanding of the relative risks of non-therapeutic laparotomy and overwhelming postsplenectomy sepsis, the concept of non-operative treatment of abdominal trauma has evolved. This concept is particularly relevant to patients with solid organ injury such as liver and spleen.

Principles

The key to success as with most therapeutic options is patient selection, and the key to patient selection is haemodynamic stability. Haemodynamic stability implies normal vital signs, in particular pulse rate and urine output $>40–50$ ml/h without need for ongoing fluid resuscitation. Patients who respond to the standard 1 to 2 L crystalloid administration of the immediate resuscitation phase of trauma assessment, and then remain haemodynamically stable can be included in this group. Repeated physical examination should not reveal signs of peritoneal irritation, thus eliminating the uncooperative, intoxicated or unconscious patient from this therapeutic option. In addition to the patient criteria non-operative management should be reserved for institutions with an interest in trauma, where adequate nursing and operating theatre facilities are available for continuous monitoring and rapid intervention if needed. In addition it requires adequate CT scanning facilities to allow serial scanning and expert interpretation.

Once established as stable and a candidate for non-operative management the next stage is to establish the presence and degree of organ injury. CT scanning provides the key to this assessment with its ability to identify both organ specific injury and severity of injury. Injury scores are both numerous and varied, but most clinicians recognize four grades of splenic injury.

Spleen
Grade I Minor capsular tear, subcapsular haematoma without parenchymal injury.
Grade II Single or multiple capsular tears with parenchymal injury not extending to the hilum.
Grade III Major parenchymal injury involving major vessels and/or hilum.
Grade IV Shattered spleen.

In an adult population Grade I and II injuries are candidates for non-operative management and some institutions would cautiously allow Grade III injuries in children to be managed non-operatively. Once the decision is made the patient should be fasting and ideally be in an intensive therapy unit (ITU) setting, although logistically this is often not possible. Vital signs should be monitored, some recommend serial haematocrits, repeated physical examination is required by an experienced clinician, at least 4–6 hourly and, a further CT scan is usually performed at 24 h to reassess the injury. Failure of non-operative management in splenic injury usually occurs within 72 h, therefore aggressive monitoring can cease at this point and the patient allowed to eat, but bed rest and ward monitoring is recommended for at least a total of 10 days postinjury. Delayed bleeding because of a liquefying haematoma, osmotic fluid shifts and capsular rupture can occur up to 4 weeks later; however, this is said to occur in less than 1% of cases. Although successful in the majority of cases, failure of non-operative management mandates emergency laparotomy and usually splenectomy, whereas initial operative intervention may well have resulted in splenic preservation. This observation was taken one stage further by Luna and Dellinger who, taking into account operative risk, transfusion risk and postsplenectomy sepsis risk, stated that the mortality risk of non-operative management was four times greater than operative. This serves to highlight that non-operative management though attractive has potentially serious consequences and should only be undertaken in a motivated and experienced practice.

Evolving management of liver injury

Despite its position of relative protection beneath the rib cage, because of its large size the liver is particularly vulnerable to injury following abdominal trauma. An estimated 20% of patients requiring laparotomy for blunt abdominal trauma have sustained liver injury and as many as 40% in penetrating injuries. As long ago as 1908 Pringle, who popularized hepatoduodenal compression for control of haemorrhage in liver trauma, recognized that in some patients with liver injury simply opening the peritoneal cavity was associated with increased blood loss. As the availability of CT scanning expanded, so the potential for accurate assessment of hepatic injury in the haemodynamically stable patient has allowed a selective non-operative management approach. Typically stable subcapsular or intrahepatic haematomas lend themselves to this approach. Some specialized centres have extended these ideas to liver lacerations and even penetrating liver injuries. For instance, haemodynamic stability and an estimated intraperitoneal blood volume of <500 ml on CT scan with any magnitude of hepatic injury initially receives non-operative intervention at Grady Memorial Hospital in Atlanta, USA.

Once again, the key to successful non-operative management of liver injury is aggressive monitoring, constant clinical reappraisal and sequential CT scans to monitor the evolution of the injury (Fig. 20.2). Development of bile collections does not mandate surgical intervention. Radiological drainage and awareness of, and close monitoring for biliary sepsis may suffice. As with most contemporary management protocols non-operative management of liver trauma is not without its critics. Some have argued the contained subcapsular and intrahepatic haematomas would have been missed on DPL prior to CT scanning and would have received a similar non-operative initial approach. Furthermore, there are a number of reports suggesting that CT assessment of liver injury does not appear to correlate with the degree of injury or degree of blood loss as assessed by laparotomy. In addition, much of the comparative literature is complicated by the lack of a universally accepted injury severity score. This inconsistency has been addressed by the American Association for the Surgery of Trauma who developed a liver injury scale that has allowed more standardized comparisons (Table 20.3). However, it

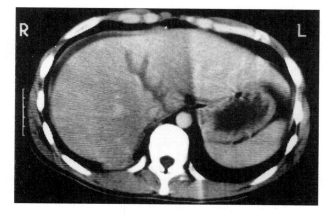

Fig. 20.2 Grade III, blunt injury to the liver. Managed successfully without intervention.

Table 20.3 Liver injury severity scale (AAST).

Grade	Type	Description of injury
I	Haematoma	Subcapsular, non-expanding, < 10% surface area
	Laceration	Capsular tear, non-bleeding, < 1 cm parenchymal depth
II	Haematoma	Subcapsular, non-expanding, 10–50% surface area; intraparenchymal, non-expanding, < 2 cm in diameter
	Laceration	Capsular tear, active bleeding, 1–3 cm parenchymal depth, < 10 cm in length
III	Haematoma	Subcapsular, > 50% surface area or expanding; ruptured subcapsular haematoma, active bleeding; intraparenchymal haematoma > 2 cm or expanding
	Laceration	> 3 cm parenchymal depth
IV	Haematoma	Ruptured intraparenchymal haematoma with active bleeding
	Laceration	Parenchymal disruption involving < 50% of hepatic lobe
V	Haematoma	Parenchymal disruption involving > 50% of hepatic lobe
	Vascular	Juxtahepatic venous injuries
VI	Vascular	Hepatic avulsion

would appear that further evaluation of these non-operative techniques are required before it is universally accepted.

Surgical management of severe life threatening hepatic injury has also continued to change. During the 1940s perihepatic packing and drainage constituted the mainstay of management. Published concerns over the introduction of infection along the drain tracts and the presence of blood and bile soaked intra-abdominal foreign material as a fine culture medium saw this approach fall into disrepute. However, the alternative management approach of radical resectional and salvage surgery for liver trauma was seen to carry an intolerable morbidity and mortality rate. Thus, with the help of improved critical care and antimicrobial agents, packing, drainage and re-operative surgery has re-emerged as the most effective treatment for severe life-threatening injury. A number of reports supported this concept, work published in 1991 from Addenbrooke's

Hospital in Cambridge, UK demonstrated a 28% mortality rate following urgent laparotomy and definitive surgery, compared to a 10% mortality following packing and re-operative surgery.

Penetrating abdominal trauma

Anatomical considerations

Although these have briefly been covered earlier in the chapter, penetrating abdominal trauma can be further classified by the site of entry.

Anterior abdomen Anterior costal margins to groin creases between anterior axillary line. *At risk*: major vessels, colon, small bowel and pancreas.

Low chest Fourth intercostal space (approximately the level of the nipple) anteriorly and seventh space (approximately the level of the inferior scapular tip) posteriorly and the

Anatomical entry site in penetrating injury		
Site	Surface boundaries	At-risk viscera and vessels
Anterior abdomen	Anterior costal margins to groin creases between anterior axillary line	Major vessels, colon, small bowel and pancreas
Low chest	Fourth intercostal space anteriorly and seventh space — approximately the level of the inferior scapular tip — posteriorly and the costal margins inferiorly	Liver, spleen, stomach, lung, and heart
Flank	Inferior scapular tip to iliac crest between anterior and posterior axillary lines	Colon, liver, spleen, and kidneys
Back	Inferior scapular tip to iliac crest between posterior axillary lines	Kidneys, pancreas and major vessels

costal margins inferiorly. *At risk*: liver, spleen, stomach, lung, and heart.

Flank   Inferior scapular tip to iliac crest between anterior and posterior axillary lines. *At risk*: colon, liver, spleen, and kidneys.

Back   Inferior scapular tip to iliac crest between posterior axillary lines. *At risk*: kidneys, pancreas and major vessels.

Although this allows accurate definition and description of entry site and identifies potential organs at risk, entry site rarely accurately predicts actual organ injury. This is particularly true of gunshot wounds where the projectile may follow a very tortuous path, ricocheting and tumbling off bony structures before exit.

Mechanisms of injury

Stab wounds

Injury tends to be dependent upon site of entry (see above), direction of the stabbing force and the length and size of the implement. Mechanisms rely simply upon slicing and tearing of the impaled tissue.

Gunshot wounds

Mechanisms of injury in gunshot wounds are more complex; they depend upon the kinetic energy stored in the projectile and on its ability to give up that energy having struck a foreign object. Furthermore, a projectile's kinetic energy is dependent upon one half its mass multiplied by its velocity squared. Thus, projectile velocity as a squared variable is critical to wounding capability and defines a classification of guns as low, medium and high velocity weapons dependent upon the muzzle velocity of < 305 m/s, $305–610$ m/s and > 610 m/s respectively. A projectile's ability to give up its energy is dependent upon its stability in flight (ruled by its centre of mass), the material from which it is made and its design. Thus, a hollow-tipped or soft, unstable bullet that gives up energy easily is significantly more destructive than a stable so-called fully jacketed bullet.

Abdominal stab wounds: three key questions
• Is there a clinical need for a laparotomy?
• If not, has the peritoneum been violated?
• If it has, does an intraperitoneal injury exist?

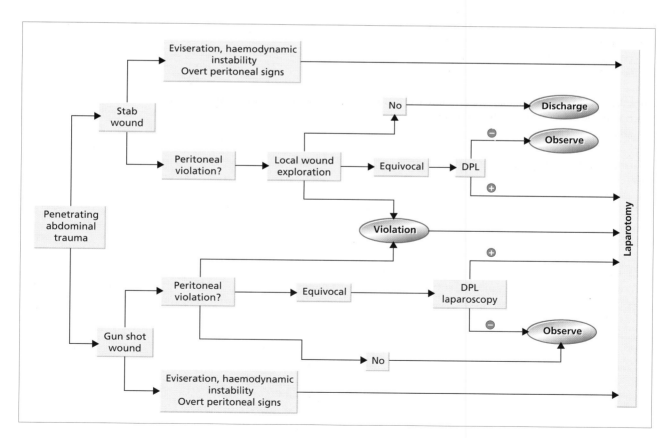

Fig. 20.3 Management algorithm for penetrating abdominal trauma (Modified, with permission from A. Read & E. E. Moore, Abdominal trauma. In: *Current Practice Of Surgery* Levine *et al.* (eds). Churchill Livingstone, Edinburgh).

Low velocity projectiles cause direct tearing and crushing injury to local tissue. Typically, only an entry wound is seen and the bullet is left *in situ*. High-velocity projectiles while also causing tearing and crushing injury to local tissue also damage tissue by cavitation. This phenomenon is caused by a rapidly expanding shock wave that follows the projectile in its path, causing crushing and tearing of tissue in a path significantly wider than the diameter of the bullet. The final extent of tissue injury produced by both these mechanisms relies upon the efficiency of energy dissipation by the projectile and the density and elasticity of the violated tissue. Liver and spleen, typically dense and inelastic are prone to more severe disruption that hollow more elastic organs such as the stomach.

Management of penetrating abdominal trauma

Anterior abdominal wall and lower chest constitute by far the most common sites of entry in penetrating trauma, and thus the next section will concentrate on these. Figure 20.3 sets out an algorithm indicating steps in the management of stab and bullet wounds.

Stab wounds

Violation of the peritoneal cavity occurs in approximately 50–70% of stab wounds to the anterior abdominal wall. Of these approximately one-half require intervention. Thus between 25 and 50% of patients with stab wounds to the anterior abdominal wall will require operation. J. A. Marx (1993) from North Carolina, USA stated that there are three fundamental questions that need addressing in an algorithmic approach to stab wounds to the anterior abdomen. (1) Is there a clinical need for operation? (2) If not has the peritoneum been violated? (3) If it has, does an intraperitoneal injury exist?

Step 1: Indications for operation

Unstable vital signs are the most likely reason for emergency intervention. It should be noted however that stab wounds to the lower chest may injure intrathoracic organs such as heart and lungs, so hypotension may not be caused by intra-abdominal blood loss. Evisceration of intraperitoneal contents carries a 60% risk of intra-abdominal injury; therefore, most units accept this as an indication to operate. Finally, patients with overt signs of peritonitis and an anterior abdominal wall stab wound should not be delayed by further diagnostic attempts, and should proceed to emergency laparotomy. In addition patients with initially benign examination but who develop signs on serial review should also proceed to laparotomy irrespective of what concurrent investigations have shown.

Step 2: Has the peritoneal cavity been violated?

Formal exploration of the abdominal wound under local anaesthetic (local wound exploration, LWE) provides the best test of peritoneal violation. A clearly negative LWE in the absence of other injury allows the patient to be discharged home following appropriate wound care. A positive or an equivocal LWE warrants further intervention or investigation.

Step 3: Is there intraperitoneal injury?

A positive LWE in most institutions is sufficient to proceed to laparotomy. However, Demetriades from South Africa pointed out that if mandatory laparotomy were performed on his patient series for anterior abdominal wall and lower chest stab wound, a 40% negative laparotomy rate would result. Confirmed peritoneal violation would result in a 28% negative laparotomy rate and positive DPL reduces this only to 28%. Clinical judgement alone, he claims, results in a negative laparotomy rate of only 7%. In view of these claims, more and more specialist institutions are refining their indications for operation in a selective approach to these patients. All patients with suspected or confirmed peritoneal violation, in the absence of unstable vital signs are subjected to DPL. Positive findings are as outlined in Table 20.2 except that if diaphragmatic injury is strongly suspected the threshold for red cell count should be reduced to 5000 RBC/ml.

More recently, if more organ specific injury is suspected, i.e. liver injury, some clinicians would advocate CT scanning. However, in a direct comparison of DPL and CT scanning in penetrating abdominal trauma, Marx and colleagues (1993) demonstrated 100% accuracy of DPL and only 25% accuracy for CT scan. Finally, laparoscopy is increasingly being used to assess intraperitoneal injury following anterior abdominal wall stabbing. It provides excellent views of the peritoneal surface of the anterior abdominal wall and equivocal peritoneal violation can be confirmed or refuted. In addition it provides excellent assessment of diaphragmatic injury.

Gunshot wounds

Gunshot wounds to the anterior abdomen result in an 80–85% peritoneal violation. If this results, intra-abdominal injury is present in between 90–95% of patients. Following a similar algorithm as that for stab wounds, the key clinical questions remain: (1) Is there a clinical need for operation? (2) If not has the peritoneum been violated? (3) If it has, does an intraperitoneal injury exist?

Indications for immediate laparotomy are the same as for stab wounds. In particular the presence of unstable vital signs and or positive signs of peritoneal irritation on physical examination. Once again serial examination is critically important as physical signs may not be apparent at the initial assessment. Indications of peritoneal violation are more difficult in gunshot wounds. LWE is less reliable because of the extent of local tissue injury. Biplanar X-rays may localize a projectile and clean entry and exit site give some indication of possible trajectory. These, however, are far from reliable signs and any suspicion of violation mandates laparotomy in most centres. Certain specialist trauma units however, would select even gunshot wounds, subjecting equivocal peritoneal violation to DPL or laparoscopy prior to laparotomy. Negative results require admission and very close clinical observation, with laparotomy at the first sign of deterioration. Most injuries missed by the DPL are to stomach and small bowel, these tend to declare themselves within 6–12 h and are associated with minimal increased morbidity and mortality. In contrast, in view of the 90–95% injury rate if peritoneal violation is confirmed, there is no place in gunshot wounding for a conservative approach and all such incidents warrant emergency laparotomy.

Penetrating injuries to the flank and back

The diagnostic dilemma of identifying serious injury following abdominal trauma is made more difficult when the 'cavity' transgressed is the retroperitoneum. Despite this difficulty, it seems clear from numerous studies that, for stab wounds to the back and flank at least, a selective policy for management is possible. Peck and Berne from USC in California reported their experience with 465 such stab wounds, entry sites being posterior to the midaxillary lines, below the tip of the scapular and above the iliac crests. Indications for laparotomy were based primarily on physical signs of peritonitis, unexplained hypotension, gastrointestinal haemorrhage and radiological evidence of genito-urinary injury. Of the 465 patients admitted only 93 (20%) underwent laparotomy. Twenty-eight had no significant injury requiring surgical repair and nine were considered negative laparotomies. Laparotomy was delayed for greater than 24 h in only two cases, yet both recovered without complication suggesting this selective approach is safe and appropriate.

Management protocols should follow the same lines as for all penetrating trauma. (1) Is there a clinical need for operation? (2) Is the wound sufficiently deep or anatomically placed such that it could potentially cause injury? (3) Is there evidence of significant organ injury?

Once again, haemodynamic instability, signs of peritonitis and gastrointestinal haemorrhage mandate emergency laparotomy. The potential for, and signs of, organ injury in penetrating injuries to the back and flank are more difficult. LWE has been advocated by some clinicians. Its usefulness being in excluding deep penetration thus allowing early discharge. Jackson and Thal reported a reliable identification of the end of the stab wound from 73 LWE allowing prompt discharge in these cases. Despite the majority of injuries

being in the retroperitoneum, DPL still plays a role in management of back and flank injury. Not surprisingly, it has had a reported false negative rate of 10% in one series, but a true positive rate of 90% suggests it may accelerate the decision to operate rather than allow early discharge. Triple contrast CT scans, with oral, intravenous and rectal contrast, have shown encouraging results, particularly in identifying colonic and genito-urinary injury.

Consequently, in a haemodynamically stable patient in whom retroperitoneal injury is suspected CT appears the investigation of choice. In patients with haematuria intravenous urography followed, if indicated, by renal angiography is seen as more specific. However, in patients in whom physical examination is unreliable because of intoxication or head injury DPL still constitutes a rapid and reliable screening procedure for significant injury.

Summary

Rapid identification of serious injury requiring intervention is the key message in this chapter. It should provide a reliable guide for inexperienced clinicians allowing safe, rapid and reliable assessment of both penetrating and blunt injury. The algorithms should be viewed as clinical guides aiding decision making rather than rigid management protocols. It is essential that clinical judgement is not clouded by over complicated diagnostic tests. The chapter pursues the therapeutic path in these patients only as far as the decision to operate, for more specific operative treatment of individual organ injuries the reader is referred to other texts.

Further reading

Catre, M.G. (1995) Diagnostic peritoneal lavage versus abdominal computed tomography in blunt abdominal trauma: a review of prospective studies. *Canadian Journal of Surgery* **38**(2) 117–122.

Larson, G.M. (1995) Laparoscopy for abdominal emergencies. *Scandinavian Journal of Gastroenterology, Supplement* **208** 62–66.

Raptopoulos, V. (1994) Abdominal trauma. Emphasis on computed tomography. *Radiologic Clinics of North America* **32**(5) 969–987.

Root, H.D., Hauser, C.W., McKinley, C.R. *et al.* (1965) Diagnostic peritoneal lavage. *Surgery* **57** 633–639.

Penetrating abdominal trauma. Emergency Medicine Clinics of North America 1993 Feb; **11**(1) 125–133.

Nonoperative management of abdominal trauma. Surgical Clinics of North America 1990 Jun; **70**(3) 677–688.

References

Davis, J.J., Cohn, I. & Nance, F.C. (1976) Diagnosis and management of blunt abdominal trauma. *Annals of Surgery* **183** 845–849.

Demetriades, D., Charalambides, D., Lakhoo, M. & Pantanowitz, D. (1991) Gun shot wound of the abdomen: role of selective conservative management. *Br J Surg* **78**(2) 220–222.

Fabian, T.C., Croce, M.A., Stewart, R.M., Pritchard, F.E., Minard, G. & Kudsk, K. (1993) A prospective analysis of diagnostic laparoscopy in trauma. *Ann Surg* 217(5) 557–564.

Ivatuary, R.R., Simon, R.J. & Stahl, W.M. (1994) Selective celiotomy for missile wounds of the abdomen based on laparoscopy. *Surg Endoscopy* 8(5) 366–369.

Jackson, G.L. & Thal, E.R. (1979) Management of stab wounds of the back. *J Trauma* 19 660–663.

Knottenbelt, J.D. (1991) Low initial hemoglobin levels in trauma patients: an important indicator of ongoing haemorrhage. *J Trauma* 31(10) 1396–1399.

Luna, G. & Dellinger, E.P. (1987) Nonoperative therapy for splenic injuries: a safe therapeutic option. *Am J Surg* 153(5) 462–468.

Marx, J.A. (1993) Penetrating abdominal trauma. *Emergency Medicine Clinics of North America* 11(1) 125–135.

McAnena, O.J., Marx, J.A. & Moore, E.E. (1991) Peritoneal lavage enzyme determinations following blunt and penetrating abdominal trauma. *J Trauma* 31(8) 1161–1164.

Peck, J.J. & Berne, T.V. (1981) Posterior abdominal stab wounds. *J Trauma* 21 298–291.

Rothlin, M.A., Naf, R. & Amgwerd, M. (1993) Ultrasound in blunt abdominal and thoracic trauma. *J Trauma* 34 488–490.

Rozycki, G.S., Ochsner, M.G., Jaffin, J.H. & Champion, H.R. (1993) Prospective evaluation of surgeons use of ultrasound in the evaluation of trauma patients. *J Trauma* 34(4) 516–526.

Strauch, G.O. (1973) Clinical findings in abdominal trauma. *Radiol Clinics N Am* 11(3) 555–560.

Thal, E.R. (1977) Evaluation of peritoneal lavage and local wound exploration in lower chest and abdominal stab wounds. *J Trauma* 17(8) 642–648.

Thal, E.R., May, R.A. & Beesinger, D. (1980) Peritoneal lavage. Its unreliability in gunshot wounds of the lower chest and abdomen. *Arch Surg* 115(4) 430–433.

Watson, C.J., Calne, R.Y., Padhani, A.R. & Dixon, A.K. (1991) Surgical restraint in the management of liver trauma. *Br J Surg* 78(9) 1071–1075.

CHAPTER 21

Head injuries

Dermot P. Byrnes

Introduction

The management of the head injured patient can be rewarding and frustrating, gratifying and disappointing, intimidating and satisfying. It carries images of death, paralysis, madness, 'missing something', litigation and, hopefully, full recovery. The immediate prospect of having to deal with an obviously severely head-injured patient is often off-putting for many who would otherwise happily and confidently care for the injured patient. The irony is that prompt, structured and confident care will often result in excellent outcome and even complete recovery in a situation which looks initially devastating.

The management of the head-injured patient is logical and has been standardized, as with other forms of major injury. Head injuries are sometimes considered to be different but this should not and need not be so. A head injury is of course any trauma to the head. A broken tooth or a penetrating eye injury are, strictly speaking, head injuries. Conventionally, however, the term is confined to damage to the scalp, skull, meninges and most importantly the brain.

When a head injury occurs certain physical events occur such as scalp laceration, fractured skull and brain-stem contusion. If the damage to the brain is sufficiently severe death will occur inevitably no matter what the management. Under such circumstances it is important that this negative

Physical events	
Primary	*Secondary*
Scalp laceration	Hypoxia
Skull fracture	Brain swelling
Brain laceration	Haematoma
Stem contusion	Infection

outcome is determined as soon as possible. With major head injuries although the patient may survive the initial impact, secondary physical events including hypoxia, brain swelling, haematoma, infection and free-radical damage create a sequence of events leading to death. It is the modification, treatment and most importantly the prevention of these secondary events which constitute proper head injury care.

Therefore, head injury management consists of providing the best possible environment for recovery if such recovery is possible.

> Management consists of providing the best possible environment for recovery—if recovery is possible.

Head injury is a common problem and approximately 150 000 people are admitted to hospital per year in the UK. A further 1 000 000 patients are seen and managed as outpatients. The vast majority recover quickly and completely, but approximately 5% can be regarded as severe and 1% will die.

The cost in social and economic terms is enormous and most are young males often at the beginning of their productive lives. Many are left either physically, intellectually or emotionally disabled. As a result, they may never work again or have the opportunity to care for their own family. In financial terms, the resources required for rescue services, medical care, rehabilitation and insurance payments are enormous. There is also a further loss to the state as the victim is no longer included as a potential tax payer. It is plain, therefore, that care must be directed not just to preservation of life but to minimizing the severity of injury and maximizing the restoration of function.

> - Up to 1 000 000 seen as outpatients in the UK per year.
> - 150 000 admitted.
> - 7500 severe (5%).
> - 1500 die (1%).

Causes

Road traffic accidents are by far the most common cause of head injuries. It is perhaps worth noting that at the depth of the 'troubles' in Northern Ireland, road traffic accident brain injuries still outnumbered those caused by civil disturbance by about 4 : 1. The victims range from the very young to the elderly and include vehicle occupants, motor and pedal cyclists and pedestrians. It should be noted that the numbers of injuries from such road traffic accidents can be greatly reduced by preventative measures such as compulsory seat belts, impact absorbing materials as well as improved highway design and drink–driving regulations.

The other major causes of head injury include domestic, industrial, sporting and criminal incidents (Fig. 21.1a–e). A common cause of head injury is falling while under the influence of alcohol. The alcohol itself may make full assessment of the patient misleading and difficult. Head injuries from assaults are common but not often severe. Sporting activities cause a small number of head injuries but they are not always from the obvious sources. This author has seen only one serious injury from boxing in some 30 years but several deaths from horse-riding accidents.

Mechanisms

Head injuries occur when the head strikes or is struck by an unyielding object (Fig. 21.1f,g). If the energy can be absorbed, dissipated or if the impact can be prolonged then no serious damage may occur. The impact of a pillow striking the head results in little injury as the force is spread and absorbed. Similarly, a well fitting crash helmet will lessen the trauma up to a point. Focal injury occurs when most of the force is imparted over a relatively small area. Local damage may be severe and even penetrating, but the patient may be surprisingly well as the rest of the brain is relatively unaffected. For example, a patient may be hemiplegic but awake and speaking normally. Such injuries are typically seen with a compound depressed skull fracture. Blunt injury, on the other hand, is caused by acceleration (Fig. 21.1h–k) or deceleration forces, as in falls or in road traffic accidents. They are often referred to as diffuse or global and the so-called diffuse axonal injury (DAI) can result. If sufficiently severe the patient may die with a surprising lack of external injury and no evidence of skull fracture. Theoretically, in such patients the whole brain is injured equally, but in fact some areas are worse than others resulting in brain swelling, contusion or even intracerebral haematoma.

Pathophysiology of head injuries

The brain is a relatively soft structure interspersed with unyielding blood vessels lying within a rigid box whose floor is rough. This explains the damage that occurs to the unrestrained car occupant in a road traffic accident. The car stops abruptly and the occupant is pitched forwards to strike the dashboard. The victim is abruptly brought to a stop and the brain pitches forward and impacts within the skull causing

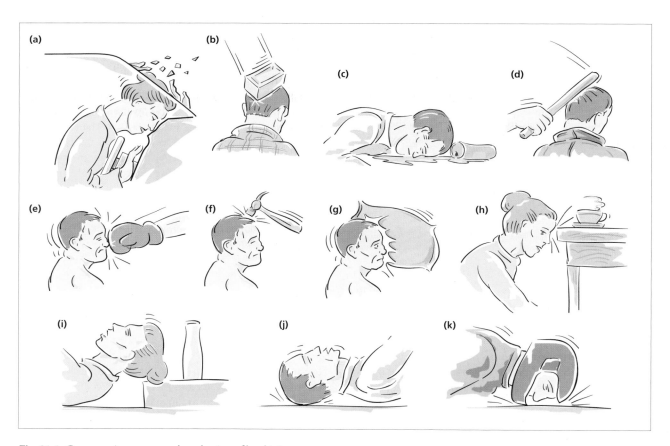

Fig. 21.1 Common sites, nature and mechanism of head injury.

damage typically to the frontal and temporal lobe (Fig. 21.2). There are also shearing forces projected towards the tentorial opening and the foramen magnum with 'cheese cutting' effects of the blood vessels, resulting in extensive and varying damage to the organ. It is perhaps surprising that the minor head injuries that occur in our daily lives such as bumping heads, playing football and minor head injuries in childhood can occur without major damage.

These events cause a so-called primary injury. Even minor forces have been shown to cause histological changes albeit of a minor nature. If repeated often enough they can cause the syndrome of 'punch drunkenness'. When these repeated minor injuries are combined with chronic alcoholism then physical and intellectual deterioration can be profound and permanent. Higher impact forces cause 'temporary brain failure', first with loss of consciousness and later with post-traumatic amnesia resulting in a postconcussional syndrome of variable duration. Greater impact again may result in physical damage to the brain such as contusions or lacerations. Blood vessels may be torn or develop spasm causing further injuries by haematoma and ischaemia.

Following this primary damage there occur within minutes, hours or even days secondary events which can be equally or even more damaging. These responses are mainly of an endogenous molecular nature and are made even more severe by the development of hypoxia. Depending on the nature of the injury a metabolic cascade may be initiated. Each cellular and catalytic event may be followed by another in a downward spiral of tissue damage and failure to improve. There may be calcium-induced damage when excitatory neurotransmitters are released locally. Similarly, during partial ischaemia and especially with reperfusion, free radicals build up causing peroxidative injury to membrane lipids. There can also be disruption of protein-bound iron and altered glutamine release. All of these interfere with cell membrane and mitochondrial function, which not only mitigates against recovery but worsens the position as swelling occurs with subsequent ischaemia, thereby initiating further damage in a vicious cycle. Modern methods of management, therefore, focus not just on oxygenation and reduction of swelling, but on attempts to address these chemical and physical events at cellular and even intracellular level. We are in an era of cerebral protection.

The concept of cerebral protection is an attempt to prevent, reduce and treat some of these secondary events following the brain insult or trauma. The requirements are complex and costly, but the potential is enormous and exciting.

Clearly, many patients who suffer head injury will also sustain other injuries. These may influence the head injury in the early stages and indeed in the subsequent days and weeks following the initial trauma. Severe blood loss from a liver laceration or the hypoxia of a tension pneumothorax will contribute to increasing cerebral damage rendering recovery from head injury less likely. Therefore, the management of head injuries also requires careful attention to other associated injury.

Immediate management

The initial care of the head-injured patient will depend on the presenting circumstances. The patient sitting in a wheelchair in an accident and emergency department with blood streaming down his face, or the child screaming because she has fallen from a swing have different needs to the unconscious trauma patient lying on a trolley or by the roadside.

In the latter case the immediate object is 'life support'. This means the maintenance or restoration of adequate oxy-

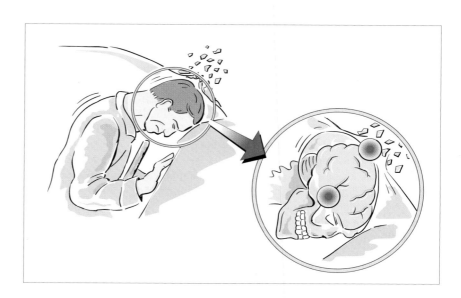

Fig. 21.2 Head impact leading to brain impact.

genation to the vital organs: the heart and the brain. This concept relates to any case of unconsciousness or life-threatening illness resulting in the familiar ABC: airway, breathing, circulation. The airway must be patent, the lungs ventilating, the heart beating, blood volume adequate and blood pressure sufficient. The initial steps, therefore, when faced with an unconscious patient from a recent head injury are to rapidly check these vital functions. Is the patient breathing through a patent airway? Is his colour normal rather than cyanosed? Is there a palpable pulse? Is he bleeding externally? An airway may be blocked by the tongue, by facial injuries or by vomited food. These must be cleared by suction and if the patient is not briskly responsive an endotracheal tube should be placed. An endotracheal tube properly placed is one of the most effective means of treating a severely affected patient. A certain expertise is required for this procedure and it may sometimes require the services of an anaesthetist. Provided the neck is not moved excessively, one need not worry about adding to a yet undiagnosed spinal injury. It is a good idea at this stage to place a support collar if the rescue personnel have not already fitted one.

During these manoeuvres a collateral history should be sought and can be done while working on the patient. How and when did the injury occur? Was the patient unconscious, driving, hypoxic or could he have had a fit or stroke?

External bleeding can be dramatic but it is normally controllable by direct pressure, and scalp bleeding is usually controlled with a support bandage. It is not necessary at this stage to be concerned about depressed skull fractures or oozing cerebral tissue as control of blood loss is the first priority.

Having established 'life support', the next steps involve the assessment of injuries and the physiological state. The former is mostly clinical and the latter involves blood tests and X-rays and in the appropriate setting these should be done simultaneously. The measurement of arterial blood gases is the first and most important blood test as the clinical estimation of adequate oxygenation is notoriously unreliable. Arterial blood gases should be measured, if time allows, prior to intubation and again following endotracheal tube placement. Blood samples should also be taken for haemoglobin, urea, electrolytes and sugar. It is also sensible to estimate the serum alcohol and carry out a relatively simple drug screen as appropriate. There is sometimes a reluctance to estimate the serum alcohol, but it is an essential part of the overall patient assessment.

The clinical examination of the patient should now proceed to decide on the severity of the head injury. An extensive neurological examination is neither needed nor indeed is it often possible at this stage. The first and by far the most important physical sign is the level of consciousness because this best reflects the brain's well-being. It is assessed by applying stimuli to the patient either by the spoken word or by inducing pain and observing the

Glasgow Coma Scale		
Eye Opening (E)	Spontaneous	4
	To speech	3
	To pain	2
	None	1
Best motor response (M)	Obeys	6
	Localizes	5
	Withdraws	4
	Abnormal flexion	3
	Extension response	2
	None	1
Verbal response (V)	Orientated	5
	Confused conversation	4
	Inappropriate words	3
	Incomprehensible sounds	2
	None	1
Coma score = E + M + V.		

From Teasdale G. and Jennett B. (1974) Assessment of coma and impaired consciousness. *Lancet* **2** 81–84.

response. This is best expressed and documented in plain English such as 'put your tongue out' or 'wriggle your toes'. The responses are measured to the Glasgow Coma Scale which is now derived from the patient's ability to open his eyes, move his limbs and speak. It is simple to use and document and can be frequently repeated. It is not a scale of head injury severity but simply scores the level of consciousness, and can be used in other conditions where the level of consciousness is affected.

Pupillary response is next assessed. In normal circumstances both pupils will constrict in response to a bright light being shone in either eye. A practical point to remember is that the environment of the casualty room may already be bright and so a strong torch may be required. If one or both pupils fail to react it does not necessarily mean there is an expanding intracranial haematoma, especially if this is noted soon after injury. It is simply the failure of a reflex mediated through the optic nerve, the mid brain and the oculomotor nerve. It could result from damage to any of these structures or damage to the eye itself. A previously blind eye, a false eye or recent use of drugs which cause pupil dilatation can cause embarrassing mistakes.

Pupils which react initially but later become non-reactive, suggests a development of an extradural haematoma. It is therefore vital that pupillary response is tested early and often. Fixed, dilated pupils are often interpreted as meaning inevitable death. However, this is not necessarily true but if they remain dilated following full and effective cardiopulmonary resuscitation the outlook is indeed very poor. Lateralizing signs are now looked for. Loss of normal symmetrical limb movement is significant. This may of course occur following a limb fracture or a brachial plexus injury but hemiparesis or hemiplegia mean that the brain is affected. It can be due to a primary injury but if it is progressive it suggests increasing ischaemia or intracranial pressure and therefore warrants rapid investigation. Accordingly, a proper documentation on admission, and at frequent intervals thereafter, is essential.

Hemiparesis from a recent cause (i.e. the head injury and not a previous stroke) will usually be accompanied by diminished reflexes even though the lesion is 'upper motor neurone' because there is loss of limb tone in the acute stage. It takes many days or even weeks for hyper-reflexia to develop. Occasionally, extreme distress will cause limb paralysis caused by hysteria but in such patients symmetrical reflexes will be present.

Thus, conscious pupillary reaction and laterality are all that are needed at this time. They should be recorded frequently and with clarity allowing a rapid and meaningful assessment and perhaps more importantly allowing a trend to be observed. The use of a 'neuro observation sheet' is now commonplace and this includes recording of blood pressure, pulse, temperature and possibly central venous pressure and intracranial pressure in the intensive care setting.

A rapid assessment for other injuries should be undertaken. Adequate air entry to the chest bilaterally is checked, obvious limb fractures should be splinted and a search made for intra-abdominal injuries. Clinical examination of the abdomen in the unconscious patient is notoriously difficult, and of course there is no patient co-operation. It is accepted that the unconscious trauma victim, especially those injured in road traffic accidents or from a fall, may require some form of invasive test for intra-abdominal bleeding. The technique of diagnostic peritoneal lavage is well established, safe and reliable and is the technique of choice in such circumstances.

Scalp injures are examined for both penetration of the skull and foreign bodies. Such wounds should be explored by the gloved finger even though skull X-rays or computerized tomography (CT) scan are planned, as it is possible to miss foreign bodies and even depressed skull fractures on X-ray. The wound should be closed as appropriate avoiding ugly scars, especially in the frontal region. Excessive bleeding from scalp wounds can be controlled by pressure dressings or sterile artery forceps until more formal closure can be carried out.

The severely injured patient should not be moved from a fully equipped, well lit, resuscitation space to a cramped dark X-ray department until at least fully resuscitated and accompanied by adequate personnel who can continue to monitor the clinical condition. Often, radiology can be performed using portable equipment in the resuscitation room because at this stage only major bony abnormalities are relevant. There is often a particular problem, however, with regard to cervical spine X-rays. Because there is a frequent association between head injury and cervical spine damage, cervical spine X-rays should be carried out routinely. The lateral cervical spine X-ray must include all seven cervical

spine vertebrae and, if normal, it eliminates most significant and unstable injuries. The X-rays are examined for evidence of fracture, malalignment and soft tissue swelling anterior to the vertebral bodies. Positive findings such as these require the addition of a neck support collar.

The next important X-ray is that of the chest. To rule out the possibility of a ruptured aorta, the examination needs to be done in the upright position to assess the mediastinal width. This may require momentarily lifting and supporting the unconscious patient. In the multiply injured patient pelvic X-rays should be carried out next.

Having completed the above examinations, the skull can now be X-rayed. It is emphasized that this is not the first X-ray in the head-injured patient. This is because skull X-rays will not reveal information which is of greater immediate importance than injuries to the cervical spine and chest. Skull X-rays are examined for evidence of fracture, foreign body and intracranial air. The views carried out are anteroposterior, lateral and the Towne's view, which is an oblique view above the horizontal directed towards the foramen magnum. A skull fracture *per se* is not life threatening but does indicate a severe injury. This can obviously result in significant complications, such as extradural haematoma or meningitis in the case of an open depressed fracture.

Fractures at the base of the skull can be difficult to diagnose radiologically. They are important however because of possibility of cerebrospinal fluid (CSF) leak caused by communication between the subarachnoid space and the outside atmosphere. A basal skull fracture may be difficult or impossible to see on a plain X-ray but CSF from the nose (CSF rhinorrhoea) or from the ears (CSF otorrhoea) makes the diagnosis. Blood from either of these orifices does not indicate a basal skull fracture. It is important to look for CSF leak and it may be necessary to sit the unconscious patient up to check this. The so-called 'battle sign', i.e. bruising behind the ear, is also thought to indicate basal skull fracture, but not necessarily CSF leak. Traditionally, CSF leak has been treated by prophylactic antibiotics; however, there is now evidence to suggest that this practice tends to promote resistant organisms and that antibiotics should be withheld until signs of meningitis become evident. This rarely develops within 24 h of injury.

The initial emergency management of the head injury patient is now complete, with resuscitation, basal neurological assessment and the relevant blood and X-ray examinations.

The next phase in the patient's management depends on the clinical state of the patient. Once resuscitation has been carried out, decisions relating to the need for admission, for a CT scan, for surgery or for consultation and/or transfer to a neurosurgical department can be made in relative calm.

There has often been confusion regarding the need for admission and transfer of head-injured patients to neurosurgical departments. Recently, guidelines have been offered which should, if properly utilized, make such decisions somewhat easier. They are, however, guidelines only and should be applied in a flexible manner. They should be displayed prominently on the wall of resuscitation rooms for easy access by junior medical and nursing staff.

Indications for skull X-ray following any form of head injury

1 Loss of consciousness or amnesia at any time.
2 Neurological symptoms, such as diplopia, vertigo, confusion or vomiting.
3 Neurological signs, such as hemiparesis, marked confusion.
4 CSF or blood from the nose or ear.
5 Suspected penetrating injury of the head.
6 Suspected alcohol or drug intoxication.

Criteria for hospital admission following recent head injury

The presence of one or more of the following:
1 Confusion or altered level of consciousness.
2 Skull fracture.
3 Neurological signs, severe headache or persistent vomiting.
4 Difficulty in assessing patient, for example due to alcohol, drugs or extremes of age.
5 Relevant medical conditions, such as epilepsy, haemophilia or diabetes.
6 Lack of appropriate adult supervision.

Criteria for consultation with a neurosurgical unit

The presence of one of the following:
1 Fracture of the skull in combination with persistent confusion, altered level of consciousness, focal neurological signs or fits.
2 Focal neurological signs or persistent confusion for more than 12 h, even in the absence of skull fracture.
3 Failure to improve from deep coma in 3 h after adequate resuscitation in patients with Glasgow Coma Scale of less than 8.
4 Suspected cerebrospinal fluid leak and/or intracranial air.
5 Depressed fracture of the skull, simple or compound.
6 Neurological deterioration.
The above are not guidelines for transfer, merely for consultation. The decision to transfer should be made jointly in discussion with the regional neurosurgical medical staff.

Indications for CT scan

There are no rigid indications for CT scan but most patients admitted to a neurosurgical department will undergo this study. The CT scan is carried out to determine whether or not intracranial haematoma exists and if so, whether the patient requires surgical evacuation. Skull fracture and loss of consciousness are the major factors associated with intracranial haematomas and any patient with this combination should have a CT scan.

In-patient management

If admission to hospital is indicated, certain procedures should now be planned. Lacerations should be sutured and other relevant injuries treated as definitively as possible. There is a temptation in the severely head-injured patient to concentrate on that injury and postpone management of other conditions until 'we see how he does'. This, however, can be quite dangerous and with modern anaesthesia and comprehensive monitoring it is quite safe to proceed to the care of other injuries such as plating of limb fractures. Of course, if the patient is unstable or moribund major surgery should not be undertaken until it is evident that the patient is likely to survive and has stabilized. Patients whose level of consciousness is below briskly responding to painful stimuli, i.e. Glasgow Coma Scale 8 or less, will usually require ventilation. Such patients will of course be nursed in the intensive care unit. If the head-injured patient is admitted to a surgical ward, the essential element of care is repeated neurological observations as previously mentioned. These observations should be initially carried out frequently (perhaps quarter-hourly) and any deterioration must be acted upon immediately. The nursing staff must be trained in such observations and appreciate the significance of deterioration. Appropriate observations allow prompt detection and treatment of complications such as extradural haematoma, progressive hypoxia, occult bleeding and fits. A pulse oximeter is also a useful tool in the monitoring of these patients. Repeat examination of arterial blood gases is also often worthwhile and may detect unsuspected hypoxia. Few drugs are indicated and steroids are not now recommended in head injuries. Mannitol should not be used without discussion with a neurosurgical unit. The role of antibiotics is controversial and may be reserved for open contaminated wounds. Similarly there is no universal agreement on prophylactic anticonvulsants and many would withhold them until fits occur. Most patients do not suffer seizures and the use of anticonvulsants can have enormous implications with regard to driving and certain occupations.

Specific types of head injury

Skull fracture

A linear skull fracture is not life threatening in itself but suggests that major force has been applied to the head.

Compound or open fractures present a risk of infection including meningitis if the dura has been breached. Depressed fractures have an even greater significance if brain laceration has occurred. The presence of cerebral tissue on the scalp near a wound does not indicate an inevitably fatal outcome, but is obviously of major significance. Such wounds need urgent debridement and the dura and the scalp should be closed where possible. This is probably best managed in a neurosurgical department. Basal skull fractures are mostly diagnosed as a result of CSF leak. These fractures often run through the petrous or spheno-ethmoid bones and suggest a compressive force which has been applied to the side of the head or face. The CSF leak or bleeding from the nose or mouth may settle following the reduction of facial fractures. Clear watery fluid issuing from the nose or ears cannot be anything but CSF and testing for sugar is pointless. Most CSF leaks will settle in 2–3 days but transfer to a neurosurgical unit will be required for spinal drainage or even craniotomy if the leak persists. It should be noted that CSF leak may start remote from the time of injury and should be kept in mind when the patient is seen at follow up clinic.

Intracranial haematoma

Haematomas can be extradural, subdural, intracerebral or a combination. Extradural haematoma classically occurs in the young patient and is usually associated with linear skull fracture which can be seen on lateral skull X-rays. Laceration by bone edges of meningeal vessels between the skull and dura causes haematoma which expands, resulting in an increase in intracranial pressure with bradycardia, hypertension and associated lateralizing signs. With an established and expanding haematoma the ipsilateral pupil will dilate and a contralateral hemiparesis develops. This may be accompanied by epilepsy and progressive deepening of the level of consciousness.

Without intervention respiratory depression occurs resulting in death. If adequate treatment is carried out speedily then complete recovery is likely to occur. Extradural haematoma is the quintessential urgent head injury and is a surgical emergency. It should be noted that the so-called lucid interval is the exception rather than the rule.

Acute subdural haematoma is usually associated with severe brain trauma and has a much worse prognosis than extradural haematoma. It is often accompanied by cerebral contusion and brain swelling and treatment is also by surgical evacuation.

Intracerebral haematoma is a blood clot within the brain substance. It may be caused by haemorrhagic contusions or pure space-occupying clot. It is simply a physical brain injury and depending on size, location and distribution it can have mild or disastrous consequences; for instance, some may rupture into the ventricular system. Occasionally surgical intervention is required but the prognosis depends on the extent of the injury rather than the size of the clot. The decision to intervene is based on intracranial pressure monitoring which usually requires neurosurgical input.

Penetrating brain wounds may be caused by low- or high-velocity missiles or stab wounds. Low-velocity by definition is below the speed of sound and includes injuries secondary to hand guns or explosions. High-velocity injuries are caused by rifles of military power. Destruction of tissue is the result of energy (E) imparted to the skull and brain according to the formula $E = \frac{1}{2}mv^2$ (where m is mass and v is velocity). Therefore, doubling the velocity of the missile quadruples the destructive power. An Armalite rifle with a muzzle velocity of 1000 m/s will have twenty-five times the force of a small revolver at 200 m/s. The injury is not just penetration, but the explosive effect of the bullet to the soft tissue of the brain. Such injuries involve massive brain destruction and are inevitably fatal and there is little point in prolonged and futile treatment. However, such decisions are best made in association with a neurosurgeon. On the other hand, penetrating wounds from knives or other sharp objects can result in apparently well patients simply because brain damage may be limited to the track of the instrument and, therefore, be relatively slight. However, if the injury involves the motor area or a venous sinus the consequences may be far greater. It should be noted in passing that surgery in the midline or behind the ears should be carried out with great care as the superior sagittal and other venous sinuses are in these areas and fatal blood loss can occur.

Indications for exploratory burr holes

There are occasions when the receiving surgeon may be obliged to perform this procedure but this is rare and should usually be done following discussion with a neurosurgeon. When faced with a rapidly deteriorating patient with probable extra or subdural haematoma, urgent treatment is of the utmost necessity. If transferring to a neurosurgical department is likely to take more than 20 min, it is preferable to proceed with exploratory burr holes. A confident diagnosis can be made in a patient who is deteriorating, is not hypoxic, has lateralizing signs and a fractured skull. In such circumstances a CT scan may not be necessary. Even if CT is available valuable time may be lost performing it. The following procedure can be undertaken. The initial burr holes are made on the side of the fracture, the dilating pupil and the side opposite the increasing weakness.

Experienced anaesthesia is required to avoid prolonged apnoea during induction as this can raise intracranial pressure still more. The head should be shaved rapidly and routine skin preparation performed. The scalp is incised approximately 7 cm above the zygoma and the temporalis

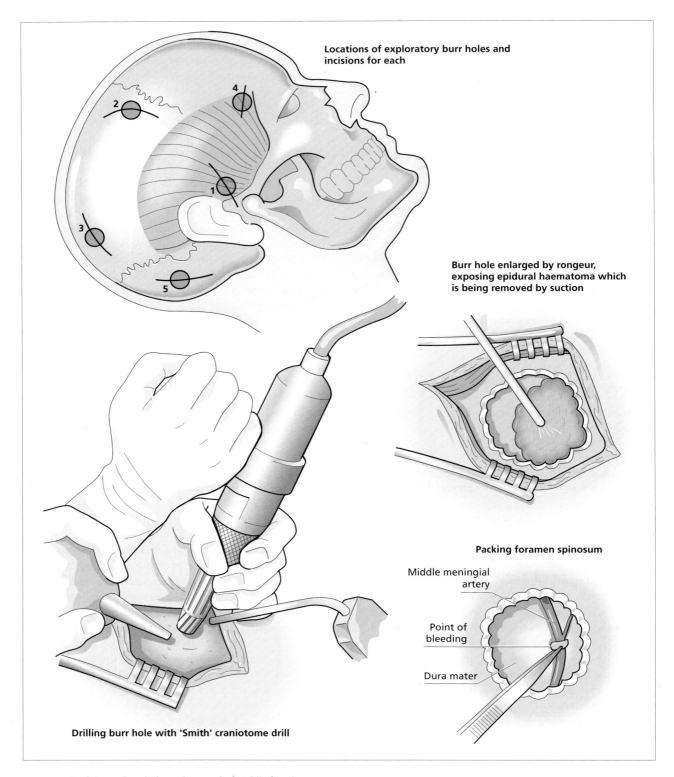

Locations of exploratory burr holes and incisions for each

Burr hole enlarged by rongeur, exposing epidural haematoma which is being removed by suction

Packing foramen spinosum

Middle meningial artery

Point of bleeding

Dura mater

Drilling burr hole with 'Smith' craniotome drill

Fig. 21.3 Exploratory burr holes and removal of middle fossa haematoma.

muscle is split vertically using coagulation diathermy to ensure haemostasis. The periosteum is scraped from the skull and a small self-retaining retractor inserted. A 16-mm perforator is set into a Hudson brace and a burr hole started. The perforator should be gently irrigated with saline and the hole inspected every few moments while sucking away the bone dust. The perforator will 'rock' when its tip has penetrated the skull, or alternatively the dura can just be glimpsed in the centre of the hole. The perforator is exchanged for the burr and the hole enlarged, again irrigating until a slight give is felt. Often the burr will jam, i.e. become difficult to rotate, on completion. If an extradural haematoma is present blood clot will be encountered. It will usually be necessary to enlarge the burr hole by nibbling the surrounding bone to expose the clot and remove it and also control the bleeding point. Evacuation of the compressing clot is the life-saving manoeuvre and, if necessary, neurosurgical assistance may be summoned to control the bleeding (Fig. 21.3). If further exposure is needed then the skin incision is enlarged to a curved flap, further burr holes are made and they are connected with a flexible saw (Fig. 21.4). Such exposure allows better access to the bleeding points. However, for the inexperienced, enlargement of the burr hole, i.e. craniectomy, is sufficient. If an extradural haematoma is not present the dura is inspected for a blue colour, suggesting subdural clot. If this is present the dura is elevated using a sharp hook, incised by a No. 11 blade, opened further and the clot washed and gently sucked out using saline. Care is exercised not to cause further bleeding from cortical blood vessels. If it does occur then these should be controlled by cautery, preferably bipolar if available. If no haematoma is found then the hole is covered and further holes made in the frontal and parietal region on the same side. The frontal is made 3 cm from the midline just behind the hairline and the parietal over the parietal eminence. If again the exposure is negative then the same exercise should be conducted on the other side.

The patient is nursed, artificially ventilated in the intensive care unit postoperatively and, if stable, transferred following discussion to a neurosurgical department.

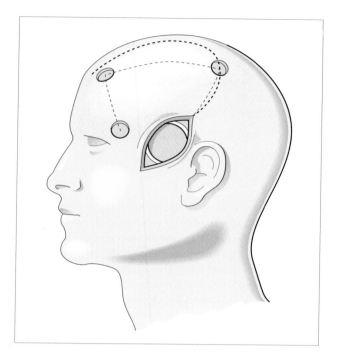

Fig. 21.4 How a small subtemporal burr hole or craniotomy is converted into a large craniotomy to facilitate complete haematoma evacuation.

Rehabilitation of the head injured

Rehabilitation of the head injured is a very topical subject. There is increasing realization that although many head-injured patients do well physically there may be major problems in relation to intellectual, emotional and even social functioning. The earlier and more effective resuscitation and early care the less these problems will supervene. It is important to involve in the first days the services of physiotherapists, occupational therapists, rehabilitation medicine, speech therapists, social workers and neuropsychologists in a bid to make recovery as complete as possible. Head injury care can be a highly rewarding experience but only with dynamic surveillance and unstinting attention to detail.

CHAPTER 22

Acute respiratory obstruction and tracheostomy

Nicholas D. Stafford & Sean R. Bennett

A tracheostomy is an opening created in the anterior wall of the trachea in order to provide an alternative airway for the patient. It can be undertaken as an emergency or as an elective procedure. An emergency tracheostomy is performed under local anaesthesia and should only be undertaken if endotracheal intubation of the patient is considered impossible. The usual indication for an elective tracheostomy is if endotracheal intubation is necessary for more than 5–7 days. The reason for this is that prolonged intubation is associated with complications which can be avoided by tracheostomy. In a patient who has an obstructing laryngeal tumour necessitating a laryngectomy it is wiser to perform a tracheostomy under local anaesthesia than to run the risk of seeding the tumour at the site of the end tracheostome by intubating the patient at the start of the laryngectomy.

> If endotracheal intubation is necessary for more than 5–7 days consider tracheostomy.

The indications for tracheostomy are numerous but can broadly be divided into three groups:

Relief of acute airways obstruction

Obviously it is essential that the clinician knows the level of the airways obstruction as there is little to be gained by performing an emergency tracheostomy above the level of obstruction. The site of the obstruction can either be above the larynx, at the level of the larynx or below the larynx. Certain pathologies may affect more than one site.

Above the larynx

Trauma

Facial fractures, e.g. Le Fort type fractures of the mid third of the face can result in airways obstruction. Soft tissue swelling from severe blunt trauma or penetrating injuries, e.g. from firearms, can also cause obstruction of the airway. In the first-aid situation a patient with an unstable middle third of face fracture can often be helped by forward manual traction on the unstable middle third fragment.

Infection

Ludwig's angina can cause marked cellulitis and oedema of the submandibular space which pushes the mobile tongue upwards and backwards and quickly progresses to airways obstruction. The patient should be commenced on a combination of penicillin and flagyl. In neglected cases a tracheostomy may then become indicated. Tonsillar hypertrophy from glandular fever may also embarrass the airway to the point where a tracheostomy is indicated. However, such a situation can often be avoided by treating the patient with a short course of high-dose steroids. A neglected quinsy can also jeopardize the airway and necessitate surgical intervention.

Foreign bodies

A foreign body above the level of the larynx is relatively unusual in that if it causes total obstruction of the airway the patient is almost always dead before they reach the hospital. A more common problem is that a fish or meat bone becomes impacted in the pharyngeal mucosa setting up local infection and a progressive cellulitis. Left untended this can lead to airways embarrassment.

Tumours

Direct encroachment on the airway by a large carcinoma of the oropharynx or hypopharynx can necessitate an emergency tracheostomy.

At the level of the larynx

Trauma

With the compulsory use of seat belts fractures of the larynx are now, fortunately, rare. However, they may still occur as the result of accidental or deliberate strangulation or as a result of martial art sports. If the airway is in jeopardy a tracheostomy should be performed under local anaesthesia and the patient's larynx then assessed under general anaesthesia by direct laryngoscopy and pharyngoscopy. Unless there is gross disruption of the architecture of the larynx with displacement of fragments of the laryngeal cartilages, surgical exploration of the larynx is rarely necessary. Another important cause of trauma resulting in airways obstruction is iatrogenic damage. Disruption of one recurrent laryngeal nerve at the time of thyroidectomy rarely precipitates such a degree of airways obstruction that a tracheostomy has to be undertaken. However, damage to both recurrent laryngeal nerves will almost always become evident on extubation of the patient. It is always prudent for the anaesthetist to assess cord movement on extubation following thyroid surgery and if both cords are immobile then significant airways obstruction in the postoperative period is very likely. In such a situation consideration should be given to re-intubating the patient and performing an elective tracheostomy at that time.

Damage to the mucosa of the larynx can occur as a consequence of smoke inhalation or the inhalation of various chemical fumes. If there is a history of such inhalation then the patient should be admitted to hospital and closely observed. Fibre-optic laryngoscopy is a valuable way of assessing the degree of oedema. Whilst a tracheostomy is rarely required it must be remembered that the effects of such chemical trauma often take several hours to reach their height.

Some patients with a relatively small (T1 or T2) carcinoma of the larynx who receive radiotherapy as a curative treatment for their tumour will develop a marked reaction to the radiotherapy. This will rarely result in acute airways embarrassment and in such a situation a tracheostomy should be performed. It is the author's view that this should be undertaken under local anaesthesia when possible. Not only will this avoid further trauma to the larynx but will also avoid the, possibly theoretical, risk of seeding of the tumour at the site of the stoma.

Laryngeal Infection

The causative organism of acute epiglottitis in children is classically *Haemophilus influenzae* type B. The symptoms and signs of acute airways obstruction are rapidly progressive and endotracheal intubation is almost always necessary. This should be undertaken by an experienced paediatric anaesthetist with an ear, nose and throat (ENT) surgeon available to perform a tracheostomy if required. Intubation is usually required for 24–48 h during which time the child is started on cerufoxime which has succeeded both chloramphenicol and ampicillin as the antibiotic of choice.

> Whilst a child with epiglottitis can almost always be intubated by the anaesthetist, the ENT surgeon should remain present.

Acute epiglottitis can also occur in adults in whom it is less likely to necessitate surgical or anaesthetic intervention. In this group, the majority of cases are caused by a variety of other bacterial agents.

Chronic perichondritis of the larynx is a well known sequela of radiotherapy. Although it is often difficult to identify a definite causative organism the patient characteristically develops airways obstruction with a sore throat and tender oedematous larynx. The onset of the symptoms can be relatively acute and if they do not settle quickly with a combination of intravenous antibiotics and steroids then a tracheostomy may become necessary. In such a situation the patient should be endoscoped following the tracheostomy as the perichondritis may herald the existence of recurrent or residual tumour within the larynx. This condition often relapses and in some instances can be controlled using long term low-dose oral antibiotics (e.g. vibramycin 50 mg o.d. for 3 months).

Very rarely, an internal laryngocele or pharyngocele may become obstructed, the mucous caught within the sac becoming infected. Such a situation will quickly give rise to gross laryngeal oedema and airways obstruction. The diagnosis can only be made with certainty following scanning of the larynx, after a tracheostomy has been performed to relieve the airways obstruction.

A viral laryngitis can be enough to precipitate respiratory obstruction particularly if the larynx is already compromised by having a unilateral vocal cord palsy or having previously undergone surgery, e.g. partial laryngectomy or radiotherapy. However, it is rare that a tracheostomy would need to be performed as the infection usually responds to steam inhalations, antibiotics and possibly steroids.

Laryngeal tuberculosis is rare but when it does occur it can mimic squamous cell carcinoma and could certainly be responsible for obstruction of the laryngeal lumen. Do not assume that all laryngeal tumours are squamous cell carcinomas: biopsy them.

Foreign bodies in the larynx

Foreign bodies in the larynx are rare. If foreign material does become impacted in the larynx this usually occurs at the level of the vocal cords. In such a situation the patient rarely gets as far as a casualty department. In the emergency situation it is best to perform Heimlich's manoeuvre in order to try and dislodge the foreign body.

Tumours

Tumours of the larynx can be neoplastic or non-neoplastic. Non-neoplastic granulomas, retention cysts or nodules can occasionally get to such a size as to precipitate airways obstruction. Such patients can usually be assessed by indirect laryngoscopy or fibre-optic laryngoscopy and it may be possible to intubate them and remove the obstructing lesion endoscopically without resorting to a tracheostomy. However, if there is any doubt about the diagnosis then the latter procedure should be undertaken and the patient then assessed by direct endoscopy, which allows biopsy of any abnormality.

The most common benign tumour affecting the larynx is the squamous papilloma. There are two types of laryngeal squamous papilloma: the juvenile type which affects children in the 0–18 age group, and the adult type which is commonly a solitary problem and can occur at any age in adulthood. The management of juvenile papillomatosis will not be discussed in detail but these children may present with airways obstruction with or without a previous history of endoscopic surgery for laryngeal papillomata. In the emergency situation each case should be treated on its own merits. If the child can be treated by laser removal of the papillomata then this should be undertaken and a tracheostomy only resorted to if a safe airway cannot be secured by any other method. One of the problems with juvenile laryngeal papillomata is that the lesions can be seeded surgically throughout the lower respiratory tract so tracheostomy will only make subsequent management of the child that much more difficult.

More than 95% of malignant tumours affecting the larynx will be squamous cell cancers. The patient usually has a history of smoking, progressive hoarseness, sore throat and possibly referred otalgia. When the tumour reaches a critical size airway compromise occurs and quickly progresses to stridor at rest. Most of the tumours that reach this stage are either stage T3 or T4 (a clinical/endoscopic/radiological staging) (Fig. 22.1). Cervical metastases may have developed on the same side as the primary tumour but this need not be the case. If a patient presents with an obstructing squamous carinoma of the larynx then the first consideration is to safely secure the airway. This can really only be achieved by performing a tracheostomy. However, it may be that the tumour itself merits a laryngectomy rather than radiotherapy as its primary treatment. In such a situation a so called emergency laryngectomy can be undertaken. Following counselling of the patient a tracheostomy and subsequent direct laryngoscopy are performed and the tumour further evaluated. Biopsies are taken and sent for frozen section. If the clinical and radiological picture is one of a T3 or T4 squamous carcinoma of the larynx then a laryngectomy can be undertaken at that time. Such management requires careful patient assessment and presurgery computerized tomography (CT) scanning of the larynx if this is feasible. The main reason for considering emergency laryngectomy is the reduction in the incidence of stomal recurrence following immediate surgery compared with those patients who undergo a tracheostomy and subsequent laryngectomy weeks later.

Obstruction below the level of the larynx

Congenital

Subglottic stenosis can be congenital or acquired. Congenital subglottic stenosis exists when a neonate or child can only be intubated with a tube two sizes smaller than the size usually required at that age. It may present coincidentally at the time of intubation, with repeated episodes of 'croup' or as an acute airways obstruction. A tracheostomy may be required and should be sited relatively low in order to leave space for a laryngotracheoplasty.

Acquired subglottic stenosis is usually the result of prolonged intubation with a cuffed tracheal tube which results in pressure necrosis and subsequent scarring of the subglottis and/or upper tracheal mucosa. Its incidence has been reduced by the introduction of low-pressure cuff tubes and a tendency to undertake a tracheostomy earlier rather than later in patients requiring long-term intubation. The stenosis may present acutely, in which case the history of recent intubation will usually alert the surgeon to the diagnosis. A tracheostomy should be undertaken below the level of the stenosis in the emergency situation. Laser therapy or dilatation of the stenosis are rarely rewarding in the long term.

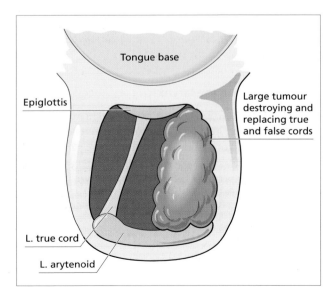

Fig. 22.1 Laryngeal tumour causing airway compromise.

> Acquired subglottic stenosis can usually be avoided by early tracheostomy and good tube care in the long-term intubated patient.

Trauma

Penetrating neck trauma can cause disruption of the trachea, which if completely severed, usually results in rapid death. When a patient has sustained a penetrating wound to the trachea it is important to consider other structures that may have been damaged at the same time. These include the major vessels in the neck, the vagus nerve, the thoracic duct and the thyroid gland. Bleeding from the latter will often cause significant haematoma formation in the neck which may lead on to airways obstruction even though the trachea itself is intact. When a haematoma develops in this area consideration will have to be given to performing a tracheostomy.

As with the larynx, the mucosa of the trachea can be damaged by toxic fumes. In a situation where there is widespread oedema of the tracheal mucosa a tracheostomy is not always the best solution as there may well be obstruction below the stoma. In such situations a preliminary bronchoscopy is often very helpful in assessing the state of the entire lower respiratory tract.

Infection

Croup

Acute laryngotracheobronchitis presents with a barking cough, hoarseness and stridor. The condition can be bacterial, but is usually viral: most commonly caused by the type I or type II parainfluenza virus. A secondary bacterial tracheitis can occur, and is characterized by ulceration of the airways mucosa.

Treatment consists of humidification, steroids and occasionally adrenaline. Intubation for a short period of time may be necessary; a tracheostomy should not be.

Foreign bodies

Foreign bodies in the trachea are almost unheard of. If a foreign body has managed to get through the glottis then it usually falls into one of the two main bronchi. At this site it can be responsible for significant bronchospasm and respiratory embarrassment but careful assessment of the airway and the patient's chest X-ray should alert the clinician to the site of the problem and rule out the need for a tracheostomy. However a bronchoscopy will be necessary.

Tumours

The most common malignant tumour affecting the trachea is a squamous cell carcinoma. Such a tumour will often have occluded more than 50% before it causes any symptoms. Again, it is very important to ascertain the precise level of the tumour. A flow volume loop performed using spirometry will allow the surgeon to avoid the embarrassing situation of performing a tracheostomy above the level of obstruction.

Protection of the tracheobronchial tree

One of the vital functions of the larynx is to prevent food, gastric secretions, saliva or blood from entering the lower airway. This airways protection is normally achieved by reflex mechanisms but under certain circumstances the larynx is rendered incompetent. In order to prevent potentially fatal aspiration from occurring either endotracheal intubation or a tracheostomy can be undertaken. The latter is preferable in a patient who is likely to require airways protection for longer than five days. The common causes of an incompetent larynx are:
- Bilateral recurrent laryngeal nerve palsies with the vocal cords both in the abducted position.
- Coma, from whatever cause, e.g. severe head injury.
- Neurological disease, e.g. Guillian–Barré syndrome, pseudobulbar or bulbar palsy, tetanus.

The necessity for a tracheostomy under these circumstances is rarely urgent and the procedure can be undertaken under controlled endotracheal intubation.

Respiratory insufficiency

Respiratory insufficiency can either be an acute problem, as in flail chest or an overwhelming chest infection, or chronic, the cause being neuromuscular weakness, or anatomical deformity of the chest which renders respiration inefficient. In either case a tracheostomy is usually undertaken after endotracheal intubation has been performed. The latter procedure should not cause any problems as there will be no lesion obstructing the upper airway. In cases of respiratory insufficiency a tracheostomy has certain advantages. These include the facilitation of positive pressure ventilation, easy access to the lungs for suction, decrease of the anatomical dead space by 10–50% and a decrease in airways resistance.

Technique of tracheostomy

Adults

In an emergency situation there will be no time for preliminary endotracheal intubation. A good light and suction are essential, as is an adequate selection of tracheostomy tubes (usually a size 7F for adult females and 8F or 9F for adult males). The patient's head is extended and the trachea palpated, the level of the cricoid cartilage being ascertained. A vertical incision in the midline of the neck is made over the trachea. The incision is carried through the subcutaneous tissues and the strap muscles separated in the midline. There is often a great deal of venous bleeding consequent upon raised intrathoracic pressure. Unless the patient has an adequate airway there is no time to arrest the bleeding until the airway is safely established. The thyroid isthmus will often overlie the trachea and if so this should be divided by sharp dissection. Although it may not be possible to fully visualize the trachea the tracheal rings will be palpable and the tracheotomy undertaken using a vertical incision through two or three rings. In order to avoid subsequent subglottic stenosis the cricoid and first tracheal ring should not be divided. A Trousseau's dilator can then be inserted into the tracheotomy and a cuffed tracheostomy tube placed into the lumen, the cuff being inflated immediately to prevent aspiration of blood. Only when the airway has been safely re-established should attention be turned to the inevitable haemorrhage most of which will be from the isthmus of the thyroid gland. The tube should be safely secured around the patient's neck with tapes. The tube flange can also be sutured to the peristomal skin.

In situations where there is time for a more methodical procedure a horizontal incision should be used midway between the suprasternal notch and the level of the cricoid cartilage (Fig. 22.2). The incision should not be too small. Once the skin and subcutaneous fat have been dissected retraction is used to expose the strap muscles. These are separated by a vertical incision in the midline and the thyroid isthmus exposed (Fig. 22.3). The tracheotomy should be performed at the level of the second to fourth tracheal rings. If the thyroid isthmus is obstructing this level of the trachea then the isthmus should be divided between clips and the ends suture ligated (Fig. 22.4). If the isthmus is not encountered then there is no value in dividing it. For the

tracheotomy a window should be excised from the anterior wall of the trachea (Fig. 22.5). This manoeuvre should be undertaken carefully, using a scalpel and toothed dissecting forceps. The inferiorly based Bjork flap whose upper margin is sutured to the skin is an unsafe alternative; if the tracheal flap becomes detached from the skin then it is quite easy for it to fall back into the trachea and obstruct the lumen. This is particularly liable to occur at the time of a tube change. In any situation where there is concern that the anatomy will not facilitate an easy subsequent tube change then it is advisable to place a stay stitch through the inferior margin of the tracheostomy and leave this available for traction should a tube change produce difficulties.

When undertaking a tracheostomy in a child, remember that the trachea is higher in the neck and is not as easy to palpate. It is a softer, smaller structure situated relatively

---

> A good light, suction and an appropriate selection of cuffed tubes are essential for an emergency tracheostomy.

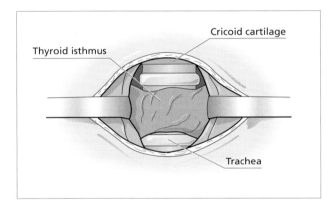

Fig. 22.3 Vertical incision in the midline exposing the thyroid isthmus.

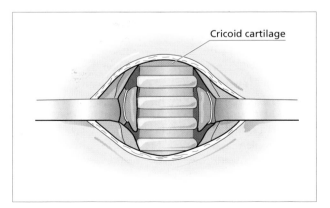

Fig. 22.4 The thyroid isthmus divided between clips.

> In adults tracheostomies remove a window of anterior tracheal wall; do not fashion a potentially lethal trap-door flap.

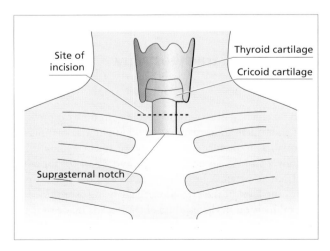

Fig. 22.2 Incision midway between the suprasternal notch and the level of the cricoid cartilage.

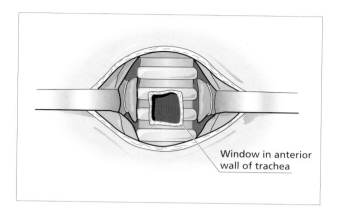

Window in anterior wall of trachea

Fig. 22.5 A window is excised from the anterior wall of the trachea.

deeper in the neck. The approach to the trachea is as described above. However, do not create a window in the trachea when performing the procedure in children. The rings are soft and flexible and can easily be retracted to allow introduction of a tube. The second, third and fourth rings should be divided vertically in the midline. An artery clip can then be used to introduce the tube tip into the lumen: Trousseau's dilators are too large to be used successfully. Cuffed tubes are not employed in children. The appropriate tube size can be calculated using the following formula:

$$\text{Tube size} = \frac{\text{age in years}}{4} + 4.5$$

If for any reason the surgeon is uncertain as to whether the structure dissected out is the trachea, the safe way to find out is to aspirate air from its lumen. No air: no tracheal lumen.

The specific complications of tracheostomy occur:

1 At the time of surgery: surgical damage to a recurrent laryngeal nerve, oesophagus or pleura can be sustained during the procedure.

2 Within 24 hours of the procedure: displacement or obstruction of the tracheostomy tube is usually evident by monitoring the patient's oximetry. Surgical emphysema in the neck can result from displacement of the tube or by trying to achieve too tight a closure of the incision around the tube (usually one suture about 1 cm from each side of the tube is enough). In patients who have sustained chronic airways obstruction their $p\text{CO}_2$ will have risen significantly. Following a tracheostomy the $p\text{CO}_2$ will drop suddenly, removing their respiratory drive and resulting in apnoea may result. This can be overcome by administering 5% CO_2 in oxygen following the procedure.

3 Late complications: these include a persistent tracheo-cutaneous fistula following extubation, stenosis of the sub-glottis or trachea and tracheal erosion with secondary haemorrhage. The latter is the most serious problem and is most likely to occur if the tube cuff is over inflated and left so for prolonged periods, or if the tube does not lie correctly in the trachea. Too big a tube will impinge on the posterior wall of the trachea: too small a tube may erode the anterior wall. The end of a tube which is too long and too curved may also cause pressure necrosis of the anterior wall of the trachea below the level of the stoma.

If a tracheostomy is undertaken for airways obstruction the patient can soon speak again by using a speaking valve attachment to the tracheostomy tube. In cases where the tube cuff has to be inflated then the tube will need to be fen-estrated to allow air to escape up into the laryngeal lumen.

When the patient no longer requires a tracheostomy the tube is removed, the wound cleaned and dressed, and an occlusive airtight dressing applied over the stoma. This will need to be redressed daily. Unless there is considerable resid-ual airways resistance above the level of the stoma closure will usually occur unassisted within 7 days. Superficial gran-ulation can be cauterised using silver nitrate.

Percutaneous dilatational tracheostomy

Tracheostomy is frequently required in the treatment of crit-ically ill patients and in patients with respiratory embar-rassment to prevent the complications associated with prolonged translaryngeal intubation. It may be performed early in an illness where long-term ventilation is anticipated or later on to aid weaning from mechanical ventilation. The general indications for percutaneous dilatational tra-cheostomy (PDT) are therefore the same as those for elective open tracheostomy. Traditionally the open procedure has been performed in the operating room using theatre time, staff and equipment. This involves transferring critically ill patients, or alternatively setting up the operating room facil-ities at the patient's bedside on the intensive care unit. Either way the open procedure is associated with certain hazards outlined above.

A PDT can be performed using one of several commer-cially available kits. The principle is either mechanical dilatation using a retractor inserted between the first and second tracheal ring (e.g. Rapi-trach) or a guide wire tech-nique in which a series of dilatations are made by using plastic dilators inserted between the first and second tracheal ring over the wire (Fig. 22.6). By gradually increasing the size of the dilators a tracheostomy tube of any size up to 9.0-mm i.d. can be inserted.

All PDT techniques can be performed at the bedside by a single operator, with minimal assistance and using the kit provided. A small skin incision is made followed by a blunt dissection so that the first and second tracheal rings can be palpated with the finger tip. The airway needs to be con-trolled by an anaesthetist managing the endotracheal tube. The endotracheal tube stays in place until the desired tra-cheostomy tube is inserted. Haemostasis is achieved by tying off visible midline veins and by the pressure exerted by the

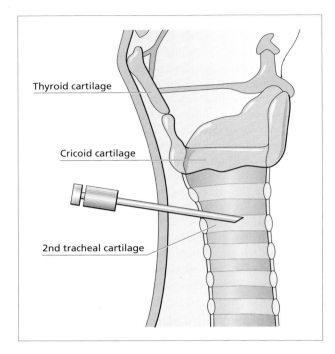

Thyroid cartilage

Cricoid cartilage

2nd tracheal cartilage

Fig. 22.6 A series of dilatations are made between the first and second tracheal rings over the wire.

tracheostomy tube in a small wound. The technique is quite different from a 'mini-trach' which is inserted through the cricothyroid membrane and is not intended for ventilation.

The technique has become widely used on intensive care units throughout Europe and the USA. There are obvious advantages of the technique which include halving of the cost, better haemostasis (it is indicated in patients with bleeding disorders), and the speed of the procedure (5–15 min being routine). However, because of the logistics a PDT can now be planned in the same way as a central line insertion. Thus the tracheostomy can play an important role in early patient management. Tracheal stenosis is less common following percutaneous dilatational tracheostomy than it is after prolonged translaryngeal intubation.

As with open tracheostomy, PDTs can be performed using local anaesthetic in the awake patient. However, it is clearly more difficult than in the anaesthetized intubated patient. Many techniques exist to provide a temporary airway whilst allowing a PDT to follow as a permanent procedure. Any attempts to use a dilatational technique as a primary emergency procedure should be performed only by those physicians with extensive experience. In the situation where an emergency tracheostomy is to be performed either in the unconscious patient, or in a patient in whom the airway has not been secured, a percutaneous tracheostomy can be performed very quickly as it is not necessary to go through all the dilatations to get up to a size 8 or 9 tracheostomy tube. In this situation, after two or three dilatations a size 5 internal diameter tracheostomy tube can be inserted: this size tube will allow inspiration and expiration in an emergency situation. This has obvious advantages over a cricoid stab which will not alleviate the problem where there is an upper airway obstruction. This is because inspiration may be achieved with high pressure through a narrow bore cannular but expiration is impossible and lung pulmonary baro trauma will result. In the slightly less critical situation, for example where a patient has failed to be intubated but can be oxygenated with a mask, then it is perfectly reasonable to proceed with a PDT tracheostomy which can be performed with the insertion of a normal size 8 or 9 internal diameter tracheostomy tube. Again, there are several aspects of the technique which may render it better than proceeding to an emergency open tracheostomy; only the kit needs to be available and it can be performed on a trolley or bed in the anaesthetic room, or wherever the patient happens to be. There is also less bleeding and the overall time from decision to insertion of the tube is shorter than with planning an open tracheostomy.

Complications

There is a learning curve so that problems such as failure to locate the trachea, malplacement of the tracheostomy tube or wire, premature extubation, haemorrhage, all occur during the physician's first few attempts.

Contra-indications

Patients in whom the trachea cannot be palpated, e.g. goitre.

CHAPTER 23

Thoracic trauma and other thoracic emergencies

William S. Walker

Thoracic trauma

Introduction

Cardiac and respiratory function are crucial to immediate survival and to the maintenance of all other body systems. Although mechanical and pharmacological circulatory and ventilatory support can be provided, it is not yet feasible to replace either function by artificial devices in the context of trauma. Approximately 60% of all cases sustaining major thoracic trauma will die instantly or before reaching hospital and thoracic trauma accounts for about 25% of all trauma-related deaths. Concurrent injury to other body regions and systems is common and associated with steeply rising mortality. For example, of those patients reaching hospital alive, overall mortality for isolated chest injury is of the order of 4–8% rising to 10–15% if one other organ system is involved and to 35% if multiple systems are involved.

Incidence

Civilian

Significant thoracic trauma (Abbreviated Injury Scale ≥ 3: Table 23.1) is present in about 10% of major trauma cases arriving at emergency units in the UK. Automotive injuries are the single greatest cause of thoracic trauma and are involved in over 80% of blunt trauma cases. Penetrating injuries, principally stab wounds, are increasing in frequency but remain relatively uncommon in UK practice at about 5–10% of all thoracic trauma although figures vary markedly between regions. In the US, however, the incidence of penetrating thoracic injury is nearly equal to road traffic related injury. This is due mainly to low (< 600 m/s) velocity gunshot wounds but knife wounds are common also. Within the civilian population blast injuries and high velocity bullet injuries are rare excepting in those areas exposed to terrorist or civil war conditions.

Military

Military experience demonstrates a remarkably consistent incidence of thoracic injury in the order of 8% of all wounds in soldiers alive at the point of reaching a major treatment facility (Table 23.2). Historical military information regarding the injury causing death probably underestimates the thorax in official accounts as bodies were labelled by non-medical personnel and in many cases damage was too severe to allow sensible categorization.

However, one medical review of 1000 World War II field corpses cited 57% with chest injuries and 40% were thought to have died from chest injury. This represents an immediate mortality rate of 70% for battlefield thoracic trauma and confirms the experience with major civilian thoracic trauma in demonstrating a very high attrition rate at the time of immediate thoracic injury. Overall somewhere between 20 and 40% of battlefield deaths are caused by thoracic injuries, probably reflecting the body surface area presented by the thorax.

The overall decline in mortality associated with severe battlefield thoracic injury (Table 23.2) is striking and reflects improved first and second line management, the development of thoracic surgical practice and the availability of antibiotics.

Philosophy of trauma management

It has been argued from US experience that death associated with trauma follows a trimodal distribution. In approximate terms, 50% of deaths occur at or immediately after injury from massive and non-survivable damage, 30% die within the first 4 h and the remaining 20% thereafter. From this observation, there has evolved the current apparatus of specialist paramedic teams and trauma centres intended to reduce particularly the middle phase deaths by expediting transfer to a receiving centre and by optimizing on site and immediate hospital care. There appears to be considerable evidence to support this hypothesis in the US but experience in the UK may not be similar. For example, one recent regional UK survey of deaths occurring within 24 h of injury (Scottish Trauma Audit Group data) found that 83% of the

Table 23.1 Synopsis of abbreviated injury scale for thorax.

Score	Injuries
x.1	Minor soft tissue injuries; simple single rib fracture.
x.2	Deep cuts >20 cm; minor soft tissue loss; lesser vessel injury with blood loss <20%; thoracic duct injury; <3 stable rib fractures; uncomplicated sternal fracture.
x.3	Great vein, pulmonary artery or subclavian artery laceration with blood loss <20%; minor vessel injury with blood loss >20%; haemopneumothorax; pulmonary contusion or laceration; incomplete bronchial injury; partial thickness oesophageal laceration; minor myocardial injury +/− tamponade; >3 rib fractures; flail chest; ruptured diaphragm.
x.4	Open 'sucking' chest wound; aortic laceration or intimal tear; great vein or pulmonary artery injury with blood loss >20%; bilateral pulmonary contusion; pulmonary laceration with blood loss >20%; bronchial rupture; bilateral 3+ rib fractures, flail chest with pulmonary contusion; oesophageal perforation.
x.5	Aortic injury with valve involvement, paraplegia or >20% blood loss; air embolism; major cardiac injury; oesophageal rupture, avulsion or chemical burn; major pulmonary air leak; tension pneumothorax; tracheobronchial avulsion; bilateral flail chest bilateral multiple rib fractures with haemothoraces.
x.6	Bilateral thoracic crush injury with massive organ damage; free aortic haemorrhage; multiple cardiac lacerations or ventricular rupture; (these are essentially unsurvivable injuries).

Adapted from 1990 Revision, Abbreviated Injury Scale, American Association for the Advancement of Automotive Medicine.

Table 23.2 Incidence and mortality of major thoracic injuries in soldiers reaching rear hospital system during war.

Conflict	Incidence† (%)	Mortality (%)
Crimean	6–8	79*
American Civil War	8	62.5*
Franco-Prussian	—	55.7
World War I	6	25–56
Spanish Civil War	12.1	—
World War II	8.2	8.3
Vietnam	—	5

* Penetrating wounds.
† Incidence does not include those who were killed in action or those who died in forward aid, collecting or clearing stations.

Surgeons Advanced Trauma Life Support (ATLS) course manual. Circumstances may occasionally dictate deviation from these strategies but such situations are rare.

Advanced Trauma Life Support in thoracic trauma

The ATLS approach represents an excellent systematic method for analysing and managing all trauma including thoracic injuries. As previously noted thoracic injuries are often encountered in a multiple injury context and the importance of a systematic approach which prioritizes therapy and which does not miss or avoid treating injuries cannot be over emphasized. Experience indicates that less than 10% of blunt thoracic trauma and only 15–30% of penetrating chest injuries will require thoracotomy. It follows therefore, firstly that the great majority of thoracic injuries are managed by the primary therapy instituted by the non-specialist and secondly that it is vital that this therapy should be correct. The ATLS approach organizes patient management through a sequence which consists of a primary injury survey, resuscitation of vital functions, a detailed secondary survey and definitive care. Complex cardiovascular, pulmonary and oesophageal injuries lie outwith the competence of a generalist and should be managed, after initial stabilization, in a regional specialty centre.

Mechanisms of thoracic injury

Structural derangement

Thoracic trauma may be divided into blunt or penetrating in aetiology. Both mechanisms can co-exist in the context of major trauma. A rib fragment may, for example, cause a severe penetrating injury from an essentially limited initial crush injury.

deaths occurred instantaneously and 3% occurred very shortly afterwards from irrecoverable injuries. Those dying with major thoracic damage did not have survivable injuries. Only 7% died within 4 h and 17% died after 4 h. In part this difference may relate to the much higher proportion of penetrating injury in the US.

The greatest opportunity to improve the mortality associated with thoracic trauma in the UK at least may, therefore, be provided by implementing measures which will reduce the incidence of this form of injury by improving primary prevention and by limiting accident damage.

Regardless of these considerations, there is no dispute, that prompt attention to the basic principles of trauma management will minimize those deaths which are avoidable following injury. In order to provide consistency with current teaching, the clinical approach described in this section is based on the strategies outlined in the American College of

Table 23.3 Relationship between zonal rib injuries and visceral injury.

Zone	Comment	Associated injuries
Upper (ribs 1–3)	Supported by the shoulder apparatus, scapulae and clavicles together with the associated large upper torso muscle groups. Fractures are indicative of major force.	Head & neck, major intrathoracic vessels, upper limb neurovascular bundle, trachea, lungs
Middle (ribs 4–9)	The majority of blunt trauma. Anterior chest compression may produce a mid-shaft break and the fractured rib end may penetrate the lung. A sideways impact may create multiple double fractures.	Pneumothorax, and/or haemothorax
		Flail segment, pulmonary contusion
Lower (ribs 10–12)	These overlie the upper abdominal viscera.	Spleen, liver, kidneys

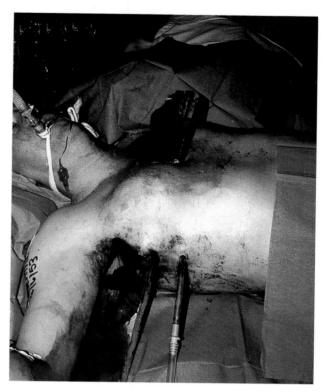

Fig. 23.1 Right chest impalement by a fence post in a young man thrown off a motorcycle. Despite the dramatic appearances he suffered no major visceral injury.

Non-penetrating injuries are frequently a combination of direct blow, crush, shear and deceleration. Specific results of these processes are discussed further in relation to the major visceral injuries. The resulting chest wall deformation is typically associated with thoracic cage fractures which may provide clues to possible underlying injuries (Table 23.3). Younger patients have a more flexible chest wall so that multiple rib fractures in this age group imply a more severe injury force than in elderly patients and gross thoracic distortion with consequent major visceral injuries may occur in young individuals without any visible fracture. Up to 15% of patients with major thoracic trauma may have no identifiable skeletal injury and the clues to injury severity may therefore be the degree and distribution of soft tissue injuries.

Penetrating injury is caused by the chest wall being pierced by a rib fragment, debris at the scene of an accident or a knife or caused by a missile such as a bullet. A penetrating wound is said to exhibit perforation when there is a traversing thoracic injury with an exit wound. The mechanism of injury in simple penetrating trauma is due to laceration of the underlying structure(s). It is remarkable how often vital structures are missed or pushed safely to the side however dramatic the initial appearances (Fig. 23.1). Low-velocity missile wounds create damage in a similar manner to direct punctures but the injuries sustained may be complicated by

deflection of the missile, flight instability, secondary fragment injury from broken bone and, very occasionally, to distant embolization of fragments entering a vascular space. The same considerations apply to high velocity missile wounds but these are further complicated by the effects of cavitation and shock wave transmission so that the injury zone will extend well wide of the apparent track. Suction caused by the cavitation effect created at the time of wounding may cause severe contamination of the wound track.

The severity of injury with missile wounds is dependant on the structures which are encountered, projectile stability and the quantity of kinetic energy absorbed. The primary determinant of missile energy is the speed and hence the distinction between high and low velocity wounds. The kinetic energy of a missile is given by:

$$\text{Kinetic energy} = \frac{\text{missile weight} \times \text{impact velocity squared}}{\text{gravity} \times 2}$$

Thus, for example, a typical 5.5 mm (3.2 g) low-velocity (245 m/s) round from a hand gun has only 6% of the kinetic energy of a similar sized 5.56 mm (3.5 g) high-velocity (972 m/s) round from an assault rifle. The energy released, however, will vary enormously depending whether the bullet traverses the chest or is retained when all the energy is dissipated in the thorax.

Physiological sequelae

Cardiac and respiratory function are impaired following thoracic trauma. A variety of negative and often simultaneous secondary pathophysiological processes occur which may cause a critical situation to degenerate into a downward and rapidly fatal spiral (Fig. 23.2).

Cardiac contusion is common and almost certainly underestimated in survivors of major thoracic trauma. Primary decrease in left ventricular function will accompany myocardial bruising and severe dysfunction will follow coronary damage, valvular insufficiency or pericardial tamponade. Low cardiac output results in tissue hypoxia with secondary metabolic acidosis which causes further deterioration in myocardial contractility. This cycle may be aggravated by circulatory volume depletion from haemorrhage which exacerbates metabolic acidosis by causing peripheral vasoconstriction and reducing atrial return. Over-zealous transfusion of crystalloid infusions may produce haemodilution thereby further reducing tissue oxygen delivery and the use of cold volume replacement fluids produces myocardial cooling and depression of cardiac function. Massive blood transfusion may contribute to acidosis and hyperkalaemia.

Pulmonary function is compromised by loss of alveolar/capillary exchange area. This may in a simple instance be a result of lung collapse from pneumothorax but is often caused by pulmonary contusion which is also generally underestimated. The resulting ventilation–perfusion (V–Q) mismatch may then cause a precipitous fall in arterial Po_2. Poor respiratory effort results in CO_2 retention and hypercarbia. Some hours following trauma adult respiratory distress syndrome (ARDS) will develop in a small percentage of cases with consequent respiratory failure.

Examples of negative interaction between cardiac and respiratory function are common. Left ventricular failure will cause pulmonary oedema with impaired gas exchange whilst the hypoxaemia associated with pulmonary dysfunction is detrimental to cardiac function. Tension pneumothorax causing mediastinal distortion and reversal of thoracic–abdominal pressure relationships embarrasses cardiac return and respiratory function simultaneously.

Immediate management of thoracic trauma

Primary survey

This survey aims to identify and treat those thoracic trauma related injuries which are imminently life threatening and therefore require immediate management. An ABC approach simplifies this process.

A: Airway management

As with all trauma it is essential to ensure a patent airway. This may require:
- Removal of oral debris including teeth or bone fragments.
- Endotracheal intubation.
- Cricothyroidotomy or tracheostomy.

Supplementary oxygen by mask is given and the patient's respiratory pattern assessed. Cyanosis is not a reliable indicator of hypoxia as haemorrhage can cause the haemoglobin to fall below the 60 g/L said to be required to demonstrate this sign. More typically, peripheral vasoconstriction, poor lighting and dirt may all make this assessment unreliable. Ear

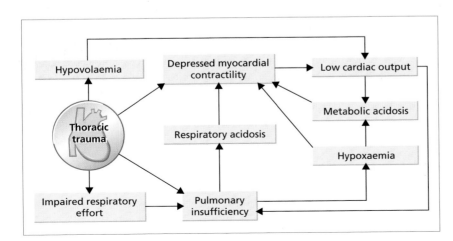

Fig. 23.2 Pathophysiological interactions following major thoracic trauma.

Initial management of thoracic trauma

Thoracic trauma is frequently associated with other serious injuries.
- Administer oxygen and establish large-bore peripheral intravenous line.
- Perform instant scan assessment of whole patient.
- Undertake primary survey — immediate life-saving corrective action.
- Undertake secondary survey — exclude and treat other life-threatening and serious injuries.
- Transfer to definitive care according to dominant pathology and life support requirement.

lobe tissue oximetry may help but the judgement may ultimately rest on clinical indicators of apparent adequacy of respiration: conscious level, vocalization, tidal excursion and chest movement. Endotracheal intubation is required when it is clear that the patient cannot adequately ventilate or protect the airway. This may be hazardous in the context of multiple trauma. The possibility of cervical spine injury must be considered and the neck handled appropriately carefully and splinted. Patients with marked cervical surgical emphysema and upper airway difficulties, often with stridor, may have tracheal disruption. Intubation should be undertaken with extreme caution under these circumstances and with bronchoscopic guidance as it is possible to completely disrupt a partially separated trachea. Emergency tracheostomy is a difficult procedure. Adequate and rapid airway access including the insertion of a small size tracheostomy tube (6 or 7 mm) can be achieved through a cricothyroidotomy approach unless laryngeal injury is present.

B: Breathing

Adequate respiration is assessed by observing the chest wall for defects and flail segments, percussing for hyper-resonance or dullness, palpating for defects and listening for air entry.

Conditions to be excluded are:
- Tension pneumothorax
- Open pneumothorax
- Haemothorax
- Flail chest.

Tension pneumothorax

Tension pneumothorax occurs when air enters the pleural cavity through a one way valve mechanism. A parenchymal defect which is occluded in inspiration by a flap of lung tissue sucked into the hole by negative airway pressure may open when the airway pressure is increased in expiration particularly in forced or grunting respiration. The effect is to create an expanding pneumothorax with complete collapse of the ipsilateral lung, deviation of the mediastinum to the opposite side and, consequently, compression of the contro-lateral lung (Fig. 23.3). The characteristic clinical findings include:
- Tracheal deviation
- Hyper-resonance to percussion over the pneumothorax
- Absent breath sounds on the affected side.

This situation severely impairs respiratory function and compromises venous return to the heart by distorting the great veins. It, therefore, requires immediate management on clinical diagnosis without waiting for a chest film. This is not equivalent to inserting a chest drain simply on suspicion. Insertion of a large bore needle into the chest on the affected side will decompress the pleural cavity, confirm the diagnosis and convert the pneumothorax into a simple pneumothorax which can then be drained.

Open pneumothorax

A defect in the chest wall allowing free communication with the external atmosphere will result in a pneumothorax as the normally negative intrapleural pressure equalizes with atmospheric pressure. If the defect is more than 2 cm in diameter air will preferentially pass through the chest wall opening on respiration rather than through the trachea thereby severely impairing respiration. Immediate management requires occlusion of the hole to cover the 'sucking' wound. If one edge of the cover is left untaped this will allow air under pressure to escape and prevent a tension pneumothorax developing. An intercostal drain should then be

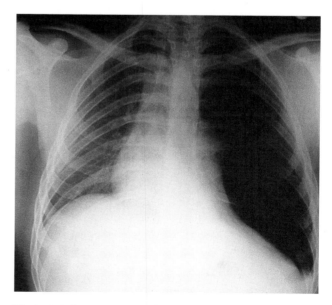

Fig. 23.3 Left tension pneumothorax: this major life threatening injury resulted from a surgically trivial knife wound to the lateral chest.

inserted and surgical repair of the chest wall subsequently performed.

Massive haemothorax

This is usually unilateral and associated with penetrating injury. The diagnosis is suggested by the combination of:

- Shock
- Dullness to percussion
- Absent or greatly diminished breath sounds.

The neck veins may be misleading as mediastinal distortion can cause fullness rather than the empty appearance which would normally be anticipated. The patient suffers from a combination of hypovolaemia with reduced cardiac output and ventilatory impairment from the space occupying effect of the intrapleural blood.

Needle aspiration should confirm intrapleural blood. Initial management is by insertion of a large calibre intercostal drain (> 32 FG), volume replacement and observation.

Flail chest

This condition occurs when a portion of chest wall is isolated from the remaining chest wall by fractures. Typically, several mid-thorax (4–9) ribs have proximal and distal fractures but a free floating sternal segment may be created by fractures of all the anterior cartilages. Proximal and distal rib fractures may be easily identified (Fig. 23.4) but some or all of the fractures may occur through cartilage and be invisible on X-ray. Flail chest must therefore be identified clinically by observation of paradoxical chest wall motion with respiration.

This greatly impairs ventilatory efficiency (Fig. 23.5). As a first aid manoeuvre, a heavy fluid bag or sand bag placed against a lateral flail portion may help improve ventilation. In many cases respiratory function declines with CO_2 retention and progressive hypoxia develops because of the collapse and contusion of underlying lung so that intubation and positive pressure ventilation are necessary. Myocardial contusion may accompany a flail sternum.

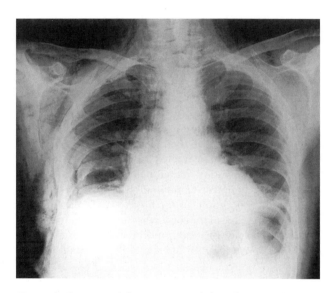

Fig. 23.4 Chest X-ray following major right lateral impact. There is gross mediastinal and subcutaneous emphysema associated with an obviously indented section of chest wall.

C: Circulation

Circulatory failure may result from primary cardiac failure, tamponade or inadequate venous return to the heart secondary to hypovolaemia or mediastinal shift.

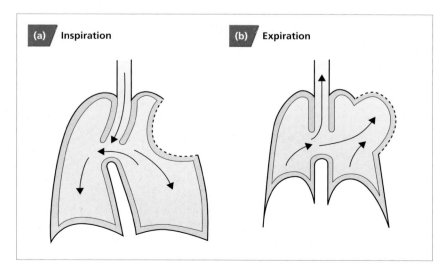

Fig. 23.5 Diagrammatic representation of flail segment. The segment is drawn in and the mediastinum swings towards the opposite side in inspiration (a). The process reverses on expiration (b). Circulatory embarrassment and ineffective ventilation result.

> ### Cardiac tamponade
>
> The diagnosis of cardiac tamponade requires a high index of suspicion and may be very difficult in the multiply injured patient with deteriorating vital signs. It is helpful to remember that:
> - The diagnosis is most likely with sharp injury in the cardiac area.
> - Low BP, raised JVP, narrow pulse pressure and tachycardia are ususal.
> - Excessive transfusion may confuse the issue or produce an iatrogenic elevation in venous pressure.
> - Needle aspiration is unlikely to be successful due to clot formation.
> - In the absence of specialist help, subxyphoid exploration offers the safest option.

Volume replacement

Replacement of blood volume by a plasma expander or blood is clearly required in all major trauma situations. The fluid should be warm and infusion monitored by clinical result and effect on venous pressure. In the initial phase of resuscitation large-calibre venous access cannulae are required. Central venous catheterization is not an immediate priority but is a particularly useful second phase measure in thoracic trauma cases as central venous pressure can be monitored and drugs which may be required to optimize failing cardiac function (inotropic agents, antidysrhythmic agents, potassium, calcium, magnesium and sodium bicarbonate) are better administered centrally. Cardiac failure may follow severe myocardial contusion but in the immediate assessment it is important to exclude cardiac tamponade as this requires immediate treatment.

Cardiac tamponade

The pericardial sac is not acutely distensible. Intrapericardial bleeding from major cardiac injury is rapidly fatal. Lesser leaks may bleed sufficiently to cause a pericardial collection and the hole may then self seal. Cardiac tamponade occurs when the accumulation of intrapericardial blood causes compression of the cardiac chambers and of the great veins in their intrapericardial portions. The result is impaired cardiac filling in diastole with consequently reduced stroke volume and reduced cardiac output. There are several immediate compensatory mechanisms which develop:
- *Elevated central venous pressure*: this improves diastolic filling against the raised intrapericardial pressure.
- *Tachycardia*: the heart rate increases in order to improve cardiac output when the stroke volume is falling in accordance with the relationship: cardiac output = stroke volume × rate.
- *Vasoconstriction*: peripheral vascular resistance rises in order to support the blood pressure in accordance with the relationship: blood pressure = cardiac output × peripheral vascular resistance.

Tamponade is most likely to be encountered in the context of penetrating trauma but may occur in association with blunt trauma due to secondary penetration by a rib fragment or due to avulsion of a great vein. Occasionally, tamponade may be an iatrogenic event resulting from cardiac massage, attempted pericardial aspiration or injudicious chest drain insertion.

Clinically, the diagnosis may be an obvious possibility in, for example, a knife wound to the anterior left chest or part of the differential explanation for low blood pressure in a multiple blunt trauma case. The diagnosis is suggested by:
- Elevated venous pressure
- Muffled heart sounds
- Low blood pressure
- Tachycardia.

Tension pneumothorax is a major differential but should be relatively easy to exclude by the relevant clinical features.

Clinical signs may be unreliable or difficult to elicit. Venous pressure can be low if concurrent haemorrhage exists and the heart sounds may be difficult to hear in a noisy resuscitation room. In doubtful cases administration of an intravenous fluid bolus may expose central venous pressure elevation and will help maintain blood pressure.

In the critically injured patient where resuscitation is failing and a high index of suspicion for tamponade exists, pericardial aspiration should be performed without delay. If the leakage has stopped aspiration will substantially improve circulatory haemodynamics provided the pericardial content is fluid. Usually, however, a substantial portion is clotted. If only clot is accessible to the needle the investigation may apparently be negative and have no effect. In such instances, against a desperate background, emergency thoracotomy may be required. A negative tap cannot exclude the diagnosis and an apparently successful tap still requires follow on thoracotomy to repair cardiac damage and to remove clot.

Thoracic bleeding

Thoracotomy is not required in over 85% of major thoracic trauma cases. Observation with appropriate blood volume replacement is indicated initially after chest drain insertion. Immediate drainage of >1500 ml is associated with a high probability that early thoracotomy will be necessary as is continued drainage >200 ml/h. Penetrating injuries medial to the nipple lines or scapulae are more likely to require thoracotomy in view of the risk of damage to the underlying heart, great vessels, hilar structures and mammary arteries. Pulmonary parenchymal bleeding usually settles. Bleeding from stab wounds to the lateral

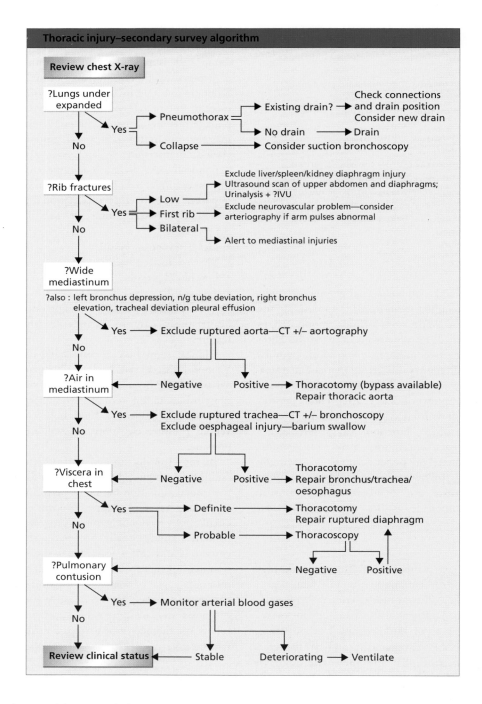

Thoracic injury–secondary survey algorithm

chest is frequently caused by injured chest wall vessels. In the case of bullet wounds, it is important to remember that the indication for surgery is clinical need not forensic convenience.

Secondary survey

During this process further physical examination and such investigations as are feasible are combined to exclude other serious and potentially life-threatening injuries.

Initial assessment of the chest X-ray

Review of the chest X-ray may suggest potential injuries, as noted in Table 23.3. Special attention should be given to fractures of the 9–11th ribs in view of the possibility of associated renal or splenic injury. It is sensible to test urine for blood and examine the spleen by ultrasound in these circumstances. Fractures involving the first ribs may suggest the possibility of neurovascular injury. Fractures involving ribs on both sides of the chest, particularly when low on one side and high on the other may indicate

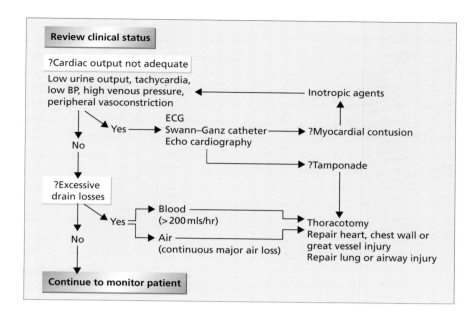

a more serious injury as they imply a trans mediastinal force. In these patients the risk of aortic and main airway injury is increased. Other features to be excluded are: haemo- or pneumothorax, subcutaneous or mediastinal emphysema, a widened mediastinum and intrathoracic bowel.

Potentially lethal injuries to be considered during this phase of assessment are:

- Pulmonary contusion
- Myocardial contusion
- Aortic disruption
- Diaphragmatic rupture
- Tracheobronchial disruption
- Oesophageal injury.

Pulmonary contusion

Contused areas of lung contain alveoli which are filled with extravasated blood and fluid. These changes prevent gas exchange and can allow shunting of desaturated blood through the damaged areas. If extensive contusions are present, ventilation is difficult due to impaired compliance and inefficient gas exchange with consequent respiratory failure.

Some degree of pulmonary contusion is associated with all rib injuries. Computerized tomography (CT) scan is more sensitive than plain chest X-ray but in severe cases pulmonary mottling may appear on the plain chest X-ray within a few hours of injury and progressive changes will develop over 24 to 48 hours.

Respiratory rate, tissue oximetry and blood gasses should be monitored. Declining respiratory function will require ventilation.

Resuscitation fluids

Thoracic trauma often involves myocardial and pulmonary contusion and, frequently, an associated coagulation disorder.

Transfusion policy should comprise:

- Warm fluid.
- Limited (<2 L) crystalloid infusion.
- Use of high oncotic pressure fluids: plasma, blood, plasma substitutes (but not Dextrans).
- CVP and/or pulmonary artery wedge pressure monitoring (after initial resuscitation).

Myocardial contusion

Severe precordial bruising, sternal fracture (Fig. 23.6) or evidence of major chest compression (Fig. 23.7) raise the possibility of myocardial contusion. The clinical features are similar to those of right ventricular infarction.

Clinical indicators include:

- Hypotension
- Tachycardia
- Irregularities of rhythm
- Elevation of venous pressure from right ventricular dysfunction.

The electrocardiograph (ECG) may demonstrate:

- Atrial fibrillation
- ST segment elevation
- Bundle branch block (usually right).

Echocardiography may show impaired anterior wall motion.

Suspicion of this condition is an indication for continuous ECG monitoring in view of the risk of dysrhythmias. These and cardiac failure are treated with standard medica-

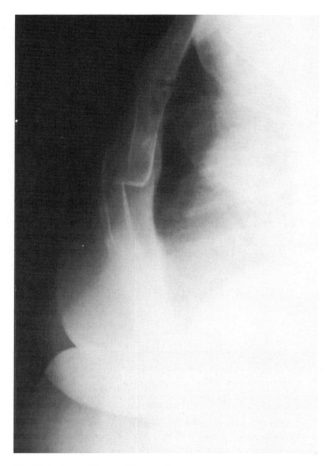

Fig. 23.6 Lateral X-ray of fractured sternum.

Clinical features. Survival to reach medical intervention requires that the rupture is contained by a combination of adventitia, haematoma and paraaortic fat and mediastinal pleura. Initial blood loss is therefore modest at about 0.5 to 1 L and hypotension associated with this injury responds well to fluid replacement. A small proportion of patients will have lower limb paralysis from spinal cord ischaemia at first presentation. The diagnosis is suggested by:

- The circumstances
    deceleration injury
    interscapular pain
    reduced left arm BP.
- Evidence of major thoracic trauma
    upper rib fractures
    transthoracic injuries, e.g. upper left/lower right rib fractures.
- Evidence of contained mediastinal bleeding
    widened mediastinum
    pleural cap (blood tracking round to the apical extra pleural space from mediastinum)
    depression of the left bronchus
    deviation of the nasogastric tube to the right
    elevation and rightward shift of right main bronchus
    loss of the separate aortic and pulmonary artery (PA) knuckles
    tracheal deviation to the left.
- Evidence of intrapleural bleeding: haemothorax.

This injury is one which should be suspected in every major thoracic trauma case. The radiographic features are variably present and may not be discernible at all particularly in the context of a multiply injured patient with poor inspiration and anteroposterior (AP) chest films (Fig. 23.10).

tions very much as with a myocardial infarction. A pulmonary artery catheter may be helpful to allow assessment of cardiac output, left atrial filling pressure and left and right ventricular stroke work indices. Serial creatine kinase (MB) enzyme estimations are elevated.

Aortic rupture
This occurs at the aortic isthmus just distal to the ligamentum arteriosum in about 85% of cases. It may rarely occur at the aortic root or in the ascending aorta. The injury usually results from upwards displacement of the lower sternum and costal margin. The heart and aortic arch are pushed upwards thereby hyper-extending the aorta at the isthmus causing an anterior tearing force (Fig. 23.8). Less commonly, a lateral impact to the left upper thorax and shoulder with fracture/dislocation of both first ribs may cause a lateral shear tear as the arch is avulsed sideways from the descending aorta (Fig. 23.9).

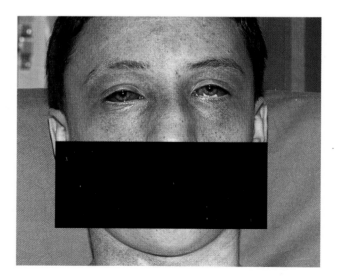

Fig. 23.7 The severity of the crushed chest injury sustained by this young man is revealed by gross petechial cutaneous and conjunctival haemorrhage.

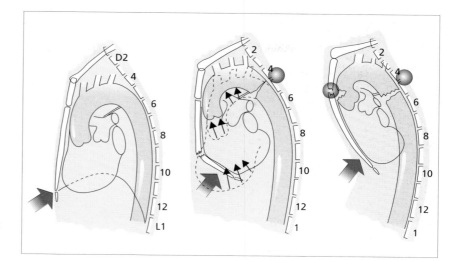

Fig. 23.8 More usual mechanism for aortic rupture: the sternum and heart are displaced backwards and upwards relative to the descending aorta. This is often a deceleration type injury where the sternum is abruptly stopped by impacting on a solid object whilst the remainder of the thorax is driven on by inertia.

Investigation. On suspicion the diagnosis is best confirmed or refuted by arch aortogram (Fig. 23.11). It is stated that, given liberal indications, 10% of these will be positive. Angiographic discrimination may be improved by digital subtraction techniques (Fig. 23.12). Contrast CT offers an alternate but less accurate screening technique. It is probably adequate if it does not show mediastinal haematoma but if it does, angiography is the better option. Transoesophageal echocardiography is potentially helpful but not sufficient to eliminate the diagnosis.

Management. Immediate treatment by a cardiothoracic surgical team is required to repair the damaged area usually by replacing the ruptured segment with a short piece of prosthetic graft (Fig. 23.13). This is usually performed with the aid of an aorto–aortic shunt or partial left heart bypass in order to minimize spinal cord ischaemia during the period when the aortic is cross-clamped. The operative mortality is about 5% and paraplegia rate similar. Missed ruptures usually burst during the first few hours in hospital but will occasionally heal as a false aneurysm and require repair in later years.

Great vessel injury

Injury to the subclavian vessels and brachial plexus may follow fractures of the first rib. Decreased pulse pressure and perfusion may be evident in the affected limb with soft tissue swelling at the supraclavicular area. There may be sensorimotor abnormalities. Extra pleural apical opacification may be apparent on the chest film.

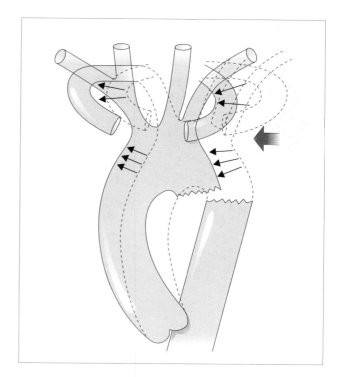

Fig. 23.9 Less common mechanism for aortic rupture caused by right lateral displacement of the shoulder girdle; e.g. landing on the left shoulder after being thrown off a motorcycle.

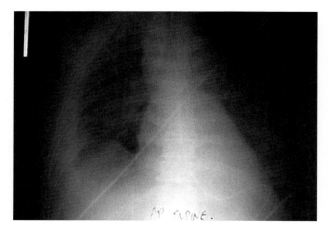

Fig. 23.10 AP chest X-ray obtained in the emergency room. As always the quality is not good but the widened upper mediastinum is obvious. The haematoma extends extrapleurally round the right chest where there are upper rib fractures. There is loss of separate aortic and pulmonary artery outlines. A pneumothorax is present on the left which is seen best at the base.

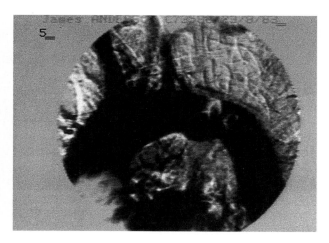

Fig. 23.12 Digital subtraction image of aortic transection. In this case a transverse partial 'crack' is clearly seen.

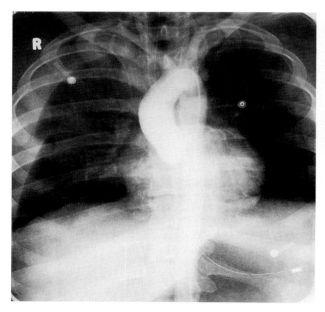

Fig. 23.11 Arch aortogram of aortic transection. Note the difference in contrast density in the upper thoracic aorta. This is the appearance when the aortic integrity is maintained by an adventitial tube after complete disruption of the intima and media.

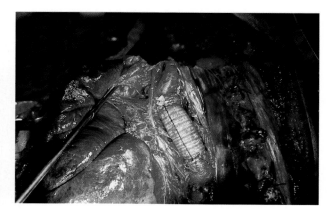

Fig. 23.13 Prosthetic repair of ruptured aorta. The left subclavian arises at the upper end of the graft.

Ruptured diaphragm

This injury results from acutely raised intra-abdominal pressure which causes the diaphragm to burst. There may be associated lower rib fractures with spleen and liver injury. The liver usually prevents herniation of the abdominal viscera through a tear in the right diaphragm so that on initial presentation the diagnosis is more frequently noted on the left.

Clinical features. The clinical findings suggesting this diagnosis are:
• Dyspnoea
• Bowel sounds in the chest
• Recovery of peritoneal lavage fluid through an intercostal drain.
Radiological findings include:
• Blurred and elevated left diaphragm

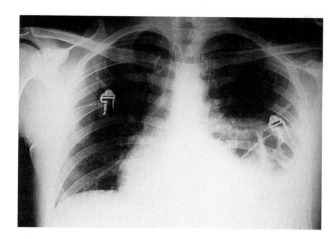

Fig. 23.14 Chest X-ray showing obscured left diaphragm with bowel shadowing in the lower left chest.

- Nasogastric tube in the left chest
- Obvious intrathoracic bowel (Fig. 23.14).

Further investigations. As follows:
- Ultrasound examination of an apparently elevated diaphragm may help differentiate between eventration of the diaphragm and rupture.
- In dubious cases thoracoscopy prior to surgery can help identify a diaphragmatic defect.

Management. Repair may be undertaken by thoracotomy (Fig. 23.15a, b, c) using multiple sutures to repair the diaphragm. Right diaphragmatic rupture may not be evident until laparotomy is undertaken for abdominal pathology. Diaphragmatic repair through the abdomen is feasible for localized defects but not for major disruption.

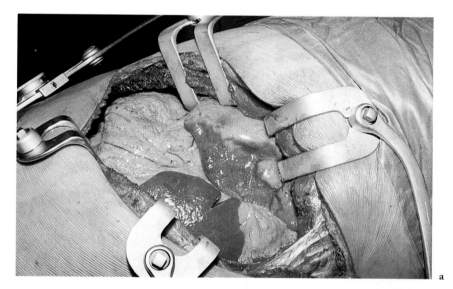

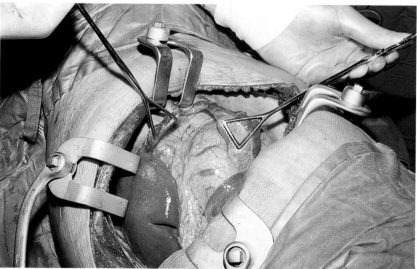

Fig. 23.15 (a) Initial appearance on opening the left chest in the above case: spleen, omentum and gut were present in the chest. (b) Abdominal contents reduced and margins of extensive diaphragmatic defect identified. (c) Repair of left diaphragm. *Continued on p. 266.*

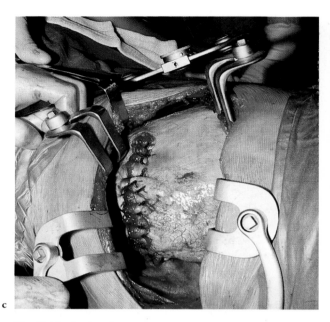

c

Fig. 23.15 *Continued.*

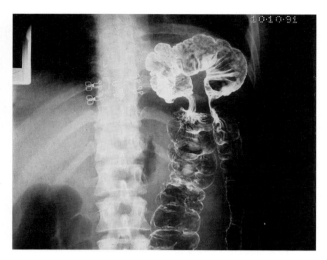

Fig. 23.16 Barium study showing colon herniated into the left chest through a previously missed left diaphragmatic defect.

There may be associated injuries to the spleen and other intra-abdominal organs. In some individuals the diagnosis is missed and they may present years later as an emergency with abdominal symptoms, often lower abdominal pain, referable to colon herniation into the chest (Fig. 23.16).

Table 23.4 Location of tracheobronchial injuries.

Site of airway injury	Frequency (%)
Trachea	15
Main bronchi	79
Lobar bronchi	6

Tracheobronchial injury

Tracheobronchial injuries collectively are rare at about 4% of all thoracic injuries (Table 23.4). They are more likely in younger patients. Major airway disruption is associated with very high energy accidents and approximately 75% of these cases die at the scene of injury.

Tracheal injury may be associated with injury to the surrounding structures, i.e. the great vessels and/or oesophagus and with other high energy injuries including aortic rupture and diaphragmatic rupture. Tracheal injury should not, therefore, be thought of as a singular phenomenon but rather as part of a group injury until proven otherwise.

Diagnosis may be difficult. While direct puncture or disruption of the airway in the neck may be immediately evident from froth at the wound site or swelling with airway obstruction, a degree of stridor and cervical emphysema may be the only clues to major intrathoracic tracheal injury.

Larynx and cervical trachea.

These injuries often result from a direct blow: such as from falling against the handle bars of a bicycle. Cervical tracheal rupture may also result from a whiplash mechanism and should be considered in the context of a patient with a severe whiplash injury.

Continuity is often maintained only by the membranous trachea so that forceful endotracheal intubation carries the serious risk of completing the tear or causing the tube to deviate into the mediastinum.

Hoarseness, subcutaneous emphysema and palpable crepitus of the laryngeal cartilages may indicate the diagnosis. Airway obstruction from laryngeal injury may require tracheostomy if endotracheal intubation is impossible. Tracheostomy is the correct method of surgical access as cricothyroidostomy would be performed through areas of collapsed architecture and may compromise laryngeal healing.

Thoracic trachea.

This injury occurs in penetrating or severe crush injuries. Laceration of the membranous tracheal wall by an endotracheal tube may also complicate resuscitation. The possibility of tracheal injury may be suggested by the nature of the injury; appropriate entry and depth of penetration or high energy impact.

Clinical features vary widely with some patients having almost no symptoms or signs. More usually, the presenting features include:

• Laboured breathing
• Stridor

- Haemoptysis
- Marked surgical emphysema at the base of the neck.
  Radiological features include:
- Transthoracic injuries
- Mediastinal emphysema
- Pneumothorax
- Possible discontinuity in air tracheogram
- CT may show loss of airway alignment.

The diagnosis is confirmed by endoscopy which should precede intubation in patients with suspected tracheobronchial injury.

Bronchus. Bronchial rupture in closed chest trauma is caused by sudden transverse widening of the thorax during a frontal crush injury. This causes lateral displacement of the lungs and severs one or other main bronchus usually within 3 cm of the carina. The right side is more frequently involved. Perhaps because the mechanism of injury requires a very supple chest cage, over two-thirds of bronchial ruptures are seen in children, adolescents or young adults. The aetiology of this injury differs from tracheal rupture and bronchial rupture is rarely found in association with tracheal injury. In 15% of cases a first rib fracture is also present. Only about 40% of bronchial ruptures are diagnosed in the first 48 hours. The diagnosis may be discovered later in the hospital admission during bronchoscopy for complete pulmonary collapse when bronchial obstruction develops. Years later, recurring infection or stridor may occur from bronchial stenosis as a result of cicatrization at the fracture site.

Clinical features which may be present in the emergency room are:
- Young patient with severe crush injury
- Haemoptysis
- Surgical emphysema
- Pneumothorax
- Gross air loss through intercostal drain.

If the diagnosis is suspected the patient should undergo endoscopy prior to endotracheal intubation. If the rate of intercostal drain air loss is catastrophic consideration should be given to inserting a double lumen endotracheal tube and selectively ventilating only the undamaged side.

Surgical repair of these injuries requires specialized facilities and knowledge. The surgical approach is via a cervical incision for the larynx and upper cervical trachea. A combined cervical and median sternotomy approach is used for a lower cervical or upper thoracic tracheal injury and a right thoracotomy for mid or lower tracheal injury or carinal injury. Bronchial rupture is approached from the relevant side. Primary repair is usually undertaken after freshening the torn ends.

Oesophageal trauma

Many more oesophageal injuries result from iatrogenic or non-accident related events than from external trauma. This section briefly outlines aspects of oesophageal injury relevant to thoracic trauma and oesophageal emergencies which are frequently managed by thoracic surgical units are discussed further under Thoracic Emergencies. Oesophageal pathology is discussed in detail in Chapter 9, 'Oesophageal Emergencies'.

Direct external oesophageal injury may be caused by penetrating trauma typically knife wounds to the neck but it is also reported with gunshot wound to the chest. As with tracheal injury, the likelihood of associated structure injury must be considered and the oesophageal injury may in fact be revealed during exploration for vascular or tracheal damage.

Blunt injury rarely results in direct oesophageal trauma excepting in injuries of such severity that aortic, tracheobronchial and spinal injuries are also present. Mortality in this group of patients is prohibitive and the oesophageal trauma is again likely to be discovered by accident. Upper abdominal compression may, however, cause forceful expulsion of gastric content into the oesophagus and, if the glottis is closed, the lower oesophagus may then rupture producing an injury which is identical to post-emetic rupture.

Oesophageal leakage produces mediastinal contamination and both chemical and bacterial mediastinitis. This contamination is slow with a simple wound to the upper oesophagus but catastrophic after a lower oesophageal rupture when gastric content is literally blasted through the lower mediastinum causing gross contamination.

Oesophageal trauma is suggested by:
- Penetrating cervical trauma
- Mediastinal emphysema
- Pneumothorax or hydropneumothorax without rib or sternal fracture
- Gastric content in intercostal drainage
- Associated injuries (trachea/aorta).

Dilute barium swallowed or instilled into the oesophagus via a nasogastric tube is diagnostic and is also useful as a localizing investigation.

Management. Direct repair is undertaken for a perforation by a knife or sharp object through an ipsilateral cervical or thoracotomy incision as appropriate.

A ruptured oesophagus may be repairable but, if the oesophagus is totally disrupted it may be more appropriate to resect the injured portion. If the patient's condition does not permit extensive surgery, mediastinal drainage with cervical oesophagostomy and gastrostomy is an alternate but much less satisfactory option. In either event thorough mediastinal debridement and drainage is an essential element in therapy.

Other thoracic emergencies

Introduction

A variety of diverse conditions may present as acute thoracic emergencies which require prompt surgical intervention by a minor or major procedure in order to manage the condition. These may conveniently be considered under the involved system. In distinction to traumatic injuries they are usually characterized by the presence of a single lesion.

Heart and great vessels

Emergencies involving the great thoracic vessels require immediate transfer to a regional cardiothoracic unit. There is no case for intervention by a non-specialist team.

Aortic aneurysm

True saccular or fusiform aneurysms can occur in the ascending, arch and descending portions of the thoracic aorta. They are often discovered as asymptomatic finding on chest X-ray but may present as acute and high mortality emergencies.

Clinical features
• Pain: may be vague thoracic discomfort or provide localizing clues: presternal with ascending aneurysms, upper sternal and neck with arch aneurysms and back with descending aneurysms.
• Shock.
• Pleural effusion (haemothorax).

Investigations
• Chest X-ray—visible aneurysm +/− mediastinal widening left pleural effusion.

• Thoracic CT—confirms presence and extent of the aneurysm (Fig. 23.17).
• Aortography—may contribute to surgical management by defining general appearance of arterial tree and exact connections to the aneurysm.

Management
In view of the risk of rupture and death surgery is advised in all patients with thoracic aortic aneurysm unless very advanced age or general medical considerations make survival highly unlikely. Aneurysms are managed by local resection and reconstruction with a Dacron tube graft. Descending aortic aneurysm is managed much as with a traumatic transection using either left heart bypass or a local shunt (Fig. 23.18). Aneurysms of the ascending aorta and arch are repaired with the aid of cardiopulmonary bypass. Aneurysms of the aortic arch pose a particular problem in that the circulation to the brain is necessarily interrupted. These are repaired using cardiopulmonary bypass to achieve total body cooling which allows hypothermic circulatory arrest during the repair process. Descending aortic aneurysms may be repaired using either left heart bypass or a local diversionary shunt. Operations on the descending aorta are associated with a risk of paraplegia (2–5%) because of inadequate perfusion of the spinal cord. Operative mortality for leaking descending thoracic aneurysm exceeds 20%. Mortality for leaking aneurysm elsewhere in the thoracic aorta is much higher.

Aortic dissection

This condition arises from a tear in the aortic intima usually located just above the aortic valve or adjacent to the left subclavian artery. This defect allows blood to enter the media

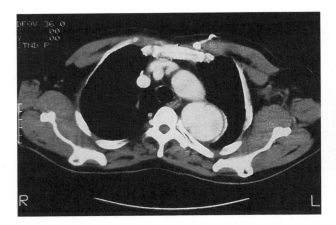

Fig. 23.17 Thoracic CT: aneurysm of descending thoracic aorta.

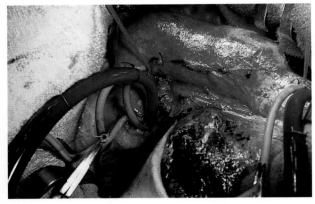

Fig. 23.18 Operative view of the descending aortic aneurysm in Fig. 23.17. An anticoagulant bonded shunt is in place to provide an alternate pathway prior to cross clamping the aorta above and below the aneurysm.

and create a false passage along the media layer which is the dissection process. The false lumen spirals around the aorta and can occlude branches of the aorta including the coronary and carotid arteries (Fig. 23.19). It may therefore cause a stroke or myocardial infarct and renal or gut infarction. The false lumen may burst into the pericardial cavity causing tamponade or into the left pleural cavity with exsanguination. Dissections are classified as Type B if the process involves only the descending aorta and Type A if it involves the ascending aorta or arch.

Clinical features
• pain, severe 'tearing' acute chest pain which may radiate through to the back
• hypotension
• variably absent pulses
• aortic incompetence
• stroke
• pericardial rub
• intra-abdominal ischaemia.

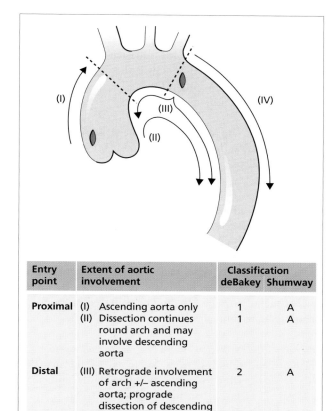

Entry point	Extent of aortic involvement	Classification deBakey	Shumway
Proximal	(I) Ascending aorta only	1	A
	(II) Dissection continues round arch and may involve descending aorta	1	A
Distal	(III) Retrograde involvement of arch +/− ascending aorta; prograde dissection of descending aorta	2	A
	(IV) Descending aorta only	3	B

Fig. 23.19 Patterns of thoracic aortic dissection.

Investigations
• ECG—helpful if it excludes a myocardial infarction but this may accompany a dissection.
• Chest X-ray—may show widened mediastinum +/− left pleural effusion.
• CT thorax contrast—should confirm the presence of two lumens.
• Aortography—helpful in showing luminal connections.

Management

Type A. The operative procedures are similar to those used with aneurysm surgery. The dissection origin is replaced together with the ascending and/or arch segments. It may also be necessary to replace the aortic valve and re-implant the coronary arteries.

Type B. The results of surgical and conservative (control of hypertension) management are similar for uncomplicated cases in this group. Conservative management is, therefore, usually advised unless there is bleeding into the left chest or the vascular branches to the abdominal organs have been compromised. Surgical technique is similar to that used for descending aortic aneurysm.

The immediate survival of those arriving alive in hospital is about 80% for each group.

Pericardial tamponade

The pathophysiology of cardiac tamponade has been discussed in Thoracic Trauma. Non-traumatic severe tamponade can occur with a large pericardial effusion. (This is a distinct process from the chronic tamponade associated with previous tuberculosis, surgery or pyogenic infection all of which may produce cardiac restriction from a fibrous encasement syndrome.)

As the effusion usually accumulates slowly there is time for the pericardial sac to distend so that it may contain up to a litre of fluid at the time of drainage.

Causes of non-traumatic pericardial effusion include:
• Malignancy involving the pericardium
• Uraemia
• Connective tissue disorders
• Myocardial infarction (Dressler's syndrome)
• Infection.

Clinical features
• History of associated condition
• Tachycardia
• Decreased blood pressure with narrow pulse pressure
• Cold peripheries
• Elevated venous pressure
• Muffled heart sounds.
• Refractory right-sided 'failure'.

Investigations
- Chest X-ray—smoothly enlarged pericardial contours in chronic cases (Fig. 23.20).
- Echocardiography—small, compressed, active heart with surrounding fluid.

Surgery

Aspiration under echocardiographic control is a useful first step as the anaesthesia is rendered safer. Continuing pericardial drainage is provided by creation of a pericardial 'window' either through a left thoracotomy with drainage into the pleural cavity or through a subxyphoid approach with drainage into the peritoneum (preferable for malignant cases). Subxyphoid drainage is entirely suitable for non-specialist use. In either case samples are taken for bacteriology, biochemical analysis, cytology and pathology.

Major vascular complications

Occasionally, major intrathoracic bleeding results from iatrogenic rather than trauma related events.

Tracheostomy related damage to the innominate artery

The innominate artery runs close to the anterior aspect of the right side of the trachea at the thoracic inlet. It may be injured in two circumstances:

1 Direct injury at the time of tracheostomy formation; this may also result in a clot-lined defect which ruptures later.

2 Late perforation from direct erosion by the tip of a tracheostomy tube.

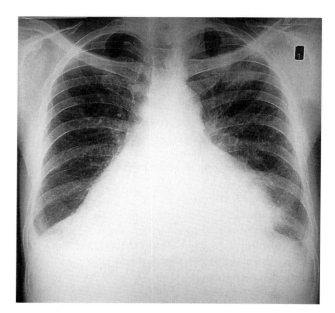

Fig. 23.20 PA chest X-ray of very large pericardial effusion.

Both of these injuries may cause major haemorrhage in the ward. This occurs around the tracheostome and into the airway.

Management. Haemorrhage around the tube can be reduced by local digital compression. Immediate control of haemorrhage into the airway may be provided by hyper inflating the tracheostomy tube cuff. If this does not work the patient will rapidly drown. In this circumstance, a last desperate measure which can be tried is to remove the tracheostomy tube and try to control the blood loss by inserting the little finger into the trachea to compress the arterial fistula.

In the event that local control can be achieved long enough to get the patient to theatre, or in the event of an innominate artery bleed created at the time of tracheostomy formation, a median sternotomy incision should be made and the innominate artery clamped proximally to provide control of the situation and allow definitive repair of the vessel. It may be necessary to have an assistant insert a finger down the side of the tracheostomy tube to compress the vessel whilst the incision is made.

Vascular injury from central venous cannulation

Although inadvertent arterial puncture or line misplacement are not uncommon during central venous cannulation, significant injury to the subclavian vein or artery during attempted central venous catheter or pacing wire insertion is remarkably infrequent.

Clinical features
- Hypotension and signs of haemorrhage post line insertion
- Pleural effusion (haemothorax)
- Rarely, collapse following line extraction (transfixion injury).

Management. Simple pleural drainage and transfusion is usually all that is required. Continued bleeding is an indication for surgical intervention preferably through a median sternotomy with lateral neck extension as replacement of the damaged segment of vessel may be required. Sternal retraction may cause the bleeding to stop by distorting the vessels so that identifying the bleeding or damaged portion can, occasionally, be difficult.

Intercostal drain insertion related vascular complications

Haemorrhage resulting from intercostal drain insertion reflects bad insertion technique. Bleeding may be immediate or delayed. Delayed bleeding is associated with chronic intercostal drainage for empyema and is caused by erosion of the underlying intercostal vessels. It is for this reason that such drains should be inserted through the bed of a resected portion of rib and the intercostal bundle ligated and divided.

Acute haemorrhage usually comes from the adjacent intercostal artery or the internal mammary artery. Less commonly a drain may be inserted into lung (Fig. 23.21) causing pulmonary parenchymal or arterial bleeding. Rarely a drain is inserted directly into the right or left ventricle.

Management. Pulmonary bleeding may stop on removal of the drain but pulmonary arterial bleeding (characterized by desaturated blood) may require surgical intervention by thoracotomy. Intracardiac placement results in immediate and catastrophic haemorrhage. This is usually an irretrievable situation because the patient exsanguinates in the time taken to recognize the situation. The only hope of survival is if the drain is immediately clamped but left *in situ* whilst the patient undergoes emergency thoracotomy.

Acute pulmonary embolism

Pulmonary embolism is normally managed by medical therapy including anticoagulation and possibly intrapulmonary arterial thrombolytic agents. Very occasionally, in a collapsed patient with minimal cardiac output, it may be appropriate to proceed to emergency pulmonary thrombectomy. The indications for this are subjective but may be summarized as:

- Young patient (< 50 years)
- Previously fit individual
- Benign disease
- Near arrested circulation
- Proximity to a unit with cardiopulmonary bypass facilities.

It is not indicated in a patient who has arrested and who has undergone cardiac massage as this causes the clot to fragment and be disseminated throughout the pulmonary arterial tree.

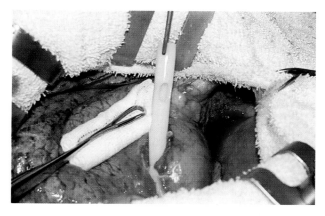

Fig. 23.21 Operative view of intercostal drain placed into right lower lobe.

Management

The patient should be fully heparinized (300 units/kg) when the diagnosis is suspected. Urgent median sternotomy is performed and cardiopulmonary bypass instituted. The pulmonary arterial trunk is then opened and clot extracted from both pulmonary arteries using suction and forceps. Forceful hyperinflation of the lungs can help to push clot fragments retrogradely out of smaller pulmonary arterial branches.

Chylothorax

Even on a nil orally regimen, at least 3 L of chyle pass through the thoracic duct each day. A major leak will therefore create a pleural effusion of rapidly serious degree. Although the accumulation of fluid may be controlled by intercostal drainage, the chylous fistula constitutes a serious continuing protein (4 g/L), fat, and extracellular fluid loss.

Causes

- Post surgical — typically oesophagectomy
- Post traumatic — particularly left upper chest wounds
- Lymphoma
- 'Spontaneous', i.e. aetiology not immediately apparent.

Clinical feature

- Relevant history
- Large pleural effusion with continuing drainage
- Obvious fat content if patient is eating meals
- Proteinaceous clots in drainage fluid
- Fluid and electrolyte loss
- Protein loss.

Management

The effusion should be drained. It may be difficult to achieve complete drainage as these effusions tend to loculate. If the rate of loss is moderate (< 2 L/day) and drainage appears satisfactory a nil orally regimen with nasogastric suction, intravenous feeding and crystalloid and plasma protein infusions sufficient to replace the lost chylous volume may be tried. Postoperative patients may find respiration difficult with this degree of fluid infusion and may require ventilation which can also be helpful in reversing the abdominothoracic pressure relationship and so inhibiting thoracic duct flow. The rate of loss should be assessed daily and electrolytes, plasma proteins, hydration and the chest X-ray appearances followed carefully.

Failure to resolve in 7–10 days or loss of control of these features should be taken as indications for surgical control of the thoracic duct. This is easiest to approach via a right posterolateral thoracotomy. The duct may be controlled by a mass ligature placed so as to include all the tissue between the aorta and azygos vein or it can be identified by dissection and specifically ligated. Recently, thoracoscopic clipping of the duct has been described.

Pleuropulmonary

Massive pleural effusion

Massive pleural effusion can cause dyspnoea with marked hypoxia. The pathophysiology is similar to tension pneumothorax with pulmonary collapse and mediastinal deviation which may interfere with venous return to the heart.
Causes include:
• Intrapleural dissemination of malignant disease (particularly bronchial carcinoma, breast carcinoma, Hodgkin's disease)
• Primary pleural mesothelioma
• Tuberculosis
• Empyema
• Liquefied haematoma
• Chylous fistula
• misplaced central venous catheter
• Connective tissue disorders
• Pancreatitis
• Ovarian tumours.

Clinical features
• Dullness to percussion
• Greatly reduced or absent breath sounds
• Features of underlying connective tissue disorder or stigmata of malignant disease.

Management
Urgent drainage is required. A basal intercostal catheter should be placed after digitally identifying that the pleural and not the abdominal cavity has been entered. Drainage should be controlled to prevent re-expansion pulmonary oedema. An initial 1 L may be drained after which the drain should be clipped. The clip should be released every 30 min releasing 500 ml aliquots until complete initial drainage has been achieved. Subsequent management will depend on the aetiology of the effusion. Clues to this may be derived from analysis of the fluid.
• Biochemistry:—protein >3 g/L = effusion, <3 g/L = transudate; amylase is diagnostic in pancreatitis related effusion.
• Culture:—type and antibiotic sensitivities of organisms (including tuberculosis).
• Microscopy—presence of bacteria; identification of malignant cells.
The post-drainage chest film may reveal a previously hidden tumour. Subsequent investigations should be based on the fluid analysis and radiological findings but may include sputum cytology, bronchoscopy, and percutaneous or thoracoscopic pleural biopsy.

Pneumothorax

Spontaneous pneumothorax may be life threatening if a tension pneumothorax is present or if the pneumothorax occurs in an elderly patient with pre-existing pulmonary impairment.

Clinical features
• Dyspneoa and tachypnoea
• Pleuritic pain
• Decreased air entry
• Hyper-resonance
• Mediastinal deviation if tension is present
• Hypoxia.

Management
As with trauma, tension pneumothorax requires decompression on clinical diagnosis. Otherwise, a chest film should be obtained to confirm the diagnosis *prior to drain insertion*. It is particularly important to exclude a large bulla being misinterpreted as a pneumothorax (Fig. 23.22) in an elderly patient as intubation of this will create a major air leak in a patient who may not be fit for thoracotomy.

Patients with long-standing chronic lung disease may develop painful surgical emphysema in association with pneumothorax. This may close the patient's eyes and can embarrass respiration. In this situation it may be helpful to insert small calibre subcutaneous suction drains in the supraclavicular area under local anaesthetic.

Sputum retention

Sputum retention is common in any situation where the patient's ability to cough is impaired by debilitation or pain. If left untreated the patient will rapidly develop airway occlusion, lobar or pulmonary collapse and severe hypoxia.

Clinical features
• At risk patient (elderly, upper abdominal or thoracic surgery, broken ribs)
• Large airway noise
• Exhaustion
• Possible lobar collapse on chest X-ray.

Management
Initial appraisal should determine whether the patient requires endotracheal intubation with toilet and ventilation. This is likely if the arterial $P\text{co}_2$ is >6.5 kPa. Otherwise there are three options:

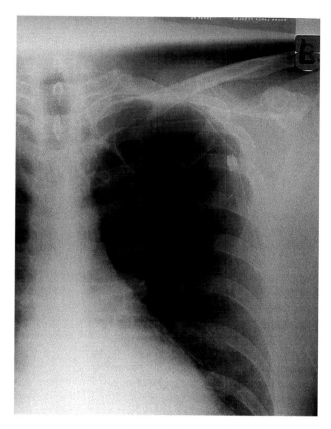

Fig. 23.22 Left upper zone bullous disease—easily mistaken on superficial inspection for a pneumothorax.

- Suction bronchoscopy
- Cricothyroidostomy ('minitracheostomy')
- Tracheostomy.

Pernasal tracheal suction is highly unpleasant, traumatizes the nasal passages and is rarely effective.

In general, formal tracheostomy is best performed as an elective procedure on an already ventilated patient as it involves an anaesthetic and is a significant operative procedure. Suction bronchoscopy is effective at removing large airway secretions but also involves an anaesthetic and does not address the issue of further sputum accumulation.

The best option in a patient who does not require immediate ventilation is, therefore, cricothyroidostomy under local anaesthesia providing that the patient has favourable anatomy and the operator is adequately experienced.

Inhaled foreign body

This is most common in very young children in whom the condition may not be apparent until pneumonic complications develop days later. Inhalation of relatively large objects such as peanuts or toy pieces may however present acutely as respiratory distress and/or stridor. In adult practice inhala-

tion is commoner in the context of trauma but peanuts, screws, pen tops or false teeth portions may also be inhaled. Distress is less likely given the larger airway.

Clinical features
- History (unlikely in a child)
- Stridor and/or respiratory distress
- Chest X-ray may show: radio-opaque object; lobar/segmental collapse.

Management
Either rigid or flexible bronchoscopy under general anaesthesia can be used to extract objects. It may be helpful to rotate an object *in situ* in order to present a better aspect for extraction. Peanuts tend to break up easily and are better retrieved using a basket snare. Occasionally a Fogarty catheter can be pushed beyond vegetable material and used to pull the material into a wider portion of bronchus. Vegetable matter causes a severe inflammatory response so that it can be difficult to identify the nature of an inhaled item beyond the swollen oedematous mucosa surrounding a bronchial obstruction. Occasionally thoracotomy and bronchotomy may be necessary to extract an embedded foreign body.

Oesophagogastric

Oesophageal perforation

Spontaneous rupture of the oesophagus (Boerhaave's syndrome)
Postemetic oesophageal rupture occurs from vomiting against a closed glottis. This results in an explosive disruption of the lower oesophagus. The mediastinum and thoracic cavity are heavily contaminated by gastric content.

Clinical features
- Sudden onset of severe lower central chest (and often back) pain
- Prostration
- Often misleading upper abdominal discomfort and tenderness
- Mediastinal emphysema +/− pneumothorax or hydropneumothorax (Fig. 23.23)
- Contrast swallow shows extravasation of medium (Fig. 23.24) and is a useful guide to planning the operative approach.

Management. Immediate drainage of any intrapleural fluid collection or pneumothorax should be performed. Intravenous broad spectrum antibiotics and an H_2 antagonist are commenced. If the condition has been diagnosed early (<24 h) thoracotomy repair is indicated. It is

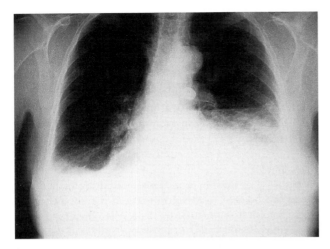

Fig. 23.23 Left hydropneumothorax in case of Boerhaave's syndrome.

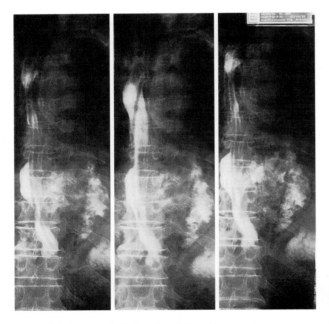

Fig. 23.24 Gastrografin leakage into left mediastinum in Boerhaave's syndrome.

important to exclude distal obstruction as there is an association with oesophageal stricture. Late presenting cases usually have a preceding misdiagnosis of myocardial infarction or upper abdominal catastrophe. In these an intrapleural drain should be inserted and consideration be given to thoracotomy for mediastinal cleansing, debridement of devitalized tissues and decortication. Primary repair is unlikely to be successful in this group but may succeed if reinforced with a diaphragm patch. Either resection and oesophagogastric

anastomosis or some form of long term drainage will be necessary. One option is to split the distal third of a chest drain, insert the limbs into the oesophageal defect and bring the end out through a rib resection. This T-tube solution provides good drainage until the lung has coalesced around the tube over the next 2–3 weeks after which the tube can be gradually withdrawn. This leaves an empyema cavity with an oesophagocutaneous fistula which will close in time. Prolonged intravenous or jejunostomy feeding will be required.

Iatrogenic oesophageal perforation
This usually occurs in the context of attempted dilatation by bouginage but may also complicate hydrostatic balloon dilatation or result from injudicious use of a rigid oesophagoscope. Perforation may be encountered from the pharynx (Fig. 23.25) to the cardia.

The clinical features are similar to those of spontaneous rupture. The degree of chest pain varies, however, and will depend on the size of the initial leak and may not be as severe initially. Radiographically, mediastinal emphysema is present but the changes may be subtle. Hydropneumothorax occurs if the parietal pleura is breached. Contrast swallow identifies the location of the leak and the extent of the defect may be gauged from the degree of extravasation.

Management. If a large leak is present mediastinitis will develop rapidly and urgent surgery is required. Patients who are not fit for surgery or those with a localized perforation with little apparent mediastinal reaction may be managed conservatively with parenteral feeding, systemic broad spectrum antibiotics and intravenous H_2 antagonist therapy. Surgery may involve simple suture repair of the oesophagus but is unlikely to be successful unless distal oesophageal

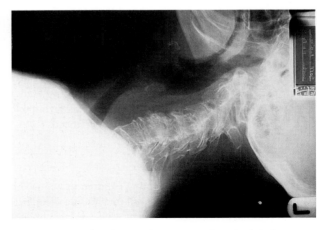

Fig. 23.25 Lateral neck X-ray showing retropharyngeal air from pharyngeal perforation.

pathology is dealt with at the same time. Therefore, concurrent resection of a carcinoma or stricture may be required.

Acute oesophageal obstruction

This is a relatively common problem. It is usually due to food bolus impaction often caused by failure to chew adequately. Less frequently, a foreign body may be swallowed, either accidentally such as false teeth, or deliberately with children or mentally defective patients. The amount of material swallowed by this latter group should not be underestimated and the author's experience includes patients who have swallowed razor blades, linoleum and, in one case, an entire pyjama jacket.

Rarely, unreported malignant dysphagia may present as apparently acute dysphagia. Food or swallowed objects tend to stick at points of narrowing: either pathological from stricture of malignancy, or physiological at the aortic arch and cardia.

A food bolus impacted at the cardia may pass when anxiety is relieved by hospital admission. It is therefore worth checking that the patient still feels obstructed before proceeding with emergency oesophagoscopy.

Clinical features
- Possible history of weight loss or dysphagia or
- History of swallowing a foreign body

Acute oesophageal obstruction

- Diagnosis should be clinically based.
- Contrast swallow is not advisable: barium will obscure subsequent endoscopic examination and gastrografin causes marked pulmonary irritation if inhaled.
- Food bolus may pass with relief of anxiety.
- If an obstructing lesion is present it should be biopsied, otherwise a contrast swallow should be obtained as a motility screening test.

- Inability to retain swallowed solids and liquids
- Regurgitation of saliva
- Lower sternal or epigastric discomfort
- Chest X-ray may reveal radio-opaque foreign body.

Management

Do *not* request a contrast swallow. This will do little to help the diagnosis, makes subsequent endoscopy and oesophagoscopy difficult and can be dangerous if the patient vomits and aspirates. Combined rigid and fibre-optic oesophagoscopy usually offers the best approach to identifying and managing an obstruction. The exact approach varies with the material concerned. A foreign body can usually be turned using biopsy forceps passed through a rigid scope and the object pulled back up to the mouth of the scope. The scope and object can then be drawn backwards so removing the foreign body. Soft, impacted food may either be picked out piecemeal using rigid instruments or gently nudged through into the stomach with a fibre optic instrument. This approach may only be used if the bolus moves easily or there is a risk of rupturing the oesophagus.

Always biopsy any abnormal areas or, if there is too much inflammation, re-admit the patient in a few days time for full examination. If no obvious cause is found consider referral for motility testing and take mucosal biopsies to test for *Helicobacter pylori*.

If a foreign body is embedded or removal appears unsafe it is better to proceed to a thoracotomy and oesophagotomy rather than cause a major oesophageal laceration and possibly even injury to extra-oesophageal structures.

The intrathoracic stomach

The stomach may be misplaced in the thorax as a rolling or sliding hiatus hernia (Fig. 23.26). This may be associated with three catastrophes:
- Intrathoracic perforation of a gastric ulcer
- Gastric volvulous
- Iatrogenic gastric puncture with a chest drain.

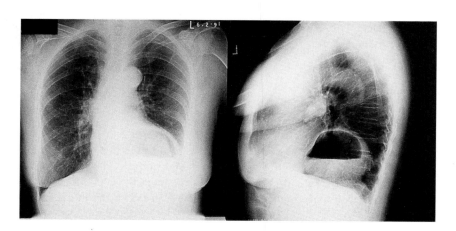

Fig. 23.26 Plain chest X-ray showing rolling hiatus hernia.

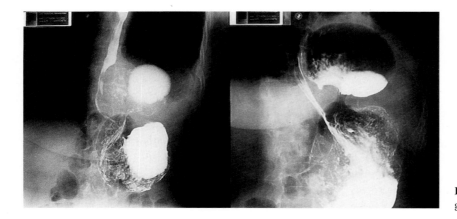

Fig. 23.27 Barium examination outlining gastric position in rolling hiatus hernia.

A sliding hernia may be associated with a short oesophagus so that the oesophagogastric junction lies in the lower mediastinum. Although the herniated stomach is covered with peritoneum, adhesions may lead to fusion of the stomach with the sac. A gastric ulcer may erode through both structures and perforate into the mediastinum or, very rarely, into the aorta or pericardium.

A rolling hernia has a relatively normally placed oesophagogastric junction with herniating stomach extending parallel to the oesophagus into the lower posterior left chest. This segment of stomach may become strangulated at the hiatus causing distension and ischaemic perforation may then result.

In massive hiatus herniae, the gastric vessels are necessarily elongated and the stomach is therefore abnormally mobile. This predisposes to gastric volvulous which may cause ischaemia, perforation and obstruction.

A further hazard with a rolling hernia is that the intrathoracic gastric bubble may be mistaken for an empyema or other localized intrathoracic collection and a drain inserted. If doubt is present a Barium swallow will demonstrate this anatomical variation (Fig. 23.27) and prevent such a mishap.

The clinical features associated with these events may include:
- Prostration
- Upper abdominal pain
- Haematemesis
- Proximal obstruction
- Pneumothorax
- Gastric content in the chest drain.

The diagnosis may be obvious when a drain has been inserted into the stomach. Contrast swallow or endoscopy may be helpful in the case of an ulcer in a hiatus hernia but often the full diagnosis is only revealed at thoracotomy undertaken because of the presence of distended stomach in the chest, hydropneumothorax and collapse. Further management by suture repair, reorientation of the stomach and/or gastrectomy will depend on the operative findings.

Surgical procedures used in the management of thoracic emergencies

Intercostal nerve blocks

Indications

- Unilateral rib fractures
- Thoracotomy wound pain.

Procedure

Use Marcaine 0.25% with adrenaline 1 in 100 000 up to 40 ml. This regimen may be repeated 12-h as required. Sit the patient up leaning on a pillow on a bed table.

Palpate the lower border of the posterior angles of the ribs. Insert the needle so as to touch the lower border of the rib and then slip the needle tip under the rib. Aspirate to exclude having entered a blood vessel. Do not advance too far or you will enter the pleural cavity and create a pneumothorax.

Deliver 2.5 ml per rib. If a chest drain is not *in situ*, obtain a chest film after administering the blocks in order to exclude a pneumothorax.

Intercostal drain insertion

Indications

- Therapeutic: pneumo-, hydro-, haemo-, or chylothorax, large pleural effusion, empyema.
- Prophylactic (all relative): patients with significant chest trauma undergoing inter-hospital transfers (particularly by

air) or about to spend a long period in scanning departments, anaesthesia for operations on other body regions, therapeutic ventilation.

Placement location

Except in extremis, a chest film should first be obtained. A lateral view will also be required when draining a fluid collection. The plain X-ray(s) will help to determine
- The location of the pathology: fluid collection/pneumothorax/empyema.
- The location of the diaphragm, where possible.
- The presence of any large bullae.
- Areas where the lung is adherent to the chest wall.

If the patient does not have a loculated or atypical air or fluid collection, the drain may be located where insertion is most convenient, comfortable and safe. An apical drain should be inserted just posterior to the lateral border of the pectoralis major. In this position the tip of the drain will naturally point towards the apex of the chest. A drain placed in the midclavicular line anteriorly will not lie as well as the drain enters the chest more perpendicularly and the AP distance at this level is relatively short. This location also offers increased risk to hitting the internal mammary artery and produces a poor cosmetic result. A basal drain should be inserted in the midaxillary line as inferiorly as safely possible.

Drains

There are two main types of intercostal drainage catheter: standard multihole catheters and those with an end hole and one or two side holes only. The second type are often supplied with a central sharply pointed rod which is intended to aid insertion. The multihole type are safer and better. There is less chance of the drain blocking and the potential risk of damaging an intrathoracic structure with the central stylet is avoided.

Technique

If the patient is conscious he should be positioned sitting up at 45° with his arm supported behind his head. Access is improved by rotating the patient away from the surgeon. Insertion is easier if the patient also leans laterally away from the surgeon as this opens the intercostal spaces. If the patient is unconscious or too ill to reposition use an assistant to expose the intended drain site as much as is possible.

In the conscious patient 5–20 ml of 1% lignocaine should be infiltrated through the layers of the chest wall, taking care to inject the immediate subcuticular and extrapleural areas as these are the most sensitive layers. The injecting needle can usefully be advanced into the pleural cavity to confirm

the presence of air or fluid as anticipated. A 3-cm transverse incision is then made and artery forceps used to separate the underlying muscle until the rib cage is reached. The chest cavity should then be entered immediately over the upper border of a rib. Air or fluid will be released and the patient will often cough. Pass one finger through the hole to confirm that the pleural cavity has been entered and that the lung is not adherent to the chest wall around the insertion site. Insert the drain and secure it with a suture. Leave a loose vertical mattress suture in the wound to close it when the drain is removed. A purse-string suture causes pressure necrosis at the wound site and should not be used.

Problems

Some of the commoner problems with intercostal drains include:

Apparently not working
Likely reasons are:
- Drain under the diaphragm: look for subdiaphragmatic air and an abnormally low drain position.
- Drain outside the chest wall: look for the position of the drain on plain chest X-ray; if it is not in the chest cavity this is easy to spot.
- Drain bottle connected the wrong way round or drain tubing clamped: check the connections.

Continuous blowing
Likely reasons are:
- Some of the drain holes are outside the chest cavity: this is easy to detect on the chest X-ray.
- Drain in the lung: it can be difficult to determine whether this is the case but clues would be a central lie to the drain and marked air leakage despite an apparently inflated lung.
- Air moving in and out of the chest around the drain: if the drain has been *in situ* for some days the hole may have enlarged; air movement may be audible, if not try compressing the drain site and seeing if the rate of air loss decreases.

Cricothyroidostomy

Indications

- Sputum retention
- Emergency airway access.

Contra-indications

- Children (risk of laryngeal damage)
- Short thick neck

- Laryngeal trauma
- Coagulopathy
- Likely need for ventilatory support: rising CO_2, multiple trauma.

Technique

Position the patient supine lying head up at about a 30° angle and extend the neck. Palpate the anterior neck to be sure that you can easily identify the cricothyroid membrane. Infiltrate this area with 5 ml of lignocaine 1%. The use of lignocaine with adrenaline 1 in 100 000 helps reduce oozing at the entry site.

Prepare the area in a sterile manner and then make a vertical stab incision through the skin and underlying membrane. Use either a commercial 'mini-trach' tube which can be inserted as a Seldinger type procedure over the supplied guide bougie. Alternatively, insert a paediatric 20 FG silver tracheostomy tube after gently dilating the track with fine artery forceps. In either case remove the guide or obturator and confirm placement in the trachea by air loss. As a double check, pass a suction catheter. Use tracheostomy tube tapes to retain the tube which should be closed with a spigot in between suction episodes in order to preserve nasal humidification of inhaled air and to maintain the concentration of inhaled oxygen.

Problems

If bleeding continues beyond a few minutes abandon the procedure and proceed to a formal tracheostomy. Otherwise the patient is at risk of developing airway obstruction from blood clot. Occasionally, patients may experience difficulty with swallowing fluids due to the tube impeding laryngeal movement.

Tracheostomy

This is a dangerous and generally underrated procedure which is often performed badly by surgeons who carry out very few tracheostomies in a year. Do not get involved in this procedure unless you are confident that you can cope with the problems it may present. Do not agree to perform this procedure without adequate assistance, operating conditions and the availability of an electrocautery. A clear dry operating field is essential. With the exception of acute laryngeal obstruction, all the indications for this procedure are relative and it can await better circumstances or a more experienced surgeon. Deciding when not to operate and when to get assistance is as much a mark of a good surgeon as performing a successful procedure.

Indications

- Laryngeal trauma/obstruction
- Prolonged ventilation/weaning
- Sputum retention.

Contra-indications

- Inadequate experience
- Possible tracheal injury.

It is safer not to paralyse the patient during this procedure so that some means of ventilation exists in the event that the tracheostomy tube is misplaced.

Procedure

Position the patient much as for a cricothyroidostomy. A sand or fluid bag between the shoulders may help by pushing the neck further forwards. Select a low pressure seal tube about 1–2 mm less in diameter than the current endotracheal tube. As a rough guide a 'normal' male would take an 8-mm tube and a female a 7-mm tube. Selecting too large a size increases the risk of traumatic insertion and of misplacement particularly in a hurried situation. Prior to starting the operation, check the tube and ascertain that the balloon cuff is functional and that the connections agree with the anaesthetist's equipment.

Make a 5-cm transverse incision about a thumb's breadth below the cricoid cartilage. Deepen the incision through the platysma. Split the deep cervical fascia in the midline from the cricoid cartilage to the suprasternal notch. The thyroid isthmus may partially overly the upper trachea in which case it can usually be pushed cranially. If not it should be divided between clamps and the ends oversewn with Vicryl or Dexon. There is debate as to the best form of tracheal incision. The options include a simple vertical incision, excising a hole and creating a flap from the anterior tracheal wall. For those with less experience a flap stoma may facilitate tube insertion. Create this by incising between the 2nd and 3rd tracheal rings and incising the 3rd and 4th rings laterally. Stay away from the first ring. Suture the flap to the deep cervical fascia inferiorly with one or two fine Dexon sutures. It may be necessary to use a cautery to control bleeding from the tracheal wall between the cut rings. The endotracheal tube should now be visible. Aspirate mucous and ask the anaesthetist to retract the endotracheal tube until the orifice of the tube lies at the upper edge of the tracheal opening. Do not use cautery at this stage as the operative field is now flooded with O_2 from the open end of the endotracheal tube. The view may be improved by getting your assistant to elevate the upper edge of the tracheal opening with a blunt hook. Insert the tracheostomy tube, inflate the cuff and connect the outer end to the anaesthetic tubing. Suction the airway and ask the anaesthetist to confirm adequate ventilation prior to securing the tube with double tapes.

Problems

Short fat or swollen neck

This may make it very difficult to palpate the cricoid cartilage. The thyroid cartilage at least serves as a midline marker unless it is disrupted. If all else fails, make the most apparently appropriate incision and palpate once the deep fascia has been opened. In these patients retraction on the cricoid cartilage with a blunt hook may be essential to get an adequate view. If the view is poor use a smaller tube and make a smaller hole in the trachea.

Can not get the tube in

- Check the balloon is properly deflated
- Consider using a smaller size of tube
- Consider using a suction catheter as a guide.

Remember to allow the anaesthetist to advance the endotracheal tube and ventilate the patient in between attempts. Ventilation is paramount; getting the tracheostomy tube in can usually wait.

Children

The neck is relatively short; beware of the innominate vein riding up into the base of the neck.

Emergency thoracotomy

Rarely, immediate thoracotomy will have to be performed by the non-specialist surgeon as a crisis intervention in the emergency room. Thoracotomy to cross-clamp the thoracic aorta as a means of theoretically improving proximal circulation and blood pressure in patients with massive lower body blood loss is a largely discredited and pointless exercise.

Access to the heart is gained by a left anterior thoracotomy, all other interventions are performed through a posterolateral thoracotomy.

Indications

Immediate thoracotomy

This procedure is limited to relieving tamponade, allowing a vascular clamp to be placed to control major haemorrhage (possibly) or providing more effective cardiac massage.
- Critical tamponade
- Rarely, massive thoracic bleeding
- Arrest in the resuscitation room.

Urgent thoracotomy

This is a planned intervention following appraisal of the patient's injuries and is carried out in an operating theatre. The interval between admission and surgery may range from nil to a few hours depending on the clinical situation.
- Subacute tamponade
- Traumatic thoracotomy, where the chest has already been opened by injury
- Excessive bleeding through drains
- Profuse air leak
- Mediastinal structure injury: trachea, oesophagus, aorta
- Repair ruptured diaphragm.

Procedures

Anterior thoracotomy

Position the patient supine with a pillow behind the left chest. Make a left submammary incision and deepen it through all layers of the chest wall. This will enter the chest through the 5th interspace. If you have a rib retractor spread the ribs otherwise get your assistant to hold them apart. Grasp the pericardium with forceps and open it vertically parallel to, but avoiding, the left phrenic nerve. If tamponade is present this will release the compression and the circulation should recover almost immediately. It may then be necessary to rapidly paralyse and anaesthetize the patient. If feasible, repair the cardiac injury or compress the bleeding point until specialist help arrives. If the heart is arrested commence massage.

If the patient recovers, the return of cardiac output will result in haemorrhage from the many vessels cut during the emergency thoracotomy. Haemostasis will therefore be required and the internal mammary artery which is often torn during emergency rib retraction will probably need ligation. Close by inserting pericardial and left pleural drains through inferior stab incisions and then loosely appose the pericardial edges with interrupted sutures. Approximate the ribs with interrupted heavy no. 2 Vicryl or Dexon and use layered Vicryl or Dexon to close the soft tissue layers.

Posterolateral thoracotomy

Place the patient in the lateral decubitus position. Make an incision starting in the inframammary crease anteriorly, curving posteriorly round the lower pole of the scapula by a margin of about 4 cm and bisecting the gap between the posterior edge of the scapula and the vertebral column. Divide the underlying latissimus dorsi and then scalenus anterior muscles. Small portions of the inferior fibres of the trapezius and rhomboid muscles may require division posteriorly. Open the chest from back to front along the upper border of the highest conveniently accessible rib, which will usually be the 5th or 6th, and insert a rib retractor.

If this procedure has been performed as an emergency for exsanguinating haemorrhage, blood and clot will have to be rapidly scooped out whilst the bleeding vessel is digitally compressed by the surgeon. It may then be possible to temporarily control the source of bleeding. In practice, this is likely to require clamping a great vein or cross-clamping either the entire pulmonary hilum or the descending aorta. These desperate measures may allow the patient to survive until specialist help is available.

Otherwise, the condition requiring very urgent thoracotomy should be corrected as effectively as possible under the circumstances. With the exceptions of massive pulmonary injury, aortic rupture and tracheal disruption most injuries require simple suture repair. Closure is by inserting two drains through inferior stab incisions. The anterior drain passes to the apex of the pleural cavity and the posterior to the base. Approximate the ribs with interrupted figure of eight heavy Vicryl or Dexon sutures and close the soft tissues in layers with Vicryl or Dexon.

Suturing cardiac wounds

Clean edged incisions such as may be created by a stab wound are relatively simple to repair. A ragged defect or a hole adjacent to a coronary artery may require a patch or detailed reconstruction on bypass. Consider, therefore, whether it may be safer to use digital pressure to control bleeding and await specialist help. Do not use cautery on the heart as it may cause ventricular fibrillation.

In general, ventricular wounds may be repaired with 3/0 Prolene and atrial wounds with 4/0 Prolene. Figure of eight or horizontal mattress Teflon pledgetted sutures may be used but in either case it is important not to overtighten the suture which could then cut through. Suturing the moving ventricle can be easier if the myocardium adjacent to the hole is stabilized by placing a finger on it. Calamitous bleeding from a major cardiac defect is usually fatal but occasionally it may be controlled by a Foley catheter inflated within the ventricle or atrium and gently retracted into the hole.

Other techniques for pericardial drainage

These techniques are described for use in the circumstance of obvious, imminent collapse of the patient from suspected tamponade in the setting of the emergency room.

Pericardial aspiration

This is often described as a first aid manoeuvre in a patient with suspected critical tamponade. In the absence of someone with appropriate surgical training it may be the only option but it is a very difficult procedure to perform effectively in the context of a major trauma case in a resuscitation room.

Under normal circumstances this procedure should be undertaken under ultrasound guidance. In extremis, a central venous cannula needle should be inserted in the angle between the xyphoid and the left costal margin and directed towards the midline. In theory this reduces the chance of ventricular laceration. Use of an ECG electrode attached to the needle as a warning device for when the needle touches the ventricular myocardium is a refinement which is of modest value and which is impracticable given the circumstances committing the attendant to this course of action. The needle should be aspirated constantly and when blood is recovered a central venous catheter passed to provide pericardial drainage. The pericardial fluid will come out under considerable pressure and as it drains the patient's haemodynamic parameters should improve. The fluid should not clot and the rate of drainage should slow after about 100–200 ml have been recovered. If it is suspected that the catheter is in the ventricle, it should be clamped and left *in situ* pending further help.

Subxyphoid pericardial drainage

This is a much safer and more effective method of providing pericardial drainage which requires only a few minutes and minimal equipment or surgical skill.

With the patient supine a vertical incision is made over the lower third of the sternum and the upper third of the epigastrium. Considerable venous bleeding will be present from the raised central venous pressure. The incision is deepened to expose the sternum and linea alba. Incise the linea alba and quickly free it from the underlying xyphoid process. Use heavy scissors to cut the xyphoid from the sternum flush with the bone. The tissue immediately below the sternum is the lower anterior pericardium. Grasp this with a forceps and make a small incision with a knife. There will be a rush of blood and the patient's circulation should improve immediately. Widen the hole with forceps and gently insert a finger. You should be able to feel the heart moving within the pericardial cavity. Make a stab incision through the skin on the right hand side of the wound and insert a large intercostal drain (36 FG) through this into the pericardial cavity. Run a simple continuous stitch up the skin wound and transfer the patient to theatre for definitive pericardial exploration.

Acknowledgement

I wish to express my thanks to Ms D. Beard, National Co-ordinator, Scottish Trauma Audit Group, Edinburgh for her help in providing National Data and access to Audit Group material.

Further reading

Advanced Trauma Life Support Course for Physicians, Chapter 4
Thoracic Trauma. pp. 111–140, 1993 Student Manual. Committee
on Trauma, American College of Surgeons.

Besson, A. & Saegesser, F. (1983) *A Colour Atlas of Chest Trauma and
Associated Injuries*, Volumes I & II. Wolfe Medical Publications Ltd,
London.

Shields, T.W. (1994) *General Thoracic Surgery*, 4th edn. Williams and
Wilkins, Philadelphia.

CHAPTER 24

The acutely swollen limb

Mary-Paula Colgan, Dermot J. Moore & Gregor D. Shanik

Oedema results from the accumulation of excess tissue fluid in the interstitial space. The interstitial fluid rather than being a static pool, is an ever changing flow of transudate from the arterial portion of the capillary bed to the tissue space and is balanced by its reabsorption by the venous portion of the capillaries and by the lymphatics. The lymphatics are only responsible for removing about one-tenth of the reabsorbed fluid but are essential for removing large protein molecules and particulate matter from the interstitial space.

The factors involved in the flow of interstitial fluid include porosity of the capillary wall, osmotic pressure, lymphatic absorption, tissue pressure and arterial and venous pressures. The main causes for increased capillary transudation include:
• Raised intracapillary pressure caused by increased venous pressure.
• Increased capillary permeability.
• Diminished reabsorption of interstitial fluid.
• Increased osmotic pressure in tissue fluid.
• Lymphatic obstruction or insufficiency.

Differential diagnosis

The distinction between pitting and non-pitting oedema is useful but not entirely reliable for distinguishing lymphoedema. A long-standing history of lymphoedema may well affect both lower extremities and may give rise to oedema, not only of the skin but also of the subcutaneous tissue, to cause the characteristic brawny swelling which does not pit easily on pressure. These appearances are easily recognizable in the chronic state (Fig. 24.1); however in lymphoedema of more recent origin, this may not be so obvious. For simplicity, oedema can be divided into three categories to aid with the differential diagnosis. These include:
• Bilateral pitting oedema
• Painful unilateral pitting oedema
• Painless unilateral oedema.
Each can then be further subdivided.

Bilateral pitting oedema

• Heart failure
• Renal disease
• Proteinuria
• Cirrhosis
• Carcinomatosis
• Nutritional.
and in rare cases
• Inferior vena caval obstruction or
• Simultaneous disease of both lower extremities.

Painful unilateral pitting oedema

• Deep vein thrombosis
• Superficial thrombophlebitis
• Cellulitis
• Injury
• Ischaemia (the chronically ischaemic limb with rest pain may show pronounced oedema caused by the patient sleeping with the leg dependent).

Painless unilateral oedema

• Post-phlebitic limb (Fig. 24.2)
• Extrinsic compression of the deep veins
• Deep venous incompetence
• Lymphoedema
• Oedema bleu
• Immobility.

Investigations

As in all areas of medicine a full history and physical examination is essential and often provides vital information to direct further investigations. Most causes of bilateral pitting oedema will be diagnosed on history and physical examination. The diagnosis will be confirmed with simple biochemical assays or radiological tests, e.g. urea/creatinine for renal failure (Table 24.1).

From the comprehensive list of differential diagnoses it becomes clear that our most important function is to outrule

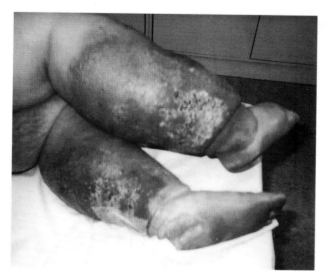

Fig. 24.1 Chronic swelling of both lower limbs secondary to lymphoedema with cellulitis and ulceration.

Table 24.1 Diagnosis of bilateral pitting oedema.

Cause	Supporting signs	Investigation
Heart failure	Sacral oedema	Chest X-ray
	Bibasal creps	ECG
	Hepatomegaly	
Renal failure		Urea/creatinine
Proteinuria		Serum proteins
Cirrhosis	Hepatomegaly	Liver function tests
	Jaundice	
Carcinomatosis	Ascites	Chest X-ray
	Organomegaly	CT scan
	Lymphadenopathy	

ECG, electrocardiograph. CT, computerized tomography.

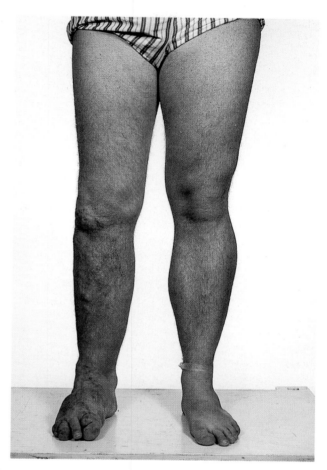

Fig. 24.2 Unilateral lower limb swelling secondary to post-phlebitic limb and varicose veins.

the presence of deep vein thrombosis (DVT) as this may have fatal consequences. The inaccuracy of clinical diagnosis of DVT has been well documented. Until recently, ascending venography has been the test of choice for diagnosing deep vein thrombosis (Fig. 24.3); however, the development of a number of accurate noninvasive tests has made venography unnecessary in the majority of cases. It should also be remembered that venography is not without complications, the most serious being thrombosis secondary to contrast medium.

Doppler ultrasound

Doppler ultrasound is the simplest and most rapid method to assess the venous system. Although Doppler pocket instruments are relatively inexpensive and thus readily available, training is essential to ensure accurate results. Many reports have compared the accuracy of Doppler ultrasound to venography and in experienced hands the overall accuracy for occlusive thrombi proximal to the calf is 87%. It is important to be aware that this test will often fail to detect thrombi that are partially occlusive and calf thrombi. Additionally, in patients with recurrent DVT the diagnosis of acute deep vein thrombosis using Doppler ultrasound is almost impossible.

Impedance plethysmography

Impedance plethysmography was developed in the 1970s and is based on Ohm's Law (Voltage = current × resistance). The voltage changes measured are the result of, and directly proportional to, the increase or decrease in blood volume of a limb. Though it is accurate in the detection of proximal thrombi (sensitivities 87–100%) sensitivities of only

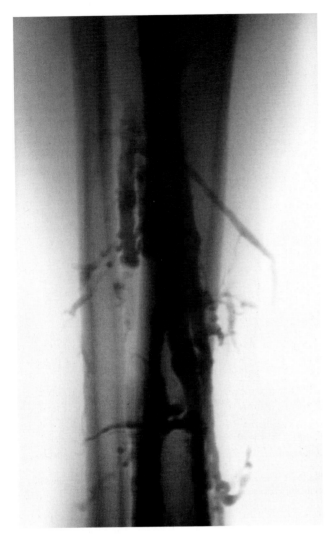

Fig. 24.3 Venogram showing filling defect in deep veins of the calf secondary to deep vein thrombosis.

17–50% have been reported for the detection of calf thrombi.

Liquid crystal thermography

Thermography detects temperature differences on the surface of the human body and is used in the diagnosis of DVT based on the observation that the skin temperature of limbs with deep venous thrombosis was frequently increased. Though the sensitivity is high the specificity is low (62%). False-positive thermograms result from ruptured Baker cysts, cellulitis and superficial thrombophlebitis while false-negative results may occur when the thrombus is greater than a week old. Thermography is a good screening tool to identify those patients who should be investigated further.

Duplex scanning

The development of real-time B-mode imaging has provided the ability to image the deep venous system, visualizing venous flow, acute thrombus and allows the differentiation of the latter from chronic thrombosis (Fig. 24.4). This is now the test of choice in diagnosing deep vein thrombosis. Sensitivities and specificities in excess of 90% have been reported. It is safe and free from side effects. It can be used in pregnancy and is easy to repeat. However it should be noted that duplex scanning is operator-dependent and requires significant training.

Duplex ultrasound can also be used in the diagnosis of superficial thrombophlebitis if there is any doubt about diagnosis. Most importantly it can localize the upper extent of the superficial thrombus as encroachment on the sapheno-femoral junction requires urgent treatment (Fig. 24.5).

Arterial assessment

Chronic ischaemia will be diagnosed on history (rest pain) and physical examination (absent pulses, dependent rubor, etc.); however, the diagnosis can be confirmed by non-invasive arterial pressure measurements. It is generally

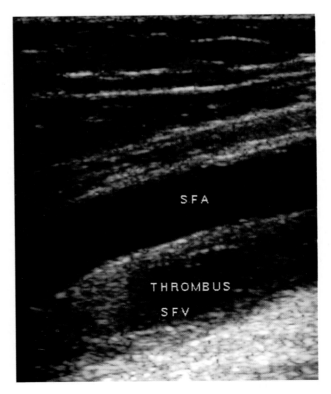

Fig. 24.4 B-mode ultrasound demonstrating thrombosis in the superficial femoral vein (SFV).

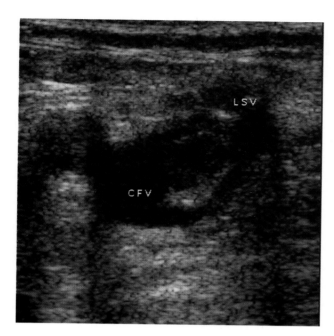

Fig. 24.5 Thrombus from the long saphenous vein (LSV) encroaching on the common femoral vein (CFV).

accepted that an ankle systolic pressure <50 mmHg or a digital pressure of <30 mmHg (in diabetics) is in keeping with the presence of critical ischaemia (European Consensus Document).

Lymphoedema

The lymphatic system returns to the vascular compartment extravascular molecules and colloids too large to re-enter directly. The rate at which a labelled protein or colloid is removed from the interstitial tissue has therefore been regarded as an index of lymphatic function and this is the basis of lymphoscintigraphy. The tracer is administered by interstitial injection, obviating the need for direct cannulation of the lymphatic channels.

Treatment

Treatment will depend on the actual aetiology of the oedema, e.g. intravenous antibiotics for cellulitis. Two areas will be discussed in detail: deep vein thrombosis and lymphoedema.

Deep vein thrombosis

Barritt and Jordan, in a landmark paper in 1960, firmly established the place of heparin and warfarin in treatment of venous thrombosis by showing a dramatic decrease in fatal pulmonary emboli. Untreated proximal DVT has a risk of

pulmonary embolization of 50%, with a fatal pulmonary embolism rate of 10%. Therapeutic anticoagulation reduces the risk of pulmonary embolism to <5%. This high efficacy may be surprising as heparin and warfarin simply inhibit the growth of new or existing clot and have little or no effect on existing clot.

To ensure optimal administration of anticoagulants one should follow these simple rules:

1 Before commencing treatment a coagulation screen and platelet count should be performed.

2 In a patient in whom there is no obvious cause or risk factor, tests for a hypercoagulable state should be performed prior to treatment as heparin and/or warfarin will interfere with the measurement of antithrombin III, protein C, protein S, anticardiolipin antibody and lupus anticoagulant.

3 Assess if there are significant contraindications to anticoagulants, e.g. ocular or intracranial surgery.

Heparinization

The goal of heparin administration is to provide immediate and potent anticoagulation to arrest the thrombotic process while oral agents take effect. Historically, heparin was administered by intermittent intravenous bolus; however, continuous intravenous infusion has been shown to have the highest efficacy with a low risk of bleeding complications. Heparin is initially administered as a bolus of 5000 to 10 000 IU while a continuous heparin infusion is simultaneously initiated at 1000 to 1500 IU/h to maintain an activated partial thromboplastin time (aPTT) between 2.0 and 3.0 times the control level. The most common complication is bleeding. Heparin-induced thrombocytopenia (HIT) is an unusual but important immune-mediated idiosyncratic reaction to heparin characterized by a decreasing platelet count and thrombosis.

Warfarin

Oral anticoagulants are used to provide long-term anticoagulation in an outpatient setting. Warfarin administration should begin as promptly as possible after administration of heparin to minimize the time required to achieve therapeutic anticoagulation. Administration is typically in a dose of 5 to 10 mg daily for 3 days depending on the size and nutritional status of the patient. The maintenance dose is calculated based on prothrombin times to obtain a ratio of 2.0 to 2.7 times the control value. Randomized trials have shown the need to maintain warfarin therapy for up to three months following a DVT. However, in practice the decision to stop anticoagulation is individualized.

The most common complication is bleeding, and it is important to remember that warfarin should not be given during pregnancy as it can cross the placenta and cause a characteristic embryopathy.

Low molecular weight heparins

These can be injected subcutaneously and have been shown to be efficacious in the prophylaxis of DVT. Some, though not all, have been licensed for the treatment of acute DVT. This could obviate the need for hospitalization and allow outpatient management of these patients. In addition, the constant monitoring required by both heparin and warfarin is not required.

Lymphoedema

Lymphoedema is, to all intents and purposes, irreversible and incurable and there are few guidelines on management. Though lymphoedema is considered a surgical condition, there is as yet no surgical solution. Recent advances in microvascular techniques and the introduction of lymphovenous anastomosis have proven to be of temporary benefit. Debulking of the grossly swollen limb is sometimes still required. The mainstay of treatment is medical and includes:
• Prevention of infection
• physical therapy
• External support
• Pneumatic compression.

External support is the cornerstone of treatment as it:
• Limits blood capillary filtration by raising interstitial pressure
• Opposes tissue expansion
• Improves striated muscle pump efficiency.
Elastic hosiery exerts a controlling external pressure and serves to maintain limb size. A garment must be well fitted and comfortable to ensure patient compliance. Lymphoedema invariably requires high compression strengths (>40 mmHg).

Further reading

Browse, N.L., Burnand, K.G. & Thomas, M.L. (eds) (1988) *Diseases of the Veins. Pathology, Diagnosis and Treatment.* Edward Arnold, London.

Nicholaides, A.N. & Sumner, D.S. (1991) *Investigation of Patients with Deep Vein Thrombosis and Chronic Venous Insufficiency.* Med-Orion, UK.

Ogston, D. (ed.) (1987) *Venous Thrombosis. Causation and Prediction.* Wiley Medical, Chichester.

Tibbs, D.J. (ed.) (1990) *Varicose Veins and Related Disorders.* Butterworth Heineman, London.

Reference

Barritt, D.W. & Jordan, S.C. (1960) Anticoagulant drugs in the treatment of pulmonary embolism: a controlled trial. *Lancet* **1** 1309–1312.

CHAPTER 25

Acute limb ischaemia

Kevin O'Malley & Neville Couse

Introduction

Acute limb ischaemia is a common surgical emergency which requires accurate assessment and urgent management to maximize limb salvage. The clinical presentation may range from a rather dramatic picture with severe pain and impending tissue loss to a somewhat more insidious but equally threatening picture. The majority who develop acute limb ischaemia are elderly and will have other manifestations of cardiovascular disease. Mental function may often be compromised, thus complicating assessment. However, a clear and precise management pathway is essential if limb salvage with minimal morbidity is to be achieved. Generally, the quicker the ischaemic limb is revascularized the more likely it is to be successful. However, it is not always essential to proceed immediately to revascularization and it may often be judged that more extensive pre-operative assessment is preferable. It is no longer acceptable to proceed immediately to an 'embolectomy' as first line management as effective treatment may well require a combination of thrombolysis, embolectomy, arterial reconstruction and attention to the cardiovascular system in general. Given the multifaceted nature of acute ischaemia and the many approaches now available to manage this condition, these patients are best treated by multidisciplinary teams including vascular surgeons, radiologists and physicians. This approach to patients with acute limb ischaemia should mean a primary amputation rate of less than 10%.

In the younger age group acute ischaemia may be related to trauma, misplaced intravenous injections, catheterization, congenital abnormalities of the peripheral vasculature and, less commonly now, rheumatic heart disease. In the older patient, atherosclerosis and cardiac rhythm abnormalities become the major factors and leg ischaemia may simply be the first manifestation of a systemic problem.

Aetiology

The common causes of acute limb ischaemia are: arterial emboli, thrombosis and trauma. Arterial trauma and peripheral embolization will frequently occur in the presence of a normal underlying vascular tree. Thrombosis, on the other hand, will most often be an acute episode occurring in an already atherosclerotic circulation (Fig. 25.1).

Embolization

An embolus may be defined as an abnormal mass carried by the blood stream from one site to another. The majority of emboli are produced within the blood stream and the heart is the source in approximately 80% of cases. Atrial fibrillation, in association with ischaemic heart disease and less frequently rheumatic heart disease, accounts for the majority of cardiac emboli. Mural thrombus secondary to myocardial infarction is an important source of embolus although the incidence of embolization following myocardial infarction is relatively low. Other cardiac sources of emboli include cardiomyopathy, prosthetic heart valves, ventricular aneurysms, paradoxic emboli through a patent foramen ovale and congenital intercardiac shunts.

Both atrial fibrillation and myocardial infarction result in compromised myocardial contraction resulting in the deposition of thrombus in the left atrium or ventricle. This may then be the source for peripheral embolization. Previously, rheumatic heart disease was a common source of atrial fibrillation with peripheral embolization to a normal circulation. However, nowadays rheumatic heart disease is less common and atrial fibrillation is more likely to be related to ischaemic heart disease. It is worth reiterating that the incidence of peripheral embolization secondary to mitral valve disease and rheumatic fever has reduced considerably. This has meant a significant reduction in the number of patients presenting with embolic ischaemia superimposed on a substantially normal peripheral circulation.

Sources of emboli in the peripheral circulation include ulcerated atherosclerotic plaques and aneurysm formation in any of the major arteries such as the aorta, the iliac,

Aetiology of emboli
• Heart
• Aneurysms
• Atherosclerotic plaques

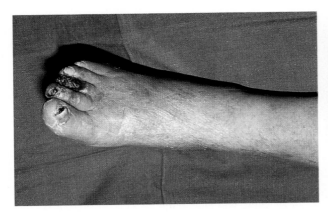

Fig. 25.1 Necrotic toe as a result of acute ischaemia on a background of chronic peripheral vascular disease.

Incidence of embolus has decreased as rheumatic fever has decreased.

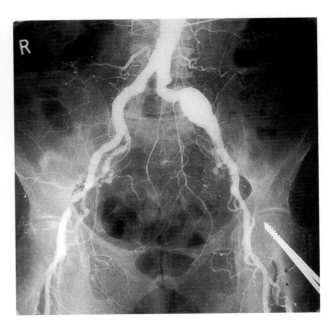

Fig. 25.2 Peripheral angiogram showing left common iliac aneurysm with occlusion of the left superficial femoral artery.

popliteal or subclavian vessels (Fig. 25.2). The final destination for peripheral emboli is unpredictable. Approximately 20% will involve the upper limbs or the cerebral vascular tree. Another 30% will involve the aorta or its branches and the remainder will involve the lower limbs. The size of the embolus will determine the site at which it lodges. However, emboli frequently lodge at the point of bifurcation of major arteries such as the common femoral artery or the tibioperoneal trunk. In the absence of pre-existing collateral circulation, a complete occlusion of a major proximal artery will result in immediate and profound ischaemia. When both lower limbs are affected simultaneously, the aorta should be suspected as a source of embolization in the absence of cardiac disease. Popliteal artery aneurysms are particularly ominous and may present with distal embolization or more proximal ischaemia due to acute thrombosis of the aneurysm.

Other causes of arterial emboli include tumour, amniotic fluid, foreign bodies and air. Iatrogenic ischaemia is seen occasionally following interventional procedures with guide wires and catheters.

Thrombosis

Arterial thrombosis may occur under diverse circumstances. Most commonly it will occur in arteries with pre-existing atherosclerotic occlusive disease and the degree of subsequent ischaemia will depend on the previous existence of collateral circulation and whether there is significant occlusive disease elsewhere in the peripheral circulation. These patients are usually elderly and have the usual risk factors for peripheral vascular disease such as cigarette

smoking, hypertension and diabetes. Pre-existing symptoms of intermittent claudication in the absence of a cardiac rhythm abnormality is a strong indicator of thrombosis rather than embolic occlusion. In such patients, thrombosis of even a relatively large artery may not be particularly significant. On the other hand in the presence of occlusive disease elsewhere in the limb it may progress a patient from relatively stable intermittent claudication to rest pain and critical ischaemia.

An increasingly common cause of acute limb ischaemia is the failure of previous arterial reconstruction such as bypass grafting. This can occur at any stage. Immediately postoperatively it is likely to be caused by technical errors or inappropriate selection of patients. During the first 2 years postoperatively, the likely cause of failure is neo-intimal hyperplasia. Occlusion of bypass grafts at a later date is likely to be caused by progression of atherosclerosis either proximal or distal to the graft.

Trauma

Arterial injuries secondary to blunt or penetrating trauma frequently result in limb-threatening ischaemia. The mechanism of injury includes partial or complex vessel transection and vessel wall contusion with secondary thrombosis and intimal damage. Blunt trauma is more likely to occur in road traffic accidents while penetrating trauma is likely to be due to knife and gunshot injuries. Patients with fractures of the long bones are particularly prone to arterial injury and the peripheral circulation should always be carefully assessed in such circumstances. Common sites of injury include supracondylar dislocations or fractures of the humerus (Fig. 25.3) or femur, tibial plateau fractures affecting the popliteal artery and, less commonly, clavicular or upper rib fractures affecting the subclavian artery.

Miscellaneous

There are many other less common causes of arterial occlusion. Occlusion of a peripheral *aneurysm* can be a particularly sinister development. Aneurysms can embolize distally with few obvious clinical consequences. However, over a period of time, this will lead to many of the smaller end arteries being occluded. Should the aneurysm itself then occlude it may prove difficult to revascularize as the run off will be compromised. This is particularly true of popliteal artery aneurysms.

Massive soft tissue swelling can lead to *compartment syndromes* and this is seen following trauma, acute massive venous thrombosis (phlegmasia cerulea dolens) and ironically following revascularization. Haematological abnormalities such as thrombocytosis, disseminated intravascular coagulopathy and polycythaemia rubor vera may also lead to acute arterial thrombosis.

Inflammatory conditions of the arterial wall such as *thromboangiitis obliterans* (also known as Buerger's disease) can also produce occlusion. *Takayasu's disease* affects the thoracic and abdominal aorta and it's major branches and is a form of arteritis which can result in severe stenoses or occlusion. The role of reconstructive surgery is controversial

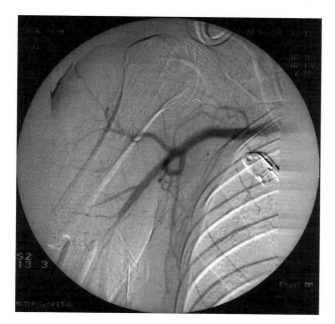

Fig. 25.3 Upper limb angiogram demonstrating acute occlusion of the brachial artery associated with a fracture of the humerus.

in the management of this condition. *Adventitial cystic disease* occurs most commonly in the popliteal arteries of young males. It usually presents as intermittent claudication but should be considered in the differential diagnosis of acute ischaemia in the younger patient. *Popliteal entrapment syndrome* produces thrombosis of the popliteal artery caused by an anatomic abnormality with the popliteal artery abnormally situated in relation to the medial head of the gastrocnemius muscle. This results in extrinsic pressure on the arterial wall leading to stenosis and post-stenotic dilatation with eventual thrombosis. A further cause of acute limb ischaemia is *aortic dissection*. The limb ischaemia may occur as the sole presenting symptom or may be part of a complex clinical picture. Systemic causes of arterial thrombosis include congestive cardiac failure with reduced cardiac output, septicaemia and disseminated malignancy.

Unfortunately, in the modern world it is becoming increasingly common to see acutely ischaemic hands or feet in intravenous drug abusers secondary to inadvertent intra-arterial injections. The mechanism is either arterial thrombosis at the site of injection, particulate embolization with obstruction of digital arteries or venous stasis and thrombosis.

Significance of ischaemia

The immediate effects of ischaemia will depend on whether the arterial circulation was previously normal or atherosclerotic. Normal arteries which are acutely occluded may lead to tissue necrosis within a matter of hours. The effects may be less severe in the presence of collateral vessels which have been already established. Profound ischaemia lasting in excess of 6 h is likely to produce irreversible muscle and nerve necrosis. Usually, soft tissues will be less vulnerable. Revascularization of ischaemic tissue carries potential systemic side effects such as acidosis and hyperkalaemia leading to cardiac dysrhythmias. Other risks include respiratory distress syndrome secondary to platelet aggregates embolizing to the lung and acute renal failure secondary to myoglobin.

Clinical assessment

All patients with acute limb ischaemia require a thorough history and physical examination with a view to establishing the cause and severity of the ischaemia and the presence of comorbid conditions. A history of cardiorespiratory symptoms, diabetes, smoking habits and drug ingestion is recorded. The classic signs and symptoms of acute ischaemia include the 'Five Ps' of pain, parasthaesia, pulseless, pallor, and paralysis. A sixth—'perishing with the cold'—is often added. Pain is a predominant feature, occurring particularly in the calf muscles and the distal extremity. In some patients, particularly diabetics, pain may not be pronounced. A motor deficit is not always reliable in assessing the degree of ischaemia as there may often appear to be muscle function in a non-viable limb because of the action of more proximal muscle groups. However, sensory deficit is an important sign to elicit and when present it indicates severe ischaemia which, if unrelieved will lead to irreversible changes within 6–8 h. Absence of capillary return and/or fixed mottling of the skin is also a firm indicator of critical ischaemia and in combination with loss of sensation generally indicates a non-viable limb. In the early stages, the acutely ischaemic limb is pale but later becomes cyanosed and mottled. Fixed skin discoloration is a late sign and usually indicates non viability of the limb.

The presence of pulses is recorded and compared to the contralateral limb. The femoral pulse is a guide to differentiation between aorto-iliac and femoropopliteal occlusion. Popliteal, femoral or abdominal aortic aneurysms are sought by palpation. The presence of atrial fibrillation is noted. In the absence of palpable pulses, the ankle pressure is easily measured with a sphygmomanometer cuff above the ankle and a Doppler flow probe. An absolute ankle pressure below 40 mmHg denotes severe or critical ischaemia.

In acute ischaemia, the main distinction is between embolus or *in situ* thrombosis. Factors pointing to an embolic aetiology include an absence of prior claudication, the presence of a cardiac lesion such as atrial fibrillation or recent myocardial infarction and palpable pedal pulses in the contralateral non-ischaemic limb.

Management

Blood is drawn for haemoglobin estimation, renal, electrolyte and clotting profiles. Blood is grouped and cross-matched. Intravenous fluids are administered to correct dehydration and a urinary catheter is passed for hourly urine estimation. A chest X-ray and electrocardiograph (ECG) are performed. A central venous line is inserted if the patient is haemodynamically unstable. Adequate analgesia, which will often include intravenous narcotics is administered.

The further management depends on the degree of limb ischaemia, and the best guide to this is the presence of a sensory deficit. In the absence of sensory deficit, there is no absolute indication for emergency surgical intervention. The patient should be anticoagulated with intravenous heparin, adequately hydrated and nursed in the vascular position with the head of the bed raised to 15°. Careful attention is paid to preventing pressure on the heels and toes

with the use of a bed cradle and heel protection. Frequent clinical review of the limb is essential to detect worsening ischaemia which would mandate immediate surgical intervention. Definitive treatment is undertaken on a semi-urgent basis and is guided by the underlying aetiology. Angiography is performed and consideration should be given to intra-arterial thrombolytic therapy (IATT). If thrombolysis is unavailable or unsuitable then revascularisation by embolectomy, thrombectomy or bypass is performed, as determined by the angiographic findings (Figs 25.4 and 25.5).

Limb ischaemia with sensory motor deficit is a surgical emergency and active intervention is urgently required. In cases judged to be caused by embolus in the absence of significant peripheral vascular disease, the patient is transferred immediately to the operating theatre with a view to performing femoral embolectomy. Angiography is not essential in clear-cut cases of embolus but this presentation is

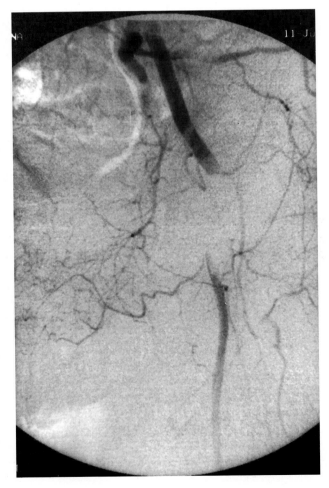

Fig. 25.4 Peripheral angiogram showing acute occlusion of the common femoral artery. Note the smooth cut off and the absence of the profunda femoral artery suggesting an embolic aetiology.

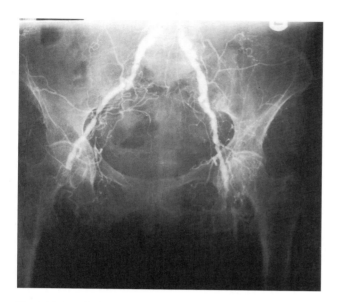

Fig. 25.5 Peripheal angiogram showing occlusion of both common femoral arteries. However, in contrast to Fig. 25.4, all vessels show evidence of chronic atherosclerosis.

increasingly rare. The type of anaesthesia to be given should be discussed at an early stage with the anaesthetist. If spinal or epidural anaesthesia is chosen, heparin is withheld until the anaesthetic has been given. If there is any delay in transferring the patient to the operating theatre heparin should be given and embolectomy is then performed either under local infiltration anaesthesia or general anaesthetic.

If the diagnosis is of *in situ* thrombosis, pre-operative arteriography is mandatory. Ideally this is performed by an experienced vascular radiologist in the radiology suite and important information regarding the inflow, the site and length of occlusion and the distal outflow tract is obtained. IATT should be considered, but unless rapidly successful treatment should proceed to thrombectomy or bypass as determined by the angiographic findings. In cases of iliac occlusion, extra anatomical bypass such as a femorofemoral bypass or axillofemoral bypass is an alternative if the patient is unfit for emergency aortofemoral bypass. Where femoropopliteal occlusion occurs, femoropopliteal or femorotibial bypass may be required.

Following revascularization of an ischaemic limb, there is always a degree of muscle swelling which is proportional to the severity and duration of ischaemia. Muscle swelling contained within the fascial boundaries of the lower limb may itself compromise arterial inflow and venous outflow and should be treated by early fasciotomy. The threshold for performing fasciotomy following revascularization should be low.

Release of myoglobin from damaged muscle may precipitate renal failure secondary to acute tubular necrosis.

Adequate hydration, mannitol induced diuresis and alkalinization of the urine will protect against renal failure.

Intra-arterial thrombolytic therapy (IATT)

Intra-arterial thrombolysis was first described by Dotter in 1974. Three thrombolytic agents are in common usage today: streptokinase, urokinase and tissue plasminogen activator (TPA). The greatest clinical experience is with streptokinase. Its major drawbacks include a relatively long half-life of 27 min and a high incidence of allergic reactions. Streptokinase is relatively inexpensive and is used at a dose of 5000 U/h intra-arterially. Urokinase is the most widely used thrombolytic agent in the United States. It is expensive compared to streptokinase but the incidence of allergy is low. The standard dose of intra-arterial urokinase is 60 000 U/h. TPA is now produced commercially following sequencing and cloning of its DNA structure. TPA acts preferentially on thrombus-bound plasminogen, with a consequent reduction in systemic effects and reduced haemorrhagic complications. It has a short half-life of approximately 6 min and has no allergic side effects. It is considerably more expensive than streptokinase. The standard dose for intra-arterial use is 0.5–1.0 mg/h. The technique of IATT has developed in concert with catheter technology. Cannulation of the arterial tree is performed at a site remote from the point of thrombolysis to minimize haemorrhagic complications at the arterial puncture site. The contralateral femoral artery is used if the occlusion is at iliac or proximal femoral level. Occlusions in the distal superficial femoral artery or popliteal artery are approached by antegrade ipsilateral femoral puncture. A guide wire is directed into the thrombus to create a short track and finally an infusion catheter is positioned into the proximal thrombus. Infusion of the thrombolytic agent is started at a predetermined dose and the patient is systemically heparinized to prevent pericatheter thrombosis. Close monitoring of vital signs and the arterial puncture site are essential. Follow up angiography is performed at 4–6 h intervals with further advancement of the catheter if successful lysis has occurred. Where no thrombolysis is observed, the infusion rate is doubled. If the leg is deteriorating or if there is no improvement within 24 h, the procedure should be abandoned.

All patients who present with spontaneous lower limb ischaemia should be considered for IATT if facilities are

Steps in thrombolysis
• Catheter placed in thrombus
• Infusion commenced
• Check angiography
• Continue to increase dose
• Surgery if not resolved at 24 hours

available. Patients most likely to benefit are those with thrombosis secondary to peripheral vascular disease, in whom there is no sensory motor deficit. Catheter thrombectomy in this situation is unlikely to be successful and intimal damage secondary to passage of the embolectomy catheter may exacerbate thrombosis. In contrast, clearance of thrombus with IATT is atraumatic to the endothelium and may reveal a stenosis amenable to angioplasty. Other indications for IATT include recently occluded bypass graft and thrombosed popliteal aneurysms although this latter indication remains controversial.

Until recently, sensory motor deficit was considered a contra-indication to the use of IATT because of the time factor involved in clot dissolution. These patients require urgent revascularization to preserve motor and sensory function. Accelerated IATT involves passage of a multiple side-hole catheter into the thrombosis and the injection of high doses of TPA (5 mg) using a high-pressure pulse spray infuser. Three bolus doses of TPA are injected at 5 min intervals and angiography repeated. If no lysis is observed after 30 min, the procedure is abandoned in favour of appropriate vascular reconstruction.

Contra-indications to the use of IATT include patients at high risk of haemorrhage. Patients who have had a recent cerebrovascular accident or surgical procedure, an active peptic ulcer or bleeding diathesis are also excluded. Complications of IATT include adverse reactions to the thrombolytic agent, usually streptokinase. Haemorrhagic complications usually occur at the arterial puncture site but there is a small risk of haemorrhagic stroke (approximately 1%).

Experience with IATT is accumulating. It offers an attractive alternative to potentially difficult bypass surgery. It is, however, labour intensive, requires close co-operation between vascular radiologist, surgeon and nursing staff and should not be seen as an easy alternative to surgery. Where facilities exist, most ischaemic limbs should at least be considered for IATT.

Femoral embolectomy

The changing aetiology of acute lower limb ischaemia has seen a decline in the use of femoral embolectomy in favour of IATT or surgical bypass. Embolectomy, however, remains the treatment for patients with acute ischaemia secondary to embolus in the absence of significant peripheral vascular disease. When the clinical history and examination point to an embolic cause angiography is not always essential, particularly if it is likely to delay the necessary embolectomy. This is particularly true in cases of severe ischaemia where urgent revascularization is required and angiography delays definitive therapy. Most patients with a femoral embolus have a palpable femoral pulse which may be enhanced because of lack of outflow. If the femoral pulse is absent,

angiography should be performed to exclude iliac thrombosis or aortic dissection.

Femoral embolectomy may be performed under local anaesthesia, but should never be performed without an anaesthetist in attendance to monitor vital signs, the ECG and oxygen saturation. We believe that femoral embolectomy is best performed under regional or general anaesthesia and is more comfortable for both patient and surgeon alike. However, some patients will present with concomitant severe cardiac disease (e.g. post myocardial infarction) and they will require surgery under local anaesthesia.

Both groins and the entire ischaemic leg are prepared. The foot is placed in a transparent isolation bag so that its appearance can be monitored. The femoral artery is approached through a vertical groin incision placed directly over the femoral artery. Careful attention is paid to haemostasis. The common femoral, superficial femoral and profunda femoral arteries are isolated and controlled with silastic slings (Fig. 25.6). Heparin is administered at this point if it has not been given previously. The controlling silastic slings are tightened around the superficial femoral artery and the profunda artery and a vascular occlusion clamp is applied to the common femoral artery. There is some debate regarding the direction of the arteriotomy incision in the common femoral artery. We favour a transverse arteriotomy just proximal to the femoral bifurcation (Fig. 25.7). This is easier to close without risk of narrowing the lumen. If subsequently a bypass is required, a transverse arteriotomy is easily converted to a diamond incision.

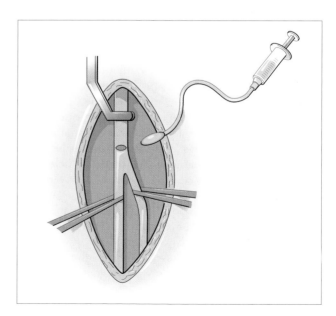

Fig. 25.6 Diagram to demonstrate exposure and control of the femoral arteries. The transverse arteriotomy in the common femoral artery is approximately 2–4 mm.

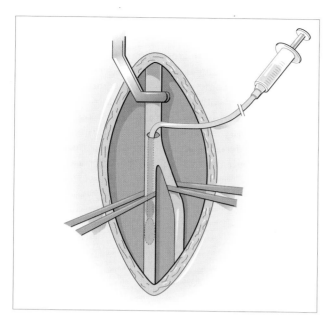

Fig. 25.7 The Fogarty embolectomy balloon catheter is passed through the embolus/thrombus and then inflated and withdrawn.

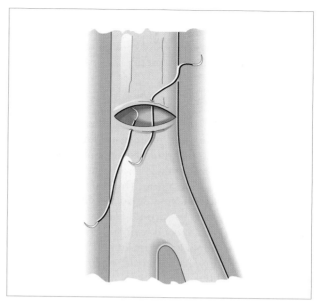

Fig. 25.8 The arteriotomy is closed using individual sutures with double needles passed from the inside of the artery out.

When the femoral artery is opened, visible thrombus is removed with a forceps. Partial release of the femoral clamp may flush out proximal thrombus. If good inflow is not established, a 4 or 5 French Fogarty embolectomy balloon catheter is passed proximally into the aorta. The balloon is inflated with saline and withdrawn gently. It is important not to overinflate the balloon as this will result in excessive intimal damage with the risk of subsequent rethrombosis. The embolectomy catheter may have to be passed several times to extract all thrombus. If the catheter fails to pass into the aorta or inflow is not established, angiography is performed. The likely diagnosis is iliac occlusion secondary to peripheral vascular disease. An extra anatomical bypass such as a femorofemoral bypass is then required.

Assuming good inflow is established by proximal embolectomy, a 4 French embolectomy catheter is then directed into the superficial, femoral and profunda arteries in turn (Fig. 25.7). The catheter is passed distally as far as possible but force should never be employed if arterial dissection or perforation is to be avoided. By filling the embolectomy balloon with contrast dye, the position of the embolectomy catheter can be monitored by fluoroscopy. The balloon is inflated and retrieved and the procedure repeated until no further thrombus is extracted.

Successful distal thrombectomy is usually followed by good backflow but this is not a reliable sign and completion angiography should be performed in all cases. If arteriography shows residual thrombus in the distal vessels, then repeat embolectomy is performed either at the same site or via a more distal vessel such as the popliteal artery. If this

fails, intra-operative thrombolysis may be considered. This is achieved by infusing 100 000 units of streptokinase in 50 ml of normal saline into the artery over a 20–30 min time period with the arterial inflow occluded. The angiogram is then repeated. The presence of persistent thrombus or occlusion necessitates popliteal exploration and possible embolectomy or bypass as determined by the operative findings.

Following successful embolectomy, the transverse femoral arteriotomy is closed with interrupted 5/0 Prolene sutures. The needles should pass from inside to outside of the artery to prevent a distal intimal flap forming (Fig. 25.8). The wound is closed in layers and wound drainage is not required. In cases of prolonged or severe ischaemia or where there is significant limb swelling, a fasciotomy of the lower limb is performed. Full anticoagulation is maintained postoperatively. Embolectomy should be undertaken only when there is the capacity to proceed to bypass if necessary.

Special considerations

Saddle embolus

A saddle embolus is a large embolus, almost invariably of cardiac origin, that occludes the aortic bifurcation. The clinical presentation is of sudden bilateral lower limb ischaemia. Such patients are often shocked with severe metabolic derangement. The differential diagnosis includes acute aortic thrombosis and aortic dissection. In the absence of femoral pulses, angiography is performed for a definitive diagnosis. Management of a saddle embolus follows the guidelines already given with aggressive resuscitation prior to urgent surgery. Surgery consists of simultaneous bilateral embolectomy via the femoral arteries.

Popliteal aneurysm

Popliteal aneurysms are prone to sudden spontaneous thrombosis which may precipitate acute limb-threatening ischaemia. The diagnosis of thrombosed popliteal aneurysm is often suspected because these aneurysms are frequently bilateral. The diagnosis is confirmed by a duplex ultrasonography or angiography. All symptomatic popliteal aneurysms require reconstruction. For acute ischaemia with sensory motor deficit, urgent surgery is required. Prereconstruction angiography determines the state of the run-off vessels. If no vessels are demonstrated, exploration of the below knee popliteal artery with thrombectomy and intra-operative thrombolysis of the distal run off may be the only option. Conventional surgery consists of aneurysmal exclusion with reverse vein bypass from the distal superficial femoral artery to the below knee popliteal artery. In cases of less severe ischaemia, IATT is often successful in recanalizing the thrombosed popliteal artery and defining the run off. If IATT is successful, aneurysm ligation and vein bypass are then performed on the same hospital admission.

Intra-arterial drug injection

Inadvertent intra-arterial drug injection is largely seen in intravenous drug abusers. The consequences of intra-arterial drug administration are dependant on the nature of the injected substance. Barbiturates cause direct endothelial damage to the vessel with resulting thrombosis and absent pulses. Fillers used to dilate drugs such as heroin cause particulate embolization with thrombosis of digital arteries and subsequent proximal propagation of clot. Early heparinization is the mainstay of treatment. Adequate hydration is important to prevent myoglobinuria. Angiography is performed where pulses are absent in order to detect a surgically correctable lesion at the injection site. IATT should be considered when distal vessels are occluded. Dextran 40 may improve the microcirculation. Early fasciotomy is performed in the presence of limb swelling to prevent further muscle damage secondary to the compartment syndrome.

Acute occlusion of the upper limb arteries

Upper limb ischaemia occurs less frequently than lower limb ischaemia. The causes of upper limb ischaemia are similar but arterial embolism accounts for 70% of cases. Atherosclerotic disease of upper limb vessels is uncommon

with a correspondingly reduced incidence of spontaneous thrombosis. Subclavian aneurysms may cause digital ischaemia secondary to micro-embolization (Fig. 25.9). The clinical findings are similar to those of lower limb ischaemia. Severe limb-threatening ischaemia is uncommon because of the well-developed collateral circulation to the arm. Clinical assessment is based on the examination of pulses and the presence of sensory motor deficit. If the nature or location of the occlusion are unclear, angiography is performed. The majority of upper limb emboli lodge in the distal brachial

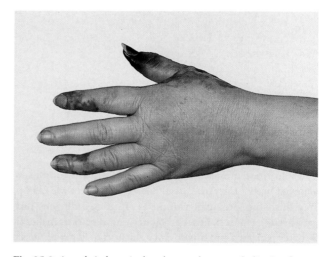

Fig. 25.9 Acutely ischaemic thumb secondary to embolization from a subclavian aneurysm.

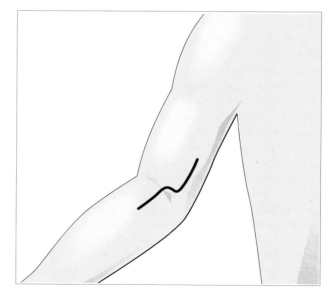

Fig. 25.10 Diagram to demonstrate the appropriate incision for brachial embolectomy.

artery. This artery is easily exposed through an 'S' incision at the anticubital fossa which also gives access to the ulnar and radial arteries (Fig. 25.10). Embolectomy is performed, as previously described. Intra-operative thrombolysis is helpful if distal thrombus is not removed by the embolectomy catheter. Occasionally, exposure of the radial or ulnar arteries at the wrist is required to remove adherent thrombus. The small brachial arteries should be opened longitudinally and repaired with a vein patch to prevent stenosis.

Thrombosis secondary to atherosclerotic disease usually requires direct exposure of the affected artery. The proximal, brachial and distal axillary artery are approached via a medial upper arm incision. The axillary artery can be readily exposed in the infraclavicular region by splitting the fibres of pectoralis major. Division of pectoralis minor gives additional exposure. Revascularization is then achieved as in the lower limb by either bypass or endarterectomy.

Summary

Although the range of treatment options for the acutely ischaemic limb has expanded considerably it remains a major challenge to limit the morbidity and mortality. This is largely because of the age group involved and the associated conditions which occur.

Further reading

Second European Consensus Document on Critical Leg Ischaemia. *European Journal of Vascular Surgery* (Supplement A) May 1992.

Bell, P.R.F., Jamieson, C.W. & Ruckley, C.V. (eds) (1992) *Surgical Management of Vascular Disease* W.B. Saunders Co., Ltd., Philadelphia.

Rutherford, R.B. (ed.) (1995) *Vascular Surgery* W.B. Saunders, Co Ltd., Philadelphia.

Reference

Dotter, C.T., Rosch, J. & Seaman, A.J. (1974) Selective clot lysis with low-dose streptokinase. *Radiology* 11 31.

CHAPTER 26

Abdominal aortic aneurysms

Roger M. Greenhalgh

Introduction

By far the commonest abdominal aneurysm which causes a surgical emergency is that of the infrarenal abdominal aorta followed by an aneurysm of the common iliac artery. Occasionally, a surgical emergency can be caused by the rupture of rare aneurysms such as splenic or renal aneurysms. In this chapter, we shall concentrate upon the common problem, ruptured aortic or ruptured aorto-iliac aneurysm. Aortic aneurysm, a swelling of the abdominal aorta, usually below the renal arteries, has a natural history of enlargement, bursting and death. The number of patients being admitted to hospital with this condition, has increased more than fivefold over the last 25 years. This can be attributed to several factors, including a more accurate diagnosis, improved surgical management and an increase in incidence. The available evidence suggests that there has been a true increase in the incidence of abdominal aortic aneurysm in England and Wales and similar trends have been observed in Australasia and North America. This increase in incidence, together with the swelling in ranks of the population most at risk (those over 60 years of age) has led to the treatment of abdominal aortic aneurysm imposing increasing burdens on the use of hospital resources. If all ruptured aortic aneurysms are taken together, the mortality rate is between 75–95%. Figure 26.1 demonstrates that some patients in the community with abdominal aortic aneurysm (AAA) have elective surgery and some elderly patients with AAA die without rupture. Others rupture, and the majority die before reaching hospital. Of those that reach hospital, some die before surgery and others are not suitable for surgery. Of those who have an operation, mortality rates of approximately 50% are reported. Bergqvist and Bengtsson reported on 212 aortic aneurysm ruptures, in whom they had good data from a population of 238 000, an incidence of 5.6 per 100 000 inhabitants. Of these, 91 were dead before arrival in hospital and a further 60 died in hospital without surgery. Only 61 were operated upon, from which 35 died. Thus, only 26 survived, 42% of those who were operated upon and 12% of those whose aortas originally ruptured, most of whom died before coming into hospital or before operation.

Diagnosis of ruptured aortic aneurysm

Aortic aneurysms are usually non-tender and asymptomatic and a decision is taken to operate upon them according to size. Most surgeons regard an asymptomatic non-tender aneurysm as requiring surgery if the diameter exceeds 5.5 cm. Otherwise, surgeons are inclined to operate urgently upon an aortic aneurysm when it is tender. Tenderness is thought to imply that an aorta is about to burst but it can also mean that there is increased inflammation in the aorta. It is easier to be certain if an aorta is tender than that symptoms are coming from an aorta. The term symptomatic aortic aneurysm is rather misleading. Many surgeons regard an aortic aneurysm associated with intermittent claudication as a symptomatic aneurysm. Others would attribute back ache or abdominal pain to an abdominal aortic aneurysm but frequently the abdominal pain or back ache can be caused by something else. Pinning symptoms on an aortic aneurysm is very difficult. The classic symptoms are of abdominal pain, back ache and diarrhoea. Diarrhoea is thought to be caused by an occlusion of the inferior mesenteric artery with consequent relative ischaemic colitis. These are the symptoms which are occasionally attributed to an abdominal aorta. Tenderness is a much more reliable finding and surgeons are inclined to attribute urgency to an abdominal aortic aneurysm in which they elicit tenderness. If the tenderness is of sudden onset, the possibility of rupture is considered and a computerized tomography (CT) scan is mandatory to see if a leak has occurred.

Any patient who is admitted urgently in a state of collapse with abdominal pain, peritonitis and abdominal rigidity should be suspected of having a ruptured abdominal aortic aneurysm. Where a leak has occurred into the peritoneal cavity, it is unlikely that the patient will have survived. The ones that arrive at hospital are the ones who have a contained leak, held by the retroperitoneal tissues. The abdominal wall is held rigid and the patient is frequently shocked, with a cold, pale, sweaty countenance. It can be very difficult to feel the abdominal aorta and a past history of intermittent claudication or of known abdominal aortic aneurysm is important. A family history of abdominal aortic aneurysm from a relative is also a useful pointer. If the abdomen is held rigidly,

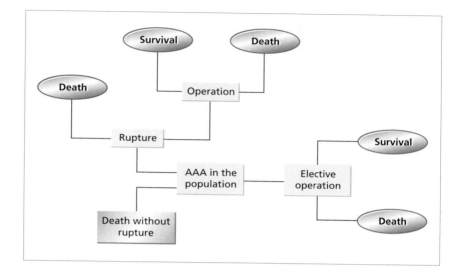

Fig. 26.1 Schematic representation of the distribution of abdominal aortic aneurysm. After Bergqvist and Bengtsson in *Emergency Vascular Surgery* (eds R.M. Greenhalgh and L.H. Hollier). W.B. Saunders, London and Philadelphia, 1992.

it can be quite impossible to be certain about an abdominal aortic aneurysm but one can be felt on some occasions. Those with an abdominal aortic aneurysm, tend to have wide arteries elsewhere and the femoral arteries should be palpated. If these are wide, this is a useful pointer also. If an urgent ultrasound of the abdominal wall in the Accident and Emergency Department is available, this could be a useful move to confirm initial thoughts of diagnosis. If the patient has a tender aortic aneurysm, a CT scan must be performed and if no leak has occurred, the patient should be admitted and operated upon, on the next convenient elective list. Where contained rupture has occurred, the patient must be made ready for the operating room as soon as is reasonably possible.

Literature review suggests the following possible contra-indications for operating for ruptured abdominal aortic aneurysm arriving alive at hospital. These are by no means absolute.

- Age, e.g. over 85 years.
- Recent myocardial infarction.
- Intractable congestive cardiac failure.
- Advanced malignancy with limited life expectancy.
- Renal failure and creatinine level above 250 μmol/L.
- Severe dyspnoea at rest and respiratory disease.
- Incapacitating mental disability and cerebrovascular events.
- Extension of aneurysmal disease above the renal arteries.
- Pre-operative circulatory arrest.

It is frustrating that even though more than 3000 aortic aneurysms are operated upon electively per year, ruptured aneurysm accounts for almost 10 000 deaths per year in England and Wales. This has led to a call for screening programmes in the community and ever more intra-abdominal ultrasound scanning in elderly patients with abdominal dis-

comfort or manifestations of atherosclerosis. The population screening studies will not be discussed further here but it should be noted that approximately 10% of patients with either myocardial infarction, carotid artery disease or peripheral arterial disease will have an abdominal aortic aneurysm on abdominal ultrasound scanning and every effort should be made for ultrasound scanning of the abdomen of such elderly patients if they come into hospital.

The UK Small Aneurysm Trial has recruited approximately 1000 patients with non-tender asymptomatic abdominal aortic aneurysm, measuring between 4.0 and 5.5 cm. These have been randomly allocated into equal groups, either for surgery or follow up.

Recruitment has now ceased and the follow up arm of the study continues and results will be announced in autumn 1998. From the study, it is expected that the size of aorta at which aneurysm should be operated upon will be determined.

Assembling the emergency team

Once the signal is given that a patient could have an abdominal aortic aneurysm, it is vital to alert the team. The patient is normally received in the resuscitation area of the Accident and Emergency Department and a senior on-call anaesthetist must be alerted to receive the patient. The surgical team of operating surgeon and first assistant and two other assistants should be standing by. The operating theatre is alerted to make preparation. The haematologist on call is alerted to receive a blood sample for haemoglobin and full blood count, blood group and sample for cross-matching the moment the patient arrives. A baseline clotting screen is helpful.

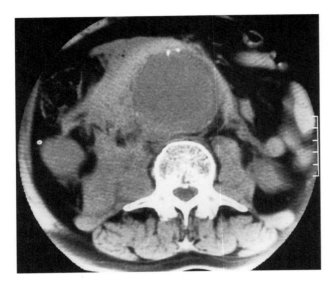

Fig. 26.2 CT scan of infrarenal aortic aneurysm showing a very thin wall and the leak posteriorly on the right into a space behind the lower pole of the kidney.

On arrival, the patient is assessed by the anaesthetic and surgical team and a brief assessment of the patient is made with a history as two large intravenous lines are set up and electrocardiogram connected to the patient for monitoring. A history of sudden abdominal pain, collapse or back ache are very pertinent. Past history of heart and lung disease and a past history of any arterial problem are sought from the relatives. It is important to determine what the quality of life of the patient has been in recent months in deciding if a life-saving operation is indicated. Central venous access is required once an acute myocardial infarction has been excluded and usually eight units of blood are requested in the first instance. Fresh frozen plasma should be available, one unit for every second unit of blood transfused. Resuscitation is limited to maintaining systolic blood pressure over 80 mmHg by slow infusion of plasma expanders. The blood is not infused until surgery is imminent. The patient is kept warm, and an oxygen mask is provided. A chest X-ray is essential to assess the diameter of the thoracic aorta and a urinary catheter is passed to measure urine output. Abdominal ultrasound is usually easy to perform but skilled interpretation is required. A decision is taken, if there is time, for a CT scan in any patient who is

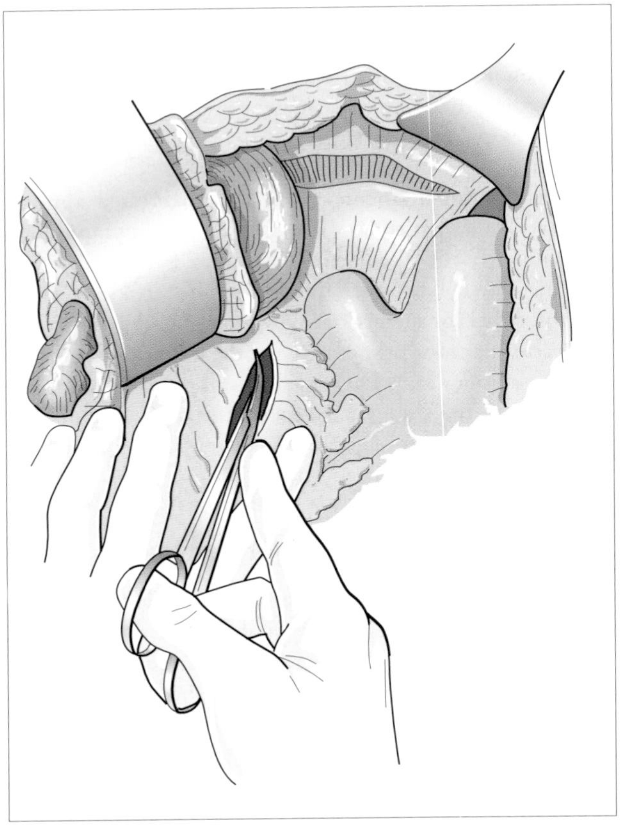

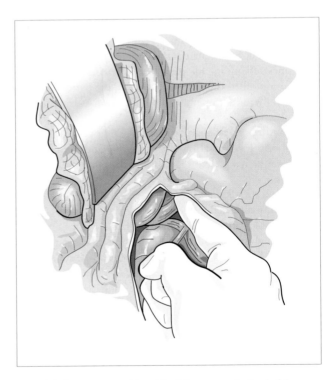

Fig. 26.3 Approaching the aorta at the level of the diaphragm. After Mannick, J.A. and Whittemore, A.D. in *Vascular and Endovascular Surgical Techniques*, 3rd edn (ed. R.M. Greenhalgh). W.B. Saunders, London and Philadelphia, 1994, p. 236.

Fig. 26.4 Fingers passes either side of the aorta at the level of the diaphragm. After Mannick, J.A. and Whittemore, A.D. in *Vascular and Endovascular Surgical Techniques*, 3rd edn (ed. R.M. Greenhalgh). W.B. Saunders, London and Philadelphia, 1994.

not absolutely collapsed. A CT scan should be performed if it can be achieved swiftly; 10-mm slices are all that are required. This can give vital and helpful information about the dimensions of the thoracic aorta and aorta around the renal vessels. A CT scan also confirms or excludes the diagnosis of ruptured abdominal aorta. In addition, vital information about the iliac arteries is provided. There are then fewer surprises at operation.

It should be remembered that the majority of patients with a ruptured aortic aneurysm will not survive long enough to reach the hospital. In addition, the criteria mentioned above, for avoiding emergency aneurysm repair should now be considered. The patient under consideration thus represents a subset of all of those whose aortas have ruptured. This patient is the lucky one to have survived thus far. The mind-set of the surgeon and team must be to recognize that if the diagnosis is a ruptured abdominal aortic aneurysm, that the rupture is likely to be contained behind the peritoneum. CT scan is very helpful in this situation to confirm or refute the diagnosis in a sick patient (Fig. 26.2).

Transfer to the operating room

The resuscitated patient is transferred swiftly to the operating suite, observed closely by a resident anaesthetist. If time permits, and if the respiratory and cardiovascular state of the patient is poor, the anaesthetist will take a decision whether epidural anaesthesia is required which could seriously reduce the need for full general anaesthetic and heavy analgesic. The majority of patients, however, can expect to have a general anaesthetic and in these, patients should be anaesthetized on the operating table, not on a trolley. It is conventional to paint the skin of the patient on the operating table and put towels in place and to use the so-called 'crash' intubation system. This is because it is desirable that there should be a very short time between the introduction of anaesthesia and relaxation of the abdominal muscles and the incision to allow control of the aortic aneurysm.

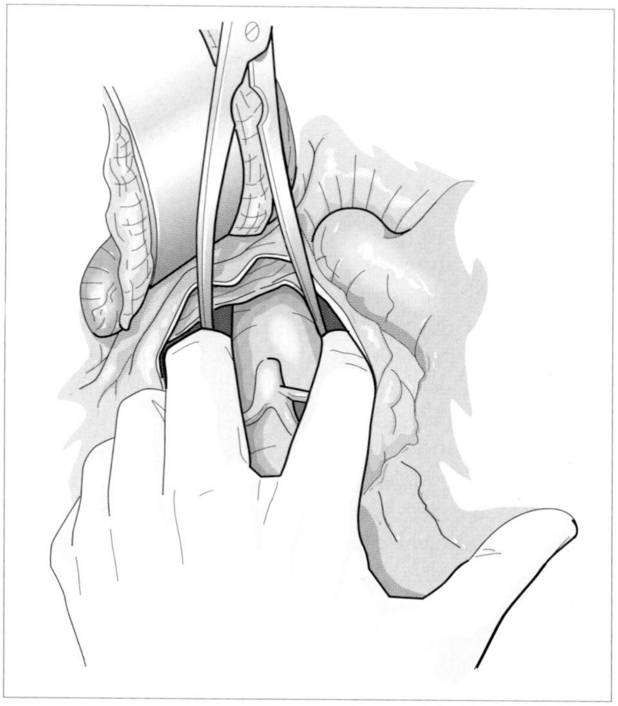

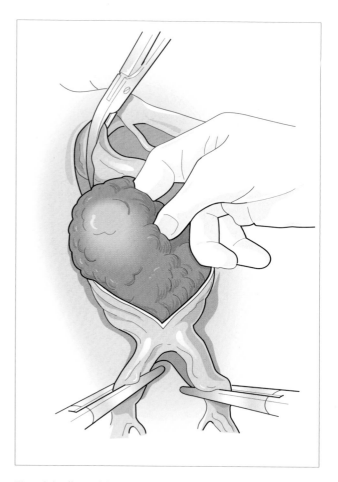

Fig. 26.5 Whilst the fingers of the left hand expose the aorta, the right hand is used to place a clamp just inside the diaphragm. After Mannick, J.A. and Whittemore, A.D. in *Vascular and Endovascular Surgical Techniques*, 3rd edn (ed. R.M. Greenhalgh). W.B. Saunders, London and Philadelphia, 1994.

Fig. 26.6 All mural thrombus and loose embolic and sclerotic debris are evacuated. After Mannick, J.D. and Whittemore, A.D. in *Vascular and Endovascular Surgical Techniques*, 3rd edn (ed. R.M. Greenhalgh). W.B. Saunders, London and Philadelphia, 1994.

Operation technique

The surgeon usually stands to the right of the patient with the first assistant opposite. At the cranial end of the patient on each side, ideally, there should be a third and fourth assistant, required especially at the beginning of the operation for retraction whilst control is achieved. The usual approach is the midline transperitoneal incision. This has the advantage of rapid access to the aorta and iliac arteries. A rapid laparotomy is performed; one would expect to see a large haematoma in the retroperitoneal tissues with staining which may lead to swelling at the root of the bowel. The aorta is approached at the level of the diaphragm by incising the attachments at the left lobe of the liver to the diaphragm and retracting the liver to the right. The lesser sac is entered and the aorta is exposed as it passes underneath the crus of the diaphragm (Fig. 26.3).

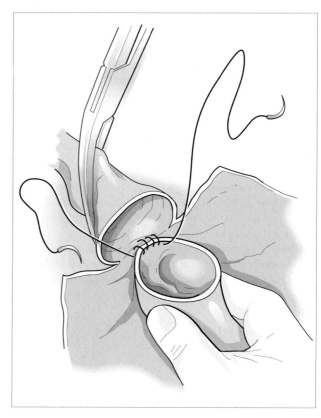

Fig. 26.8 Anastomosis of the infrarenal aorta. After Mannick, J.D. and Whittemore, A.D. in *Vascular and Endovascular Surgical Techniques*, 3rd edn (ed. R.M. Greenhalgh). W.B. Saunders, London and Philadelphia, 1994.

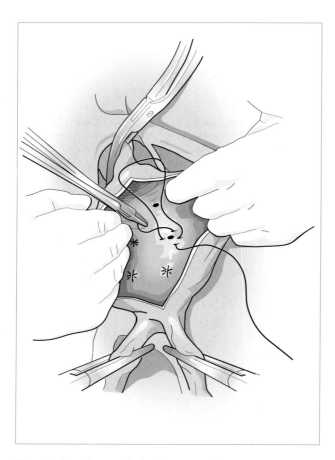

Fig. 26.7 Transfixion of the lumbar vessels. After Mannick, J.D. and Whittemore, A.D. in *Vascular and Endovascular Surgical Techniques*, 3rd edn (ed. R.M. Greenhalgh). W.B. Saunders, London and Philadelphia, 1994.

With finger dissection, the crus of the diaphragm can be stretched and split enough so that the fingers can be placed either side of the aorta at the level of the diaphragmatic hiatus where the aorta is usually of normal calibre and without branches (Fig. 26.4). A traditional slightly curved aortic clamp is then placed alongside the fingers between the diaphragm and the coeliac axis (Fig. 26.5). No attempt is made to put the fingers behind the aorta. A useful clamp to use is the so-called Mattox clamp. This is a conventional DeBakey clamp with the handles bent backwards out of the way of the operator. Once in place, the large retractors are moved so as to expose the infracolic portion of the abdominal aorta. The next move is to find the plane alongside the iliac arteries and apply clamps. The angled DeBakey type are suitable. Care must be taken not to injure the common iliac veins behind: these are often adherent to the arteries. No dissection behind the iliac arteries is necessary and slings should not be used. The angled DeBakey clamps are merely placed alongside the iliac arteries and applied.

At this point, it is sometimes difficult to recognize the infrarenal abdominal aorta because of the haematoma. With the inflow and most of the back-bleed controlled, it is best to approach the abdominal aorta directly and clear the peritoneum off it. If the infrarenal neck cannot be found easily and without damage to neighbouring structures, a knife incision is made into the aneurysmal sac which is opened with curved Mayo scissors. Back-bleeding is quite little and the aortotomy is taken up to the neck of the aneurysm above and to the bifurcation below. Horizontal cuts are made so as to open the aorta like the leaves of a book. With a finger of the left hand in the neck of the aorta above, fingers of the right hand find the plane outside the aorta and an aortic clamp is then placed below the renal vessels. At this stage, the suprarenal clamp can be released. One needs to note the time of warm ischaemia to the kidneys: it is usually less than 10 min. Thrombus is removed from the aortic sac, as for elective surgery (Fig. 26.6) and lumbar vessels are transfixed from within the aorta (Fig. 26.7). If the inferior mesenteric

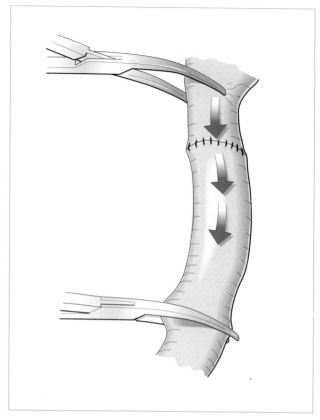

Fig. 26.10 Checking the aortic suture line. After Mannick, J.D. and Whittemore, A.D. in *Vascular and Endovascular Surgical Techniques*, 3rd edn (ed. R.M. Greenhalgh). W.B. Saunders, London and Philadelphia, 1994.

artery bleeds back, it is transfixed similarly from within the aortic sac. Care is taken not to ligate the inferior mesenteric artery outside of the aorta. Heparin is usually not used for leaking abdominal aortic aneurysm although a small amount of heparin, say 2000 units intravenously can be given, once the clamps are in place; this discourages intra-arterial thrombosis below the clamps if it is thought that the procedure might, for some reason, be delayed. Normally, no heparin is required. The aim is to use a straight woven Dacron tube if at all possible. To determine this, the site of the rupture should be found. Usually the rupture is easy to find and more often than not it is on the left side of the aorta, towards the lower end. Occasionally, rupture can be into the vena cava and occasionally it is a common iliac aneurysm which ruptures. If the iliac arteries are significantly aneurysmal, these should be opened with the scissors down to the point where the aneurysmal disease is less marked. Usually, this will be at the bifurcation of the common iliac arteries.

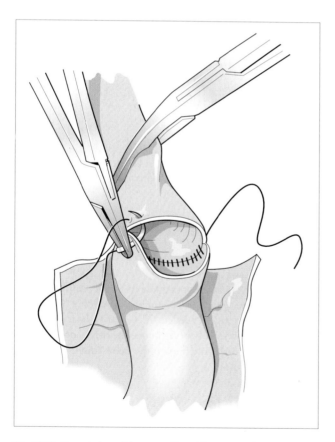

Fig. 26.9 Completion of the suture line. After Mannick, J.D. and Whittemore, A.D. in *Vascular and Endovascular Surgical Techniques*, 3rd edn (ed. R.M. Greenhalgh). W.B. Saunders, London and Philadelphia, 1994.

A tube graft is usually possible (about 70%) although occasionally, as mentioned, a bifurcation graft is required. Woven Dacron is ideal for emergency aneurysm surgery; it does not leak and does not require to be pre-clotted. A 3.0 polypropylene suture with double arm is used for anastomosis (Fig. 26.8) and the suture is carried around from each side of the neck of the aneurysm and tied at the front (Fig. 26.9). The Dacron is divided with straight scissors and the proximal suture line is checked (Fig. 26.10). This is usually achieved by applying a cloth-covered clamp to the Dacron and releasing the infrarenal aortic clamp. Following this, anastomosis of the lower end is performed with double-armed polypropylene 3.0 suture (Fig. 26.11) using a similar technique at the upper end. The aneurysmal sac is closed over the Dacron for bowel protection using a suitably strong absorbable suture such as polyglycolate (Fig. 26.12). For more extensive disease involving the iliac vessels, a bifurcation graft is used

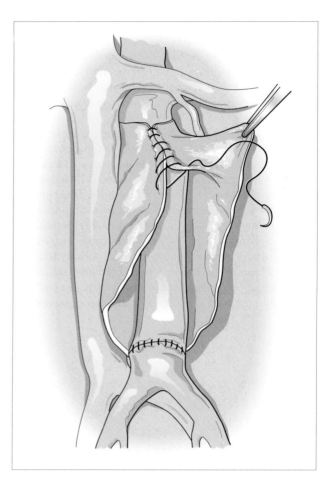

Fig. 26.12 Closing the aneurysm sac for bowel protection. After Mannick, J.D. and Whittemore, A.D. in *Vascular and Endovascular Surgical Techniques*, 3rd edn (ed. R.M. Greenhalgh). W.B. Saunders, London and Philadelphia, 1994.

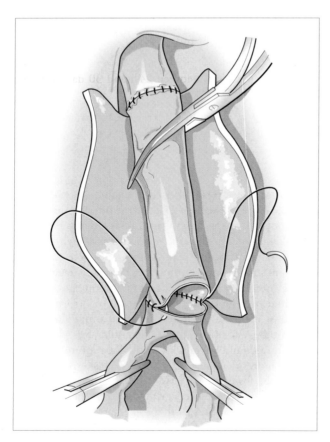

Fig. 26.11 The lower anastomosis. After Mannick, J.D. and Whittemore, A.D. in *Vascular and Endovascular Surgical Techniques*, 3rd edn (ed. R.M. Greenhalgh). W.B. Saunders, London and Philadelphia, 1994.

(Fig. 26.13). Every attempt is made to do the simplest emergency procedure which is the straight tube inlay operation. If a bifurcation graft is needed, it is vital to anastomose at least one limb, preferably both, above the origin of the internal iliac arteries to ensure flow to the pelvis and especially to the lowermost colon.

Autotransfusion

A variety of cell-saving autotransfusion devices are available and the enthusiasm for surgeons to use these is mixed. In an enthusiastic centre, the autotransfusion device can be set up rapidly and the patient's own blood returned to the patient which significantly reduces the need for banked blood being used.

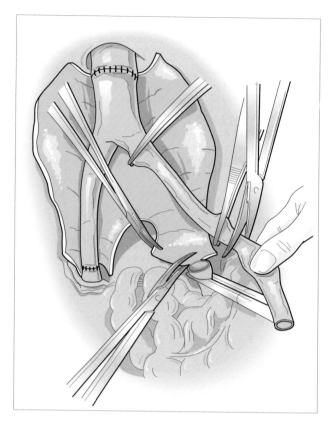

Fig. 26.13 Use of a bifurcation graft. After Mannick, J.D. and Whittemore, A.D. in *Vascular and Endovascular Surgical Techniques*, 3rd edn (ed. R.M. Greenhalgh). W.B. Saunders, London and Philadelphia, 1994.

Postoperative care

The patient will almost always require ventilation for some time, usually until the temperature is satisfactory. This virtually implies that the patient needs to be recovered in an intensive care environment, although some high-dependency units and recovery units can be used to great advantage. My personal inclination is to press for extubation as soon as is reasonably possible so that the patient can cough and be alert and to do as much for themselves as possible. It is always gratifying to see a patient able to move around and be encouraged to avoid venous thromboses and other postoperative complications by being able to enter into an active recovery programme. There is an inclination among some anaesthetists to delay extubation and to continue the intensive care regimen for rather longer than is absolutely required. To achieve the optimal extubation timing, surgeons must take a very detailed interest in the postoperative management of the patient and not leave this entirely to the specialists in critical care: a partnership is required.

In my own series of patients who undergo aortic surgery for ruptured aortic aneurysm, the mortality rate is approximately 11% at 24 h but with regret, this rises to 42% after 30 days. The average age of the patient is approximately 70 years and the cardiovascular and pulmonary complications between 24 h and 30 days are very significant.

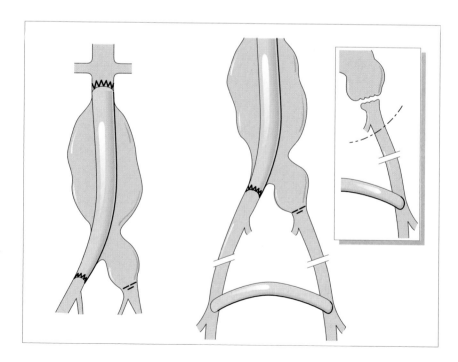

Fig. 26.14 The aorto-uni-iliac stent–graft system with femorofemoral cross-over graft. After Mannick, J.D. and Whittemore, A.D. in *Vascular and Endovascular Surgical Techniques*, 3rd edn (ed. R.M. Greenhalgh). W.B. Saunders, London and Philadelphia, 1994.

The future of the endovascular stent graft technique for ruptured abdominal aortic aneurysm

Yusef and Hopkinson have reported (letter in *Lancet* 1994) that it is feasible to use an aorto uni-iliac stent graft technique for the correction of abdominal aortic aneurysm. They have now performed the procedure several times and although the technique is in its infancy, results are encouraging. This can only be applied in patients in whom the rupture is contained. However, it is plain to see how this approach could produce an enormous advance and improvement in the mortality figures. First of all, the abdomen is not opened, nor is a general anaesthetic required. A stent–graft system is introduced through a small incision in the femoral artery at the groin. Such patients absolutely must have CT scan to assess the dimensions of the aorta, and if there is a neck of 1–2 cm below the renal arteries, it is feasible for an aortic stent to be fixed below the renal vessels above and in one of the iliac systems below. On the opposite side, using a radiological technique, the iliac system is occluded by blowing up an appropriate detachable balloon (Fig. 26.14). The procedure is completed with a femorofemoral crossover via small incisions in the groin.

It is too early to tell precisely what the impact will be of this novel system but it is entirely possible that the value of the system could be proved first in the emergency situation.

Reference

Yusuf, S.W., Whitaker, S.C., Chuter, T.A., Wenham, P.W. & Hopkinson, B.R. (1994) Emergency endovascular repair of leaking aortic aneurysm (letter). *Lancet* **344(8937)**, 1645.

CHAPTER 27

Acute mesenteric ischaemia

Daryll M. Baker & Averil O. Mansfield

Introduction

Acute mesenteric ischaemia (AMI) was first reported by Virchow in 1852. It is the sudden cessation of mesenteric capillary blood flow resulting ultimately in intestinal necrosis. As the superior mesenteric vessels are always involved resultant ischaemia affects all or part of the small bowel and right colon. Very rarely the coeliac axis is also involved, affecting the stomach, duodenum and liver as well. Although a relatively rare disorder (0.1–0.36% of all hospital admissions), the seriousness of AMI lies in the general failure to diagnose the condition early enough to prevent the terrible 90% mortality. AMI affects men as often as women in the older generation, the average patient being in their 70s.

Demographics
• Rare disorder
• 90% mortality
• Old age
• Equal between sexes

Aetiology

Acute mesenteric ischaemia has either an arterial or venous cause. Arterial causes are embolic occlusion, acute thrombosis and non-occlusive mesenteric ischaemia.

Almost half of the cases result from emboli which originate predominantly from the left atrium due to a supraventricular arrhythmia or from the left ventricle following myocardial infarct. Rarer sources of superior mesenteric artery (SMA) emboli include complications of angiography, aortic aneurysm resection or cardiac valve disease. The emboli may lodge at the origin of the SMA or at points of normal vessel narrowing, usually just distal to the origin of a major branch such as the middle colic, right colic or ileocolic. The presence, at laparotomy, of a pulse in the root of the SMA proximal to its first major branch is suggestive of an embolic cause. There may also be sparing of the proximal jejunum.

Aetiology	
Arterial:	
Embolic	50%
Atherosclerotic occlusion	25%
Low flow	5%
Venous	10%
NB: In practice actual aetiology difficult to determine premorbidly in 50%	

Acute atherosclerotic SMA occlusion accounts for a quarter of all AMI cases. Most occur from progressive stenoses at the origin of the SMA. Consequently, up to half of this patient group give a history of previous chronic mesenteric ischaemia including postprandial abdominal pain, and weight loss. There may be an associated history suggestive of diffuse atherosclerotic disease including ischaemic heart disease, cerebrovascular disease and peripheral vascular disease. At laparotomy none of the small bowel is spared from the ischaemic event and there is no pulse in the SMA even at its root.

Non-occlusive mesenteric ischaemia is responsible for 5% of AMI cases. Most of these patients are severely ill prior to the onset of AMI. It results from a major reduction in cardiac output as occurs during cardiac disease (e.g. myocardial infarction, congestive cardiac failure) or severe hypovolaemia (e.g. sepsis, pancreatitis, haemorrhage, burns) causing marked splanchnic vasoconstriction. Vaso-active drugs used to support a failing myocardium can exacerbate splanchnic vasoconstriction. The incidence of non-occlusive AMI has fallen markedly as the result of improved haemodynamic care of the seriously ill patient in the intensive care unit.

Ten per cent of AMI cases are attributable to mesenteric vein thrombosis. Predisposing conditions are either local or systemic. Local precipitating conditions include portal hypertension, abdominal inflammatory processes (e.g. pancreatitis, diverticular disease, peritonitis) and abdominal trauma. Systemic causes include congenital hypercoagulation states such as protein C and protein S deficiencies and acquired hypercoagulopathies as precipitated by the oral contraceptive pill, polycythemia vera and thrombocytosis. The location of the initial thrombus varies with the aetiology. In local causes it is at the site of trauma precipitating vein obstruction, but in hypercoagulation states it starts in the smaller branches and propagates into the larger ones. Actual bowel infarction is rare, and only occurs when the thrombosis is extensive and involves several vessels. However, patchy full thickness necrosis may occur.

Although the aetiologies of AMI appear to be clearly separable, in practice in almost half the cases it is not possible to identify the causative factor.

Clinical features

There is no single symptom, sign or investigation which conclusively diagnoses AMI, and only a very high index of suspicion helps make the rapid and early diagnosis vital to ensure survival. Too often the presentation is one of a patient in extremis as a result of sepsis secondary to bowel infarction.

By this stage there is little that can be done to save the patient's life. It is therefore necessary to make the diagnosis early and then attempt to determine the cause, prior to surgery.

Abdominal pain occurs in most patients (75–98%). Although it can vary in severity, nature and location, it is often of sudden onset. In the early stages of AMI it is markedly out of proportion to the physical signs, usually constant, and referred to the anterior midpoint of the abdomen. In the remaining patients, pain may be absent, especially in those with non-occlusive disease. Nevertheless, if abdominal pain is present for more than 2 h and more common diagnoses such as obstruction or perforation of a hollow viscus have been excluded, the diagnosis of AMI has to be assumed or at least considered.

The sudden onset of abdominal pain is often associated with a rapid and forceful bowel motion, which is loose in a third of cases and may contain either frank (dark or bright red) or occult blood. Over half the patients with AMI report

> A high index of clinical suspicion is needed to make an early diagnosis and save lives.

Clinical features
History   • Abdominal pain: sudden onset, severe, constant   • Bowel movement: forced, blood stained   • History of chronic mesenteric ischaemia   • Associated atherosclerotic cardiovascular diseases   *Examination*   Early: minimal   Late: peritonitis

nausea and vomiting and a third develop acute confusional states.

It is important to consider the whole clinical picture. Causative risk factors will raise the level of suspicion of AMI, such as a potential source of embolization, for example supraventricular arrhythmias, a recent myocardial infarction and previous or synchronous arterial emboli. A history suggestive of chronic mesenteric ischaemia (postprandial abdominal pain, weight loss) may be suggestive of an atherosclerotic cause for the AMI. The presence of atherosclerotic disease elsewhere in the cardiovascular system is common, with up to 75% of patients having ischaemic heart disease, 15% cerebrovascular accidents and 10% peripheral vascular disease.

Initially, although the patient has abdominal pain, often on examination their overall distress is disproportionately minimal and not indicative of the abdominal catastrophe suffered. The pulse may be elevated and they appear a little dry with a slight pyrexia. Early profuse sweating probably due to sympathetic nervous activity is sometimes present. The abdomen is tender, but soft and bowel sounds are hyperactive. However, as bowel infarction occurs, the patient becomes more dehydrated from 'third space' fluid losses, develops a tachycardia and pyrexia which subsequently drops as the septic shock progresses. The abdomen distends and signs of localized and then general peritonitis become obvious. Bowel sounds disappear once peritonitis is established.

Investigations

Laboratory investigations

No laboratory investigation is pathognomonic and several suggested markers are indicative of advanced intestinal necrosis and sepsis rather than AMI.

Blood sample analysis

Three-quarters of patients have a white cell count in excess of 15 000 cells/mm^3 which in the early stages is often out of proportion of the clinical findings. A metabolic acidosis is present in half the cases with AMI. This, however is often not markedly different from that which occurs with any other intra-abdominal catastrophe and may be a late development.

Investigations
• White cell count: raised   • Blood gases: metabolic acidosis   • Amylase: raised   • Inorganic phosphate: raised   • Abdominal X-ray: no other pathology

Elevated serum amylase is found in up to 50% of cases, and can result in a misdiagnosis of pancreatitis. The rise in serum levels of enzyme considered suggestive of ischaemic and thus gut ischaemia has been extensively investigated in various animal models. Enzyme markers considered including creatinine kinase, alkaline phosphatase, lactate dehydrogenase, aspartate transferase and their co-enzymes. However, no single enzyme or combination of enzymes has proved sensitive or specific enough to enable an earlier diagnosis of AMI to improve morbidity and mortality rates.

Serum inorganic phosphate levels are often clinically raised in AMI and although some consider this to be an early marker of bowel ischaemia others believe it to be the result of extensive injury and associated with a poor outcome. In the correct clinical setting a raised phosphate level strongly suggests AMI but normal levels do not exclude it.

Peritoneal fluid analysis

Peritoneal lavage fluid, obtained by methods similar to those used in assessing abdominal trauma have shown that intestinal ischaemia is associated with a raised white cell count, raised inorganic phosphate levels and raised cellular enzymes such as lactate dehydrogenase. Its main limitation is the inability to differentiate AMI from other acute abdominal pathologies. This method of investigation is unlikely to gain clinical acceptance and can not be recommended.

Other investigations

Radioisotope studies using [99]technetium or [111]indium bound to leucocytes or platlets have failed to be clinically of any diagnostic significance.

Imaging investigations

Plain abdominal X-ray

The plain abdominal X-ray is of no help in making the diagnosis of AMI, but with the chest X-ray, it serves to exclude other causes of an acute abdomen, such as a perforated or obstructed viscus. In the early stages of AMI the abdominal X-ray is usually normal. It only alters when irreversible bowel necrosis has occurred to show formless loops of small bowel, 'thumb printing' of ischaemic bowel and free intraperitoneal gas. Unfortunately such signs develop late and are already present in two-thirds of AMI cases at presentation.

Angiography

Significance
Mesenteric angiography is the investigation of choice. It will distinguish arterial from venous causes and differentiate occlusive from non-occlusive causes. Angiography should be undertaken immediately the diagnosis of AMI is considered. Such an aggressive approach resulting in angiography for all presumed AMI causes leads to a 30–50% negative examination rate. However, the diagnosis will usually have been excluded. Unfortunately, in practice, despite the value of early angiography being recognized for many years there is still a reticence by most surgeons to order it. This may indicate the management of the disorder being undertaken by general or gastrointestinal surgeons rather than vascular surgeons, as well as the practical problem of actually obtaining an angiogram. Significant management delays must be avoided if mortality rates are to be improved.

Method
Before proceeding to angiography, a history of allergy to contrast and the coagulation status of the patient is noted. A 5F pigtail catheter via a transfemoral approach is used to obtain a biplane aortogram. These views exclude extramesenteric causes for the abdominal pain such as renal and splenic emboli and aortic aneurysms. The patency of the SMA is identified as is the extent of the collateral circulation from the coeliac and inferior mesenteric artery. If the SMA os is patent it is selectively catheterized often using a cobra curved catheter. If subsequent vasodilator agent infusion is planned a catheter without side holes reduces pericatheter thrombosis.

Findings

Emboli. On the angiogram, SMA emboli are sharp rounded filling defects which may show proximal and distal propagation or distal fragmentation along the mesenteric arterial tree. Emboli occlude the SMA origin in a fifth of cases making differentiation between embolic and atherosclerotic aetiologies difficult. The distal vessels are poorly visualized as collateral flow is inadequate and vasospasm is often very intense. There are usually minimal atherosclerotic changes in other vessels. Angiography of lower limb vessels at the same time is wise as concomitant embolization occurs in 20% of cases.

Thrombosis and atherosclerotic disease. On a flush angiogram an acute SMA thrombosis appears as a complete occlusion of the SMA at or within 2 cm of its origin, usually as an abrupt vessel cutoff. There are few or no visceral collaterals and the SMA distal to the occlusion fills exceptionally sluggishly. Atherosclerotic narrowing in other vessels, as well as considerable vasoconstrictive spasm is often present. Large collaterals from the coeliac axis or inferior mesenteric artery in the presence of an occluded proximal SMA, but with adequate filling of the distal SMA suggests an acute on chronic disorder (Fig. 27.1).

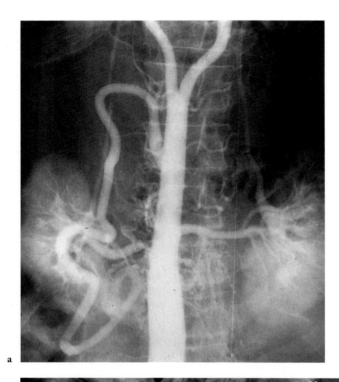

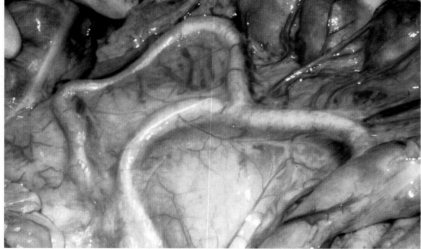

Fig. 27.1(a) and (b) Half the patients suffering from an acute atherosclerotic occlusion of the superior mesenteric artery give a previous history of chronic mesenteric ischaemia. Angiographically this is suggested by enlarged collateral circulation. In this angiogram the marginal artery of Drummond is prominent. At laparotomy the enlarged vessel is easily visible. However, if the clinical and laparotomy findings do not make the diagnosis of acute mesenteric ischaemia, another pathology should be sought as generalized atherosclerosis commonly affects the aged population and a chronic superior mesenteric artery stenosis could be a coincidental finding.

Non-occlusive AMI. In the absence of complete SMA occlusion and other causes of mesenteric vasoconstriction such as shock, pancreatitis and vasopressor drugs, radiographic signs of vasospasm are diagnostic of early non-occlusive AMI. These signs include narrowing of SMA branch origins; irregularities in the outlines of intestinal branches and arcades and impaired filling of intramural vessels.

Mesenteric vein thrombosis. Radiographic signs suggestive of mesenteric vein thrombosis include the presence of thrombus in larger veins (superior mesenteric and portal vein) causing their partial occlusion or failure to be visualized. The thrombosis causes a prolonged blush in the involved segment and arterial spasm with the arterial arcades failing to empty and contrast reflux into the artery.

Bowel contrast studies are not indicated in AMI as they contribute little and hinder the interpretation of angiography.

Computerized tomography (CT) scanning

Although CT may assist in excluding other causes of an acute abdomen such as a symptomatic aortic aneurysm, it is unable to diagnose early AMI. Signs of complete arterial thrombosis and necrotic bowel are late events. CT scanning will detect 90% of mesenteric venous thromboses, by identifying the thrombus in the vein, venous collateral circulation and abnormal segments of intestine, but is of most use in chronic rather than acute venous thromboses. In AMI its use can not be recommended.

Duplex scanning

Duplex scanning can accurately detect flow in both the superior mesenteric artery and vein. However the wide range of normal SMA blood flow values (300–600 ml/min) which vary with food intake reduces the sensitivity of the technique. The deep location and many anatomical variations of the mesenteric vascular bed makes the process time consuming and requires considerable operator skills. Nevertheless, it can be assumed that in the SMA, the presence of a normal waveform, a normal peak systolic and a normal end-diastolic velocity makes haemodynamically significant stenoses very unlikely.

Management

Ideally, the patient is first resuscitated and an abdominal X-ray performed in order to help exclude other pathologies. Angiographic imaging of the mesenteric vessels is then undertaken to make the diagnosis and allow for selective SMA vasodilator infusion to be started before surgery.

Resuscitation

Initial resuscitation is aimed at relieving causative factors such as hypovolaemia, or congestive cardiac failure. Accurate fluid balance management requires careful monitoring including a urinary catheter, central line and at times a Swan–Ganz catheter on an intensive care unit. Antibiotics aimed at covering bowel flora, such as cefuroxime and metronidazole are administered once the diagnosis has been entertained. The use of oxygen free radical scavengers such as allopurinol or mannitol, although possibly of some help, are rarely used. Intravenous administration of vasodilators thought to be specific to the mesenteric vessels, such as glucagon, have in isolated reports been suggested to be of benefit to patients. However, despite experimental evidence of improved intestinal viability, its use in patients with AMI is not recommended.

Endovascular procedures

Selective vasodilator infusions

Selective SMA catheter infusion of visceral vasodilator, such as papaverine (initial 60 mg bolus then 30–60 mg/h infusion, given diluted in saline 1 mg/ml), markedly reduces the

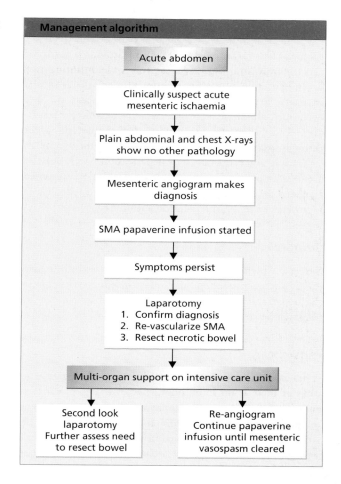

Management algorithm

Acute abdomen

↓

Clinically suspect acute mesenteric ischaemia

↓

Plain abdominal and chest X-rays show no other pathology

↓

Mesenteric angiogram makes diagnosis

↓

SMA papaverine infusion started

↓

Symptoms persist

↓

Laparotomy
1. Confirm diagnosis
2. Re-vascularize SMA
3. Resect necrotic bowel

↓

Multi-organ support on intensive care unit

↓

Second look laparotomy Further assess need to resect bowel

Re-angiogram Continue papaverine infusion until mesenteric vasospasm cleared

visceral vasoconstriction present in all forms of AMI. Although no controlled clinical trials have been performed, its use, if possible, is recommended as it appears to be associated with few side effects and improved survival rates. The selective papaverine infusion is started when the preoperative angiogram is performed, continued throughout surgery and for 24 h postoperatively. Normal saline is then infused for 30 min before a repeat angiogram is performed. If there is residual vasoconstriction, infusion is continued for a further one to five days until it has cleared. The papaverine line must not also be used for heparin infusion as this causes precipitation.

Local complications associated with intra-arterial infusion of vasodilator are those found in any intra-arterial infusions and include pericatheter thrombosis and local puncture site haematomas. The systemic effects of papaverine are minimal as most is removed in the first passage through the liver. Any sudden changes in systemic pressure indicates that the catheter has fallen out of the SMA.

Other vasodilators such as phenoxybenzymine, prostaglandin E_1, tolazoline and adenosine triphosphate have been selectively injected into the SMA, but have not been used as extensively or as successfully as papaverine.

Angioplasty and thrombolysis

Endovascular management of SMA occlusions is at present experimental and with no clear way of monitoring end-organ ischaemic injury is not recommended outside specialist units. Percutaneous transluminal angioplasty of SMA occlusions although reported, is rarely technically feasible (Fig. 27.2). Successful infusion of thrombolytic agents through selectively placed catheters to clear superior mesenteric artery and vein (via a transhepatic route) occlusions has also been reported. We believe this is a logical management provided that lysis times are kept minimal and failed lysis is followed by surgical intervention within 2 h.

Surgery

Surgery, which is almost always necessary, is indicated to exclude other intra-abdominal catastrophes, to revascularize the bowel following arterial occlusion and to remove any infarcted bowel.

Laparotomy

A full laparotomy is vital to exclude other pathologies, especially if there is no frank bowel necrosis. The presence of an occluded SMA may be a long-standing coincidence and the abdominal symptoms from another cause. Initially the whole gut is carefully examined from oesophagus to rectum. The extent and severity of ischaemic changes are then assessed (see below) and extrinsic causes of the ischaemia such as an adhesion band or internal volvulus are excluded. Attempts are made to determine or confirm the aetiology. This includes examining the aorta to exclude an aneurysm and assess the degree of atherosclerotic disease, palpating the root of the mesentery for a pulse and assessing the degree of SMA collateral circulation (Fig. 27.1b). A large marginal artery of Drummond may indicate an acute on chronic atherosclerotic disorder rather than an embolic cause. Mesenteric vein thrombosis, in the extreme form, presents at laparotomy with serosanguineous peritoneal fluid, dark red to blue black oedematous bowel, a thickened mesentery with good arterial pulses in the involved segment and thrombus in cut mesenteric veins.

Revascularization

As with any surgery for ischaemia it is necessary to undertake revascularization procedures before resecting necrotic tissue. Revascularization of the gut should, however, only be attempted when there is a real prospect of reversible ischaemia to a good proportion of the gut (see Fig. 27.4). Extensive bowel necrosis requiring resection leaving residual viable healthy small bowel will not benefit from revascularization.

Surgical exposure of the superior mesenteric artery

A midline incision from xiphisternum to umbilicus or lower is made. The chest is not opened. The proximal SMA is exposed by retracting the transverse colon superiorly and the small bowel inferiorly and to the right. At the point in the root of the transverse mesocolon where the middle colic artery ascends, the small bowel mesentery is incised and the proximal SMA dissected free between the pancreas and the fourth part of the duodenum. Adequate exposure of at least 2 cm of SMA proximal and distal to the middle colic artery origin is important (Fig. 27.3). Use of magnification helps preserve the small branches coming off this segment of the SMA; the superior mesenteric vein, which lies to the left and the several other smaller veins around it. Vascular control is obtained by placing fine soft slings around the artery.

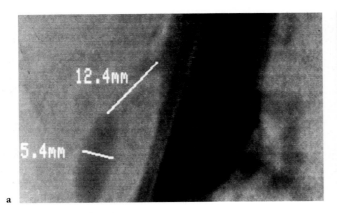

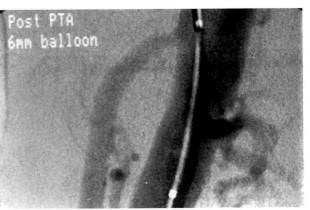

Fig. 27.2(a) and (b) A short atherosclerotic occlusion at the origin of the superior mesenteric artery has been successfully angioplastied to relieve symptoms of mesenteric ischaemia. Although not often a feasible procedure in the acute situation, once performed, very careful clinical patient observation are undertaken to ensure that no distal embolization or restenosis has occurred.

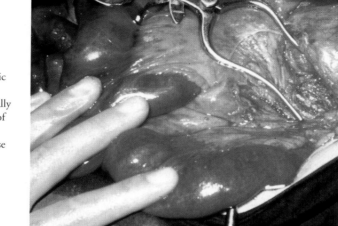

Fig. 27.3 To expose the superior mesenteric artery near its origin the transverse colon is drawn superiorly and the small bowel laterally and inferiorly. The peritoneum at the root of the small bowel mesentery near where the middle colic artery arises is divided to expose the vessel. The superior mesenteric artery is displayed here between the teeth of the self retaining retractor. Note also that the small bowel to the right of the patient appears ischaemic, but not infarcted (see Fig. 27.6 and 27.7).

Clamps are avoided as they increase the likelihood of fracturing the atheroma or embolus and dislodging fragments into distal branches.

To expose both the SMA and the coeliac axis, the lesser omentum is opened lateral to the oesophagus whose displacement to the left is aided by a firm nasogastric tube. By dividing the median arcuate ligament the anterior surface of the supracoeliac aorta is displayed, care being taken to avoid bleeding from the small phrenic arteries. The aorta is not fully mobilized; only a segment of vessel suitable for clamping is revealed. The aorta is exposed caudally until the coeliac axis is reached. The anatomy of the coeliac axis is variable; it may arise from the aorta at right angles and branch after a centimetre, or it can arise under the median arcuate ligament and run some distance into the abdomen before dividing. The SMA is exposed by continuing the dissection under the upper border of the pancreas and dividing the nerve plexus around it.

The posterior approach is a useful exposure of the SMA, coeliac and renal vessels in cases of previous surgery or joint pathology. The table is tilted left side up and the left colon mobilized along its peritoneal reflection. The splenorenal ligament is divided and the left and transverse colon, spleen and tail and body of pancreas reflected to the right until the left adrenal and left renal vein are fully exposed. The visceral vessels are then exposed along the anterior border of the aorta.

The distal SMA is easily exposed in the mesentery, but the smaller calibre of the vessel can make subsequent patency a problem.

Management of specific AMI types

SMA embolus. With the SMA exposed, the site and extent of the embolus is determined by direct palpation of the pulse or by using the hand-held Doppler where the monophasic thud of flow down a distally occluded vessel gets louder as the probe is passed along the vessel, until the occlusion is met and Doppler recordings are lost. Vascular control is obtained by placing fine soft slings around the artery proximal and distal to the embolus and 5000 units of heparin are given intravenously. The embolus is removed via a longitudinal arteriotomy over it. Part of the embolus is sent for culture and part for histology. Residual clots are washed out by releasing the slings. A small embolectomy balloon catheter is passed proximal and distally through the SMA. It is difficult to clear the thrombus distally and the vessel is easily damaged. The arteriotomy is closed with a vein patch to prevent narrowing.

Acute superior mesenteric artery thrombosis. It is often difficult to differentiate between an embolic and a thrombotic cause of AMI. In such cases the patient is initially treated as though they have an embolic cause.

Acute SMA revascularization procedures for thrombosis are similar to those used for chronic mesenteric ischaemia (bypass, re-implantation, and endarterectomy). A short side-to-side bypass graft from the aorta to the SMA distal to the obstruction is the simplest and recommended procedure in emergency surgery.

There is debate as to the optimal inflow site for the graft, because the great mobility of the SMA within the mesentery is thought to induce graft kinking and early failure or stimulate further atherosclerosis and thus late failure. The actual proximal inflow site selected is often determined on practical grounds; extensive aortic atherosclerosis may preclude its use and the iliac vessels, including the internal iliac can be used as these may be spared the disease. Alternatively the supracoeliac aorta may be used. Autogenous reversed long saphenous vein is the most suitable conduit, particularly in the presence of sepsis or necrosis. As it has to be at least 5 mm in diameter the long saphenous vein is retrieved proximal from the saphenofemoral junction and not from the ankle. If the long saphenous vein is not suitable polytetrafluoroethylene (PTFE) or Dacron (8 mm) are adequate conduits.

Re-implantation of the SMA into the aorta has been used, but is not recommended. The artery distal to the occlusion is transected and anastomosed directly to the aorta. This is technically difficult as the SMA is short and in spasm and the aorta usually has an atherosclerotic thick hard wall.

Endarterectomy either through the diseased SMA or via an eversion method through the aorta is potentially hazardous as emboli may be dispersed distally and atheromatous flaps may be raised at the edge of the endarterectomy which are not always visible, especially with the transaortic eversion method. The transaortic endarterectomy is carried out through a left thoracoretroperitoneal approach and this along with suprarenal aortic clamping makes it a major operation, not usually suitable for the emergency situation. Results in the acute situation are poor, with up to 50% rethrombosing within 48 hours.

Non-occlusive mesenteric ischaemia. The diagnosis is made when pre-operative angiography has revealed signs of mesenteric vasoconstriction in a patient who has clinical features of mesenteric ischaemia and is neither shocked nor receiving vasopressor drugs. The initial treatment is a SMA papaverine infusion. Should peritonism be present or pain persist, with the vasodilator infusion running, laparotomy is performed. The SMA is not manipulated at all and necrotic bowel resected.

Mesenteric vein thrombosis. Surgical thrombectomies of mesenteric veins are difficult and rarely successful or indicated. Local vasodilator therapy is helpful and full heparinization is required. Surgery, is however, usually required to resect necrotic bowel.

Managing end organ (bowel) ischaemia

Operative assessment of bowel viability

Determining the viability of the bowel is vital. If necrotic gut is left it will perforate and sepsis will follow. However, removing excessive amount of viable bowel and producing a short bowel syndrome is not acceptable.

Visual means. Once maximum vasodilation has been stimulated by leaving the gut in warm saline soaked packs for 20 min, traditionally, gut viability is assessed according to its colour, sheen, peristaltic activity and presence of pulses. Such assessment is unreliable. The bowel is a dark purple colour when venous obstruction has produced venous

Methods of assessing bowel viability
• Visual
(a) Bowel colour
(b) Bowel sheen
(c) Bowel peristalsis
(d) Mesenteric pulses
• Vital dyes (fluorescein)
• Doppler
• Other (experimental)

engorgement, but is often viable, unlike early arterial obstruction when there is little colour change and the bowel is not viable. Arterial arcade vessel pulsations may be present when the ischaemia is caused by a low flow state or following successful revascularization, despite irreversible bowel changes occurring. Peristaltic activity may persist after the onset of irreversible AMI.

Vital dyes. To aid determination of bowel viability, the distribution of the vital dye, fluorescein, through the bowel wall is determined within 10 min of a 100 mg intravenous injection using an ultraviolet light. Three patterns of fluorescence are seen: a homogeneous yellow–green pattern of normal bowel, a hyperfluorescent hyperaemic pattern and a finely granular reticular pattern. Patchy fluorescence or areas of non-fluorescence are not viable. The technique is practical, quick and cheap with sensitivities and specificities of 95% having been claimed. However, experience in detecting the reduced fluorescence of questionable viability is needed and most theatres are not equipped with the ultraviolet light necessary to perform the test.

Doppler. Intra-operative Doppler ultrasound probes are inexpensive and simple to use, being able to detect flow in arteries and veins within the mesentery. Anastomoses within 1 cm of the last audible Doppler signal will heal, but at 2–3 cm beyond the last audible Doppler signal will break down and necrose. The major draw back is that infrequent use of the intra-operative Doppler can result in incorrect positioning of the probe in relation to the vessel and thus ambiguity in determining the presence or absence of Doppler pulses.

Others. Several other investigations have been tried experimentally, but have to date proved to be of little practical value. Serosal pH and $P\text{co}_2$ levels depend on blood flow rather than intestinal viability and so have no role in theatre. Experimentally, bowel serosal surface oxygen tension ($P_s\text{o}_2$) correlates well with ability of the bowel to survive anastomosis. However, at present the probes are small and areas of patchy necrosis are missed. Infrared photoplethysmography wave forms have failed to show any correlation with subsequent bowel viability. The presence of intestinal wall smooth muscle contractile activity when electrically stimulated correlates well with subsequent tissue viability. This has not been confirmed clinically.

In conclusion, intestinal viability remains difficult to determine. A combination of visual assessment with fluorescein dye fluorescence and bowel wall Doppler pulses to date gives the best results.

Management of ischaemic bowel

Management of infarcted bowel depends on the degree and extent. There are three situations. Firstly, if only a single short segment of small bowel is non-viable it is resected and a primary anastomosis performed.

Secondly, if the ischaemia appears to involve several regions of bowel, but the extent and degree of ischaemia is unclear, then only obviously necrotic areas are resected. A 'second-look' laparotomy is performed 24 h later to assess bowel of questionable viability (Fig. 27.4). In the interim the bowel ends are either brought out as stomas or simply oversewn. A decision to perform a 'second-look' laparotomy is made during the first operation and is performed irrespective of the clinical condition as it gives time for supportive measures to take effect. In 20% of cases where a second look is undertaken it will contribute to the patient's survival. This is especially true for mesenteric vein thromboses where the dusky blue colour of the venous engorged bowel can be difficult to distinguish from necrotic bowel. At a 'second-look' laparotomy, following a period of heparin and possibly vasodilator infusion the venous congestion may have cleared or its extent clarified.

Diagnostic or 'second look' laparoscopy has been reported. However, laparoscopy only examines the bowel

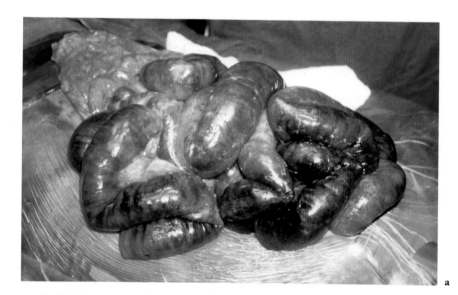

a

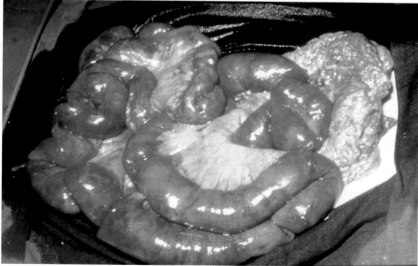

b

Fig. 27.4 It is often difficult to determine the extent of irreversible bowel necrosis during acute mesenteric ischaemia. Extensive areas of the bowel may appear ischaemic to varying degrees. In such cases only frankly necrotic regions are excised and a 'second look' laparotomy performed 24 h later. In this case at the first laparotomy (a) most of the small bowel appears ischaemic to varying degrees. Following revascularization and full multi-organ support on the intensive care unit at the 'second look' laparotomy (b) the regions of ischaemia had improved sufficiently not to require further bowel resection.

serosa and there are theoretical risks involved in raising the intraperitoneal pressure in the presence of an already decreased SMA blood flow. A negative observation does not exclude AMI, or its progression. Therefore at present it can not be recommended in place of angiography and exploratory laparotomy.

The third situation occurs when there is extensive obvious small bowel infarction. *The decision to perform a massive bowel resection is made on the merits of each individual case* and depends on the likelihood of the patient surviving. Vital information pertaining to the patient's premorbid medical condition will have been obtained from the pre-operative consultation with the patient and their relatives. In general, patients with other manifestations of atherosclerotic disease, such as severe ischaemic heart disease, heart failure and debilitating cerebrovascular episodes are not candidates for extensive bowel resections. Indicators that the AMI has progressed to a point where survival is unlikely include bowel perforation, septic shock and multi-organ failure. These are also factors against massive bowel resection. The length of unaffected bowel, taken in isolation, should not be the sole reason for refraining from extensive resection. Although there is always the worry of a resultant short bowel syndrome with long-term total parenteral nutrition (TPN) and probably reduced quality of life especially in the older age group, it must be remembered that as little as 12–18 cm of residual unaffected small bowel will result in only 20% of patients requiring long-term TPN.

In practice, at laparotomy only about 5% of cases have segments of the bowel which are ischaemic but viable. More often (35% of cases) a limited segment of small bowel is infarcted and needs resection. Most commonly, however, (60% of cases) the bowel is extensively infarcted from proximal small bowel to right or transverse colon. Surgical resection is only likely to be indicated in about half of these patients with extensive bowel infarction.

Postoperation for AMI

Postoperative management

Careful postoperative management of patients with AMI on an intensive care unit is important to prevent and support multi-organ septic failure. Anticoagulation reduces the number of postprocedural thromboses, especially in venous cases. Thus despite the risk of haemorrhage, it is recommended that intravenous heparin be commenced immediately after surgery to obtain an activated partial thromboplastin time (aPTT) clotting ratio of 2.0, even if a second-look laparotomy is planned. Intravenous heparin is continued until the patient is able to start oral warfarin.

The broad-spectrum antibiotics started pre-operatively should be continued until the patient is fully recovered, only being changed to more specific ones if directed by positive blood cultures.

Fluid balance remains vital and careful monitoring of both fluid input and output in the form of urine output, nasogastric aspirates and fistula losses must be rigorously undertaken. Postoperative serum electrolytes can easily become deranged and need to be carefully watched.

As with any bowel operation, alimentation is reintroduced after successful revascularization once the surgeon is happy that a paralytic ileus is unlikely. The exact timing and the type will depend on the procedure undertaken and the residual bowel remaining. There is often delay in returning to a normal dietary intake, and parenteral nutrition, be it only as a temporary measure must be introduced early. Management of patients whose intake remains a problem and long-term parenteral nutrition is likely are best managed on a specialist metabolic unit. This may involve transferring the patient to another hospital.

If an embolic cause to the AMI is suspected a cardiac echo will identify a cardiac source. If intraventricular thrombus is extensive, depending on the patient's overall condition surgical evacuation may be considered.

Postoperative complications

The commonest event following AMI surgery is development of multi-organ failure secondary to septicaemia, when the pathology has not been identified and treated early enough.

Early complications of revascularization include thrombosis at the arteriotomy site when an embolectomy was performed, or of the jump graft when a bypass procedure was undertaken. Thrombosis occurs in up to 20% of cases in which a pulse was restored usually within two weeks of surgery. The resultant clinical picture is similar to the original presentation and should be treated aggressively as good secondary patency rates can be achieved. Thus any early recurrence of symptoms while the patient is still in hospital must be assumed to be a result of failure of the revascularization procedure and full investigations, with angiography and then re-exploration, is required.

Another complication of revascularization is haemorrhage from the arteriotomy or graft anastomosis site. Secondary haemorrhage should always be assumed to be the result of infection and is a major problem.

Postoperative persistent diarrhoea, including in those who do not have a short bowel syndrome is common. Mucosal ulceration and intestinal bleeds also occur. Major postoperative gastrointestinal haemorrhage can occur occasionally at the site of revascularized bowel or rarely from a SMA intestinal fistula.

A late complication is the development of arterial strictures at the site of arteriotomy or anastomosis as the disease progresses or intimal hyperplasia develops.

Outcome

If the diagnosis of AMI is made early and treatment started promptly a mortality of 50% can be expected, falling to 10% if abdominal pain but not peritonitis is present when treatment is established. Unfortunately, this is rarely the case and bowel infarction has usually already occurred by the time treatment is initiated. Consequently the mortality for arterial AMI has remained between 70–90% for the last 30 years, tending to be higher in atherosclerotic than embolic causes and higher if resection alone rather than revascularization and resection are undertaken together. Non-occlusive AMI has a very grave outcome, because of the underlying precipitating disorder. Mesenteric venous thrombosis has a better prognosis with a mortality around 50%.

If the patient survives following massive bowel resection the average hospital stay is 2 months. Of patients who leave hospital assuming parenteral nutrition is not required, most will return to their premorbid level of independent life. A risk of suffering further atherosclerotic induced events exists, especially cerebrovascular accidents. Recurrent arterial-caused AMI is rare, 10% occurring at a median of 18 months postsurgery. Recurrence of symptomatic mesenteric vein thrombosis is 15%, rising to 25% if the patient is not anticoagulated.

Conclusions

AMI is a rare, but catastrophic acute surgical emergency, occurring in the older generation and associated with a very high mortality. A high index of clinical suspicion is needed to make the diagnosis as there are no clear symptoms, signs or investigations to suggest the disorder. In the absence of more common diagnoses, the presence of severe persistent pain, coming on suddenly and out of proportion to abdominal signs often associated with a forceful bowel motion, a raised white cell count, a raised serum amylase and a metabolic acidosis is sufficient suspicion to obtain a mesenteric angiogram from which the diagnosis is suggested and a selective SMA papaverine infusion can be initiated. Surgery is almost always required. Revascularization should be attempted before bowel resection is undertaken.

Further reading

Kaleya, R.N., Sammartando, R.J. & Boley, J.J. (1992) Aggressive approach to acute mesenteric ischemia. *Surgical Clinics of North America* **72** 157–181.

Geelkerken, R.H. & van Bockel, J.H. (1995) Mesenteric vascular disease: a review of diagnostic methods and therapies. *Cardiovascular Surgery* **3** 247–260.

Mansfield, A.O. (1992) Mesenteric ischaemia. In: *Surgical Management of Vascular Disease* (eds P.R.F. Bell, C.W. Jamerson & C.V. Ruckely). Chapter 53, pp. 767–780. W.B. Saunders Company Ltd., London.

CHAPTER 28

Vascular trauma

Aires A. B. Barros D'Sa

Introduction

Vascular injuries through the millenia demanded attention solely to arrest haemorrhage and only during the early part of the twentieth century did the concept emerge of vascular repair aimed at preserving organ and limb. The difficult operational conditions of World War I which presented a dismal testing ground for new vascular anastomotic techniques and vein grafting in injuries caused by high explosives and missiles led to an amputation rate of 72.5%. During World War II, vascular repair was observed to be demonstrably superior to ligation, and although casualties were often treated 10 hours after injury, the amputation rate fell dramatically to 35.8%. In the Korean War the time lag before vascular repair had dropped to 6 h and the amputation rate fell to 13%. That incidence remained virtually unchanged at 12.7% during the Vietnam War and improved long-term results recorded by the Vietnam Vascular Registry were attributed to helicopter evacuation for treatment within 3 h of injury and specialist care in well-equipped operating theatres by vascular surgeons experienced in vein grafting. Experimental studies on the wounding capacity of missiles contributed significantly to optimal care of the injured tissues.

Although the second half of the twentieth century may not have witnessed wars on a global scale, they still recur along with civil wars and flashpoints of endemic terrorism. Simultaneous with penetrating trauma, the endless toll of accidents sustained on the road and in industry inevitably account for a proportion of vascular injuries. In many cities and conurbations violence associated with a mounting culture of gangsterism and traffic in illicit drugs, once inflicted by knives and handguns, is now being caused by automatic assault weapons, often by juveniles. The portrayal of gratuitous violence as if it were a 'normal' ingredient of human existence, and the glamorization of brutality in the media and films may well have a part to play in influencing the young mind. Democratic societies and governments deservedly place importance on free expression and libertarian values but they also have a responsibility to ensure that those ideals are tempered by the tenets of a universal sense of morality enshrined in appropriate legislation.

Indiscriminate assault by terrorists armed with sophisticated weapons, massive bombs and incendiary devices over a period of 25 years in Northern Ireland has accounted for approximately 3500 deaths, 37 000 maimed and an estimated 1500 injured vessels treated. The people have endured physical suffering and grief with resilience and dignity, even as the fabric of their lives was blighted by the systematic destruction of their homes and their places of work and leisure. Belfast's largest university hospital, the Royal Victoria, often assumed the main responsibilities of a front-line evacuation centre for casualties from major disasters. Vascular injuries caused by shrapnel from bombs, mines, mortar shells and rockets, and by high- and low-velocity bullets, were treated. This experience led to innovations in management in which these victims of inhumanity have been the key contributors. Simultaneously with this penetrating vascular trauma, deceleration accidents on the roads and injuries sustained in industry and elsewhere were also responsible for many cases of complex vascular injuries.

The vast majority of patients sustaining severe, often penetrating, injuries to major vessel trunks in the chest and abdomen succumb at the scene or in transit from exsanguination and the sequelae of associated vital organ injury. Those who are fortunate to be admitted to well-equipped trauma centres arrive in hypovolaemic shock and may stand a chance of survival. Immediate resuscitation, recognition of the true extent and complexity of the trauma and prompt operative intervention for vascular control and repair continue to challenge the acumen of the vascular surgeon.

Amputations	
World War I	72.5%
World War II	35.8%
Korean War	13%
Vietnam War	12.7%

Mechanisms of vascular injury

Penetrating trauma

Vessels in the neck, upper extremity and chest are most vulnerable to a stabbing attack which generally lacerates or divides a vessel cleanly, possibly injuring adjacent nerves and other organs in its path. Posteriorly placed vessels in the abdomen may be injured depending on the length of the blade and the force of impact. The classic self-inflicted butcher's injury by a boning knife in the vicinity of the common femoral artery may result in fatality. The wounding force of a missile depends on its mass, muzzle velocity and the distance it travels before impact. While a low-velocity bullet ordinarily damages a vessel lying directly in its path (Fig. 28.1), a high-velocity missile dissipating its energy at right angles to its trajectory produces a cavitational effect, in the process destroying all tissues including bone which fragments into secondary missiles (Fig. 28.2), but the extent of damage may be concealed by apparently benign wounds. Similarly, a shotgun discharged at close range produces a concentrated 'spread' of damage (Fig. 28.3), the depth of

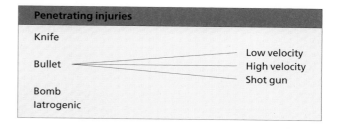

Penetrating injuries	
Knife	
Bullet	Low velocity / High velocity / Shot gun
Bomb	
Iatrogenic	

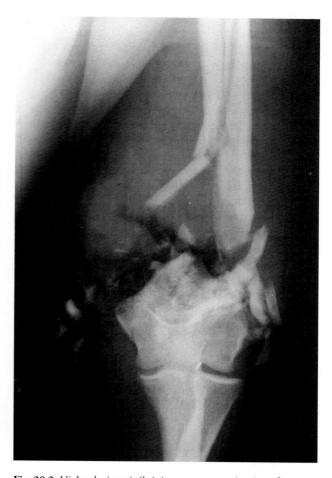

Fig. 28.1 Penetrating injury to lower superficial femoral artery. Distal pulses present but reduced in volume, not by spasm but by mural damage which progressed to thrombotic occlusion. Thrombus visible on angiogram and on excised segment (inset). (With permission from Barros D'Sa, A.A.B. (1981) A decade of missile-induced vascular trauma. *Annals of the Royal College of Surgeons of England* **64** 37.)

Fig. 28.2 High velocity missile injury: gross comminution of humerus, transection of brachial artery and ulnar nerve. (Reprinted from Barros D'Sa, A.A.B. (1992) In: *Arterial Surgery* (ed. H.H.G. Eastcott), p. 358, by permission of the publisher Churchill Livingstone.)

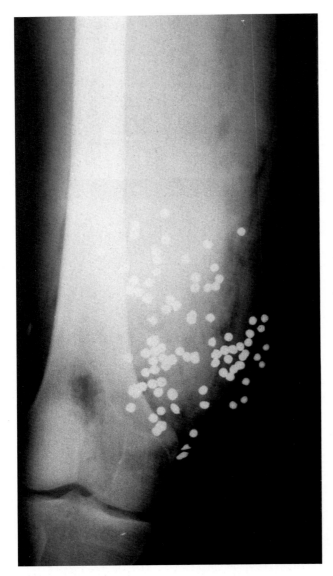

Fig. 28.3 Shotgun blast at close range: widespread soft tissue destruction, nerve damage and 15 cm segments of adjacent femoral and popliteal artery and vein required vein graft replacement. (Reprinted from Barros D'Sa, A.A.B. (1992) In: *Arterial Surgery* (ed. H.H.G. Eastcott), p. 358, by permission of the publisher Churchill Livingstone.)

which is often underestimated on inspection. In bomb explosions, shrapnel (Figs 28.4 and 28.5) and secondary missiles cause widespread internal trauma, while injuries from falling masonry lead to the crush syndrome. Iatrogenic sources of penetrating vessel trauma are most commonly observed during arterial diagnostic and interventional catheterization procedures daily undertaken by cardiologists and radiologists.

Blunt trauma

Significant forces are responsible for vascular injury as a consequence of blunt trauma, most resulting from sudden deceleration in road traffic accidents, falls, rail, air and mining disasters. The severity of the injuries may exceed that caused by penetrating trauma (Fig. 28.6). The immense shearing forces generated by the sudden violent angulation and fracture of long bones may damage adjacent vessels directly by sharp bone fragments or indirectly at points of relative fixity. The avulsive forces which operate in posterior dislocations of the knee result in the tearing of all tissues during which process the layers of the popliteal artery beginning with the intima disrupt progressively, an injury which may easily be missed because a dislocated knee tends to reduce spontaneously. In the severe Type IIIc open fractures, comminution with periosteal stripping and severe muscle and skin loss may accompany injury to long segments of popliteal and crural vessels as well as collaterals, features further compounded by contamination. In the proximal upper limb arterial trauma is often accompanied by traction injury of the brachial plexus (Fig. 28.7).

Sudden deceleration places inordinate strains on certain vessels in the chest or abdomen which are either relatively fixed or form the pedicles to organs of substantial mass. This can result in traumatic rupture of the isthmus of the thoracic aorta (Fig. 28.8) or the origin of the innominate artery, and less frequently the origins of the left subclavian and left common carotid arteries. The renal artery, particularly the left, is similarly vulnerable, as are the branches of the superior mesenteric artery and the tributaries of the portal vein. Direct damage to vessels in the torso is uncommon although the subclavian artery is occasionally torn in fractures of the clavicle and upper ribs, and the abdominal aorta may be crushed in the rare instance of seat belt trauma.

Blunt injuries
• Road traffic accident
• Falls
• Rail and air accidents
• Mining disasters, etc.

Irradiation

While acute traumatic necrosis and rupture of the wall of an artery was observed in the past following excessive dosages of irradiation, in most cases the damage caused becomes apparent many years after the insult. Injury to the endothelium and internal elastic lamina followed by fibrosis of the media and inflammation of the adventitia may with the passage of time become indistinguishable from the appearances of atherosclerosis and in some cases may progress to critical

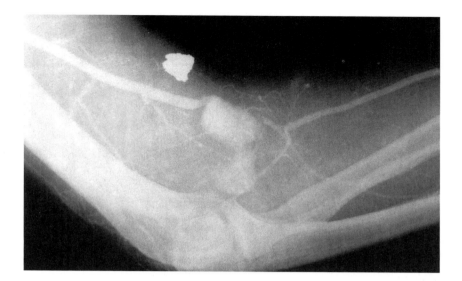

Fig. 28.4 Shrapnel injury to the lower brachial artery resulting in false aneurysm. (With permission from Barros D'Sa, A.A.B. (1997) In: *Emergency Vascular Practice* (eds A.D.B. Chant & A.A.B. Barros D'Sa). Arnold, London.)

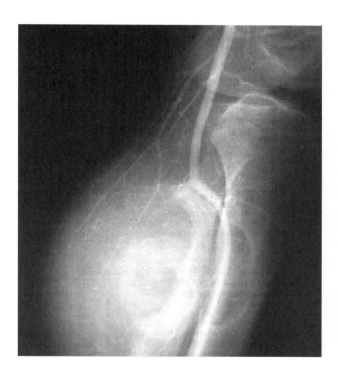

Fig. 28.5 Shell fragment injury of tibioperoneal trunk with a massive pulsatile false aneurysm in the calf; a healed tibial fracture with a large defect is also seen. (With permission of Barros D'Sa, A.A.B. (1997) In: *Emergency Vascular Practice* (eds A.D.B. Chant & A.A.B. Barros D'Sa). Arnold, London.)

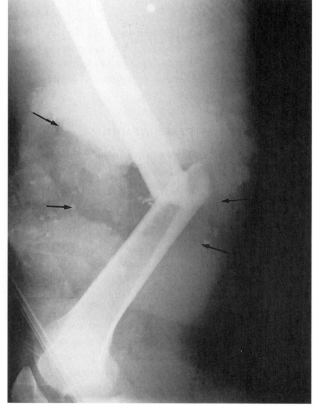

Fig. 28.6 X-ray shows virtual dismemberment at midfemoral level. Gap in soft tissues between arrows. (With permission from Barros D'Sa, A.A.B. and Moorehead, R.J. (1989) *European Journal of Vascular Surgery* **3** 578.)

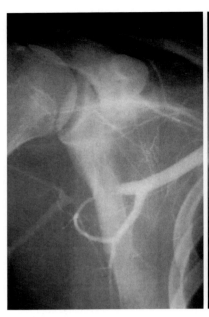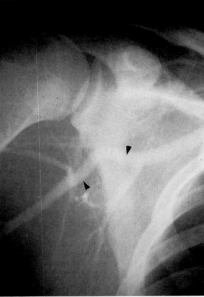

Fig. 28.7 Injury to right shoulder caused by a falling tree, producing crush injury of the axillary artery and brachial plexus and a humeral fracture. Pre-operative angiogram shows defect in the midaxillary artery. Postoperative angiogram shows interposed vein graft (arrows) deliberately left lax enough to permit safe adduction. (Reprinted from Barros D'Sa, A.A.B. (1992) In: *Arterial Surgery* (ed. H.H.G. Eastcott), p. 396, by permission of the publisher Churchill Livingstone.)

limb ischaemia. Injury of the carotid vessels may complicate irradiation of tumours and nodes in the neck, the subclavian–axillary arterial system is vulnerable to adjuvant therapy for breast cancer, while the iliofemoral arterial segment may be affected following treatment of tumours of the ovary, cervix and testis.

Morphology of vascular injury

A diagnosis of true traumatic spasm is rare and when presumed, tends to engender inactivity which may threaten a limb when an arterial injury is actually present; at least some endothelial damage and contusion of the adventitia is usually found in these cases. Arterial injury caused by blunt trauma or proximity to the path of a bullet may permit flow transiently before it progresses to thrombotic occlusion (Fig. 28.1). More frequently, an intimal fracture may develop into a flap, leading to dissection, intramural bleeding and eventually occlusion particularly if the tear is circumferential.

Laceration of an artery may lead to swift exsanguination because the vessel is unable to contract circumferentially. Internal bleeding may present as an enlarging haematoma which in a limb will raise compartment pressure. Arterial injury in the chest may cause bleeding externally, into the pleural cavity or confined within the mediastinum. In the abdomen an arterial laceration may either form a pulsatile retroperitoneal haematoma or result in intraperitoneal haemorrhage. When a laceration in a limb or elsewhere forms a haematoma, blood usually forces its way into the organizing haematoma to create an endothelialized false aneurysm (Figs 28.4 and 28.5) within which thrombosis tends to occur. This false aneurysm expands to compress surrounding venous channels and eventually it may rupture.

Morphology
• Spasm
• Intimal fracture/flap
• Dissection
• Thrombosis
• Laceration
• False aneurysm
• AV fistula
• Transection or avulsion

Simultaneous penetration of artery and vein results in an arteriovenous fistula (Fig. 28.9) which compromises flow to a limb and in occasional cases brings about a high output cardiac state.

Transection of a vessel, whether cleanly by a knife or by shrapnel or missile, usually allows the free ends to constrict, retract and become sealed by a plug of thrombus. This process of constriction and thrombosis is best observed in traction injuries, classically in posterior dislocations of the knee in which, seen in slow motion, the intima stretches relentlessly until it fractures and curls back on itself to be followed similarly by disruption of the media and adventitia.

Pathophysiology of vascular injury

Arterial injury which results in arrest of distal flow is followed by ischaemia, tissue hypoperfusion and hypoxia, further compromised by hypovolaemic shock and vasoconstriction. Cell membrane permeability increases, which predisposes to interstitial and cellular oedema (Fig. 28.10). In particular, striated muscle does not tolerate continued warm ischaemia extending beyond 6–8 h, depending on the

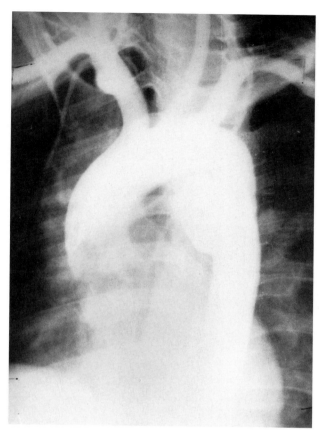

Fig. 28.8 Road traffic accident leading to partial ischaemic rupture of thoracic aorta, resulting in false aneurysm and haematoma which at operation extended from the root of the aortic arch down to mid-descending aorta. Femoral artery and left atrium were cannulated for bypass, the aorta was cross-clamped proximal and distal to rupture, and after excising the edges a Dacron graft was successfully interposed. (Reprinted from Barros D'Sa, A.A.B. (1992) In: *Arterial Surgery* (ed. H.H.G. Eastcott), p. 387, by permission of the publisher Churchill Livingstone.)

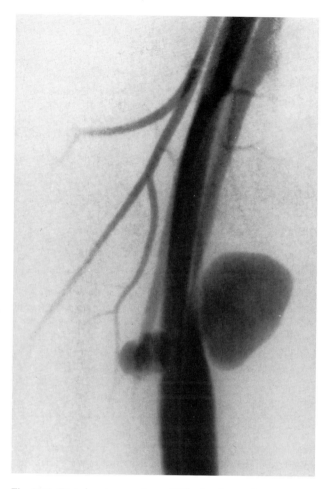

Fig. 28.9 Digital angiogram shows AV fistula of upper femoral vessels with associated false aneurysms. (With permission from Barros D'Sa, A.A.B. (1997) In: *Emergency Vascular Practice* (eds A.D.B. Chant & A.A.B. Barros D'Sa). Arnold, London.)

Pathophysiology
• Ischaemia → hypoperfusion → hypoxia
• Hypovolaemic shock and vasoconstriction
• Ischaemia–reperfusion injury
• Wound contamination

degree of injury and availability of collateral flow, which in the majority leads to myonecrosis and amputation. The restoration of flow paradoxically brings about ischaemia–reperfusion injury (IRI) which represents a further assault on cell membranes manifested by muscle oedema, necrosis and loss of function, and is directly proportional to the duration of preceding ischaemia. The complex biochemical and cellular pathophysiology of IRI has only been appreciated over the last decade. The generation of oxygen-derived free radicals (ODFRs), activation of neutrophils and the production of arachidonic metabolites play a central role in mediating IRI which has wider systemic implications for the lungs, liver, heart and kidneys. These complex interactions produce exudation, oedema and rising interstitial pressure within the inelastic fascial confines of muscle compartments, further aggravated if an injured vein has to be clamped or ligated, or if bone and soft tissues are also injured. Compartment pressure may rise to levels which even obliterate the main arteries, inviting sequelae of compartment syndrome, microvascular stasis and thrombosis, aseptic muscle necrosis, ischaemic nerve palsy, Volkmann's contracture with fixed plantar flexion (Fig. 28.11) and amputation.

Contamination by a wide spectrum of organisms may aggravate the adverse effects of IRI. Some Gram-positive cocci and Gram-negative cocci and bacilli acting synergisti-

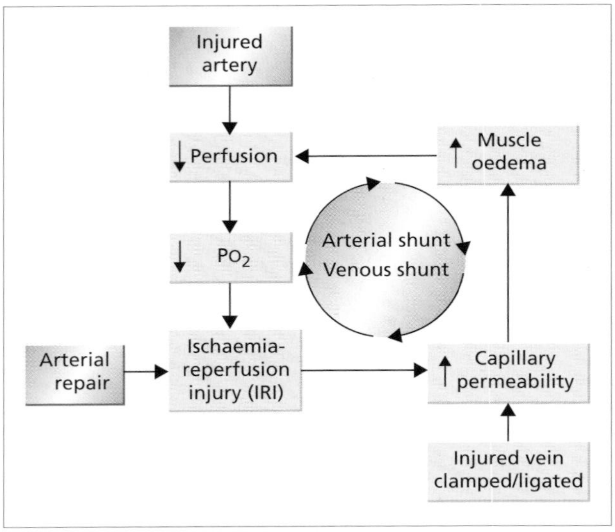

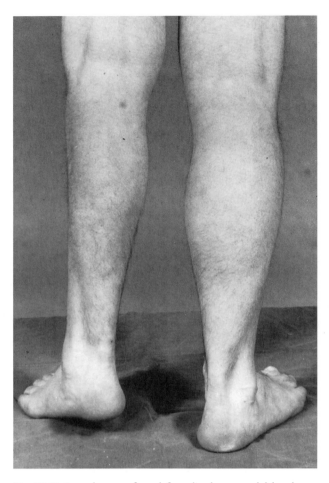

Fig. 28.10 Diagram depicts the pathophysiological sequelae of arterial injury and repair, and the influence of ligating a concomitantly injured vein. The beneficial effect of adjuvant early arterial and venous shunting in countering that process is illustrated.

cally, may cause cellulitis or necrotizing fasciitis, while an anaerobic environment in ischaemic tissue facilitates the regeneration of clostridial spores, some of which may be responsible for gas gangrene (Fig. 28.12). Conditions which favour such an outcome are varied: prolonged ischaemia, delayed diagnosis and exploration, defects in the essentials of wound care, ligation rather than repair of vessels and unrelieved compartment hypertension. Fasciotomies which alleviate the effects of IRI are open to superinfection, particularly by *Pseudomonas aeruginosa* which further heightens the possibility of amputation.

Limb vascular injuries

Early management

External bleeding is immediately controlled digitally and by the use of pad and bandage, avoiding the use of arterial forceps or clamps which are liable to cause damage to vessels and nerves. A tourniquet is ill-advised, especially as it is often poorly applied and may actually accelerate the bleeding; if inadvertently left unreleased, tissue and nerve damage may be irreversible. Standard resuscitative measures are employed, particularly in the multiply injured patient, to ensure an adequate airway, ventilation and the correction of hypovolaemic shock. Information about the nature of the wounding agent, blood loss and time interval since injury will be helpful. Tetanus toxoid, prophylactic cefuroxime and metronidazole, and analgesia are routine measures.

Fig. 28.11 Lateral suture of torn left popliteal artery and delayed fasciotomy led to Volkmann's ischaemic fibrosis and fixed plantar flexion at ankle. (Reprinted from Barros D'Sa, A.A.B. (1992) In: *Arterial Surgery* (ed. H.H.G. Eastcott), p. 367, by permission of the publisher Churchill Livingstone.)

Diagnosis and assessment

Sound clinical assessment is required. If bleeding is continuous is it mainly arterial or venous? If a haematoma is present is it expanding or pulsatile? Is there a thrill or audible bruit? Are the 'hard' signs of ischaemia such as absent distal pulses, pallor, mottling, coolness and numbness present? If not, are the 'soft' signs of transient ischaemia, mild neurological deficit or a small non-expanding haematoma detectable? In the multiply injured patient the signs of arterial injury may be obscured until circulatory recovery reveals one limb lagging behind the other. In most long bone fractures, resuscitation and correction of alignment restore distal flow. Arterial injury caused by dislocation of the knee is a notorious pitfall in examination because spontaneous reduction of the knee is fairly common and restores the normal contour

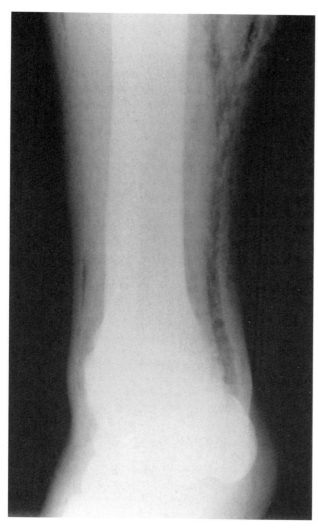

Fig. 28.12 Gas gangrene (Reprinted from Barros D'Sa, A.A.B. (1992) In: *Arterial Surgery* (ed. H.H.G. Eastcott), p. 367, by permission of the publisher Churchill Livingstone.)

will give the surgeon the confidence not to intervene and thereby limit the incidence of worthless exploration. Controversy surrounds the use of angiography in penetrating wounds in close proximity to the femoropopliteal system and trifurcation. Other factors, however, should influence the need for angiography, namely a high-velocity missile which may injure an artery well outside its path, the presence of 'soft' signs of arterial injury and not least the potential medicolegal consequences of limb loss resulting from missed injury. Should ischaemia persist after reduction of a femoral fracture, particularly in the elderly atherosclerotic patient, timely angiography may avert disaster. The high incidence of occult arterial injury associated with dislocations of the knee is a clear recommendation for a policy of routine angiography in such cases. If angiography facilities do not exist the surgeon is compelled to rely on meticulous and repeated clinical examination.

The non-salvagable limb

The success in recent times of improving salvage in critically injured limbs may have induced overoptimism in managing the very mutilated limb. This sometimes induces inappropriate zeal, committing both patient and surgeon to a protracted series of operations with serious complications and often eventual amputation of an insensate appendage. It might be preferable and indeed prudent to resort to primary amputation and early rehabilitation with a prosthesis. Various scoring systems can be of assistance in making a clinical judgement in the difficult case, and an additional experienced opinion is worthwhile in such cases. These considerations obviously do not apply when primary amputation represents no more than the completion of a traumatic amputation or the excision of a severely crushed limb.

The crucial importance of time

In order to shorten the period of ischaemia and to minimize IRI, particularly in complex limb vascular injuries, control of haemorrhage, resuscitation and definitive surgical treatment ought to be overlapping rather than sequential stages of management. In the multiply injured patient, injuries of the head, chest and abdomen which are life threatening, deserve priority, while repair of a limb vascular injury would have to be delayed, in which case the duration of ischaemia

of the leg and there may be no sign of bleeding within the tissues.

An audible Doppler signal is not as helpful as the evaluation of the pulse waveform, Doppler pressures and the ankle–brachial pressure index, which, if below 0.90, ought to be viewed with suspicion. Duplex scan imaging is being used increasingly to exclude potential injuries of the femoropopliteal system lying in proximity to the path of a bullet or knife. Ultrasound examination, however, may be impracticable in severe open injuries and may delay intervention.

The competence of angiography in delineating an arterial injury or in excluding it is well established, particularly in penetrating leg injuries. A positive angiogram will define the injury clearly (Figs 28.1, 28.7 and 28.9) while negative films

would influence outcome. However expeditious surgical intervention may be, a finite and sometimes unacceptable period of time is required for exposure, wound care, bone fixation and repair of artery and vein.

An understandably acute awareness of the passage of time and a wish to intervene swiftly may in turn introduce lapses in operative principles and technique. In particular, care of the wound may be cursory, leading to sepsis and complications in a downward spiral to amputation. The sense of urgency to restore flow encourages repair of the artery often before a fracture is stabilized, using less than satisfactory techniques such as lateral suture causing stenosis, end-to-end anastomosis under tension or vein grafting which is either too short or too slack. In addition, a vital venous channel might be ligated to save time, causing venous hypertension which simply compounds IRI and compromises an adjacent arterial repair. The robust manipulations required to reduce a fracture can disrupt a delicate vascular repair. If, however, fixation of the fracture precedes vascular repair, damage to soft tissues and vessels by bone fragments is averted and in addition an ideal length of vein is used to repair the artery. This prolongs ischaemia time and the orthopaedic surgeon, consciousness of this fact, may resort to a hurried, less than ideal or even defective fixation which potentially raises problems in bone union.

The management of the crucial factor of time in these complex vascular injuries demands an approach which eliminates the necessity to cast a constant and anxious eye on the clock. The placement of intravascular shunts in both artery and vein at the outset (Fig. 28.13), a policy which has been in force for nearly two decades at this centre, provides the solution to these dilemmas. These shunts, which imme-

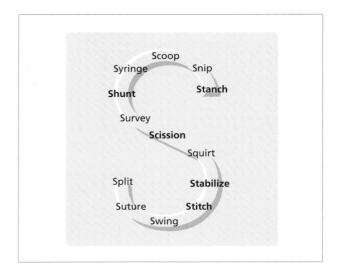

Fig. 28.14 *Aide-mémoire* for the Sequence of Steps in the operative management of complex limb vascular injury: *stanch* the bleeding, *snip* damaged ends of vessels, *scoop* out clot, *syringe* in heparinized saline, *shunt* both artery and vein, *survey* the wound and identify nerve injury, perform *scission* of non-viable soft tissue, *squirt* saline to irrigate wound, *stabilize* fractured bones, *stitch* or repair both artery and vein, *swing* tissue for cover, *suture* the wound (delayed primary if contaminated) and, if necessary, *split* fasciae (fasciotomy). (With permission from Barros D'Sa, A.A.B. (1992) Editorial. Complex vascular and orthopaedic limb injuries. *Journal of Bone and Joint Surgery* **74-B** 178.)

diately restore both perfusion and drainage, limit ischaemia and IRI (Fig. 28.10), and introduce a considered and logical operative plan which in turn has fostered a harmonious multidisciplinary approach to such injuries. The manoeuvres taken in correct sequence (Fig. 28.14) have improved technique, reduced the need for fasciotomy, lowered the rate of sepsis, ischaemic nerve palsy and amputation, and promoted early discharge. Following the recognition of these dividends an ideal design for a shunt specifically intended for limb vascular trauma was conceived at this centre which has stimulated experimental studies by armed forces medical establishments in the development of a temporary shunt.

Initial operative steps

The vessels in the limbs are approached through standard incisions and controlled initially by digital pressure and secured by exposing a segment on either side and applying a vessel clamp. The damaged ends are trimmed back sufficiently, the upper clamp is released to allow thrombus to be washed out, clot from the distal vessel is retrieved by a balloon catheter, assisted in delayed cases by milking the limb upwards, following which heparinized saline (20 U/ml) is perfused into the distal limb.

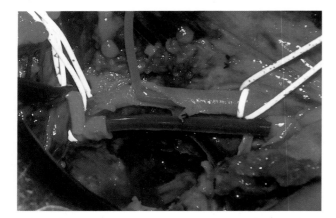

Fig. 28.13 Intravascular shunts: Brener in torn popliteal artery above and Javid in transected popliteal vein below preparatory to vein graft replacement of each vessel. (With permission from Barros D'Sa, A.A.B. (1988) In: *Limb Salvage and Amputation in Vascular Disease* (eds R.M. Greenhalgh, C.W. Jamieson & A.N. Nicolaides), p. 143. W.B. Saunders, London, UK.)

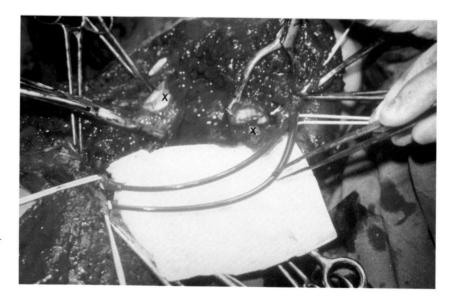

Fig. 28.15 A virtually dismembered leg at mid-thigh: Javid shunt bridging lengthy gap in femoral artery and perfusing distal limb; another such shunt bridging adjoining femoral vein and draining the limb. Ends of a fractured femur (XX) being manipulated prior to fixation. (With permission from Barros D'Sa, A.A.B. & Moorehead, R.J. (1989) *European Journal of Vascular Surgery* **3** 579.)

Shunting and operative discipline

The restoration of flow by means of an indwelling shunt in a transected femoral or popliteal artery (Fig. 28.15) arrests ischaemia and reduces IRI and consequently keeps compartment pressures within a safe range and buys time for a precise operative approach. An outlying shunt is sometimes necessary when lengthy segments of vessel are destroyed in the midst of extensive wounds (Fig. 28.16). The placement of a shunt in a severed adjacent vein (Fig. 28.15) will re-establish venous drainage and discourage thrombosis; the alternative of clamping the vein will cause an acute and unacceptable rise in compartment pressure and increase the likelihood of fasciotomy. Occasionally a vascular surgeon, working alongside others undertaking life-saving surgery in the head or torso, may be able to place these shunts in wounds of the lower limb until definitive repair is possible. Various commercially produced shunts are available for use but in their absence silicone elastomer or plastic tubing of suitable consistency, length and calibre may be used as long as the ends are carefully tailored to prevent intimal damage. The side-arm of a shunt placed in an artery (Fig. 28.13) provides a convenient portal for blood gas and other tests or for injection of saline or contrast for angiography. Such a shunt

Revascularization
• Mobilization of vessels
• Debridement
• Establish inflow and backflow
• Heparin
• Shunting
• Repair or reconstruction

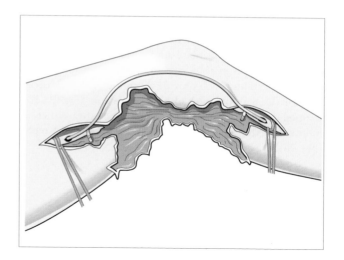

Fig. 28.16 In extensive injury outlying shunt picks up flow proximal to the injured segment and revitalizes the limb distally. (With permission from Barros D'Sa, A.A.B. (1989) In: *Vascular Surgical Techniques* (ed. R.M. Greenhalgh), p. 54. W.B. Saunders, London, UK.)

placed in a vein permits stagnant blood to be flushed out via the side-arm, thereby protecting the myocardium from a sudden bolus of blood rich in potassium and the products of reperfusion.

The surgeon has ample time to inspect the wound, identify nerve injury, remove debris and irrigate the tissues. Precise debridement and haemostasis is possible when re-established circulation allows sharper demarcation between dead and viable tissue. Removal of bone fragments and foreign bodies followed by copious irrigation, will lower the

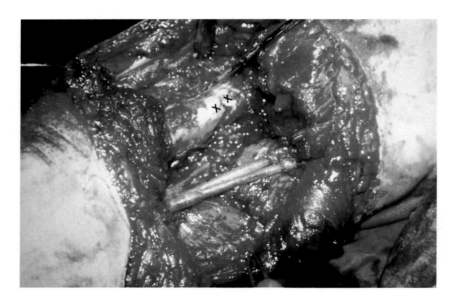

Fig. 28.17 After stabilization of fracture (XX) three interposed vein grafts restore flow through femoral artery and vein and the deep femoral vein. (With permission from Barros D'Sa, A.A.B. & Moorehead, R.J. (1989) *European Journal of Vascular Surgery* **3** 579.)

concentration of the bacterial innoculum. In the critically injured limb, temporary restoration of flow may be helpful in deciding whether primary amputation may be preferable to futile attempts at reconstruction. The insertion of long intravascular shunts will provide the amount of slack necessary for the manipulation of bone fragments (Fig. 28.15). Reduction and restoration of skeletal integrity either by internal or external fixation sets the scene for vascular repair (Fig. 28.17).

Arterial repair

It may not be necessary to explore every minor lesion discovered on angiography. On the other hand, a non-operative approach to mild or occult injuries may require protracted supervision, possibly further angiography and other studies, and sometimes delayed surgical treatment, all of which raise management costs. An interventional approach using stents to repair more modest injuries has been employed in a few centres.

When both artery and vein are concomitantly injured and shunts have not been used, arterial repair should be undertaken first, but with shunts in place, the order of repair is immaterial. The presence of a shunt eliminates the pressure to use expedient and perhaps flawed techniques such as lateral suture and direct anastomosis as ample time is available for vein graft reconstruction. In general, vein is harvested from the contralateral limb, a requirement which becomes absolute if the deep vein is injured. Long saphenous vein is usually of adequate calibre as an arterial interposition graft. It may be drawn over a shunt which acts as a stent preventing purse-stringing at the anastomoses, particularly if fine everting interrupted sutures are used.

A vein graft of much smaller diameter than the host artery may re-establish arterial flow for a short time but often undergoes thrombotic occlusion. A shunt bridging the gap removes the constraint of time and allows the construction of a compound vein graft of suitable diameter which holds better prospects of long-term patency. A well tried method has been to use two, and if necessary three equal segments of vein of suitable length opened longitudinally to form panels which after excising any valves are sewn together side by side to create a panel compound vein graft (Fig. 28.18). This graft may either be fashioned over a shunted vessel or prepared on the bench and then slipped over the shunt. An alternative technique is to produce a spiral compound vein graft (Fig. 28.19) in which a longitudinally slit length of vein bereft of valves is wound spirally over a bridging shunt and the adjoining margins of artery and vein are sutured. In severe injuries which damage lengthy segments of an artery, which may well be atherosclerotic, an outlying shunt will maintain flow, providing time for reconstruction using an extra-anatomic vein bypass graft tunnelled through clean tissues (Fig. 28.20).

The use of prosthetic grafts such as polytetrafluorethylene (PTFE) is effective in closed vascular injuries and even in those caused by knives and low-velocity missiles but one should not complacently use such grafts in contaminated wounds caused by bomb explosions. The calibre of the artery may itself call for the use of a prosthetic graft and unlike a vein graft which is liable to break down under the action of bacterial collagenase, it is fair to observe that the former is immune to such action except at the anastomoses with the host vessel.

Most false aneurysms of the femoral artery are catheter induced, and until recent success with ultrasound-guided compression therapy, repair was effected with a couple of transversely placed sutures or a patch graft. Arteriovenous fistulae are frequently missed, most notoriously in shotgun wounds, not only at initial examination but even on exploration; if angiography is unavailable intra-operative use of a sterile stethoscope may be helpful. In most cases reconstruction takes the form of lateral suture or patch angioplasty.

Peroperative evaluation of the quality of any repair is simply achieved by simulating a pulse in the distal artery by pumping heparinized saline from a syringe. Intra-operative use of a Doppler ultrasound probe or on-table angiography will determine the adequacy of repair and reveal defects for immediate correction.

Vein repair

Repair of a damaged vein will ensure free venous drainage and thereby enhance the patency of an adjacent arterial repair. Secondarily, a number of complications such as thromboembolism, chronic oedema, venous insufficiency and remotely of venous gangrene and amputation are averted. There is little evidence to support certain isolated but well-held views either that vein repair is followed by thrombosis, or that ligation is not necessarily harmful or that venous collaterals are perfectly adequate to keep the limb alive. Ligation of a large vein, however, is an entirely legitimate procedure in life-endangering situations.

A vein is usually of larger calibre than its companion artery and better able to tolerate lateral suture. It is also less tolerant of a small diameter interposition graft and therefore if a shunt is in place a compound vein graft ought to be constructed (Fig. 28.21). If time allows, a recently ligated vein confirmed to be free from thrombus by venography, can be shunted to relieve venous hypertension immediately prior to appropriate repair.

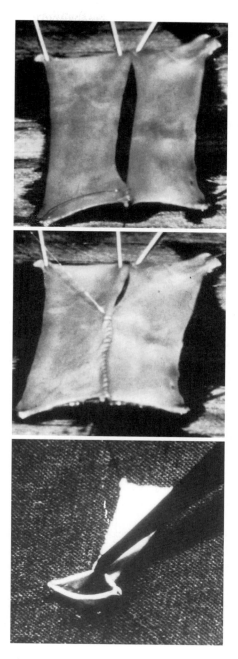

Fig. 28.18 Steps in construction of panel compound vein graft.

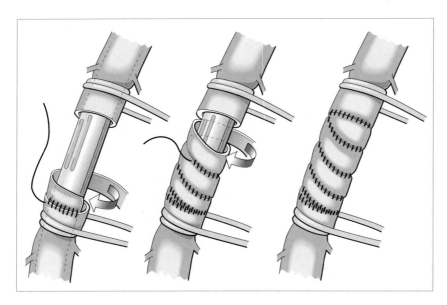

Fig. 28.19 Steps in construction of a spiral compound vein graft. (With permission from Barros D'Sa, A.A.B. (1989) In: *Vascular Surgical Techniques* (ed. R.M. Greenhalgh), p. 60. W.B. Saunders, London, UK.)

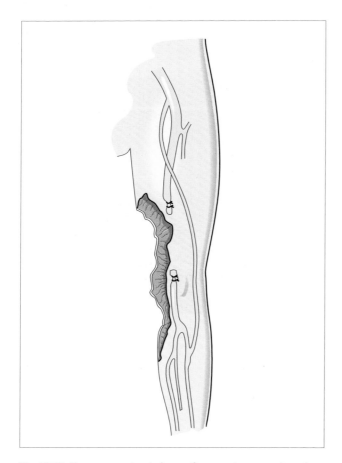

Fig. 28.20 Extra-anatomic vein bypass for extensive contaminated wound. (With permission from Barros D'Sa, A.A.B. (1989) In: *Vascular Surgical Techniques* (ed. R.M. Greenhalgh), p. 59. W.B. Saunders, London, UK.)

Fasciotomy

The use of intravascular shunts in an artery and in a concomitantly injured vein not only decreases the degree of IRI and its consequences but also significantly limits the requirement for fasciotomy. During the first 24 h mannitol is of value in accelerating the inactivation of ODFRs and reducing IRI.

In the upper limb the muscle compartments of the forearm and palm, and in the lower leg the anterior compartment which lies within rigid osseous and fascial boundaries are particularly vulnerable to raised compartment pressure. The indications for fasciotomy as a definitive procedure, usually inapplicable when shunts are employed, include: delay of 4–6 h after vessel injury, concomitant injury of main artery and vein, significant soft tissue injury, oedema and paralysis of muscle with patchy muscle necrosis, plantar flexion of the foot after completion of vascular repair, compartment pressures in excess of 40 mmHg.

Indications for fasciotomy
• Delay after injury
• Arterial and venous injury
• Soft tissue injury
• Muscle oedema
• Plantar flexion of foot
• ↑ Compartment pressures

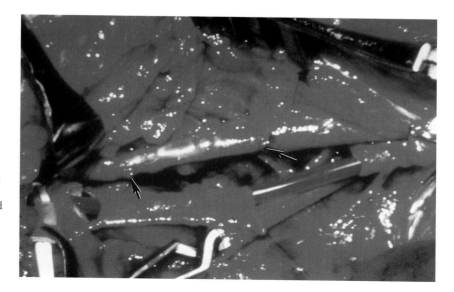

Fig. 28.21 Popliteal artery above (previously shunted) repaired using reversed interposition vein graft (between arrows). Popliteal vein below (also previously shunted) being repaired by panel compound vein graft. (With permission from Barros D'Sa, A.A.B. (1996) In: *Emergency Vascular Practice* (eds A.D.B. Chant & A.A.B. Barros D'Sa). Arnold, London, UK.)

A number of techniques for lower limb fasciotomy have been suggested, but the standard two-incision approach is both simple and effective: the lateral decompressing the anterior and peroneal compartments and the medial decompressing the superficial and deep posterior compartments. Decompression of the arm is achieved by a longitudinal centrally placed incision over the extensor compartment and by a further curvilinear incision on the flexor aspect commencing in the antecubital fossa, care being taken to identify and preserve the cutaneous nerves of the arm, crossing the wrist and extending distally into the palm along the thenar crease.

Wound closure

The quality of vessel cover and elimination of dead space afforded by adjacent soft tissue and muscle strongly influences the success of vascular repair. Shunting of severed vessels provides time for proper wound care at the end of which the quality and viability of tissue can be relied upon. A vein graft left open to desiccation, particularly in a contaminated field, will break down and cause secondary haemorrhage. Superficial muscles such as the sartorius and gracilis may be freed with their blood supply intact and swung over in such a way as to ensheath a graft. The skills of a plastic surgeon may have to be sought in the construction of free vascularized musculocutaneous flaps to cover both vessel repair and exposed bone (Fig. 28.17). In suitable cases the construction of an extra-anatomic vein bypass through clean viable tissue eliminates the need for these measures (Fig. 28.20). Skin closure is contra-indicated in contaminated

wounds; a policy of delayed primary suture 5–7 days later has been borne out by experience at this centre. Further inspections, if necessary under anaesthesia, should be undertaken until final closure is considered to be safe.

Postoperative care

The injured limb is nursed in the horizontal position. Restoration of fluid balance is necessary to ensure satisfactory perfusion of the distal bed. Low-dose heparin may be of value in aiding graft patency, while at the same time preventing deep vein thrombosis, although caution may be required in the multiply injured patient. Close vigilance of pulses, capillary refill time, Doppler pulse waveforms and pressures will register an early fall in distal flow. Thrombotic occlusion of a vessel repair usually reflects the use of less than optimal methods of reconstruction, often in response to the exigencies of time. Suspicions of impaired flow and graft failure should be confirmed by urgent angiography and if necessary the defective repair should be revised immediately. The defects which were often observed prior to the introduction of a policy of shunting include: constriction at the site of

Postoperative care
• Horizontal position
• Fluid balance
• ? Heparin
• Monitor circulation

lateral suture, purse-string constriction of a direct anastomosis, inadequate excision of damaged vessel, anastomotic tension when the vein graft is too short or kinking when too long. The latter circumstance is more likely to prevail when vessel repair precedes bone fixation. The incidence of re-exploration and revision of grafts fell sharply after shunting became routine policy.

Brachiocephalic vascular injuries

Early management

In the resuscitation room, compromise of the airway, breathing difficulty or evidence of cerebral hypoxia requires immediate endotracheal intubation, checking cord function if possible. The cuff should be inflated below the level of a tracheal tear accompanying injury to the carotid artery (Fig.

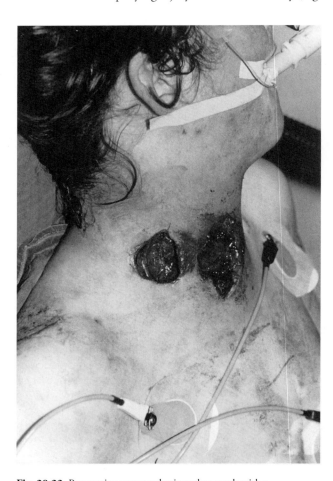

Fig. 28.22 Penetrating entry and exit neck wounds with a haematoma and probable tracheal injury. The vital first measure was to insert an endotracheal tube, inflating the cuff beyond the assumed site of injury, thereby preventing blood from entering the lungs. (Reprinted from Barros D'Sa, A.A.B. (1992) In: *Arterial Surgery* (ed. H.H.G. Eastcott), p. 390, by permission of the publisher Churchill Livingstone.)

28.22) and, if necessary, a tracheostomy should be performed and ventilation instituted. External bleeding and sucking wounds can usually be controlled by direct pressure. Administration of fluids, and O Rhesus negative blood if required, through large calibre i.v. lines, avoiding the side of presumed subclavian vessel trauma, will replace losses and maintain life-saving organ perfusion.

Major losses from a chest drain inserted for haemothorax are a signal for immediate operation. A high pressure mediastinal haematoma should be treated without delay as precipitate rupture into the pleural cavity may occur as a terminal event. Pericardiocentesis is indicated in cardiac tamponade (Fig. 28.23) but if time permits direct pericardiotomy may be more effective, especially if immediate median sternotomy is required to deal with injuries of the great vessels. A nasogastric tube may predispose to mediastinitis by entering unsuspected injuries of the upper respiratory and alimentary tract; endoscopy and contrast studies are usually unhelpful in locating them.

Diagnosis and assessment

Penetrating injury of the main brachiocephalic arteries may result in exsanguination externally, into the pleural cavity,

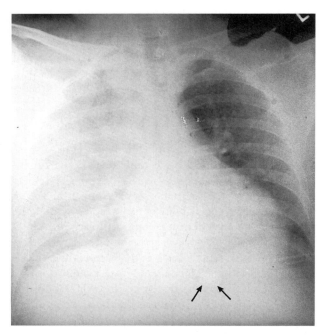

Fig. 28.23 Attempted assassination. Patient presented with shock and signs of cardiac tamponade. Chest X-ray shows bullet (arrowed) which penetrated right lung, liver, intrathoracic and subdiaphragmatic inferior vena cava and right ventricle, and classic features of haemopericardium and haemothorax. Victim survived. (Reprinted from Barros D'Sa, A.A.B. (1992) In: *Arterial Surgery* (ed. H.H.G. Eastcott), p. 385, by permission of the publisher Churchill Livingstone.)

the lungs or remain confined at high pressure in a mediastinal haematoma. Small entry and exit wounds often belie the gravity of internal injuries. In blunt arterial injury the patient may complain of dyspnoea, hoarseness or dysphagia. On examination there may be a haematoma or surgical emphysema at the root of the neck, pulses in the neck or upper limb may be weak or impalpable, a thrill or bruit may be present and there may be evidence of cranial nerve deficit, Horner's syndrome or signs of hemispheric ischaemia. Injuries of the oesophagus and lower trachea are generally below clavicular level.

Carotid artery injury may present with bleeding through the neck wound, an expanding pulsatile haematoma, hoarseness, stridor, thrill or bruit. Concomitant damage to the jugular vein may be associated with a caroticojugular fistula (Fig. 28.24) recognized by a machinery murmur. Associated laryngotracheal injury places the respiratory tract in danger from extravasated blood at high pressure. Bruises and abrasions from direct blunt carotid trauma may be apparent but rotation–hyperextension injury to the carotid artery leaves little external evidence. The duration, extent and progress of a neurological deficit are of great importance in management. In the absence of a closed head injury a neurological deficit must be presumed to be associated with carotid artery trauma, especially if the patient is fully conscious.

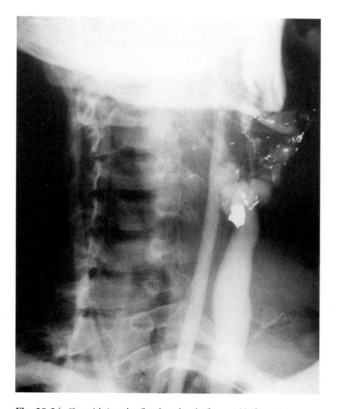

Fig. 28.24 Carotid–jugular fistula at level of carotid bifurcation.

Injury to the *vertebral artery* is rare and should be suspected when bleeding continues from a posterolateral neck wound despite pressure on the carotid artery. Alternatively, a false aneurysm or arteriovenous fistula may occur with co-existing damage to adjacent nerves. The third part of the vertebral artery which lies beyond the scope of the vascular surgeon may be injured, sometimes fatally, in a fist fight.

Injuries of the *subclavian vessels* by knife or bullet may penetrate the lung and sever elements of the brachial plexus. They present with torrential bleeding externally or into the neck or chest, and if of mild degree may present much later as a false aneurysm, possibly with episodes of thromboembolism. In blunt injury the presence of fractures of the clavicle and upper ribs should raise suspicions of coincidental subclavian artery damage recognizable by a pulseless, pallid and cold hand accompanied by paraesthesia and arm weakness, a subclavian bruit or an expanding pulsatile haematoma.

Chest films following blunt trauma may reveal the classical widened mediastinum and possibly fractures of the clavicle, first and even the second rib. In penetrating injury the signs of mediastinal emphysema and haemopneumothorax may be present. The path of a bullet or shrapnel fragments seen on a chest film (Fig. 28.23) is not necessarily linear, and speculation as to its presumed track may be misleading. In the stable patient angiography and enhanced spiral computerized tomography (CT) scans accurately define arterial injury, exclude coincidental heart or proximal thoracic aortic trauma which falls within the premise of the cardiac surgeon, and assist in planning surgery for control and repair.

The neck can be divided into three convenient zones to facilitate assessment and selection of patients for angiography and surgery: Zone I—inferior to the clavicle and anterior chest wall; Zone II—the neck between the clavicle below and the angle of the mandible above; and Zone III—between the angle of the mandible and the base of the skull. In general, angiography is of value in Zone I and Zone III carotid injuries as long as the patient is stable haemodynamically. In penetrating injuries within Zone II pre-operative angiography in the stable patient may not be essential but it is undoubtedly helpful in that the vascular surgeon will know exactly what to expect at operation (Fig. 28.25). Certainly in blunt trauma early angiography will define a carotid artery injury while the condition is still remediable. In vertebral artery injuries, pre-operative angiography not only locates the site and nature of the injury but it also establishes the existence of a patent contralateral vertebral artery, aplasia of which is most commonly observed on the left side. Transfemoral angiography will, of course, help to delineate the exact site and nature of subclavian artery injury so that the incisional approach is accurate.

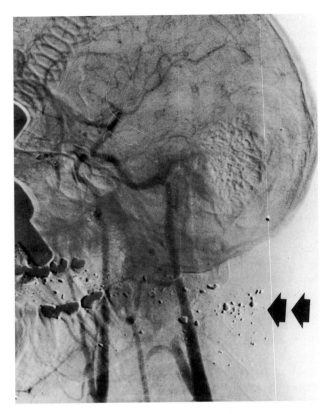

Fig. 28.25 Penetrating high velocity missile injury of the neck, its path traced by fragments traversing mandible, mouth and maxilla. Pharyngeal haemorrhage necessitated immediate endotracheal intubation with cuffed tube. Arch angiography revealed a transected external carotid artery as the source of bleeding. (With permission from Barros D'Sa, A.A.B. (1981) A decade of missile-induced vascular trauma. *Annals of the Royal College of Surgeons of England* **64** 37.)

Operative management

A median sternotomy which can be extended laterally into the intercostal spaces and supplemented upwards by oblique cervical and supraclavicular incisions permits complete access to any injured artery in the cervicomediastinal region. Median sternotomy is also a useful approach for relieving cardiac tamponade, suturing the heart wall or undertaking direct cardiac massage. Inability to secure swift control of a major bleeding artery in the chest is the commonest cause of intra-operative mortality. The superior vena cava may be sutured while the left innominate vein may be clamped and divided with impunity to gain access to arterial bleeding beneath. A partially occluding aortic C-clamp is used to control bleeding from a tear or avulsion at the origin of the great vessels. Lacerations within the innominate or left common carotid arteries are controlled by simple proximal and distal clamping.

Shunts are not necessary routinely but it is wiser to use at least one shunt when the innominate and left common carotid artery are simultaneously injured. As ligation of these vessels can cause fatal cerebral ischaemia it would seem logical to assume that clamping is also unacceptable, therefore, flow should be maintained until reconstruction is complete, particularly in the hypotensive patient. Ligation of the left subclavian artery is undesirable but it can be undertaken within the chest without seriously compromising upper limb flow. Lateral suture may be quite effective for lacerations of these large vessel trunks, and alternatively prosthetic patch graft angioplasty may be necessary. For simple transections, end-to-end anastomosis may appear possible but in fact vessel retraction introduces tension and a prosthetic graft usually has to be interposed. For injury at the origin of the innominate artery, especially if it exists in a contained haematoma at the arch, a fresh aortotomy from the ascending aorta may be used as an inflow site for an aorto-innominate bypass before finally closing off the injury, if necessary by means of a prosthetic patch. Such a graft may be bifurcated to restore flow in both the innominate and left common carotid arteries, with jump grafts if necessary taken to the subclavian arteries.

Urgent intervention is obviously necessary in cases of haemorrhage from the neck but wounds which fail convincingly to penetrate deeper than the plethysma need not be explored. A policy of selective exploration of the carotid artery is sharpened by good angiographic delineation of the carotid system. In practice, routine neck exploration, except for superficial injuries, is both cost effective and achievable with minimal complications and no mortality. In patients with developing neurological signs a CT scan is of little value in excluding cerebral infarction and to defer a decision to repair a carotid artery until the scan becomes conclusive will be too late.

The decision to repair a carotid artery in the neurologically intact patient or in the presence of mild neurological deficit presents no difficulty, but in those with a severe deficit the mortality rate may be high. While ligation may be quite justifiable in a patient with established neurological deficit and complete thrombotic occlusion of the entire carotid, the consensus of opinion now firmly favours carotid reconstruction in these cases as long as antegrade flow is present. Distal clot from an injured carotid must be removed by balloon catheter prior to repair or insertion of a shunt. Evidence of back flow, especially if above 60–70 mmHg, is regarded as evidence of satisfactory cerebral perfusion. An injured internal jugular vein calls for immediate head-down tilt to a level below that of the heart and control of the open vessel in preparation for repair. Ligation is entirely acceptable as long as the opposite internal jugular is intact. Lateral suture is acceptable for puncture wounds of the carotid but vein patch repair will prevent constriction and in a few cases end-to-end anastomosis may just be possible without tension. In instances where graft interposition is necessary, a long saphenous vein graft slipped over an intraluminal shunt may be used. Alternatively, a damaged proximal internal carotid artery may be replaced by a detached proximal external carotid artery.

Exposure of the vertebral artery through the neck is difficult but manageable, and ligation within its bony canal on either side of the injury may be necessary as long as the contralateral vertebral artery is present and intact. An occluding balloon may be inserted most appropriately in cases of vertebral arteriovenous fistula.

For subclavian artery repair, lateral suture or end-to-end anastomosis may be achieved without tension but PTFE interposition grafts have been used successfully. Adequate tissue cover for this rather delicate artery is often difficult, especially in high velocity penetrating injuries.

Postoperative management

Patients with injuries of the great vessels are usually monitored in the intensive care unit. If a neurological deficit preceded surgery, then ideally the patient should be allowed to regain full consciousness. Systemic administration of heparin is acceptable in the isolated carotid artery injury, even when signs of cerebral ischaemia are present. Adequate cerebral perfusion must be ensured by fluid and blood replacement. Consideration may be given to a nimodipine infusion as a means of countering cerebral arterial spasm. If neurological deterioration is suspected, Duplex ultrasound imaging or angiography may identify a possible source of thrombosis which calls for revision of repair. A similar clinical approach is called for if upper limb flow diminishes following subclavian or axillary artery.

Abdominal vascular injuries

Early management

Standard resuscitative measures including volume replacement must commence at the scene and continue en route to hospital. The military antishock trousers (MAST) or G suit is used in some countries but the application of this device requires skill and must be regarded as a waste of time when a trauma centre is close at hand. As blood pressure rises, bleeding from a vascular injury, temporarily contained by tamponade at low pressure, may resume. The possibility of intrathoracic injury in the form of an unrecognized haemothorax or cardiac tamponade (Fig. 28.23) must be considered, particularly if the patient fails to respond to volume replacement. Precious time should not be wasted on fruitless resuscitation and instead laparotomy and, if necessary, thoracotomy should be undertaken immediately.

Operative placement of clamps to control bleeding represents an intrinsic component of the resuscitative process and therefore should be undertaken in concert with other measures. In some well-equipped trauma centres, emergency room thoracotomy to cross-clamp the descending thoracic aorta has proved rewarding in a percentage of patients who are moribund or in a state of incipient or recent cardiac arrest.

Diagnosis and assessment

A dramatic external wound (Fig. 28.26) should not distract the clinician from a less conspicuous but possibly vital injury elsewhere. The fully undressed patient's abdomen, chest, axillae, back and perineum are inspected carefully for other wounds, keeping in mind the fact that the abdominal cavity extends from the level of the nipple line above to that of the gluteal crease below, and also that concomitant chest injury may be present. The stable patient may be examined further for evidence of an abdominal bruit or asymmetry of femoral pulses. Lacerations and bruises may provide a clue to injuries of underlying organs.

Investigations are undertaken only if the patient is stable. Diagnostic peritoneal lavage and a CT scan will assist in allaying doubts of internal injury. In the stable patient who

Abdominal investigations
• Peritoneal lavage
• Angiography
• CT scan
• IVP

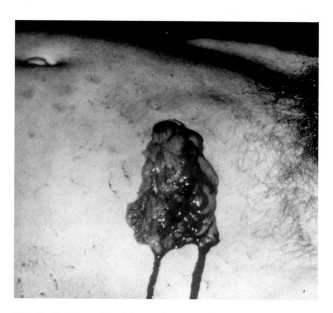

Fig. 28.26 Penetrating abdominal injury with omentum extruding through entry wound. (With permission from Rowlands, B.J. & Barros D'Sa, A.A.B. (1997) In: *Emergency Vascular Practice* (eds A.D.B. Chant & A.A.B. Barros D'Sa). Arnold, London.)

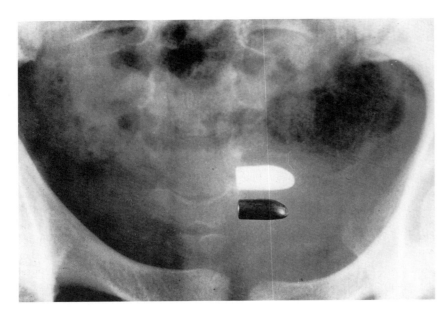

Fig. 28.27 Plain X-ray shows bullet in abdomen; superimposed is the missile, which was removed. (With permission from Rowlands, B.J. & Barros D'Sa, A.A.B. (1997) In: *Emergency Vascular Practice* (eds A.D.B. Chant & A.A.B. Barros D'Sa). Arnold, London.)

has sustained penetrating injury, X-rays of the torso may reveal shrapnel or bullets (Fig. 28.27). Angiography is of little value in penetrating trauma and delays operative intervention but in blunt injury it usually pinpoints the exact site of damage in the aorta or its branches. A CT scan is much more helpful than a pyelogram in confirming injury to a kidney because, complemented by contrast enhance-ment, it demonstrates loss of function and even reveals damage to the renal artery itself (Fig. 28.28a). Failure to demonstrate any enhancement or sign of excretion suggests renal artery injury; angiography will define the clas-sical abrupt 'cut-off' at the origin of the renal artery and importantly will establish the presence of a functioning contralateral kidney (Fig. 28.28b). A renal artery injury

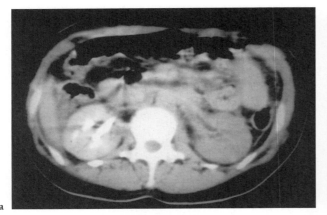

a

b

Fig. 28.28 Deceleration injury to left renal pedicle. (a) CT scan with enhancement shows a non-functioning left kidney. (b) Angiogram shows sharp cut-off of left renal artery and confirms satisfactory flow in right renal artery. (With permission from Rowlands, B.J. and Barros D'Sa, A.A.B. (1997) In: *Emergency Vascular Practice* (eds A.D.B. Chant & A.A.B. Barros D'Sa). Arnold, London.)

requires immediate repair, especially if it supplies a solitary kidney.

Operative management

In the hypotensive patient light anaesthesia is employed and the muscle relaxant withheld until the moment preceding incision so as to sustain the tenuous tamponade offered by the tone of the abdominal wall. A standard midline incision enables easy extension to a median sternotomy or anterolateral thoracotomy. Subdiaphragmatic aortic control by clamp or compressor may be required in cases of active haemorrhage. Rapid delivery of bowel outside the abdominal cavity and evacuation of blood and clots using large abdominal packs will expose the main sites of injury and bleeding. Solid organs are checked and tears in small and large bowel mesentery are temporarily controlled with light bowel clamps. In the presence of bowel perforation and faecal soiling from a lacerated colon these clamps will reduce further contamination. Cleansing and profuse irrigation are essential in lowering the concentration of the bacterial innoculum. Adequate collateral channels facilitate cross-clamping of the abdominal aorta and mesenteric arteries for a time but that does not hold true for the renal artery as kidneys have a low tolerance of warm ischaemia. In the stable patient, a contained retroperitoneal haematoma is left alone until proximal and distal control has been secured and only after first attending to obvious intraperitoneal injuries. An expanding pulsatile haematoma requires more urgent attention.

Injuries of the inferior vena cava tend to be rapidly exsanguinating, especially as the system is devoid of valves and receives the entire flow from the systemic circulation below the diaphragm as well as from the portal venous system and the liver itself. Injuries of the rather inaccessible retrohepatic cava are the most challenging of all. The application of cross clamps will abruptly deny venous return to the right heart and in the shocked patient can precipitate terminal arrest. Two helpful steps are temporary clamping of the aorta and Pringle's manoeuvre in which the border of the lesser omentum is compressed to occlude the hepatic artery and portal vein. These are rather ineffective measures in injuries of the retrohepatic cava. Packs and pressure will contain losses while the coronary and triangular ligaments are divided to allow the liver to be mobilized forward and downwards to expose the upper part of the retrohepatic cava. Many elegant techniques have been proposed to isolate the injured cava while still maintaining venous return. The concept of atriocaval shunting is worth considering. An Argyle drain is inserted through a purse-stringed opening in the right atrial appendage, exposed through a median sternotomy, and is guided down the inferior vena cava to the level of the renal veins. The snugged and isolated damaged section is controlled while venous return continues unhindered. This procedure is not easily accomplished and in common with other such ingenious methods has not been met by more than limited success.

Exposures for control and repair

All the main vessels are retroperitoneal in position and the exposure deemed to be the most appropriate has to be achieved.

Infrarenal

A vertical incision from the root of the mesocolon distally and to the right, similar to that employed for abdominal aortic aneurysms, will permit exposure of the infrarenal aorta, the origins of the renal arteries, the left renal vein and the inferior vena cava below it. The site of confluence of the common iliac veins can best be exposed by dividing the right common iliac artery and mobilizing the aortic bifurcation to the left; after repair of the injured vein the iliac artery is reconstructed. To expose the iliac vessels distally, the peritoneum is incised lateral to the caecum reflecting the bowel to the left, or lateral to the sigmoid colon reflecting the bowel to the right.

Left suprarenal

The splenic flexure and left colon can be mobilized and reflected to the right via a left paracolic incision to reveal the entire suprarenal aorta giving access to the coeliac axis, the splenic artery, the proximal superior mesenteric artery, the left renal artery and the tributaries of the portal vein.

Right suprarenal

An extended Kocher manoeuvre mobilizing the duodenum, head of pancreas and right colon provides remarkable exposure of the suprarenal inferior vena cava, the right renal vein and the suprarenal aortic segment and its coeliac, superior mesenteric and right renal branches, and the portal vein as far as the porta hepatis.

Vascular repair

The healthy young *aorta* must be handled carefully and sutures on the edge of a puncture wound or laceration should be placed without tension. For through-and-through puncture wounds the anterior opening is extended to enable repair of the posterior wall before closing the anterior aortotomy. A larger defect may be closed by means of a prosthetic patch, and if a segment is crushed or transected a Dacron tube graft should be interposed.

Should there be coincidental colonic injury with faecal soiling a prosthesis is very likely to become the seat of chronic sepsis complicated later by secondary haemorrhage; in such cases the ends of the aorta should be oversewn and a temporary axillobifemoral bypass graft constructed. If a small defect is present in association with peritoneal soiling a further option would be the use of autologous internal iliac artery as donor patch material.

These basic principles are also applicable to repair of the *iliac arteries*. If both internal iliac arteries are intact, conceivably one could be sacrificed as an autologous graft in reconstructing the common or external iliac artery. A simpler alternative would be to ligate the free ends of the iliac artery and to establish an extra-anatomic femorofemoral crossover bypass. If the proximal common iliac artery is injured at the aortic bifurcation a further option may be possible: the aorta is oversewn and the ipsilateral distal common iliac artery is mobilized across for anastomosis to the distally detached contralateral proximal internal iliac artery thus re-establishing crossover flow.

Deceleration injury of the *renal artery* may be represented by anything from an intimal fracture and thrombotic occlusion to complete avulsion, in each case infarcting the kidney. Minimal flow through collaterals might preserve the viability of the kidney, especially if the renal vein is intact. It is always worth reconstructing the renal artery if the CT scan demonstrates some renal function and particularly if that artery supplies the patient's only kidney. A minor tear may develop into a false aneurysm which can enlarge insidiously and therefore early intervention is indicated. Control of the renal artery is often best achieved by means of a partially occluding aortic clamp. The origin of the renal artery may be ligated and a new opening created for an aorto-renal bypass using either vein or prosthesis. A spleno-renal anastomosis is a further alternative which achieves the same objective.

A localized *coeliac artery* injury can be approached directly through the gastrohepatic omentum and repaired. The *hepatic artery*, once considered indispensable to the viability of the liver, may be ligated with impunity as long as portal blood supply is intact. The ligature should be applied proximal to the origin of the gastroduodenal artery to ensure collateral supply from the superior mesenteric artery. Fullen's anatomical classification of *superior mesenteric artery* injuries into three zones, with suitable operative approaches for each, takes into consideration relationships with the pancreas and concurrent pancreatic injury. Thus, a proximal superior mesenteric artery injury can be reconstructed with a vein graft or the stump re-implanted into the infrarenal aorta; an injury distal to the middle colic branch requires an aortomesenteric vein or prosthetic bypass. Attention to pancreatic injury must be meticulous in minimizing continued enzyme release which would be hazardous to any vascular repair. The inferior mesenteric artery may be ligated except in the rare instance of simultaneous damage to the other two mesenteric arteries. In all these cases, and particularly if the viability of the bowel is in doubt, a 'second look' procedure within 24 h is mandatory.

In injuries of a large venous trunk such as the *vena cava* lateral suture or patch vein grafting is quite effective. The cava may have to be ligated in a life-threatening situation but it should be reconstructed if the defect lies suprarenally. This can be done by means of a compound spiral graft fashioned from a length of saphenous vein wound over a shunt of suitable calibre; less desirably a free graft of suitable length taken from the infrarenal cava may be used to bridge the gap. A compound spiral graft can also be used in reconstructing an iliac vein but ligation may be the only option available. Ligation of the injured left renal vein, unlike the right, is of limited significance.

An injured *portal vein* should be repaired if subsequent portal hypertension is to be avoided; if the hepatic artery has had to be ligated, portal vein reconstruction would be essential in averting hepatic ischaemia. While *superior mesenteric vein* ligation is compatible with survival, gross intestinal venous pooling and hyperaemia of the splanchnic bed will ensue, increasing the chances of thrombosis and bowel infarction. Repair, if necessary by means of a vein graft, should be encouraged or alternatively a splenomesenteric vein bypass may be possible.

Postoperative care

Patients sustaining abdominal vascular injury are transferred to an intensive care unit where blood and fluids are replenished and abnormalities of coagulation corrected. A prophylactic antibiotic regimen of at least cefuroxime and metronidazole is required when contamination has occurred. Renal and hepatic and, if necessary pancreatic function, should be monitored. Urinary output provides a reasonable estimate of kidney function following renal artery repair in the solitary kidney but more reliable verification of the outcome requires angiography or isotope excretion urography. A 'second look' operation is essential when bowel has been resected against a background of vascular injury or when mesenteric arteries or elements of the portal venous system have been repaired; it also provides an opportunity to remove packs, inspect individual vascular repairs and re-irrigate the peritoneal cavity.

Further reading

General

Barros, D'Sa, A.A.B. (1992) Arterial injuries. In: *Arterial surgery* (ed. H.H.G. Eastcott), pp. 355–411. Churchill Livingstone, Edinburgh.

Barros, D'Sa, A.A.B. (1995) Editorial: Twenty five years of vascular trauma in Northern Ireland. *British Medical Journal* **310** 1–2.

Barros D'Sa, A.A.B. (1996) Adjunctive use of intravascular shunts in management of arterial and venous injuries. In: *Vascular Surgery: Twenty years of Progress* (eds S.J. Yao & W.H. Pierce). Appleton Lange, Connecticut.

Barros, D'Sa, A.A.B., Hassard, T.H., Livingston, R.H. *et al.* (1980) Missile-induced vascular trauma. *Injury* **12** 13–30.

Bergentz, S.E. & Bergqvist, D. (1989) *Iatrogenic vascular injuries.* London Springer Verlag, London.

Chant, A.D.B. & Barros D'Sa, A.A.B. (eds) (1997) *Emergency Vascular Practice.* Vascular trauma section. Arnold, London.

Feliciano, D., Mattox, K.L., Graham, J. & Bitondo, C. (1985) Five year experience with PTFE grafts in vascular wounds. *J Trauma* **25** 71–82.

McCormick, I.M., & Burch, B.H. (1979) Routine angiographic evaluation of neck and extremity trauma. *J Trauma* **19** 384–387.

Rich, N.M., Baugh, J.H. & Hughes, C.W. (1970) Acute arterial injuries in Viet Nam: 1000 cases. *Journal of Trauma* **10** 359–369.

Limb vascular injuries

Barros, D'Sa, A.A.B. (1992) Editorial: Complex vascular and orthopaedic limb injuries. *Journal of Bone and Joint Surgery (Br)* **74** 176–178.

Barros, D'Sa, A.A.B. (1994) Upper and lower limb vascular trauma. In: *Atlas of Vascular and Endovascular Techniques*, 2nd edn, (ed. R.M. Greenhalgh). W.B. Saunders, London.

Gregory, R.T., Gould, R.J., Peclet, M. *et al.* (1985) The mangled extremity syndrome (MES): A severity grading system for multisystem injury of the extremity. *J Trauma* **25** 1147–1150.

Menzoian, J.D., Doyle, J.E. & Cantelmo, N.L., *et al.* (1985) A comprehensive approach to extremity vascular trauma. *Arch Surg* **120** 801–805.

Mubarak, S.J. & Owen, C.A. (1977) Double-incision fasciotomy of the leg for decompression in compartment syndromes. *J Bone Joint Surg (Am)* **59A** 184–187.

Walker, A.J., Mellor, S.G. & Cooper, G.J. (1994) Experimental experience with a temporary intraluminal heparin-bonded polyurethane arterial shunt. *Br J Surg* **81** 195–198.

Brachiocephalic vascular injuries

Barros, D'Sa, A.A.B. (1996) Brachiocephalic artery injury. In: *Arterial Surgery: Management of Challenging Problems* (eds S.J. Yao & W.H. Pierce). Appleton Lange, Connecticut.

Brawley, R.K., Murray, G.F. & Crisler, C. (1970) Management of wounds of the innominate, subclavian and axillary vessels. *Surg Gynecol Obstet* **131** 1130–1140.

Johnson, R.H., Wall, M.J. & Mattox, K.L. (1993) Innominate artery trauma, a thirty year experience. *J Vasc Surg* **17** 134–140.

Mitchell, R.L. & Enright, L.P. (1983) The surgical management of acute and chronic injuries of the thoracic aorta. *Surg Gynecol Obstet* **157** 1–4.

Monson, D.O., Saletta, J.D. & Freeark, R.J. (1969) Carotid-vertebral trauma. *J Trauma* **9** 987–999.

Abdominal vascular injuries

Courcy, P.A., Brotman, S., Oster-Granite, M.L., *et al.* (1984) Superior mesenteric artery and vein injuries from blunt abdominal trauma. *J Trauma* **24** 843–845.

Fullen, W.D., Hunt, J. & Altemeier, W.A. (1972) The clinical spectrum of penetrating injury to the superior mesenteric arterial circulation. *J Trauma* **12** 656–664.

Graham, J.M., Mattox, K.L. & Beall, A.C. (1978) Portal venous system injuries. *J Trauma* **18** 419–422.

Kudsk, K.A., Bongard, F. & Lim, R.C. (1984) Determinants of survival after vena caval injury: analysis of a 14-year experience. *Arch Surg* **119** 1009–1012.

Sankaran, S., Lucas, C. & Walt, A.J. (1975) Thoracic aortic clamping for prophylaxis against sudden cardiac arrest during laparotomy for acute massive haemoperitoneum. *J Trauma* **15** 290–296.

CHAPTER 29

Urological emergencies

Thomas H. Lynch & John M. Fitzpatrick

Introduction

Investigation and management in the accident and emergency department of the more common urological problems are dealt with in this chapter. The commonest problems presenting to the Accident and Emergency (A&E) department are urinary tract infections (including epididymitis), acute urinary retention, stone related symptoms and testicular torsion.

Urinary tract infections

Although the normal urinary tract is sterile and does not contain bacteria or white cells urinary tract infection is the most common bacterial infection of all ages. Acute urinary infection is caused mainly by aerobic Gram-negative rods (*Escherichia coli*, *Proteus mirabilis*) and Gram-positive cocci (e.g. staphylococci, enterococci) but occasionally may be caused by anaerobic organisms.

Bacteriuria can occur with or without pyuria and may be symptomatic or asymptomatic. Significant bacteriuria refers to a bacterial count greater than 10^5/ml and signifies a urinary tract infection (UTI). Patients may have irritative symptoms with counts as low as 10^2/ml.

Urine culture is the only way of diagnosing a urinary tract infection. In acute infections one infective pathogen is usually found whereas two or more pathogens may be found in chronic infections. One hundred thousand bacteria per ml is accepted as the diagnostic criterion. The probability of true bacteriuria being present with this finding is about 80%. Conversely when the bacterial count is less than 10^5/ml there is about a 5% chance of an infection being present.

The presence of pyuria correlates poorly with the definitive diagnosis of UTI. In children, urine culture should be used as the diagnostic criterion, as pyuria can be seen after immunization and gastroenteritis. Clinical differentiation between upper and lower urinary tract infections is generally unreliable, but lower bacterial counts associated with pyuria in a symptomatic patient almost certainly indicates a lower urinary tract infection.

Most community acquired infections are caused by coliforms and generally respond to a short course of oral antibiotics. A single high dose is adequate but as symptoms often persist for 2–3 days patients feel better being treated for the duration of their symptoms. Antibiotics with minimal effect on bowel or vaginal flora are to be preferred. Nitrofurantoins and trimethoprin are suitable in this regard and are excreted well in the urine.

Hospital acquired infections often include resistant organisms such as *Pseudomonas aeruginosa* and may require broad-spectrum intravenous antibiotics such as augmentin and gentamicin.

Acute pyelonephritis

This is defined as an infectious inflammatory disease involving both the parenchyma and the pelvis of the kidney but the diagnosis is made on clinical grounds.

Patients usually present with chills, fever, vomiting and flank pain accompanied by bacteriuria. These so-called upper tract symptoms are frequently accompanied by urinary frequency and urgency. The urine is usually cloudy and malodorous.

Relevant laboratory investigations include a urinary sediment showing white and red blood cells and positive bacterial cultures. A polymorphonuclear leucocytosis is often present and rarely creatinine may be elevated because of renal impairment.

The microbiological pathogens most commonly include: *Escherichia coli*, *Klebsiella*, *Proteus*, *Enterobacter*, *Pseudomonas*, *Serratia* and *Citrobacter*. Of the Gram-positive organisms *Streptococcus faecalis* and *Staphylococcus aureus* are important.

Immediate radiological investigation is not usually warranted in suspected upper tract infection. Plain films are generally normal. An intravenous urogram will show some renal enlargement in the acute phase in about 20% of patients due to inflammation and congestion. There may be delayed uptake and excretion of contrast or changes of chronic pyelonephritis (Fig. 29.1). Dilatation of the ureter and renal pelvis may be seen without any obstructive cause and this has been attributed to paralysis by bacterial endotoxins but is usually seen with chronic inflammation.

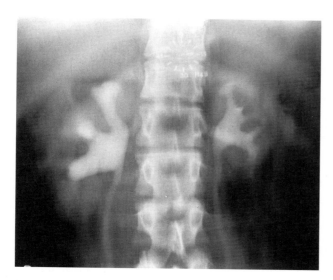

Fig. 29.1 Patient presenting with loin pain and fever; intravenous urogram shows evidence of chronic pyelonephritis with thin parenchyma and loss of cupped calyces.

Renal ultrasound although helpful in demonstrating renal size and obstruction gives little additional information to the IVU. Computerized tomography (CT) is very rarely justifiable in acute infections. The differential diagnosis of acute pyelonephritis is shown in Table 29.1.

Management

Mild acute pyelonephritis is characterized by mild loin pain with a low grade fever and usually responds to oral antibiotics. In patients requiring hospitalization, urine and blood cultures should be obtained before antimicrobial therapy is commenced. This is generally started on an empirical basis until the results of urine culture are known. Aminoglycosides (e.g. gentamicin) and ampicillin or augmentin have proved effective against *Enterobacter*, *Pseudomonas* and other Gram-negative organisms.

Analgesia is usually required with more severe infections. The patient should receive fluids intravenously and orally to maintain adequate hydration and upper tract imaging

Table 29.1 Differential diagnosis of acute pyelonephritis.

Pancreatitis
Basal pneumonia
Cholecystitis
Appendicitis
Diverticulitis
Acute pelvic inflammatory disease
Ureteric colic
Lower urinary tract infections

should be performed to exclude obstruction. If the kidney is shown to be obstructed then management usually involves upper tract drainage either percutaneously or by internal stenting depending on the underlying cause.

In general, 48 h of intravenous antibiotics is adequate before commencing oral antibiotics. If the clinical response is poor then re-evaluation is necessary to determine whether upper tract obstruction has occurred or whether the antibiotic is appropriate once sensitivities are available.

Repeat urine cultures are indicated during and after treatment because in about 30% of patients symptoms improve despite persistence of the bacterial pathogen. Therapy in acute pyelonephritis should be continued for at least two weeks.

Approximately 30% of patients relapse in spite of 14 days of therapy but most are cured with a further course and a minority will require a 6 week course.

Other less common causes of upper tract infection

Emphysematous pyelonephritis

Emphysematous pyelonephritis is a relatively rare life-threatening illness. It manifests as an acute necrotizing pyelonephritis caused by gas-forming organisms and is almost exclusively seen in diabetics. If initial management with antibiotics fails then nephrectomy may be indicated.

Renal abscess

A renal abscess is a collection of purulent material confined to the renal parenchyma. Infection may be by haematogenous spread (staphylococcal) from distant sites or from ascending infections (Gram-negative organisms) secondary to urinary tract obstruction. A perinephric abscess may develop from rupture of an intrarenal abscess into the perinephric space. Patients generally do not present acutely but have symptoms for 2–3 weeks.

The patient may present with fever, chills and loin pain. If there is no communication with the collecting system then lower urinary symptoms are rare. Investigations will typically reveal a leucocytosis. Ultrasound may be helpful although the features can be confused with a renal tumour. CT scan with and without contrast is the most accurate investigation but this is generally not indicated in the A&E setting.

Optimal management involves surgical drainage either percutaneously or open in addition to antibiotic therapy.

Papillary necrosis

Papillary necrosis results from ischaemic necrosis of the papillary tip or the entire pyramid and is usually associated with a UTI. It may present in the acute phase with symptoms caused by the sloughing of papillae which may mimic ureteric colic. If associated with infection the patient may experience chills, fever and haematuria. Management depends on the presentation and may be expectant, with antibiotics and occasionally endoscopic removal of the sloughed papillae from the ureter.

Bacteraemic and septic shock

Gram-negative septicaemia is a serious and often life-threatening condition. The organisms involved are listed in Table 29.2. Urethral and intravenous catheters and ventilatory equipment are the most frequent sources of Gram-negative infections. The clinical manifestations and management are dealt with elsewhere in this book (Chapter 6).

Cystitis

Although cystitis is not an emergency as such, it presents so frequently to casualty that it warrants discussion. It is a bacterial infection of the bladder with accompanying irritative symptoms. The urine typically shows pyuria and bacteriuria. The infection usually ascends the urethra to the bladder and is consequently more common in females than males. The onset in women frequently follows sexual intercourse, thus it is called honeymoon cystitis. The patient rarely has a temperature or feels systemically unwell. Most cases of cystitis are managed by the general practitioner but some occasionally present to the A&E department. The differential diagnoses are given in Table 29.3.

A simple community acquired infection can be treated with the cheapest most appropriate antibiotic and the patient is often better before the results of sensitivities are available.

Table 29.2 Genito-urinary pathogens involved in Gram-negative septicaemia.

Escherichia coli
Proteus
Klebsiella
Pseudomonas

Table 29.3 Differential diagnosis of cystitis.

Vulvovaginitis
Acute urethral syndrome
Acute pyelonephritis
Prostatitis

Bacterial prostatitis

The infecting organisms are those that cause urinary tract infections.

Acute bacterial prostatitis is often associated with acute cystitis and acute urinary retention. The patient complains of deep perineal pain and an exquisitely tender prostate on examination. A leucocytosis is often present and generally there is a positive urine culture. Acute bacteraemia with septic shock is a potential complication of acute bacterial prostatitis.

Patients often require admission for intravenous antibiotics and depending on the clinical setting may be continued for up to 5 days. Aminoglycosides and ampicillin are generally appropriate for both Gram-negative bacteria and enterococci. Oral antibiotics are generally continued for 30 days. If in acute urinary retention a suprapubic catheter should be employed to allow drainage of prostatic secretions from the urethra. Patients may develop chronic prostatitis or a prostatic abscess.

Prostatic abscess

In the past, prostatic abscesses were caused by gonococci, whereas these days they are caused by coliforms and are generally a complication of acute bacterial prostatitis. They present usually in the fifth or sixth decade. The clinical features are often indistinguishable from prostatitis but fluctuation is an important diagnostic clue. Patients frequently need to be catheterized and transurethral incision usually suffices.

Acute urethritis

Although patients generally present to a sexually transmitted disease clinic they may be seen in the A&E department.

Acute urethritis is characterized by dysuria and urethral discharge and is usually caused by a sexually transmitted disease. It is classified as gonococcal or non-gonococcal (non-specific) urethritis (NSU). NSU is caused by *Chlamydia* and common urinary pathogens.

The usual incubation period for N-gonorrhoea after sexual intercourse is 2–6 days whereas for NSU it is 1–5 weeks. If no secretions from the urethra are apparent they may be facilitated by urethral or prostatic massage. Specimens can be obtained from the distal urethra with calcium alginate swabs and then rolled over a slide rather than streaked. The slide is air dried and heat fixed. NSU can be differentiated from gonorrhoea by the absence of *N. gonorrhoea.*

Management

All patients should be referred to a sexually transmitted disease clinic for full microbiological screening and proper contact tracing in order to prevent serious sequelae. Treatment of gonococcus is now with cephalosporins because of the emergence of multiresistant strains. *Chlamydia* is the most common causative organism of non-gonococcal urethritis. Tetracyclines or erythromycin for 10 days are the drugs of first choice. Other organisms are treated depending on sensitivities.

Renal and ureteric stones

Renal stones

Renal stones generally form in a calyx where they may remain and be asymptomatic. Stones more frequently pass into the pelvis where they either become trapped or pass down the ureter. In the acute phase patients with renal stones may present to the A&E department with loin pain or with features of acute pyelonephritis with loin pain and fever. These stones occasionally cause obstruction giving rise to loin pain radiating to the groin. Staghorn calculi rarely present acutely but they may cause septicaemia and pyonephrosis.

Many renal diseases do not cause pain because they do not cause capsular distension. However, when there is sudden distention of the renal capsule from back pressure, such as in pyelonephritis or acute ureteral obstruction renal pain is prominent.

Ureteric calculi

Ureteral pain may be seen as a result of the passage of a stone or blood clot or more rarely a sloughed papilla, transitional cell carcinoma of the renal pelvis or ureter, or a fungus ball in drug addicts.

The pain experienced is generally colicky in nature, sudden in onset and very severe. It may radiate from the costovertebral angle down along the course of the ureter. In men it may also be felt in the bladder or scrotum and in women in the vulva. It is typically associated with nausea and vomiting.

Paradoxically the smallest stones seem to cause the greatest pain and stones under 0.5 cm in diameter usually pass spontaneously. Women who have experienced a difficult childbirth have often said that they would prefer another labour to another stone.

Urinalysis invariably reveals microscopic haematuria but of course this may be absent in cases of complete ureteric obstruction.

It can be difficult to differentiate ureteric colic from other intra-abdominal pathology and the differential diagnosis includes most other causes of acute abdominal pain.

Management

An intravenous urogram (IVU) should be performed in the A&E department on admission to confirm the diagnosis of suspected ureteric colic (Figs 29.2, 29.3, 29.4). Renal ultrasound is sometimes indicated to exclude obstruction. Treatment in the acute phase is symptomatic with analgesia and antibiotics for infection as required.

In uncomplicated ureteric colic diclofenac sodium is given intramuscularly or as a suppository. Occasionally, opiate analgesics are required but this should not be used as first line treatment.

A very important situation is where there is proximal obstruction with infection as in this case there is a high risk of sometimes fatal septicaemia. Obstruction with infection may also lead to renal deterioration. In these situations the upper tract needs to be decompressed and drained either percutaneously or internally with a stent.

Acute urinary retention

Acute urinary retention is the commonest acute problem associated with benign prostatic hyperplasia and carcinoma of the prostate. It is the sudden onset of the total inability to void. It is most commonly caused by benign prostatic hyperplasia (Table 29.4). Acute urinary retention occurs at any time in the natural history of the development of benign prostatic hyperplasia and it is usually an indication for surgery.

Although in most patients no definite precipitating factor is ascertained it may be associated with alcohol intake, infection, constipation leading to faecal impaction, anticholinergics, antidepressants or tranquilizers.

Clot retention of urine may be caused by bleeding from the prostate gland but can also be caused by other underlying pathology such as a bladder tumour. Occasionally patients may bleed profusely 2–3 weeks after transurethral

Table 29.4 Causes of acute urinary retention in males.

Benign prostatic hyperplasia
Carcinoma of the prostate
Prostatitis
Bladder neck stricture following previous surgery
Clot retention
Urethral strictures
Phimosis
Chronic retention with or without overflow

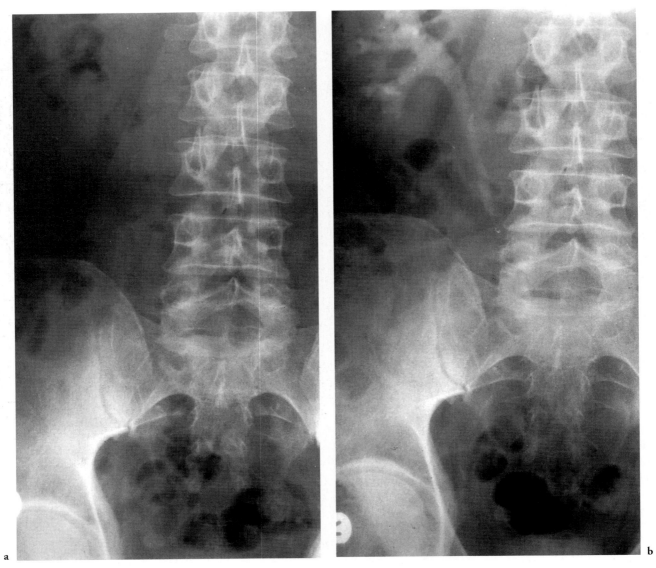

Fig. 29.2 Patient presenting with right ureteric colic with stone at the level of L4 on right. (a) Plain film, (b) after intravenous contrast.

prostatectomy and require admission because of clot retention of urine.

Patients generally present with suprapubic pain and the inability to void.

If a patient gives a history of recent onset of back pain or weakness in his legs, anal tone and perianal sensation should be assessed to exclude cord compression from metastatic prostate cancer. Cord compression can present with acute urinary retention and if diagnosed early the patient can benefit from a laminectomy (or radiotherapy) to decompress the spinal cord.

The abdomen should be examined to establish if the patient has a palpable bladder. If a patient is passing some urine but has a painless palpable bladder with a normal serum creatinine then catheterization is not generally necessary. This is chronic rather than acute retention and the prostate can usually be dealt with on the next convenient operating list.

If the patient has overflow incontinence or has renal impairment then they should be catheterized. Following catheterization the patient may have a marked diuresis. This leads to dehydration giving a falsely high haemoglobin which will 'fall' when the patient is rehydrated. In the past the excess urinary output was replaced with intravenous fluids however this is not necessary after the first 24 h. A jug of water by the bedside will suffice. Prostatic surgery is best

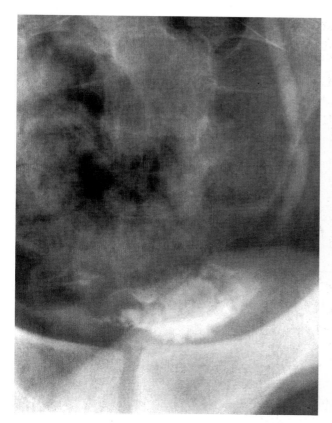

Fig. 29.3 There is a column of dye in a distended ureter extending down to the level of a lower ureteric calculus. This demonstrates the importance of emptying the bladder prior to delayed films.

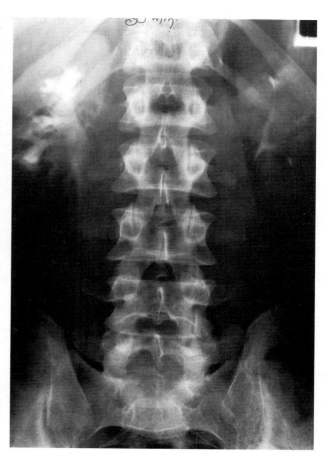

Fig. 29.4 A twenty-four-year-old presented to the accident and emergency department with a right ureteric colic. Intravenous urogram demonstrates calyceal rupture on the right secondary to acute obstruction from a stone which has passed before IVU was performed.

delayed in these patients until renal function improves with an indwelling urinary catheter.

Catheterization in acute retention

Urethral catheterization is the treatment of choice and if haematuria is not expected a 16 or 18Ch Foley catheter is adequate (see note on catheterization). A coude tip catheter can safely be used to negotiate the bladder neck — the commonest site of obstruction when introducing a catheter in acute urinary retention. If urethral catheterization fails then a suprapubic catheter can be passed, and in some centres urologists prefer their patients to have a suprapubic catheter inserted initially. Experience has shown that most patients with acute urinary retention will require some form of treatment for bladder outflow obstruction.

Haematuria and clot retention

Haematuria is usually not an indication for emergency admission to hospital but is an indication for urgent referral to a urologist. If a patient has concomitant fever, clot retention or is passing large amounts of blood then admission is required. It is rare to find a drop in the haemoglobin attributable to haematuria. A diagnosis of bladder tumour should always be considered in the older patient but bleeding is more commonly caused by the prostate or a urinary tract infection.

In the case of clot retention a large 22Ch catheter should be passed and the bladder washed out. It is advisable to give intravenous prophylactic antibiotics if the patient has a fever or a surgical prosthesis. After catheterization the bladder should be washed out with a 66 ml bladder tip syringe with either water or saline and this should be continued until all the clots have been evacuated. If all of the clots are not evacuated the patient may continue to bleed. If the catheter continues to block off or evacuation of clots proves impossible then the patient may need to be brought to theatre for clot evacuation under general anaesthetic using the resectoscope sheath.

Acute urinary retention in females

Acute urinary retention in the female is far less common than in the male. Ovarian and uterine pathology, a retroverted gravid uterus or a neuropathic bladder may cause acute retention. As in the male infection, constipation leading to faecal impaction, anticholinergics, antidepressants or tranquillizers may also cause retention. Catheterization in the female is generally easier and if haematuria is not expected then a 14Ch Foley catheter should be adequate.

Conditions of the testes and scrotum

In acute conditions of the testes and scrotum the most important diagnosis to exclude is testicular torsion (see Table 29.5).

Testicular torsion

Testicular torsion is a true urological emergency and is most common between the ages of 12 and 18 years but may occur at any age. Typically, the patients will give a history of previous attacks of pain which resolved spontaneously.

The classical symptoms of local pain, nausea, vomiting, high testes with a tender spermatic cord are diagnostic. Urinary symptoms are unusual. Abnormal urinalysis is more common with epididymitis. A twisted appendix testes may be seen in boys 7 to 14 years of age and in some reported series this was more common than true torsion of the testes. The tenderness of a torted appendix testes is localized to the upper pole and a blue tinge may be seen through the scrotal skin. This preoperative differentiation may prevent unnecessary scrotal exploration but if there is any doubt the scrotum should be explored without delay. Other testicular appendages which may become torted are appendix epididymis, para-epididymis and vas deferens.

Radionucleotide scans and colour flow Doppler ultrasound have been used as an aid to diagnosis but are not 100% accurate; thus, surgical exploration remains the gold standard in investigation and treatment of suspected testicular torsion.

Table 29.5 Acute painful scrotal conditions.

Testicular torsion
Torsion of testicular appendages
Epididymitis and its complications
Scrotal haematoma with or without testicular fracture
Acute hydrocele
Incarcerated hernia
Testicular tumours (rare cause)
Trauma

Management

Manual detorsion can be considered in adolescent boys if the operating theatre is not immediately available. The cord can be anaesthetized with lignocaine and the testes is rotated from within outwards and if successful the patient will notice instant relief. This detorsion is not suitable for babies whose torsion is extravaginal.

If unsuccessful, a suspected diagnosis of testicular torsion warrants immediate surgical exploration. If true testicular torsion is explored early 100% salvage rates can be obtained. Exploration within 6 h: 100% testicular salvage
6–12 h: 70% testicular salvage
> 12 h: 20% testicular salvage
In the case of a twisted appendix testes many surgeons would only explore the affected side. We would suggest routinely exploring both sides as the appendages are found bilaterally in about two-thirds of patients and contralateral exploration adds little to patient morbidity.

Table 29.6 gives the general principles involved in testicular fixation.

Epididymitis

Epididymitis is the most commonly encountered intrascrotal inflammatory condition. It may be associated with inflammation of the testes causing epididymo-orchitis. Isolated inflammation of the testes is uncommon. Bacterial epididymitis caused by coliforms and *Pseudomonas* are most commonly seen and are often associated with underlying urological pathology. This is the most common form in children and older men. Sexually transmitted epididymitis is most commonly seen in young men and is usually caused by *C. trachomatis* or *N. gonorrhoea*. A relevant history of sexual exposure can be anything from 1 day to 6 weeks. Epididymitis may also be caused by trauma or may arise by blood-borne dissemination from other sites or rarely may be due to brucellosis or tuberculosis.

The patient complains of a painful scrotal swelling, usually unilateral, which may be of acute onset (1–2 days) or

Table 29.6 Principles of testicular fixation.

- Tunica vaginalis is opened behind the testes to obliterate the potential hydrocele sac.
- Fixation by dartos pouch or non-absorbable suture.
- For suture fixation sutures are placed either two medially, or else one medially, laterally and inferiorly.
- It is advisable to remove testicular appendages as these can become torted in the future despite testicular fixation.
- Open the contralateral side of the scrotum and fix the other testes in the same way.
- Contralateral side should not be explored if infection is found to be the cause of scrotal pain.

Table 29.7 Management of acute bacterial epididymitis.

Antibiotics for both aerobic Gram-negative rods and aerobic Gram positive cocci
Scrotal support and bed rest
Analgesics
Surgery may be indicated for the management of complications such as drainage of an abscess

more insidious. There may be a history of sexual exposure, recent urethral instrumentation or indwelling catheter. The epididymis which is posterior to the testis is characteristically tender. Early in the course of the infection the swelling may be localized and the testicle palpable separate from the epididymis. With involvement of the testes the swelling may be larger. Patients may have a fever and feel systemically unwell.

Outpatient treatment may be appropriate for patients with less severe disease; however, hospitalization is advisable for local complications or systemic signs. We usually give intravenous gentamicin and augmentin for five days for severe cases followed by a further two weeks of oral antibiotics (Table 29.7).

The complications of epididymitis are given in Table 29.8.

Table 29.8 Complications of epididymitis.

Testicular infarction
Scrotal abscess
Chronic draining scrotal abscess
Infertility
Chronic epididymitis

Orchitis

Orchitis is significantly less common than epididymitis and differs from other genito-urinary tract infections in two aspects: the haematogenous route is most common and viruses are an important aetiological factor. Management is the same as for epididymitis.

Mumps rarely cause orchitis in prepubertal boys but is the cause of orchitis in about 30% of postpubertal boys. The onset of symptoms appears 4–6 days after the onset of parotitis. Treatment includes bed rest and scrotal support only. Mild cases resolve after about 5 days and more severe cases last up to 4 weeks. Infertility as a sequel is not as common as once thought.

Priapism

Priapism is a prolonged erection (generally greater than 4 h) not associated with sexual stimulation. It is not relieved by

ejaculation and may lead to impotence. It can occur at any age, having been described in both neonates and the elderly.

It is due to a failure of detumescence most commonly as a result of decreased venous outflow. It is rarely caused by increased arterial inflow seen occasionally after trauma. Veno-occlusive priapism results from persistent obstruction of lacunar space venous outflow and once the corporal bodies have been fully expanded the arterial inflow is impeded leading to ischaemia and pain.

Causes (Table 29.9)

Before the use of vaso-active drugs for erectile dysfunction in 1984 the cause of priapism was unknown in most cases. Today almost 80% of the cases of priapism seen are as a result of intracorporeal vaso-active agents such as papaverine and, less commonly, prostaglandin E_2.

The diagnosis is easily made by history and physical examination. Enquiries should be made as to whether the patient had intracorporeal vaso-active agents. Corporeal pain and tenderness are characteristic. Colour flow Doppler studies and corporeal blood gas analysis may rarely be required to determine the degree of ischaemia. Arteriography and embolization may be required in high flow priapism resistant to medical therapy.

The aim of all priapism management, medical or surgical, is to re-establish arterial blood inflow to the erectile tissue by augmenting drainage from the corpora cavernosa. In the era of vaso-active drugs first-line therapy includes cavernosa aspiration, and the injection of an α-adrenergic agent.

Aspiration technique

Use a large butterfly-type needle and insert it into one corpus cavernosum and aspirate as much blood as possible. If necessary the corpora may be irrigated with saline to assist with washout and drainage. In otherwise healthy patients an injection of an α-adrenergic agent after aspiration to pharmacologically contract the corporal smooth muscle is more

Table 29.9 Some of the causes of priapism.

Drugs
Idiopathic
Anaemia
Leukaemia
Sickle cell disease
Multiple myeloma
Gout
Renal failure
Penile or perineal trauma

effective. Relative contra-indications are heart block and bradycardia. Our agent of choice is phenylephrine because it is a pure α_1 agonist with low β_1 activity.

Mixing instructions

1 With a 10-ml syringe withdraw 9 ml of saline.
2 Withdraw 1 ml of phenylephrine with the same syringe, making it up to 10 ml (1 ml = 100 µg)
3 This mixture can be injected in 1-ml aliquots with an insulin syringe.

If arterial inflow is not re-established as evidenced by persistent or recurrent dark corporeal aspirates, then medical management should be considered unsuccessful. In this case surgical shunting to the glans or corpus spongiosum should be performed.

If the patient was initially diagnosed as having the rarer high flow priapism as evidenced by bright red blood on corporeal aspiration then early transcatheter embolization should be considered.

Bladder stones

Bladder stones are seen almost exclusively in men with bladder outflow obstruction. They are occasionally seen in women associated with foreign material such as a stitch from incontinence surgery. In general they are clearly seen on a plain X-ray (Fig. 29.5).

In addition to outflow obstruction the patient will often have bladder irritative symptoms with haematuria. He will often experience pain which may be referred to the tip of the penis.

Examination of the urine

Examination of the urine in patients with acute urological symptoms is often very rewarding and helpful. Freshly voided specimens analysed within 1 h are most reliable whereas urine left standing for a few hours becomes alkaline thus causing lysis of red blood cells, disintegration of casts or rapidly multiplying bacteria.

Method of collection

Specimens collected at home by the patient are generally useless and should always be discarded.

Men are instructed to retract the foreskin and after passing the first part of the stream (approx 20 ml) to collect the next part of the stream in a sterile container. It is virtually impossible for a woman to obtain a satisfactory clean voided specimen without help. In practical terms she is asked to separate the labia and give a midstream specimen and if the urinalysis is completely normal then no further efforts are

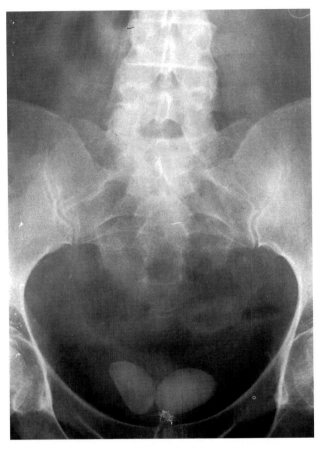

Fig. 29.5 A seventy-three-year-old man presented with symptoms of a urinary tract infection superimposed on a history of bladder outflow obstruction. Plain X-rays shows two previously undiagnosed bladder stones.

required to get a sample. If a clean sample is mandatory she may be placed in the lithotomy position and catheterized under aseptic conditions.

Dipstick urinalysis

Urine dipsticks can be used to determine specific gravity, pH, protein, glucose, ketones, bilirubin, urobilinogen, blood, nitrites and leucocytes. The reagent areas on the dipstick must be immersed in a fresh, uncentrifuged urine specimen and then withdrawn immediately to prevent dissolution of the reagent in the urine. When removed it should be held horizontal to prevent mixing of the reagent chemicals leading to a false reading.

Nitrites

Normal urine does not contain nitrites. Many species of Gram-negative organisms can convert nitrates to nitrites (Table 29.10). The specificity (true negatives) lies between 95 and 100% but unfortunately the sensitivity (true positives) is about 50%. The only major cause of false positives is specimen contamination. When the nitrite test is positive it suggests the presence of greater than 100 000 organisms/ml.

White blood cells (pyuria)

Although this test is a good indicator of pyuria it does not necessarily detect bacteria. Leucocyte esterase tests for the presence of leucocytes in the urine which are a surrogate for bacteria. Many patients with bacteriuria do not have pyuria. Sensitivity (true positive) is about 80% and specificity (true negative) is about 70%. This test combined with the nitrite test is as predictive as microscopic urine analysis. The major cause of a false positive result is contamination (Table 29.11).

Blood

The dipstick detects intact erythrocytes, free haemoglobin from lysed erythrocytes and myoglobin. Analysis is based on the peroxidase like activity of haemoglobin but false positive results can occur (Table 29.12). The sensitivity is about 90% (low false negatives) with a low specificity (high false positive).

Table 29.10 Causes of false negatives results for nitrites.

Non-nitrite reducing organisms
Frequent voiding, i.e. short bladder dwell time (<4 h) with insufficient time for reduction of nitrites to occur
Not using first morning specimen
Dilute urine
Acidic urine
Large dietary intake of vitamin C
Presence of urobilinogen

Table 29.11 Causes of false negative results for pyuria.

Glycosuria
Urobilinogen
Nitrofurantoin therapy
Vitamin C therapy
Rifampicin therapy

Table 29.12 Reason for false positive results for haematuria.

Urine contamination
Menstruating females
High specific gravity (dehydration)
Exercise

Urine microscopy

The ability to perform microscopic examination of the urinary sediment is very helpful in the presence of urinary tract symptoms. Early morning voided urine is best and analysis can be done within minutes of collection. Depending on the method of collection the finding of bacteria on a freshly voided specimen is indicative of infection and empirical treatment can be initiated while waiting for results of culture and sensitivity.

Preparation

1 10 ml urine centrifuged at 2000 r.p.m. for 5 min.
2 Decant the supernatant of which approx 0.2 ml will remain.
3 Resuspend the sediment in the remaining supernatant.
4 Place one drop on microscope slide and cover with a cover slip.
5 Examine under low power ($\times 10$) and high-power ($\times 40$) lens. In a fresh uncontaminated specimen the finding of bacteria is indicative of a urinary tract infection. Each high power views between 1/20 000 and 1/50 000 of a millilitre thus each bacterium seen per high-power field (HPF) signifies a count of more than 20/1000 ml; thus 5 per HPF gives a count of approximately 10^5/ml.

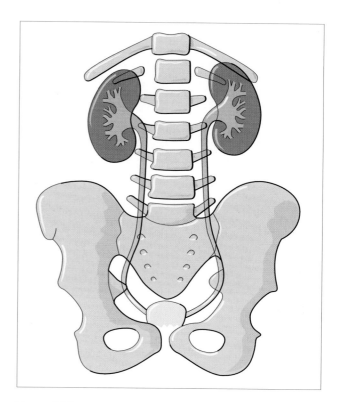

Fig. 29.6 The anatomical arrangement of kidneys, ureters and bladder as seen on X-ray.

Imaging techniques

A urinary tract infection associated with possible urinary tract obstruction must be evaluated.

Plain film of the abdomen

A plain film of the abdomen may show calculi or an absent psoas shadow suggesting a perirenal or renal abscess.

Intravenous urography

An intravenous urogram should be performed in the acute setting if upper tract pathology is suspected. In particular, if ureteric calculi are suspected then the intravenous urogram should be performed in the A&E dept and not delayed until the next day. If there is a delay a stone may pass and it may then be impossible to make a definitive diagnosis.

It is a useful test to determine the exact site and extent of urinary tract obstruction and the line of the ureters can be examined for opacities (Fig. 29.6). It is essential to obtain an initial plain X-ray of the kidneys, ureter and bladder (Fig. 29.7). After obtaining a negative allergy history a bolus of 50–60 ml of iodine-containing contrast material is injected intravenously. Films are taken at timed intervals (5, 10, 15 and 30 min as an example) and delayed films may be required if there is poor opacification of the kidney. The bladder is often filled with contrast medium at 5 min. It is important to obtain a postvoid film to help establish the integrity of the urinary tract.

Renal ultrasound

It is non-invasive, easy to perform and offers no radiation or contrast risk to the patient. It is particularly useful in determining the presence of upper tract obstruction, pyonephrosis or perirenal abscess.

Computed tomography

This is the radiological modality which in general offers the best anatomic detail but its cost and radiation exposure prevent it from being an initial investigation.

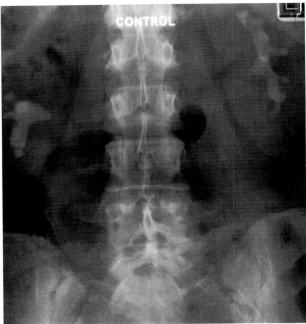

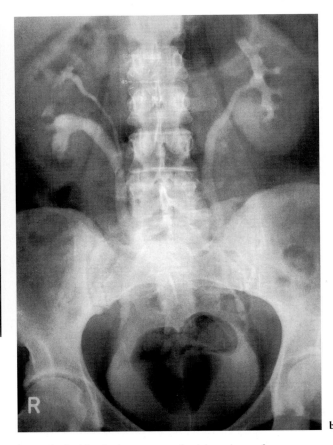

Fig. 29.7 The importance of a control film (a) demonstrating bilateral staghorn calculi with a duplex system on the right and seen after intravenous contrast (b).

Serum analysis

Results of serum analysis may give clues as to the severity of the underlying renal condition.

Serum creatinine

Creatinine is the end product of the metabolism of creatine in skeletal muscle and is normally excreted by the kidneys. Serum creatinine concentration is very helpful for measuring renal function and depends on two factors: rate of production within the body and the rate of excretion through the glomeruli. Creatinine is produced at a relatively constant rate and if the lean body mass does not change appreciably and there is no change in renal function the serum creatinine should remain fairly constant. The normal level of creatinine will vary depending on the age and muscle mass of the patient.

A patient requires only 30% of renal reserve to maintain a normal level of creatinine; thus, any elevation generally signifies underlying renal impairment. A single creatinine value cannot determine whether the insult to the nephron is acute or chronic. If the creatinine is elevated then an intravenous urogram is unlikely to give a good result unless high doses of contrast are used and this is rarely warranted in the A&E department.

Urea is the primary metabolite of protein catabolism and is excreted entirely by the kidneys; thus, its serum level is influenced by glomerular filtration rate. Although its estimation is simple it is the crudest and most imprecise method of determining renal function and its levels can be influenced by dietary protein, hydration status and gastrointestinal bleeding.

Full blood count

Normochromic normocytic anaemia is often seen with chronic renal insufficiency. The determination of the white cell count can often add helpful additional information and one would expect it to be elevated in the presence of acute infection.

Urethral catheterization

Many types of catheters are available and the choice of a specific type depends on the reason for catheterization (Fig. 29.8). Regular Foley catheters are used for patients in acute urinary retention or where urine output is to be monitored. Generally an 18Ch (14Ch for females) is adequate. Where haematuria is expected then a larger 20Ch to 24Ch catheter should be used. Three way catheters can be used when bladder irrigation and drainage is necessary. Occasionally a coude tip catheter is required to negotiate areas of the male urethra or the bladder neck. Catheter introducers should be used *only* by an experienced urologist.

Catheter size is usually referred to using the French (Fr.) scale whereby 1 Fr = 0.33 mm in diameter. Catheter sizes refer to the outside circumference and not the luminal diameter. If long-term catheterization is anticipated then silicone catheters rather than latex should be used.

When a patient is catheterized for acute urinary retention the amount of urine drained on catheterization should be measured and recorded.

Any patient with risk factors for bacterial endocarditis must be treated with systemic antibiotics when a catheter is inserted or removed. In addition, patients with prostheses such as hip or knee replacement should also have antibiotics.

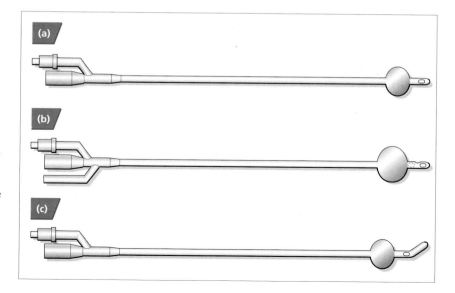

Fig. 29.8 (a) Foley balloon catheter with one pair of opposed eyes available with 10- or 30-ml balloons. (b) Triple lumen catheter. The third lumen is for continuous irrigation of the bladder. The eyes at the tip of the catheter are generally bigger than the standard catheter. (c) Coude tip catheter with one drainage eye. The angled tip can be useful to negotiate a high bladder neck in patients with acute urinary retention.

Asymptomatic bladder bacteriuria, funguria or pyuria in catheterized patients should not be treated so long as the patient remains asymptomatic and is not immunocompromised. Approximately 40% of patients with indwelling catheters for longer than 4 days will have catheter-associated infections. All symptomatic patients with indwelling catheters should receive antimicrobial treatment. It is important to determine that neither the catheter nor the urinary tract is infected and it may be wise to change the catheter if it has been in place for longer than 3 weeks.

When urethral catheterization has failed, a suprapubic catheter can usually be passed without difficulty.

Suprapubic catheterization

Important points are:
1 That the bladder is palpable.
2 That bladder cancer is not suspected.
3 Special care must be taken where previous lower intraabdominal surgery has taken place with resultant adhesions.

If the bladder is not full and urethral catheterization has failed then the bladder can be filled by passing a 14Ch Foley into the fossa navicularis and inflating the balloon with 2 ml and filling the bladder in a retrograde fashion.

Technique

Whatever catheter is used the same basic technique applies but the Bonnano catheter is safer in the relatively inexperienced hand rather than the trocars with a Foley catheter.
1 Prepare the skin in the suprapubic area with antiseptic solution.
2 Infiltrate the skin and deeper tissues with local anaesthetic two finger breadths above symphysis pubis in the midline.
3 Incise the skin and deeper tissues down to the rectus sheath.
4 Place an 18 G needle on a 10-ml syringe and pass it 40° from the vertical in the direction of the bladder. If urine is aspirated then continue with catheterization.

CHAPTER 30

Acute urological trauma

Thomas H. Lynch & John M. Fitzpatrick

Introduction

With the exception of the external genitalia the genitourinary tract is well protected from trauma by musculo skeletal structures, viscera and by its hypermobility. Despite this protection approximately 10% of all injuries presenting to the Accident and Emergency Department involve the genito-urinary tract to a greater or lesser degree. Following initial resuscitation subsequent urological management depends on the nature and extent of the injuries. Most injuries are minor and require limited investigations but for the purposes of triage, injuries may be divided into two groups: those with penetrating injuries requiring exploration and those with blunt injuries who may be managed conservatively. The latter group often require the greatest clinical judgement as less than 5% will have a major injury requiring exploration whereas penetrating injuries cause serious underlying trauma in about 80% of patients. An observed drop in blood pressure or gross haematuria is strongly suggestive of serious underlying trauma and the need for radiographic studies.

Lower urinary tract injuries should be suspected in the presence of blood at the meatus, pelvic fracture or perineal discoloration. If the patient is unconscious and no such features are obvious it may be prudent to perform retrograde urethrographic studies.

In general, bladder and urethral injuries are best investigated by urethrography and cystography whereas upper tract injuries are best assessed by intravenous urography (IVU) and, if indicated, by computerized tomography (CT).

If an IVU demonstrates an excretory urogram one can be 95% sure that there is no significant renal artery injury present. This is not true of CT scanning because even in the presence of severe arterial injury a collateral vessel on the parenchyma of the kidney may show up as the cortical rim sign. This may be seen even in the presence of a kidney-threatening arterial injury and selective renal arteriography is very helpful in this case.

McAninch and Carroll (1989) have suggested that contrast studies should be reserved for patients with a history of a drop in blood pressure and/or gross haematuria and reported that such a policy would have missed only one serious renal injury out of 1671 patients studied. Our policy is to perform, at the very least, an IVU on all patients with a history of trauma and haematuria.

Renal trauma

In spite of the fact that the kidneys are well protected they are the most common site of urological injury. The kidneys are protected by the lumbar muscles, vertebral bodies, ribs and the viscera. The kidney may be penetrated by fractured ribs or lumbar transverse processes, gunshot or stab wounds or a variety of other sharp objects. Because of their greater participation in contact sports injuries occur more commonly in men and young boys. Injuries are also more common in kidneys with underlying pathology such as hydronephrosis. Isolated adrenal injury is rare but iatrogenic injuries have been reported. For management purposes injuries are classified as penetrating or blunt. Penetrating wounds as a rule need to be explored as associated visceral injuries are present in about 80% of cases.

Renal injuries were classified by Moore in 1989 as follows (Fig. 30.1):

1 *Minor renal trauma* (85% of cases). Renal contusions often associated with subcapsular haematomas. A laceration would also be considered a minor injury.

2 *Major renal trauma* (15% of cases). Deep lacerations of the kidney may extend through the parenchyma into the collecting system. This injury may lead to a large retroperitoneal haematoma and extravasation of urine and multiple such lacerations may cause complete disruption of the kidney (Fig. 30.2).

3 *Vascular injury.* There may be total avulsion of the artery or vein or damage to segmental branches. Stretching of the renal artery may lead to thrombosis. In general, vascular injuries are difficult to diagnose and often result in total destruction of the kidney.

Presentation

The degree to which haematuria is present does not always correlate with the degree of renal injury, as it may be completely absent in cases of renal artery injury. However,

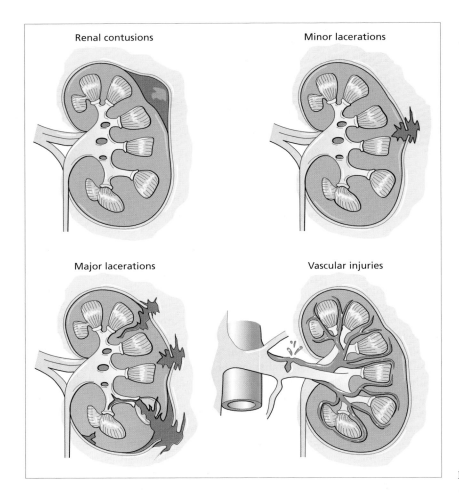

Fig. 30.1 Classification of renal injuries.

if the haematuria is disproportionate to the injury one should always think of pre-existing disease such as a renal tumour.

Abdominal injury is usually clinically obvious and if it has caused a large retroperitoneal haematoma this may result in ileus formation with abdominal distention, nausea and vomiting.

Features which increase the suspicion of underlying renal injury are:

• History of injury to the flank or abdomen.
• Ecchymosis in the flank or upper abdomen.
• Fractured ribs especially the lower ribs.
• Patients with gross or microscopic haematuria.
• Penetrating injury associated with haematuria either gross or microscopic.
• A palpable mass which may be due to a large retroperitoneal haematoma or extravasation of urine. Remember however that if the retroperitoneum is torn there may be free blood in the peritoneal cavity and no retroperitoneal mass will be felt.

Blunt renal trauma

Two injuries are associated with sudden deceleration and can occur in both adults and children. These are *arterial intimal tears* and *pelvi-ureteric disruption*. Both these injuries are seen more commonly in children because of the greater mobility of the renal pedicle and sparse perirenal fat.

Parenchymal fractures with preservation of the blood supply may also result from blunt trauma (Fig. 30.3a–c). These patients can be observed with serial CT scans although some authors advocate exploration and the bringing together of the fragments with collagen nets. We feel that this policy results in greater blood loss without any significant saving of renal units.

One group of patients in the blunt injury group that do benefit from early surgery is the small subset with a devascularized polar avulsion (Fig. 30.4). If these kidneys are not explored early over 80% will require delayed surgery greatly prolonging the patient's hospitalization. Various reports have shown that about 85% of blunt renal injuries require

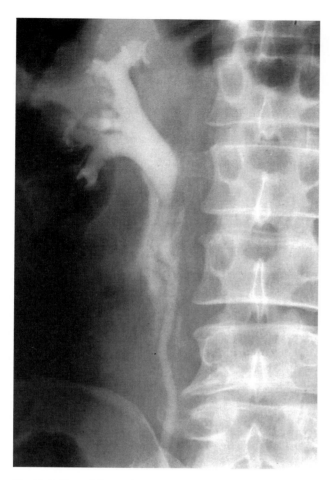

Fig. 30.2 Blunt abdominal trauma in a 40-year-old man showing extravasation of contrast on IVU.

no surgery, 5–10% require judgement and surgical exploration and about 5% require nephrectomy.

Indication for renal exploration

Those patients with minor or major lacerations associated with limited urinary extravasation or bleeding who are clinically stable may be managed expectantly.

Absolute indications

1 Intra-operative finding of an expanding or pulsatile retroperitoneal mass.
2 Renal bleeding rendering the patient haemodynamically unstable.
3 Pedicle injury in a solitary kidney.
4 Urine extravasation alone is not an indication for exploration. Both intracapsular and extracapsular extravasation may subside spontaneously; however, more significant extravasation particularily associated with evidence of active internal bleeding should be explored.
5 Penetrating injuries associated with haematuria in a haemodynamically unstable patient.

Relative indications

1 Major lacerations.
2 Non-viable renal tissue.
3 Laparotomy for associated injuries.
4 Incomplete clinical or radiographic staging.

Surgical principles for open renal exploration

1 All patients should be explored through a generous laparotomy incision. After an exhaustive search for other intra-abdominal injuries the pedicle of the kidney must be controlled before the kidney is explored. This is probably the single most important point in surgery for renal trauma and cannot be overemphasized. The small bowel is reflected superiorly and the inferior mesenteric vein is identified (Fig. 30.5). An incision is made in the peritoneum medial to this overlying the aorta and should be extended superiorly to the left renal vein, as it crosses the aorta. The inferior mesenteric vein is a particularly helpful landmark where a large retroperitoneal haematoma prevents easy identification of the aorta. The left renal artery is identified above and behind this. The right renal artery is identified between the aorta and inferior vena cava and the right renal vein is identified lateral to the inferior vena cava (IVC). Vessel loops should be placed around the vessels supplying the side to be explored before opening Gerota's fascia. Medial mobilization of the kidney may be required on the right side. If the inferior mesenteric artery needs to be sacrificed this can generally be done without any longterm sequelae; however, it may have effects in children under 2 years of age and in the elderly with evidence of atherosclerosis.
2 If the patient's condition demands immediate laparotomy imaging studies should be obtained on the operating table with a one shot intravenous bolus of contrast medium. The main purpose of this is to establish the presence of a functioning contralateral kidney.
3 If a polar nephrectomy is necessary the remaining capsule acts as a better cover than an omental patch or fascial free graft.
4 If a lower pole nephrectomy is required fat should be placed between the kidney and the pelvis (Deming procedure) to prevent secondary pelvi-ureteric junction (PUJ) obstruction.
5 After partial nephrectomy a nephropexy should be performed by fixing the kidney to the psoas. This manoeuvre will help prevent a Dietl's crisis (abdominal pain and vomiting) or renal infarction from a possible torsion of the pedicle.

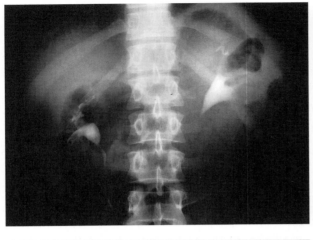

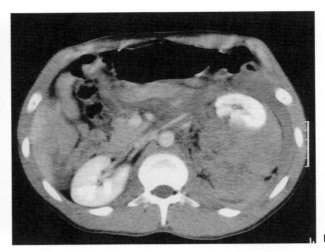

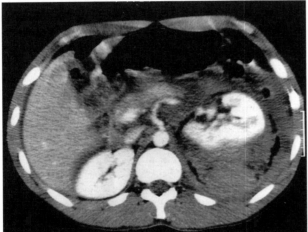

Fig. 30.3 (a) Left blunt renal trauma in a 28-year-old male rugby player. IVU shows bilateral functioning kidneys with the suspicion of a mass in the left lower pole. (b, c) A retroperitoneal haematoma is easily seen on CT scan. Haemoglobin was recorded at 9 g/dL.

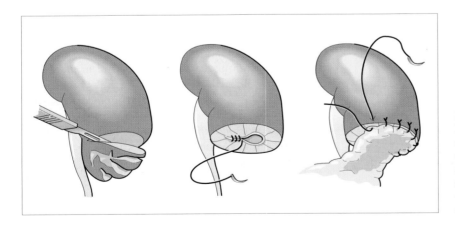

Fig. 30.4 Technique for partial nephrectomy. Partial nephrectomy is indicated with a devascularized polar avulsion. The kidney is completely exposed and non-viable tissue is removed by sharp dissection. The collecting system is closed with absorbable sutures and the defect is covered with either the remaining capsule or an omental patch.

6 Non-viable tissue should be debrided by sharp dissection. Bleeding from the cut ends indicates viability despite a dusky appearance. 30% of function of one kidney is usually sufficient to obviate the need for dialysis—a useful guideline when determining whether renal salvage should be undertaken.

7 If warm ischaemia time is expected to exceed 60 min then ice slush should be used.

8 Always use absorbable suture material around a kidney. Non-absorbable material may predispose to later stone formation. Vascular injuries can be repaired with 5-0 or 6-0 Prolene sutures.

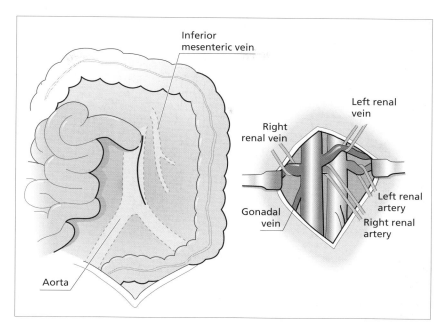

Fig. 30.5 The pedicle of the kidney must be controlled before the kidney is explored. The small bowel is reflected superiorly and the inferior mesenteric vein is identified. An incision made in the peritoneum medial to this, overlying the aorta, should be extended superiorly to the left renal vein as it crosses behind this. The right renal artery is identified between the aorta and inferior vena cava, and the right renal vein is identified lateral to the IVC. Vessel loops should be placed around the vessels supplying the side to be explored to gain control before opening Gerota's fascia.

9 A spatulated repair of injuries to the pelvis or upper ureter with 4-0 chromic catgut over a double pigtail catheter gives good results. It is probably best to avoid any form of nephrostomy drainage to prevent further damage to the kidney. In addition to an internal drain it is best to have an external drain and a closed free drainage system gives satisfactory results.

10 Some time after initial exploration if it is felt that the patient has further devascularization of the kidney or may have developed a urinoma then early re-exploration gives the best results.

Renal exploration and reconstructive techniques

By employing the above principles the kidney can be salvaged in the majority of cases.

Nephrectomy

It is very important to gain control of the renal vessels in the midline prior to opening Gerota's fascia. The kidney should be exposed completely. Nephrectomy is indicated for extensive parenchymal damage, vascular injuries not amenable to repair or life-threatening associated injuries. Contrast studies are mandatory to confirm the presence of a contralateral functioning kidney.

Partial nephrectomy

Partial nephrectomy is indicated for deep laceration of the upper or lower poles where devitalized tissue results. A patch of capsule as described above can be used and it is important to separate the repair and the upper ureter for lower pole nephrectomies.

Renorrhaphy

After exposure of the kidney any perirenal haematoma should be evacuated and any non-viable renal tissue debrided. Intrarenal vascular injuries or collecting system injuries can be repaired with 4-0 chromic catgut (Fig. 30.6). The renal capsule can be repaired with 2-0 chromic catgut and if necessary a patch of omentum can be employed.

Vascular injuries

These injuries require special attention as these patients are at higher risk of renal loss and complications than patients with parenchymal injury.

Incomplete injury to the main renal artery can be repaired with 5-0 Prolene sutures. Repair of complete disruption is difficult, however, it should be attempted in patients with bilateral renal disease or in a solitary kidney. Patients with a delayed diagnosis of renal artery thrombosis can have a nephrectomy if there is another indication for exploration; however, they do not need immediate nephrectomy and this should not be the sole indication for surgery. Most of these kidneys will atrophy but the onset of hypertension may be an indication for later nephrectomy. Even if early revascularization of a thrombosed kidney is performed often only minimal function is restored.

Segmental veins can be ligated without difficulty because there is an extensive intrarenal collateral venous drainage.

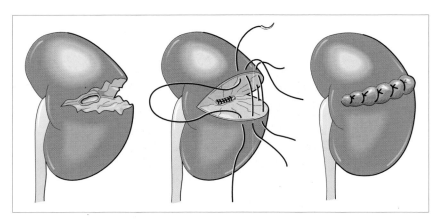

Fig. 30.6 Technique of renorrhaphy. The kidney is fully mobilized and debrided. The collecting system is closed with absorbable suture material and the parenchymal edges are approximated.

On the right the renal vein should be repaired if possible and cannot be ligated near the vena cava because of its lack of collateral drainage. On the left the renal vein can be ligated as venous run-off is also provided by the gonadal, lumbar and adrenal vessels.

At the Parkland Memorial Hospital in Dallas, Texas, the mortality rate from renal pedicle injuries was 37% (44% nephrectomy rate) and was caused more by associated injuries. By contrast, death occurred in 12 (10%) of 115 patients admitted with blunt renal trauma and associated injuries. Over 95% of patients with blunt renal trauma recover following expectant management only.

Sequelae of renal injuries

Urinoma

Lacerations resulting in urine leak may give rise to a perinephric mass and eventually hydronephrosis and abscess formation. In general this complication requires prompt surgical drainage.

Hydronephrosis

Large haematomas may result in fibrosis giving rise to ureteric obstruction and hydronephrosis. Intravenous urograms should be performed 3–6 months after initial injury to rule out this complication, which may require surgical correction.

Arteriovenous fistula

Arteriovenous fistula is uncommon but may be a late feature of penetrating injury.

Renal vascular hypertension

The blood flow in injured tissue may be compromised resulting in non-viable tissue which can lead to renovascular hypertension in about 1% of cases. Fibrosis around the renal artery may also cause constriction of the artery leading to hypertension. This complication may require vascular repair or interval nephrectomy.

Ureteric injuries

Ureteric anatomy

A clear knowledge of the anatomy of the ureter makes the understanding of the mechanism of injury and its repair much easier. Anatomically, the ureter is divided into three parts: upper, middle and lower but, for practical purposes it can be divided into two parts: abdominal and pelvic ureter.

The abdominal ureter lies on the psoas muscle and, as it descends it becomes closely adherent to the posterior peritoneum. It is often elevated with the latter when the colon is being reflected medially. It enters the pelvis by crossing the iliac artery medially as it bifurcates. It tracks along the curvature of the pelvis down to the levator ani musculature and crosses under the superior vesical artery to enter the postero-inferior aspect of the bladder. In the female the ureter courses below the broad ligament and uterine vessels.

The ureteral blood supply is variable and is derived from the aorta, renal, gonadal, iliac, middle haemorrhoidal, vaginal and superior vesical arteries. In general to avoid damage to the blood supply dissection should be lateral to the ureter above the pelvic brim and medial to the ureter below the pelvic brim. As its blood supply courses through the adventitial layer dissection of this layer should also be avoided.

Aetiology of ureteric injuries

Ureteric and renal pelvic injuries resulting from external violence are rare and account for less than 1% of urological injuries. Rapid deceleration injuries may avulse the ureter from the renal pelvis. Injuries may occur during gynaecological or colorectal surgery, endoscopic stone manipulation, or during surgery either open or endoscopic to the lower urinary tract. Rarely injuries to the intramural ureter may occur during transurethral resections. The incidence of gynaecolgial ureteric injuries during abdominal surgery is about 10 times that of vaginal surgery. In a review of 1093 gynaecological operations 16 were reported to have ureteric injuries.

Mechanism of ureteric injuries
• Ligation
• Crush injury
• Transection (partial or complete)
• Ischaemic injury
• Avulsion (PUJ)
• Fulguration
• Contusion
• Resection

Clinical features of ureteric injury

After trauma a high index of suspicion is warranted rather than depending on any specific clinical signs.

Intra-operative recognition of ureteric injuries provides the best opportunity for successful ureteric repair. Direct inspection of the site looking for presence of normal peristalsis and normal calibre affords the best chance of assessing ureteric integrity.

Delayed diagnosis may be made on the basis of prolonged ileus, urinary leakage, urinary obstruction, anuria or oliguria and sepsis.

Radiological investigations

IVU may not demonstrate the injury in the early stages but if the patient has a penetrating injury then retrograde pyelography is probably the best investigation (Fig. 30.7).

Intra-operative recognition of an injury may be facilitated by intravenous injection of methylene blue or indigo carmine. In a poorly perfused patient either may be injected directly into the ureter with a 25 gauge needle. If all these fail then retrograde pyelography remains the most sensitive means for identifying extravasation. This may, however, be absent in the early stages of crush or ischaemic injury which may not become apparent for several days to weeks later.

Management

In general, injuries from trauma, or those detected intra-operatively and those detected within a week in an otherwise stable patient should be repaired immediately.

If the injury is recognized after 7 days then attempts at placement of a ureteric stent should be made. This can be

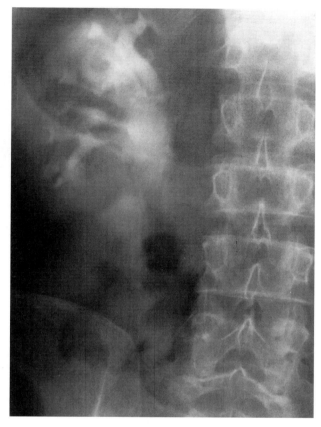

Fig. 30.7 Blunt abdominal trauma with extravasation from right renal pelvis.

placed either by antegrade or retrograde means and done only under fluroscopic control. If stent placement fails or is felt to be inappropriate then proximal drainage via a nephrostomy drain in addition to percutaneous drainage of a urinoma may suffice. Definitive repair can be performed 6 to 8 weeks later.

Surgery

The type of repair depends on the site of injury and any associated injuries as well as the condition of the patient. The right ureter is exposed by incising the peritoneum over the bifurcation of the common iliac vessels and the left ureter is exposed by mobilizing the colon medially. The ureter above and below the area of damage should be exposed without dissecting too close to the ureter.

Surgical techniques

- Primary repair
- Re-implantation of ureter into bladder
- Uretero-ureterostomy

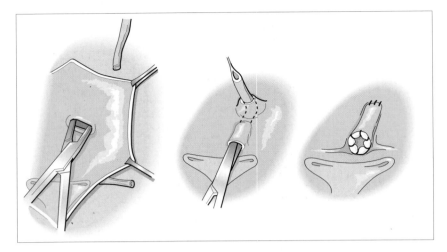

Fig. 30.8 Re-implantation of the ureter by a modified technique of Palitano and Leadbetter. The ureter is brought through the posterior wall of the bladder medial to the ureteric orifice on the same side. The ureter is tunnelled submucosally, spatulated and sutured over a pigtail catheter to the bladder mucosa with 3-0 chromic or Maxon sutures.

- Transureteroureterostomy
- Ureteric replacement
- Autotransplantation

For lower ureteric injuries the ureter should be re-implanted into the bladder. The modified technique of Leadbetter and Politano is demonstrated in Fig. 30.8. The ureter is brought through the posterior wall of the bladder medial to the ureteric orifice on the same side. Placement of the ureter in the more mobile lateral wall may predispose to kinking. The ureter is tunnelled submucosally (a ratio of length to diameter of 3 : 1), spatulated and sutured over a pigtail catheter to the bladder mucosa with 3-0 chromic sutures or maxon. The bladder should be closed in two layers with 2-0 absorbable sutures and the pelvis should be drained with closed non-suction drainage. The ureteric catheter is left in place for 10 days and cystography should be performed before its removal. If the ureter cannot be brought to the bladder without tension then a psoas bladder hitch or Boari flap may be required.

Psoas hitch

The bladder is stripped of peritoneum and is dissected off the cervix and uterus in the female and the rectum in the male (Fig. 30.9). Division of the ipsilateral obliterated umbilical ligament in addition to the contralateral supravesical vessels may be necessary. The bladder is hitched up to the psoas minor tendon or the psoas major if the former is absent (10% of individuals). These sutures are tied after the ureter has been re-implanted into the bladder.

A Boari flap can be used when greater length is required than that obtainable from a psoas hitch. In addition a psoas hitch is relatively contra-indicated in cases with a small contracted bladder or previous pelvic surgery where the blood supply to the bladder may already be compromised.

Boari flap

The bladder should be fully mobilized and this includes division of the umbilical ligaments. A flap over the superior vesical pedicle (Fig. 30.10) or one of its branches with a base of approximately 4 cm is created—a shorter segment may cause stenosis when closed over. The ureter can be sutured to the end or tunnelled submucosally as an antirefluxing anastomosis. Up to 12 cm in length can be obtained and the flap should be closed with 2-0 absorbable sutures.

Repair of abdominal ureter

If the abdominal ureter is damaged an end to end ureteric anastomosis may be achieved (Fig. 30.11). This must be done without tension and with clean-cut spatulated ends of ureter. Occasionally the ureter may need to be brought across to the contralateral ureter (Fig. 30.12), or bowel may have to be interposed. In very rare circumstances the kidney may need to be 'autotransplanted' down to the iliac fossa in the same manner as a cadaveric renal transplant.

General principles of ureteric repair

- Debridement of non-viable tissue.
- Tension free anastomosis.
- Spatulated mucosa to mucosa anastomosis.
- An end to end anastomosis without spatulation should never be performed.
- Internal and extraperitoneal drainage.
- The earlier the recognition and repair of a damaged ureter the better the outcome.
- If there is evidence of infection the repair may be isolated with fat or omentum.

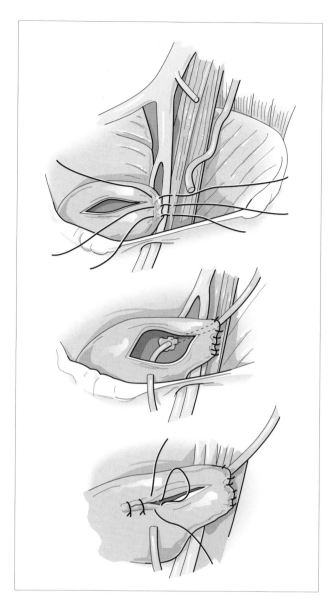

Fig. 30.9 Psoas hitch. The bladder is mobilized and hitched up to the psoas minor tendon or the psoas major if the former is absent. These sutures are tied after the ureter has been re-implanted into the bladder.

Bladder trauma

The bladder is infrequently injured because of the protection afforded by the bony pelvis; however, in children it is an abdominal organ rendering it more vulnerable to injury. Whether the injury is intra- or extraperitoneal often depends on the volume of urine in the bladder at time of injury.

Aetiology of bladder injuries (Table 30.1)

Blunt trauma

Blunt trauma accounts for up to 80% of all bladder injuries. Up to 70% of these patients will have an associated pelvic fracture, and 90% will have concomitant organ injury. Approximately 15% of patients with pelvic fractures sustain trauma to the bladder. 90% of patients with both abdominal and bladder injury will have a pelvic fracture.

Penetrating trauma

The most common injury results from surgical misadventure either endoscopic or open surgery. 60% of those with penetrating injury will have a concomitant organ injury.

Diagnosis

Clinical features

Haematuria is present in 90% of patients and over 60% will have abdominal pain. Although intraperitoneal extravasation of urine may lead to ileus and abdominal distention this may not be apparent at presentation, especially if the urine is sterile. Patients may have features associated with other injuries such as a fractured pelvis.

X-ray findings

The cystogram (see description of technique) is the only study that will definitely diagnose bladder rupture (Fig. 30.13 a&b). Great care must be taken to rule out urethral trauma before a catheter is passed to fill the bladder. Upper tract studies with an IVU is indicated in all cases where the cystogram demonstrates extravasation.

Table 30.1 Aetiology of bladder injuries.

Operative injury	Open or transurethral surgery
External violence	Gun shot or knife wounds
	Bony spicule from fractured pelvis
	Blunt injury secondary to road traffic accident
Internal migration	Surgical drains or hip prosthesis
	Long-term indwelling Foley catheters (rare)
Spontaneous bladder rupture	Spontaneous bladder rupture associated with bladder outflow obstruction is extremely rare.

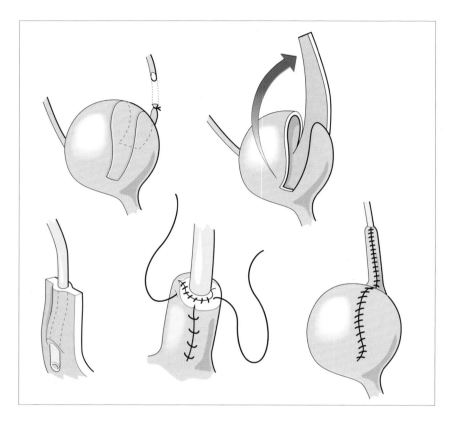

Fig. 30.10 Boari flap. The bladder should be fully mobilized and a flap over the superior vesical pedicle or one of its branches is elevated. The ureter can be sutured to the end or tunnelled submucosally as an antirefluxing anastomosis. The flap should be closed with 2-0 absorbable sutures.

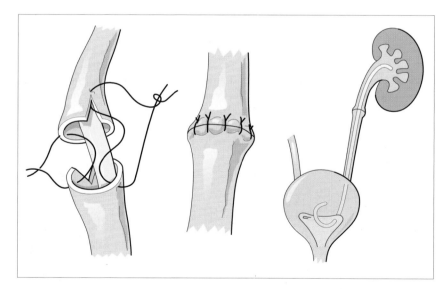

Fig. 30.11 Primary anastomosis of the abdominal ureter. The end-to-end anastomosis must be achieved without tension. The ends of the ureter must be fresh and spatulated.

Management

The shocked patient must be stabilized in the usual manner.

All patients with penetrating injuries should undergo exploration of the abdomen. Even if the injury is felt to be entirely extraperitoneal, the peritoneal cavity should be opened and inspected. The bladder should be repaired in two layers with a 3-0 absorbable suture (e.g. chromic catgut or vicryl). A large-bore suprapubic catheter is brought out through a separate incision. These are generally better tolerated than urethral catheters and give rise to less problems such as epididymitis. A closed non-suction drain should be placed in the extravesical space. In addition to penetrating injuries all patients with intraperitoneal

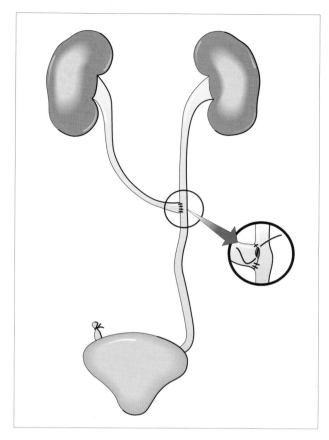

Fig. 30.12 Technique for transureterureterostomy if indicated.

ruptures should undergo laparotomy and formal repair. Morbidity is considerably lower with formal repair when compared to conservative management with catheter drainage.

If the condition of the patient allows, an extraperitoneal rupture due to blunt trauma may be managed conservatively with a urethral catheter for 1 to 5 weeks and cystogram done before catheter removal.

If a bladder tear is noticed intra-operatively then the defect should be repaired with a two-layer absorbable 3-0 suture. A careful inspection of the bladder should be made as a common mistake made is that a second tear is missed.

If the bladder is injured during endoscopic surgery and the leak is extraperitoneal these patients can be managed with a large urethral catheter as long as their condition does not deteriorate. Minor contusion is safest dealt with by a few days drainage.

In general 10 days catheterization is adequate for bladder tears to heal and cystography prior to catheter removal is recommended.

Acute urethral trauma

The outlook for the patient with trauma to the urethra has improved considerably in the last decade. Because of the rarity of this injury it is impossible for one urologist to gain sufficient experience and to draw firm guidelines about management. Consequently, the early management of traumatic urethral injuries remains controversial but the general principle of alignment of the distracted urethra is fundamental to a satisfactory long term outcome.

Anatomic considerations

The male urethra is made up of four components and extends from the bladder neck to the external meatus (Fig. 30.14).

The anterior urethra extends from the inferior aspect of the urogenital diaphragm to the external meatus and is

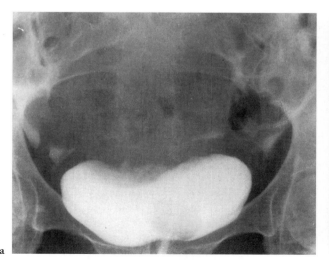

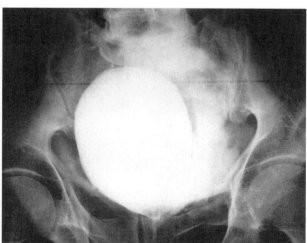

Fig. 30.13 (a) Intraperitoneal bladder rupture. (b) Extraperitoneal bladder rupture.

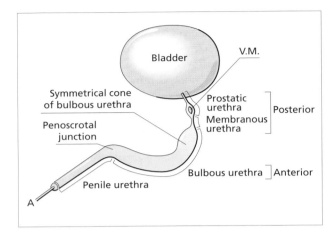

Fig. 30.14 The anatomy of the male urethra.

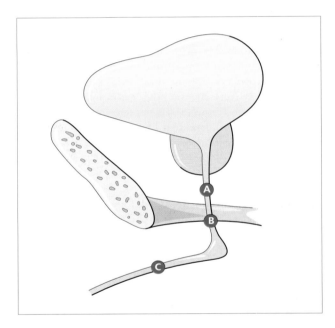

Fig. 30.15 The sites of urethral injury. A, Injury to membranous urethra from a fractured pelvis. B, Perineal contusion. C, Injury to penile urethra from falling astride.

divided into two parts by the penoscrotal junction, anterior to which is the penile urethra extending to the corona. Above this junction is the bulbar urethra which continues to the urogenital diaphragm.

The posterior urethra has a membranous and prostatic portion and extends from the urogenital diaphragm to the bladder neck. The urethra may be injured in three different sites, as shown in Fig. 30.15. The female urethra is about 3.5 cm long and is entirely protected behind the bony pelvis.

Aetiology of urethral injury

- Blunt perineal injury
- Penetrating injury
- Urethral instrumentation
- Pelvic fracture
- Fractured penis

Anterior urethral injuries

Complete anterior urethral rupture with distraction of the two ends is relatively uncommon and can be diagnosed when the continuity of the urethra is completely disrupted. Incomplete rupture may occur where some continuity of the urethra remains.

Anterior urethral injuries typically occur as the result of a straddle injury such as when the patient falls astride on the cross-bar of a bicycle or on a fence or sustains a kick in the groin. The injury may result in anterior urethral contusion or complete or partial rupture of the bulbar urethra as a result of crushing against the inferior aspect of the pubic ramus. A pelvic fracture is generally not present. Contusions are associated with normal urethrograms and are occasionally associated with stricture formation. The clinical triad of acute urinary retention, blood at external meatus and scrotal haematoma may be present. Injuries to the anterior urethra may also occur from penetrating trauma or be self-inflicted. During transurethral procedures the mucosa may be denuded by the to and fro movement of the instrument at narrow areas such as the meatus, penoscrotal junction and the membranous urethra. Catheterization may also cause injury in the same locations.

If the urethra has been ruptured then extravasation of contrast will be demonstrated. If Buck's fascia is intact then the injury will be limited to the space between Buck's fascia and the tunica albuginea of the corpus spongiosum. If Buck's fascia is disrupted then the contrast may be extravasated within the confines of Colles' fascia and extend into the scrotum or perineum.

Management of injuries to the anterior urethra

Injuries to the anterior urethra can be managed by careful catheterization after performing a urethrogram. If unsuccessful the placement of a suprapubic catheter alone may be all that is required as more than 70% will heal without stricture. More damage is done by trying to do a primary closure than by cystostomy alone and if a stricture develops it can be treated by internal urethrotomy. Formal urethroplasty may be considered if the stricture requires repeated urethrotomies.

Occasionally partial and complete ruptures can be managed by a trial of micturition with repeat urethrography 10 days later.

If complete transection of the urethra occurs then primary repair is required. This can be performed within a few days of the injury and a primary anastomosis after debridement can be done. Tension relieving sutures between the urethral adventitia and adjacent Buck's fascia will avoid anastomotic tension should postoperative erections occur.

Urethral injury following pelvic fracture

Incidence

The incidence of urological injuries varies from series to series and this may be because of the fact that most reviews are retrospective and may only include those referred for evaluation and care, thereby missing many less severe cases. About 10–15% of patients with a pelvic fracture will have urological trauma and between 10 and 20% of male patients with an injury to the posterior urethra will also have an injury to the bladder.

Clinical and radiological features

The diagnosis of rupture of the membranous urethra is often made on the basis of blood at, or bleeding from the external urethral meatus, in addition to the inability to void and a palpable bladder. Secondary clinical features include a high riding prostate in association with a perineal haematoma. An IVU may reveal the bladder to be high in the pelvis with compression of its lateral walls by haematoma, giving it an inverted teardrop appearance.

Although these features are helpful in diagnosing urethral trauma they are unreliable in determining the degree or actual site of injury. Their absence does not preclude the possibility of injury thus urethrography is essential when urethral trauma is suspected.

Bleeding

Blood at the meatus is just as likely to indicate a contusion or minor rupture as it is a complete rupture. There may be absence of blood in complete rupture as the urogenital diaphragm may go into spasm, thus preventing blood from entering the anterior urethra.

Inability to void

The bladder may have been empty at time of trauma or may be slow to fill following trauma. The bladder itself may be ruptured without any damage to the urethra. Inability to void may indicate rupture of the urethra and conversely the ability to void does not exclude rupture.

Rectal examination

Although a high-riding dislocation of the prostate is relatively rare, it is diagnostic of a urethral tear. This is important to recognize as difficult strictures inevitably develop if it remains unreduced. As the majority of these injuries occur in young men with smaller prostates, assessment can be very difficult. Tenderness in the presence of a pelvic haematoma following a fracture may also make interpretation difficult.

Rectal examination is also important to exclude a rectal tear. Coincidental rectal fistula may be found in about 8% of patients with features of complex fracture urethral injuries. These rectal injuries need to be protected by defunctioning colostomies. The majority resolve without any long-term complications.

Intravenous urography

An inverted tear drop bladder is often considered diagnostic of posterior urethral rupture but this may also occur with a pelvic haematoma without urethral injury.

Perineal or genital haematoma

Although perineal and genital haematoma are commonly found in association with urethral injuries this finding may not yet be present at the time the patient attends the accident and emergency department.

Initial management

The method of immediate management is determined by the condition of the patient, facilities and resources of the receiving hospital and the experience of the surgeon. Most pelvic fractures and the associated urethral injuries are relatively minor causing only a contusion or partial rupture. These patients can be managed expectantly and allowed to pass urine spontaneously with the passage of a suprapubic tube if unable to void.

The problem lies with patients with more serious injuries. As a urologist is not always present it is helpful to have a set of guidelines for emergency room staff. Following initial assessment and patient stabilization a urethrogram (see description) should be done in patients with:
• Pelvic fracture and gross haematuria
• Blood at the meatus
• Genital or perineal swelling
• Haematoma or contusion
• Free floating prostate on rectal examination.

Catheterization

If the urethrogram is normal a catheter can be passed into

the bladder. If there is some extravasation of contrast but some also enters the bladder or on initial assessment there is no blood at the meatus then one gentle attempt at catheterization may be made. Such partial tears rarely require further treatment after successful catheterization however this placement does run the risk of completing a partial tear and introducing infection.

If one gentle attempt at urethral catheterization is unsuccessful then suprapubic drainage should be attempted.

In all cases of gross haematuria and in those with a ruptured urethra who have been catheterized a cystogram with a full and empty bladder should be performed as between 10 and 20% of these patients will have a bladder tear.

The passage of the full length of a catheter into a urethra does not necessarily indicate that it has passed into the bladder. It may pass out of the urethra and inflation of the balloon may cause further damage.

It is essential that catheters should not be placed on traction in an effort to reduce a dislocation, because the bladder neck — the only remaining sphincter mechanism — may be damaged in this way.

Routine IVUs are not indicated in all patients with pelvic fracture but should be performed in all patients with associated rib fractures, evidence of upper abdominal trauma or rapid deceleration injuries.

Traumatic rupture of the female urethra

Because of anatomical differences urethral injuries are more common in males than females and children. The short course of the female urethra behind the pubic arch, its mobility in the pelvic floor and its relative lack of exposure afford adequate protection from pelvic trauma. Female urethral injuries are associated most commonly with instrumentation, vaginal operations and obstetric complications. They occur infrequently with pelvic trauma and in a review of 160 female patients with pelvic fracture six (4.6%) had a ruptured urethra. A review of 381 patients with traumatic rupture of the urethra included only seven female patients all of whom had incomplete tears.

The mechanism of urethral injuries in the female is different to that of the male and commonly involves vaginal injuries.
1 The anteroposterior diameter of the bony pelvis may be increased by lateral compression at the time of injury displacing the bladder upwards resulting in avulsion of the bladder neck or proximal urethra.
2 Upward displacement on the femur and hip joint may cause displacement of the pubis resulting in traction injuries.
3 Sudden diastasis of the pubic symphysis or symphysiotomy may tear the urethra. The urethra may also be lacerated by a bony spicule.

4 Similarily, anteroposterior compression forces produce traction on the proximal urethra.

Blood in the vagina or at the introitus is the most reliable early physical finding suggesting injury and similarly successful urethral catheterization does not eliminate the possibility of injury. Coincidental bladder rupture will be present in two-thirds of patients and this should be repaired to provide the chance of maintaining continence.

Injuries to the penis

Amputation

Self-mutilation or emasculation during a psychotic episode is the most common amputation injury to the penis. Despite the obvious self-mutilation there is only about a 5% relapse rate among those patients who have had a successful re-implantation. The penis appears unique in that it is relatively resistant to ischaemic injury when compared to other organs. Succesful re-implants have been reported after 16 h of warm ischaemia and after 24 h of hypothermic ischaemia. Microsurgical techniques are required for the vasculature and neuro-attachment of the penis.

Principles

1 Amputated part should be cleansed with sterile saline and placed in sterile salt solution surrounded by ice. A tourniquet should be placed on the proximal part of the penis to arrest haemorrhage.
2 Place suprapubic catheter to divert the urine.
3 Patient should be operated on in a centre with microsurgical facilities.
4 Meticulous debridement is required prior to repair.
5 Place a Foley catheter into the bladder to stabilize the penis. The urethra is the first to be approximated with a standard two-layer spatulated anastomosis.
6 Anastomosis of the cavernosal artery is then performed with 10-0 Prolene.
7 Tunica albuginea is then approximated with 4-0 Dexon.
8 Dorsal artery, vein and nerve are approximated with 10-0 nylon.
9 The dartos is closed with 5-0 absorbable suture.
10 The skin can be re-anastomosed with absorbable sutures. Lymphodema rarely occurs if the lymphatic channels of the penis are disrupted by the amputation.

Penetrating penile injury

Knife or gunshot injuries are the most common causes of penetrating penile injuries. A low threshold for surgical exploration, debridement of devitalized tissue, closure of the tunica and repair of the urethra should be the mainstay of treatment. In most cases it is wise to obtain a retrograde urethrogram prior to surgical exploration. Patients should be warned that permanent impotence may result from the injury.

Traumatic rupture of the corpora cavernosa

Rupture of the corpora may be the result of blunt trauma during sexual intercourse. Unilateral transverse tear of the tunica albuginea is the most common injury although injury to the corpus spongiosum, tears to Buck's fascia and urethral injury may also occur. The diagnosis is usually easy to make based on the history and the swelling of the penis. Cavernosography is rarely required to establish a diagnosis; however, a urethrogram is mandatory as 20% will have some degree of urethral injury. Although the patient can be managed conservatively with pressure dressing, Foley catheter, analgesia and antibiotics, we feel that surgical exploration provides the most satisfactory result. The foreskin should be incised circumferentially as with circumcision and the penis degloved and the defect repaired with absorbable sutures.

Degloving injury of the penis

The loose skin of the penis may be torn off when clothing is caught in machinery. The skin of the penis is loosely attached to the underlying areolar tissue above Buck's fascia.

Principles

1 Debride as little as possible to save as much skin as possible.
2 The skin and its underlying areolar tissue carry the lymphatics therefore if there is a circumferential injury the distal skin should be removed because if this is left *in situ* it will become oedematous and non-functional.
3 The defect can be covered with a thick or split-thickness skin graft. If potency can be sacrificed the penis can be buried in the scrotal skin with the glans exposed.

Scrotal injuries

Management of scrotal trauma is directed towards maintaining spermatogenesis and hormonal functions in addition to restoring cosmesis of the scrotum.

Superficial lacerations may be debrided and closed primarily however when there is loss of the scrotal skin covering the testicles a few principles must be observed:
1 Placement of the testes in the superficial thigh is preferable to subcutaneous abdominal placement due to the lower temperature of the former. Later reconstruction of the scrotum can be considered.
2 If a small amount of scrotal skin remains, flaps can be mobilized from the perineal area.

3 If a patient has multiple other injuries and the scrotal injury is not a priority then the testicles can be dressed daily with saline soaks until scrotal granulations are adequate for the application of a skin mesh or skin graft.
4 If there is a laceration through the tunica the testes should be meticulously debrided with a primary closure with absorbable sutures to prevent the extrusion of testicular contents.
5 A drain should always be placed in the scrotum but never placed beneath the tunica albuginea of the testes as it will provide an exit for the seminiferous tubules.
6 Broad-spectrum antibiotics should be used.
7 Re-implantation of the amputated testes with microsurgical techniques should be considered in cases seen within 8 h of injury.

Blunt scrotal trauma

The patient generally has sudden onset of excruciating scrotal pain often associated with nausea and vomiting. If the tunica albuginea is ruptured and the tunica vaginalis remains intact, the patient may suffer only minimal swelling or ecchymosis. Extreme tenderness will be elicited because of the compression of the seminiferous tubules. If the tunica vaginalis is also ruptured then a scrotal haematoma will also be present. Minimal trauma causing severe symptoms should raise the suspicion of pre-existing disease (see Table 30.2)

Testicular ultrasound is accurate in about 90% of cases in demonstrating fracture of the tunica albuginea. Once testicular torsion has been ruled out the decision on operative or conservative management has to be made. Early exploration is advised but if the injury is longer than 24 h then a more conservative approach can be adopted. The testes should be explored through the midline raphe, haematoma evacuated, devascularized tubules excised and the tunica albuginea repaired with absorbable sutures. The scrotum should be drained through a separate stab incision. The above principles should be applied to penetrating scrotal injuries.

Table 30.2 Differential diagnosis of testicular pain after blunt scrotal trauma.

Fractured testicle
Testicular torsion
Reactive hydrocele
Torsion of the appendix epididymis or appendix testes
Epididymitis
Injury to the testicular vessels (including rupture of a varicocele)
Haematocele
Haematoma of the cord or epididymis
Testicular tumour

Radiological investigations

Intravenous urography

An initial plain X-ray of the kidneys, ureter and bladder is obtained. After obtaining a negative allergy history a bolus of 50–60 ml of iodine containing contrast material is injected intravenously. Films are taken at timed intervals (5, 10, 15 and 30 min as an example) and delayed films may be required if there is poor opacification of the kidney. The bladder is often filled with contrast medium at five minutes. It is important to obtain a postvoid film to help establish the integrity of the urinary tract.

Computerized axial tomography (CT scan)

CT scanning in abdominal injuries is preferred because:
1 It defines associated visceral injuries more precisely than the IVU.
2 It may show minute extravasation of urine often missed by IVU.
3 It gives more information on an ectopic or absent kidney which might be interpreted as a non-functioning kidney on IVU.
4 It may be very helpful in delineating injuries to the bony pelvis and its contents.

If time allows both non-contrast and contrast studies should be performed to allow for a more complete evaluation of the urinary tract. Non-contrast scans are particularly helpful if haemorrhage or extravasation are suspected. Administering the contrast medium by a bolus is preferred for the assessment of renal anatomy and aortorenal transit. After a bolus injection renal arterial opacification is followed by immediate enhancement of the renal cortex. The nephrogram phase is reached in about 60 s with excretion into the ureters after 2–3 min.

Cystogram

The cystogram is the only study that will definitely diagnose a ruptured bladder. If two rules are rigidly adhered to: (1) adequate filling of the bladder; and (2) postdrainage films,
then the cystogram is a very accurate investigation. After a plain film to identify a pelvic fracture, the bladder should be filled via a foley catheter with about 300 ml of contrast medium and a plain film obtained from the anteroposterior, oblique and lateral projections. The bladder should then be allowed to drain freely and a further film taken to see if there is extraperitoneal extravasation not seen on the full bladder film. An intraperitoneal rupture will be seen on the full film.

Ascending urethrography

To obtain maximum information dynamic studies should be done. A 14 F or 16 F non-lubricated catheter should be placed into the urethral meatus for about 2–3 cm with 1–2 ml in the balloon to anchor it in the fossa navicularis. The length of the catheter allows the investigator to keep hands well clear of the X-ray beam. The patient should then be placed approximately 35° in lateral tilt rather than being laid flat as this causes the bulbous urethra to be superimposed on itself. Generally 20–30 ml of contrast is sufficient. Fluoroscopic control is favoured in order to observe the progress of posterior urethral filling and the onset of extravasation of contrast medium. In the patient with multiple injuries this may not be possible and in these cases the injection is done in small increments of 10 ml. If a Foley catheter has already been successfully placed in the urethra then it should not be removed as this almost certainly excludes a complete rupture. A cystogram should be performed to exclude bladder rupture.

Further reading

McAninch, J.W. & Carroll, P.R. (1989) Renal exploration after trauma; indications and reconstructive techniques. *Urology Clinics of North America* **16** 203.

Dixon, C.M., Carroll, P.R. & McAninch, J.W. (1994) The management of renal and ureteric trauma. In: *Clinical Urology* (eds R.J. Krane, M.B. Siroky & J.M. Fitzpatrick), p. 399. JB Lippincott & Co., Philadelphia.

Lynch, T.H. & Fitzpatrick, J.M. (1995) Acute urethral trauma. *European Urology Update* **4** 122–127.

CHAPTER 31

Emergency conditions affecting the breast

Philip J. Drew & Michael J. Kerin

Acute non-malignant afflictions of the breast are rarely life threatening. Nonetheless, they remain a source of severe discomfort for many women and, if not treated promptly and appropriately, can lead to significant physical and cosmetic morbidity. Acute painful infections of the breast (mastitis) are by far the commonest cause of emergency presentation. Trauma to the breast can also cause discomfort and concern. The majority of problems relate to non-malignant disease. However, aggressive cancers such as inflammatory breast cancer can mimic acute infection and deserve separate consideration.

Acute mastitis and breast abscess

In general, acute infection of the breast is much less common than in the past. However, it remains most common in the physiologically active breast, i.e. between the ages of 8 and 50 years. It must be remembered that infection in the breast may arise from common skin conditions such as sebaceous cysts as a secondary event as well as from within the breast itself. Infection of the breast and its sequelae is classified into lactational and non-lactational.

Non-lactational breast infection

Improvements in general health and maternal and infant hygiene have led to a marked reduction in the incidence of lactational breast infection. In fact, non-lactational breast abscesses now make up greater than 90% of the total. Non-lactational breast infections can be sub-classified into central or peripheral.

Aetiology

It remains unclear as to whether the presence of periductal mastitis or blocked secretion filled ducts is more important in the development of breast abscesses. Whilst nipple inversion and resultant problems with nipple hygiene have traditionally been thought to be related to the development of non-lactational infections less than 10% of women with primary subareolar abscesses and less than 20% of women with recurrent abscesses are afflicted by nipple inversion. It

Non-lactational breast abscess

- Most common type
- Subareolar usually associated with periductal mastitis
- Recurrence associated with anaerobic infections and cigarette smoking
- 20% develop mammary fistulae
- Peripheral abscess associated with immunocompromise and systemic illness

Lactational breast abscess

- Less common in antibiotic era
- Usually settles on conservative therapy
- Rarely recurs
- Not as frequently associated with smoking
- *Staphylococcus* most common organism

may of course be the infection that leads to the nipple inversion and therefore the nipple inversion may represent the chicken rather than the egg.

However, periductal mastitis appears to be a separate clinical entity from duct ectasia and tends to affect younger women who smoke. Therefore its association with acute and chronic infections of the breast is considered to be much stronger. The organisms isolated from non-lactational breast abscesses are somewhat different from those found in pregnant or lactating women. Staphylococci and streptococci are the commonest aerobic organisms encountered but a variety of anaerobic species are also frequently implicated. The presence of anaerobic organisms correlates with recurrent abscess formation and is more common in women who smoke.

Clinical presentation

In peri-areolar infections the patients may give a history of periductal mastitis (Fig. 31.1). This condition is much more commonly seen in smokers and is associated with central 'letter box' nipple retraction, and nipple discharge. If there is already an established abscess the patient usually presents with the classic signs: localized tenderness, fluctuance,

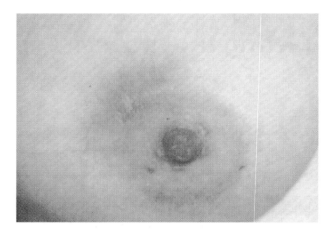

Fig. 31.1 Periductal mastitis; note the periareolar inflammation.

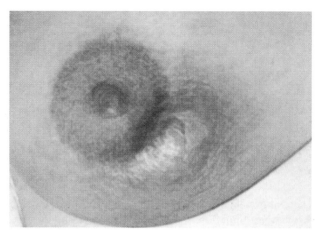

Fig. 31.2 Non-lactational breast abscess.

erythema and induration (Fig. 31.2). There may be a significant associated cellulitis with signs of systemic upset.

Peripheral non-lactational breast infections are more commonly related to underlying conditions such as diabetes, trauma and steroid treatment. Generally, cellulitis is more common in this group than with peri-areolar infections. In particular, infections associated with granulomatous lobular mastitis tend to be associated with multiple synchronous breast abscesses and extensive cellulitis.

Rarely, the patient may present with full-blown sepsis, although this is more commonly seen in the immunocompromised.

Treatment

When presenting as an acute emergency cellulitis and localized infections should be treated with an appropriate course of antibiotics to cover both aerobic and anaerobic organisms. If necessary, the woman should be admitted to hospital and antibiotics administered intravenously until the infection is under control; although in general the majority of women can be successfully treated on an outpatient basis.

Whenever possible the traditional approach of incision and drainage of breast abscesses should be avoided. The accepted modern management of breast abscesses involves broad-spectrum antibiotics and repeated aspiration with regular ultrasonographic review. If an abscess is obviously about to point, or the abscess fails to resolve, formal incision and drainage should be performed and only with the smallest effective incision. In younger women with recurrent breast abscesses the cosmetic turmoil rendered by the over-enthusiastic use of the knife can be catastrophic in addition to being inappropriate. A chronic mammary duct fistula may develop following treatment of peri-areolar breast abscesses (Fig. 31.3). This occurs whether primary therapy is open surgery or aspiration. If an infection fails to settle on antibiotics the diagnosis of inflammatory breast cancer must be considered and the appropriate fine needle aspiration cytology, core biopsy or surgical biopsy obtained. Whenever possible patients with acute breast infections should be managed by a specialist in breast disorders as recurrent episodes will require specific treatments. In patients with peri-areolar disease recurrent episodes of sepsis can treated by excision of the diseased duct under antibiotic cover. Mammary fistulae can be managed by excision of the fistula tract and major duct complex under antibiotic cover.

Lactational mastitis and abscess

Lactational mastitis refers to the development of cellulitis in the lactating breast. Its incidence has markedly decreased because of general improvements in maternal health and hygiene. The phenomenon of staphylococcal hospital-acquired epidemic lactational mastitis has now largely disappeared, principally because of shortened hospital stays, improved hygiene and prompt treatment of individual cases. In the more common sporadic cases infection is most frequently seen within the first 6 weeks of breast feeding

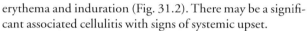

Treatment
• Aspiration as outpatient
• Ultrasound follow up with serial aspiration if required
• Pus for culture and sensitivity
• Broad-spectrum antibiotics for 2 weeks
• Incision and drainage rarely required

Remember
• Inflammatory cancer
• Aspiration and broad-spectrum antibiotics
• Recurrent abscess — biopsy and culture

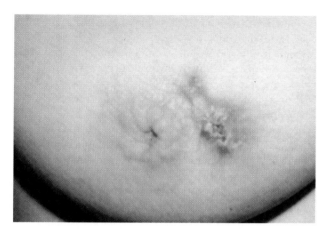

Fig. 31.3 Mammary duct fistula.

although there is a double incidence peak with problems also occurring during weaning. The condition has been reported to affect 1–9% of women and is often associated with irritated or cracked nipple skin which may act as a portal for infection.

Clinical presentation

Typically a woman will present within the first few weeks of breast feeding with a segment of one breast that is erythematous, indurated and tender. There may also be signs of an underlying abscess although this is actually far less common than isolated cellulitis and this should be born in mind when attempting an aspiration of a suspected abscess without prior ultrasound confirmation. Non-infectious inflammation and milk stasis are for all practical purposes clinically indistinguishable from infectious mastitis. Some authors have suggested that conditions can be separated by assessing the leukocyte count in the breast milk. However, most clinicians would agree that antibiotics should be administered in either case and therefore the matter is of diagnostic interest only.

Treatment

Unlike epidemic lactational mastitis the suckling infant is not thought to be the source of bacterial infection and therefore weaning is not recommended in sporadic lactational

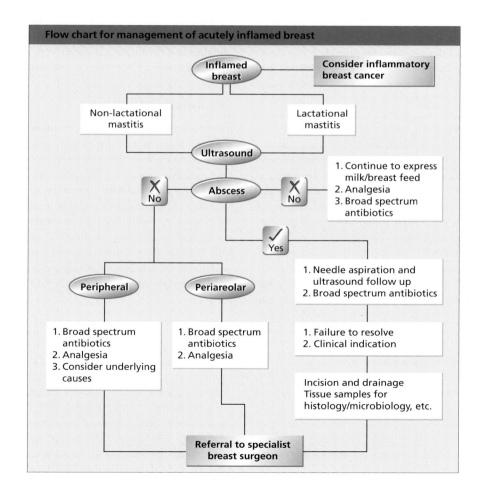

mastitis. In fact, it has been shown that the regular emptying of the duct system facilitated by continued breast feeding actually shortens the duration of symptoms. However, in addition to the discomfort it may cause, women are often anxious about feeding their child from an obviously infected breast and, therefore, at least should be encouraged to express their milk from the affected side until the infection settles. Patients with lactational breast abscesses are best treated with broad-spectrum antibiotics and repeated aspiration with ultrasound review. Unlike non-lactational abscesses the development of fistulas is rare. Of course, care must be taken not to prescribe antibiotics that may harm the infant. As such, co-amoxiclav (amoxycillin with the β-lactamase inhibitor clavulanic acid) represents an example of an antibiotic with sufficient streptococcal, staphylococcal and anaerobic cover that only appears in trace amounts in breast milk.

Skin-associated and uncommon breast infections

A primary staphylococcal cellulitis or fungal infections of the skin of the breast are most commonly seen in overweight women with larger breasts. There may also be an underlying medical condition such as diabetes, but in general these infections are related to poor personal hygiene. Treatment of bacterial cellulitis and abscesses is as for primary breast infections. However, these conditions tend to be recurrent and often a diplomatic referral to a sympathetic breast care nurse for advice on personal hygiene, the use of non-perfumed soaps and powders, etc. can prove to be the most effective form of treatment, especially for candidal intertrigo.

Sebaceous cysts are common in the skin of the breast and have the same natural history as sebaceous cysts elsewhere on the integument. The risk of infection should be balanced against the cosmetic problems associated with removal although in general removal prior to the onset of infective complications should be advised. Once infection is apparent incision and drainage of the cyst is required.

Hidradenitis suppurativa can lead to acute presentations with cellulitis and abscess formation in the inframammary fold or the axilla. Treatment involves controlling the infection with the appropriate broad-spectrum antibiotics and the drainage of any pus. Once settled conservative excision of the affected skin prevents recurrent infection in about 50% of patients.

Tuberculosis, actinomycosis, blastomycosis, sporotichosis and syphilis represent rare causes of breast infection that may present in the emergency setting. Tuberculosis may be primary or more commonly secondary. Obviously the patient's ethnic background should be considered when making the diagnosis, as the reported incidence in India is 1–4.5% of all breast problems requiring operation, whereas in the West it is practically unheard of. The most common presentation is with a painful solitary breast mass with associated lymphadenopathy. The diagnosis is difficult to make pre-operatively and is most commonly obtained following excision biopsy. Treatment involves surgery and antituberculous therapy.

Primary and secondary infection of the breast by *Actinomycosis israelii* tends to mimic inflammatory breast cancer and the diagnosis is most commonly made postoperatively. Abscess drainage and debridement of necrotic tissue along with high-dose tetracycline treatment is required.

Primary syphilis of the breast is a sexually transmitted disease. Patients present with a chancre which heals within 2–6 weeks and then secondary syphilis develops with associated gummas of the breast. *Treponema pallidum* can be isolated from the primary chancre to confirm the diagnosis. High-dose penicillin remains the mainstay of treatment.

Blastomycosis and sporotrichosis are extremely rare and result either from primary infection of from direct extension through the chest wall. As would be expected diagnosis is rare prior to abscess drainage and specific fungal stains and cultures are required in addition to serological examination. Amphotericin B is the treatment of choice although potassium iodide may be effective for cutaneous disease.

Wegener's granulomatosis of the breast is an extremely rare condition that can mimic breast infection and should be considered if the history is suggestive of an autoimmune disorder although it is most commonly diagnosed on biopsy.

Neonatal infection

Suppurative mastitis may occur in neonates and infants. Culture of any nipple discharge is required to differentiate between an infective problem or physiological neonatal mastitis, which is related to transplacental passage of maternal hormones and resolves spontaneously after birth. The majority of infections are related to *Staphylococcus aureus*, although *Escherichia coli* is also commonly implicated. Once confirmed appropriate antibiotics, aspiration or incision, and drainage of any ultrasonographically confirmed abscess will result in resolution. If an incision is required it should be placed peripherally in order to avoid damaging the breast bud.

Trauma

Whilst trauma to the breast is in itself a non-life-threatening condition its presence can be used as indicator of more serious thoracic injuries. Blunt trauma results in ecchymoses, erythema and oedema with penetrating trauma causing associated soft tissue disruption. Seat belt injuries make up the largest aetiological group. Subcutaneous rupture of the breast has been reported following such trauma, with the mechanism of injury related to compression and shearing forces acting on the breast tissue. The breast may actually be divided at the line of impact of the seat belt. The resulting injury will normally resolve spontaneously although widespread fat necrosis with associated deformity may require plastic surgery. Rupture of breast implants may also occur. This may not be obvious clinically at the time of injury but ultrasonongraphy and magnetic resonance imaging (MRI) of the breast will help confirm the diagnosis.

Breast haematoma is the most common sequelae of trauma to the breast. These haematomas are usually self-limiting and no specific treatment is required. Patients present with echymosis and a palpable tender mass soon after the trauma. Any residual mass should be fully evaluated as, while fat necrosis remains the most likely diagnosis, 9–20% of women with breast cancer have a history of recent trauma.

Treatment

Primary breast haematomas should not be treated operatively as they will resolve. Analgesia and a supportive bra will help alleviate any discomfort. The basic surgical principles of debridement and primary or secondary closure according to the nature of the injury should be applied to the management of penetrating trauma. If there is extensive loss of breast tissue a myocutaneous flap may be required to achieve closure of the defect with an acceptable cosmetic outcome.

In both blunt and penetrating trauma to the breast due consideration should be given to the possibility of damage to intrathoracic structures.

Mondor's disease

Described in detail by Mondor in 1939 superficial thrombophlebitis of the lateral thoracic or superior thoraco-epigastric veins now holds his eponym. Patients usually present with a tender subcutaneous cord in the breast without systemic signs of infection. It is related to trauma to the breast, including surgery and radiotherapy, and other benign conditions such as infection, excessive physical strain and rheumatoid arthritis. Breast cancer is associated with up to 13% of cases and therefore careful assessment is required. The process is self limiting and normally resolves within 2 to 10 weeks. Local application of heat and non-steroidal agents may give some systemic relief.

Warfarin-induced breast necrosis

This is an extremely rare phenomenon with only 32 cases ever reported. Massive necrosis of the breast occurs 3–5 days following the initiation of warfarin therapy. The exact mechanism of damage remains unclear. Wide debridement or simple mastectomy is the only effective treatment.

Inflammatory breast carcinoma

This rare sub-type of breast cancer accounts for less than 1% of all cases of breast malignancies. Classified into types I and II according to whether an underlying palpable tumour is present, the characteristic erythema and peau d'orange associated with this type of tumour mimics the clinical signs of breast infection (Fig. 31.4). Histologically tumour is seen to be invading the cutaneous lymphatics with subsequent inflammation and oedema. Fine needle aspiration, cytology, ultrasound, mammography and, more recently, MRI of the breast may help in the diagnosis. Inflammatory breast carcinoma must be regarded as a systemic disease at the time of presentation and the prognosis is worse than most other types of breast cancer making neo-adjuvant chemoradiotherapy the treatment of choice. MRI of the breast may be able to predict those women able to undergo less extensive surgery following neoadjuvant therapy. The diagnosis of inflammatory breast carcinoma must always be considered when a women presents with an acutely inflamed breast especially if it fails to respond to antibiotic therapy.

Summary

Incision and drainage of breast abscesses is now considered unnecessary as primary therapy in the majority of cases. Simple aspiration and ultrasound follow up with appropriate aerobic and anaerobic antibiotic cover will lead to complete resolution in the majority of cases. Underlying disorders such as diabetes and inflammatory carcinoma should always be considered.

Whether presenting with an acutely inflamed breast or following trauma patients that fail to respond or are left with a residual mass should be fully evaluated by a specialist breast surgeon.

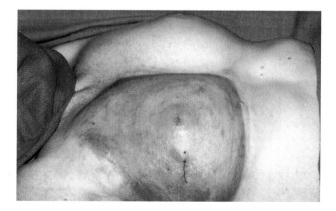

Fig. 31.4 Inflammatory breast carcinoma: note the scar from an inappropriate attempted incision and drainage performed in the casualty department. Inflammatory carcinoma should always be excluded in patients presenting with an inflamed breast.

CHAPTER 32

Gynaecological emergencies

Kevin Hickey, Peter McKenna & Malachy Coughlan

Introduction

Acute gynaecological presentations to a casualty department usually involve a combination of lower abdominal pain and vaginal bleeding or discharge. Non-menstrual vaginal bleeding is abnormal—whether it arises before puberty, after the menopause, between periods except for slight ovulatory spotting, after coitus, or during pregnancy. In women under the age of 40 years the cause is usually benign, but cancer of the cervix must be excluded. In women with post-menopausal bleeding atrophic vaginitis caused by lack of local oestrogen is the leading cause, but it is essential to rule out endometrial cancer. The characteristics of each symptom should be explored, including their relationship to menstruation, coitus, or genital tract trauma. Details of previous gynaecological procedures, last menstrual period and likelihood of pregnancy, last cervical smear test, and use of contraceptive pill or hormone replacement therapy are of particular importance. In sexually active women a gravidex test is wise, irrespective of contraceptive use and certainty regarding last menstrual period. Vaginal bimanual examination should be performed by the gynaecology team, if available, and helps to define the position (ante/retroverted), size, mobility, and tenderness of the uterus as well as any tubal or ovarian adnexal mass. Normal sized ovaries are only palpable in thin people. Bimanual recto-abdominal examination in children and virgins can detect a foreign body in the vagina or a pelvic mass. Cusco's bivalve speculum examination in the dorsal position allows inspection of the cervix and vagina for local lesions, as well as permitting the collection of vaginal and endocervical bacteriological swabs or the removal of aborted products from the cervical os. Examination of the premenarchal child in casualty should be limited to inspection of the external genitalia.

Acute clinical presentations/differential diagnoses

Vaginal bleeding

The volume and duration of blood loss should be gauged by enquiry into the number of sanitary towels used per day and whether the pads were stained or soaked. It is vital to ascertain the date of the last menstrual period, coital and contraceptive history, and any past history of gynaecological procedures or bleeding diathesis.

Non-pregnant

Menstrual bleeding

> **Menstrual bleeding**
>
> - Dysfunctional uterine bleeding
> - Uterine fibroids
> - Adenomyosis

Dysfunctional uterine bleeding is heavy and irregular bleeding where no local cause is found. It is caused by an imbalance of gonadotrophins, ovarian hormones, or uterine prostaglandins. It is commonest in adolescence and nearing the menopause. In women of less than 35 years of age uterine curettage is usually uninformative and unnecessary, and menstrual cycle control is effected with oral norethisterone 5 mg b.d./t.d.s. or a low-dose combined oestrogen/progesterone contraceptive pill. In older women, or those with a history of polycystic ovarian disease or tamoxifen usage, it is important to rule out endometrial pathology by hysteroscopy and endometrial curettage before considering medical or surgical treatment options. For regular, heavy menstrual loss tranexamic acid, an antifibrinolytic agent, 1 g t.d.s. orally from day 1 to 5 of the period is the most effective medical treatment. Oral progestogens in the form of norethisterone 5 mg t.d.s. or duphaston 10 mg b.d. on days 5–25 of the menstrual cycle can be used for more irregular bleeding. When the progestogen-releasing intra-uterine contraceptive device (IUCD mirena coil) becomes licensed for use in menorrhagia it will serve a dual purpose of providing effective contraception and decreasing menstrual blood loss. Surgical options include endometrial ablation/resection or hysterectomy.

Uterine fibroids/leiomyomata are benign tumours of smooth muscle and fibrous tissue arising in the uterine wall. They develop in 25% of women over the age of 35 years. These firm growths can lie wholly within the uterine wall (intramural), or can protrude into either the uterine cavity (submucous) or the peritoneal cavity (subserous). The submucous form are more commonly associated with menorrhagia, while the subserous growths can become pedunculated and occasionally undergo torsion. The centre of a fibroid may degenerate and even calcify if of long standing ('womb stones'), but malignant sarcomatous change only occurs in 0.2% of cases. Fibroids are more common in nulliparous women, and may cause no symptoms or present with menorrhagia or abdominal swelling and discomfort. Rarely, acute pain may arise if a pedunculated fibroid undergoes torsion, or a bleed occurs into a degenerating fibroid (red degeneration). The latter is a more common event in pregnancy, when conservative management with analgesics is advisable. Fibroids are oestrogen-dependent tumours which tend to grow in size during pregnancy and regress after the menopause. Medical treatment in the form of gonadotrophin releasing hormone (GnRH) analogue treatment makes use of a pseudomenopause to induce shrinkage. However, the osteoporotic effects of this treatment with greater than 6 months' use limits its administration to symptomatic patients nearing a natural menopause or in younger women to diminish the size and vascularity of bulky growths prior to surgery. If future pregnancies are contemplated resection of the bulky fibroids is carried out (myomectomy) either by laparotomy or more recently by laparoscopic 'coring' from the uterus. Smaller submucous fibroids can be removed hysteroscopically by diathermy loop resection, while those greater than 2 cm in diameter should be shrunk with monthly GnRH analogue treatment for 3 months before resection. Recent use of intramyometrial vasopressin at laparotomy for these vascular growths has proven useful in decreasing operative blood loss. In the USA and France management of uterine fibroids by selective uterine artery embolization has yielded promising results and the procedure is now carried out in a few UK centres.

Endometriosis is the existence of active endometrial tissue in locations outside the endometrial lining of the uterus. The commonest sites are ovarian, pouch of Douglas, and pelvic peritoneum. Pelvic deposits are felt to arise by retrograde spill of menstrual fluid through the uterine tubes and implantation of these deposits on the adjacent peritoneal and ovarian surfaces. Adenomyosis ('internal endometriosis') is more common in parous women and refers to painful deposits of endometrial tissue within the uterine muscle causing dysmenorrhoea and often a tender, bulky uterus. Endometriosis arises after puberty and regresses during pregnancy and after the menopause. The main symptoms are pelvic pain, dysmenorrhoea, and dyspareunia as the

---

Endometriosis

- Pelvic pain
- Dysmenorrhea
- Dyspareunia
- Uterine bleeding
- Infertility

---

ectopic endometrial implants are stimulated by the cyclical ovarian hormones. Infertility and low parity are common associations. Menorrhagia does not usually occur, but an irregular vaginal bleeding pattern may arise if ovarian tissue is compromised by the disease. In constrast, the congested uterus which develops with adenomyosis can give rise to heavy periods. The severity of symptoms in endometriosis is no guide to the extent of the disease. Findings on examination can range from mild pelvic tenderness to a fixed pelvic mass when adhesions or large ovarian 'chocolate' cysts are present. Laparoscopy confirms the diagnosis. Treatment is hormonal or surgical and depends on the patient's age, fertility wishes, and disease extent. Hormonal treatments suppress menstrual activity and include high-dose progestogens, androgens (danazol, gestrinone), and GnRH analogues (buserelin, goserelin). These are highly effective at both disease clearance and symptom relief, although they are limited in their use by masculinizing (androgens) or menopausal-type (GnRH analogues) side effects. Surgical options include laser or diathermy cautery to endometriotic lesions, and abdominal hysterectomy with bilateral salpingo-oophorectomy in women whose families are complete. Oestrogen-based hormone replacement therapy can be given to the latter group of women who undergo a surgical menopause as reactivation of any residual peritoneal deposits of endometriosis seems to be rare in the absence of the cyclical peaks in oestrogen secretion associated with normal ovarian function.

Non-menstrual bleeding

Lesions of the urethra, vulva, vagina, or cervix may present with intermenstrual or post-coital bleeding. There may be an associated vaginal discharge.

Non-menstrual bleeding

- Urethral caruncle
- Cervical lesions: ectropion, polyp, carcinoma
- Edometrial polyp, carcinoma
- Rare causes—vaginal atrophic change or carcinoma

Urethral caruncle is a red protrusion of the posterior urethral wall which is commonest in older women and can be treated by excision.

Cervical lesions include ectropion, polyp, and cancer.

Cervical ectropion refers to an eversion of the vascular, mucus producing columnar epithelium of the cervical canal out onto the vaginal ectocervix, which is normally covered with non-secreting stratified squamous epithelium. The older term of cervical erosion to describe this physiological process is best avoided as patients are inclined to suspect cancer, despite reassurances. The condition predominates in high oestrogen states such as puberty, pregnancy, and with the combined oral contraceptive pill. It causes no pain or dyspareunia, but may be associated with a mucoid vaginal discharge or light intermenstrual/postcoital bleeding. An ectropion should be treated only if symptomatic, and not if found incidentally when taking a cervical smear. Acijel ointment vaginally will lower the local pH and promote metaplasia of the everted columnar cells to squamous epithelium. Thermal, cryo-, or laser cautery are alternative modes of treatment.

Cervical polyps arise from the cervical canal and may cause postcoital or intermenstrual bleeding. They can generally be avulsed by twisting off without anaesthetic, and then sent for histological examination. An endometrial polyp or a submucous fibroid are similar in appearance and presentation when extruded through the cervix, but the pedicle is usually wider and removal under general anaesthetic is wiser if cautery or suture ligation of the stalk is a possibility.

Cervical cancer is the most serious cause of postcoital or intermenstrual bleeding. The lesion may be polypoidal, ulcerated, or infiltrative. It is important to appreciate that cervical smear cytology can be normal in the presence of a cervical carcinoma and any suspicious looking cervix should be biopsied. Advanced local spread of tumour can give rise to vesicovaginal fistulae, ureteric obstruction, or back pain from sacral nerve root involvement or boney metastases. Urgent referral to a gynaecologist is advisable for clinical staging, biopsy, and cystoscopy under general anaesthesia, as well as ruling out ureteric obstruction by renal tract imaging with ultrasound or intravenous urography (IVU). Occasionally heavy bleeding from a vascular, friable tumour requires hospitalization to insert a vaginal pack and urinary catheter as a temporary measure. Definitive treatment of cervical cancer depends on the stage of the tumour. If cancer has spread to the pelvic side wall, lower two-thirds of the vagina, or is obstructing a ureter then radiotherapy is the first line treatment. In earlier disease radical abdominal hysterectomy with pelvic lymphadenectomy is more usual, although primary radiotherapy for patients of poor anaesthetic risk yields equivalent cure rates. It is worth remembering that precancer of the cervix (cervical intra-epithelial neoplasia; CIN) is asymptomatic and the cervix looks normal. Colposcopy is mandatory, and diathermy loop excision of the abnormal cervical epithelium under local anaesthesia is a highly effective treatment.

Endometrial polyps may be single or multiple, and can cause irregular vaginal bleeding or discharge. They are frequently diagnosed by transvaginal ultrasound, which also yields valuable information on the endometrial thickness. In postmenopausal women an endometrial thickness of greater than 4 mm should be regarded as abnormal and further investigated by hysteroscopy and endometrial curettage. Endometrial polyps are easily removed using an ovum/polyp forceps at the time of hysteroscopy.

Endometrial carcinoma usually presents in a similar manner or with postmenopausal bleeding. Total abdominal hysterectomy and bilateral salpingo-oophorectomy with peritoneal washings for cytology is the standard treatment, following the diagnostic curettage. The precise role of pelvic lymphadenectomy is still to be determined and is the subject of a current Royal College of Obstetricians and Gynaecologists trial. For poorly differentiated tumours, and those invading cervix or more than half of the myometrial wall thickness, either pelvic lymphadenectomy at the time of hysterectomy or adjuvant pelvic radiotherapy after the hysterectomy are advisable. Most endometrial cancers present at an early stage and carry a good prognosis. For those women with advanced cancers a combination of radiotherapy, surgery, and progestogens are used.

Rare causes. Vaginal cancer appears as an irregular nodule or ulcer and those involving the proximal or distal one-third are usually managed by radical surgery with regional lymphadenectomy, while midvaginal tumours require radiotherapy. Cervical carcinoma can spread to the vaginal wall, and less commonly endometrial, ovarian, or choriocarcinomata. Uterine tube cancer presents in older women with a light vaginal bleed or watery discharge.

Bleeding in early pregnancy

Any young woman with irregular vaginal bleeding should have pregnancy excluded by a urine pregnancy test, vaginal examination and ultrasound scan. Bleeding in pregnancy can be life threatening, and because of the increased circulating blood volume shock can be a late development. In the recent triennial report on confidential enquiries into maternal deaths in the United Kingdom there were eight deaths from ectopic pregnancy and a further eight deaths following abortion, with evidence of substandard care in all but one of these cases. In patients with heavy blood loss aggressive fluid resuscitation and early blood transfusion are necessary, together with post-operative care in an intensive care setting. In severe cases group O Rhesus negative blood may need to be administered. After estimating blood loss and instituting resuscitative measures, it must be determined by clinical and ultrasound assessment whether the patient in early pregnancy is aborting or has an ectopic pregnancy. In either case RhD negative patients should receive 250 IU anti-D i.m. within 72 h of presentation to prevent isoimmunization.

Ectopic pregnancy

A gestation outside of the uterine cavity occurs in about 1% of pregnancies, and risk factors include a history of pelvic inflammatory disease, infertility, tubal surgery, previous ectopic pregnancy, or current IUCD use. The commonest site of ectopic pregnancy is in the ampulla of the fallopian/uterine tube. In unruptured cases there is generally a history of 6–8 weeks amenorrhoea, lower abdominal pain, and light vaginal bleeding. White tissue may be passed vaginally as a decidual cast from the uterus. Complaints of either shoulder tip pain referred from the diaphragmatic irritation of an intraperitoneal bleed or of syncopal episodes are particularly suggestive. Lower abdominal and pelvic tenderness are usually found, although an adnexal mass from the small tubal swelling is not often apparent. Moving the cervix laterally with the vaginal examining finger puts the distended uterine tube on stretch with resulting pain and tenderness ('cervical excitation'). The urinary pregnancy test is invariably positive. A confirmatory pelvic ultrasound may not always show a tubal swelling, but an empty uterus on scan in the presence of a positive pregnancy test and pelvic tenderness is highly suggestive of an ectopic pregnancy and requires a diagnostic laparoscopy.

Conversely, a scan showing an intra-uterine pregnancy virtually excludes an ectopic as the two rarely occur simultaneously ('heterotopic' pregnancy, 1 : 30 000 cases). At the time of laparoscopy no instrumentation of the uterus should take place until the distended tubal ectopic has been visualized in order not to disturb a possible early intra-uterine pregnancy. In most cases of ectopic pregnancy a salpingectomy or salpingostomy with extraction of the gestational sac can be readily performed laparoscopically using diathermy scissors. Extensive tubal adhesions or a significant tubal haemorrhage may necessitate a laparotomy via a suprapubic transverse incision to carry out the salpingectomy. Less commonly, tubal rupture and the associated heavy bleeding intraperitoneally results in hypovolaemic shock at presentation with a rigid, tender abdomen. In such cases urgent volume replacement and laparotomy are essential, and even vaginal examination should be abandoned. In doubtful, clinically stable cases, serial serum human chorionic gonadotrophin (HCG) levels 48 h apart can help to distinguish an early intra-uterine gestation from a non-viable pregnancy. Prior to discharge from hospital patients should be informed of the ×6-fold increased risk of an ectopic pregnancy occurring in their other uterine tube, and of the importance of booking early in any future pregnancy to exclude this eventuality by transvaginal ultrasound scan.

Abortion/miscarriage

This refers to delivery of a pre-viable fetus, generally < 24 weeks gestation, and occurs in 15% of pregnancies. Most occur in the first trimester, and over two-thirds of these are due to a chromosomal defect in the zygote. The clinical presentation is usually one of crampy lower abdominal pain and vaginal bleeding. There may be a history of passing white tissue or membrane (gestational sac) per vagina. On pelvic assessment the uterus feels slightly enlarged. If the cervical os is open (admits a finger) the abortion is 'inevitable' or 'incomplete' and the patient generally requires uterine evacuation by curettage. If bleeding is profuse in these cases ergometrine 500 µg intramuscularly decreases haemorrhage by contracting the uterus, and a blood transfusion may be required. Products of conception trapped in the cervical os can give rise to a vasovagal shock and should be promptly removed using a sponge forceps. If the cervix is closed the vaginal blood loss is usually not excessive, and the diagnosis is either 'threatened', 'complete', or 'missed' abortion. An ultrasound scan distinguishes between a live and a dead fetus. With threatened abortion a viable pregnancy is confirmed on scan and managed conservatively with a few days of bed rest. In cases of missed abortion there is typically no pain or vaginal bleeding and the diagnosis of a non-viable pregnancy is made on scan. In this situation using the term 'silent miscarriage' is preferable to 'missed abortion' in talking to patients. If the pregnancy is not on-going and less than 12 weeks gestation uterine evacuation by curettage is performed. For second trimester miscarriages induction of delivery using vaginal prostaglandin E_2 is more usual. More recently the traditional method of managing first trimester miscarriage by surgical evacuation of the uterus is being increasingly challenged by medical treatment or even expectant management in selected cases. Sepsis can follow spontaneous or surgically-induced abortions. Blood cultures and vaginal/endocervical microbiological swabs should be taken prior to commencing broad-spectrum antibiotics. After 24 h of antibiotic cover an evacuation of the uterus by curettage is advisable if any retained products of conception are visible on scan.

After any pregnancy loss the two principal questions which patients have are: 'why did it happen?' and 'will it

---

Ectopic pregnancy

- Amenorrhoea
- Lower abdominal pain
- Vaginal bleeding
- Shoulder-tip pain
- Positive urinary HCG
- Ultrasound/empty uterus
- Laparoscopy/diagnosis and treatment

happen again?'. It is important to convey that in over two-thirds of early pregnancy losses a basic defect is present and the pregnancy would not be healthy were it to carry on. In terms of future pregnancies, it should be emphasized that miscarriage tends to be a sporadic event and that, while a small number of women do suffer recurrent abortions, over 85% will go on to have a normal pregnancy following a miscarriage.

Pelvic pain

Vulval and lower vaginal pain is carried by the somatic pudendal nerves (S2,3,4), and hence, is well localized. However, the pain from pelvic viscera is poorly localized because it is transmitted by the autonomic nervous system (uterine T10,L1). In differentiating between likely causes of pain enquiry should be made regarding the onset of the pain (acute/gradual), and its characteristics (site, severity, relation to menses and coitus, and associated symptoms such as vaginal bleeding). Sudden onset of sharp pain may suggest ovarian cyst rupture, torsion, or bleed. Protracted pain is more in keeping with pelvic inflammation or a neoplastic process. Backache may accompany gynaecological disease, but is more frequently musculoskeletal, especially in the absence of other gynaecological symptoms.

Acute pelvic pain

Menstrual pain
Primary dysmenorrhoea, which is usually crampy in nature and of varying severity, is related to the production of prostaglandins. It characteristically occurs in teenagers at the start of a period. Prostaglandin synthetase inhibitors such as mefenamic acid and the combined contraceptive pill provide relief. A 'congestive'-type secondary dysmenorrhoea with a more constant aching pain occurs in mid-late reproductive years in association with endometriosis, chronic pelvic inflammatory disease, or pelvic venous congestion.

Ovulation pain/mittelschmerz
Midcycle pain lasting up to 2 days can occur at the time of ovulation caused by the ruptured follicle releasing prostaglandins and a small volume of extravasated blood which irritates the peritoneal lining.

> **Acute pelvic pain**
> - Menstruation
> - Ovulation
> - Ovarian cyst — Torsion / Rupture / Bleed
> - Pelvic inflammatory disease

Ovarian cyst complications
Ovarian cysts can undergo torsion, rupture, or bleeding. Benign functional cysts such as follicular or corpus luteal cysts are usually <5 cm in size and resolve spontaneously. Repeat assessment by pelvic examination and ultrasound scan 4 to 6 weeks after diagnosis is advisable, and for growing or persistent cysts laparoscopy is warranted.

Neoplastic ovarian cysts originate from the surface epithelium (80%), germ cells (15%), or gonadal stroma (5%). Mucinous or serous cystadenomata are the commonest types. The most frequent germ cell tumour is the dermoid cyst, which is the commonest pathological ovarian cyst during the reproductive years and is bilateral in 15% of cases. Torsion is particularly characteristic of dermoid cysts and fibromata. Benign ovarian fibromata may present with ascites and a pleural effusion (Meig's syndrome).

Ovarian cancer
Ovarian cancer is usually of epithelial origin and in over 75% of cases presents late with abdominal swelling or discomfort. In such advanced cases surgical debulking of tumour by total abdominal hysterectomy, bilateral salpingo-oophorectomy, and infracolic omentectomy is usually followed by platinum or taxotere-based chemotherapy. The role of pelvic and para-aortic lymphadenectomy is uncertain, and is the subject of a current European multicentre trial. Another trial is addressing whether patients with extensive intra-abdominal disease would be better managed by initial chemotherapy to shrink the tumour and render it more resectable by later surgery.

Ultrasound scanning is invaluable in defining the likely benign or malignant nature of ovarian cysts based on the morphology (cyst wall thickness, septation, solidity, surface papillary projections) and the blood flow on colour Doppler imaging.

Serum tumour markers, although non-specific, give additional information: principally the glycoprotein CA125, which is elevated to >35 U/ml in over 85% of clinically apparent ovarian epithelial cancers. Unfortunately, CA125 is only raised in 50% of early ovarian cancers, and many other conditions such as endometriosis or PID can give a small rise in the serum levels. Alphafetoprotein (germ cell tumours) and βHCG (choriocarcinoma) are tumour markers which should be requested in addition to CA125 in young patients with suspicious ovarian cysts on scan.

If a cyst is persistently painful or >5 cm in diameter laparoscopy or laparotomy is necessary. Often cystectomy and ovarian reconstitution are possible, and this should be attempted especially in younger women. In patients over 45 years of age oophorectomy is more usual, often in conjunction with total hysterectomy.

Acute pelvic inflammatory disease (PID)
Usually presents with diffuse lower abdominal and pelvic

pain, accompanied by purulent vaginal discharge and pyrexia. The fact that the pain is in both iliac fossae and associated with cervical excitation on pelvic examination helps to differentiate the condition from an acute appendicitis. Laparoscopy may be required to clinch the diagnosis by seeing hyperaemic uterine tubes, often with surface exudate or even a pyosalpinx.

Chronic pelvic pain

Menstrual

Dysmenorrhoea secondary to pelvic disease is most frequently caused by endometriosis, chronic pelvic inflammatory disease, or pelvic venous congestion. Pelvic tenderness is usual, and laparoscopy provides the definitive diagnosis. Analgesics may help to alleviate symptoms, but frequently pelvic clearance by total abdominal hysterectomy and bilateral salpingo-oophorectomy is necessary in cases of severe pain to provide a cure, especially if the woman's family is complete. *Premenstrual tension* is a syndrome of pelvic discomfort, bloating, breast tenderness, and mood changes preceding periods. Norethisterone 5 mg b.d. or duphaston 10 mg b.d. orally in the second half of the menstrual cycle (days 10–25), pyridoxine 100 mg daily, or evening primrose oil may help. *Haematocolpos* is a condition where menstrual blood accumulates in the vagina due to an obstructed genital tract outlet. Usually a teenager presents with primary amenorrhoea, cyclical pelvic pain, and pelvic or abdominal swelling. An imperforate hymen is often found, or less commonly a transverse vaginal septum or vaginal atresia. Surgical drainage is required.

Non-menstrual

Chronic PID, endometriosis, ovarian cysts, or uterovaginal prolapse can give rise to a chronic pelvic or low back ache throughout the month. Non-gynaecological causes must be borne in mind, including irritable bowel syndrome, diverticulitis, or urinary tract pathology.

Dyspareunia. Pain with intercourse can be felt at the introitus or deeper within the pelvis. Superficial pain results from vaginal conditions such as inflammation or atrophy and vulval disorders such as candidal infection, dystrophy, carcinoma, ulceration, or Bartholin's cyst. Genital ulcers may arise in Behçet's syndrome in association with arthralgia and iritis. Primary herpes simplex causes extremely painful and tender shallow vulval ulcers which may even give rise to urinary retention. After taking viral swabs for culture, saline washes and topical analgesics (lignocaine gel, EMLA cream) should be given as well as oral acyclovir if herpetic vesicles are present for less than 6 days. Referral to a genito-urinary clinic should be arranged. A Bartholin's cyst typically causes swelling of the posterior labium minus, and can be marsupialized by incising the cyst just inside the vaginal introitus and suturing the cyst wall to the vaginal skin. It is best to avoid incising and draining these cysts on the vulval aspect as a troublesome discharge can occur necessitating the wearing of sanitory towels for a protracted period of time. Deep dyspareunia is more commonly associated with endometriosis, chronic pelvic inflammatory disease, or pelvic venous congestion.

Vaginal discharge

The history should include details of the amount, colour, and odour of the discharge and any accompanying symptoms such as vulval irritation, dyspareunia, or vaginal bleeding. An enquiry must be made about genito-urinary symptoms in the patient's partner, any recent sexual contacts, and use of barrier contraception. Examination should begin with careful inspection of the vulva for local lesions such as condylomata accuminata (genital warts). A swab should be taken from any discharge arising from the urethral orifice or Bartholin's ducts. Cusco's bivalve speculum examination allows collection of specimens and visualization of vaginitis/cervicitis which appear as congested red epithelium.

Laboratory evaluation includes
• Wet slide preparation and direct microscopy
• High vaginal swab from the posterior fornix for *Trichomonas vaginalis*, aerobes and anaerobes
• Lateral vaginal wall swab for *Candida* species
• Vaginal pH testing (normal is mildly acidic)
• Urethral and endocervical swabs specifically for *Chlamydia* (in enzyme immuno-assay kit (EIA) kit) and *Gonococcus* (in general transport medium)
• Cervical smear with an Aylesbury spatula

More sensitive chlamydial screening by polymerase chain reaction (PCR) or newer, molecular-based techniques will soon become standard.

Pelvic inflammatory disease (PID)

PID refers principally to salpingitis which has usually ascended from the lower genital tract, and in < 1% of cases

Chronic pelvic pain
• Endometriosis
• Chronic PID
• Pelvic venous congestion
• Non-gynaecological causes

> Most cases of acute PID will resolve with antibiotics and will not require surgery.

may spread locally from adjacent inflamed bowel (diverticulitis or a pelvic appendix) or via the bloodstream. It is little wonder that the Americans describe the condition as 'hot tubes'. In the acute form the uterine tubes become inflamed and oedematous, with exudate and later adhesion formation within and on the surface of the tubes. Pus may accumulate within the tube lumen as a pyosalpinx or loculated in the pelvis as an abscess. In its acute form the patient is clinically toxic with a pyrexia, tachycardia, severe lower abdominal pain and tenderness, a vaginal discharge, and marked pelvic tenderness on vaginal examination. A pelvic mass may be felt, and should be confirmed by ultrasound scan. Lower genital culture swabs should be collected and tetracycline and metronidazole antibiotics commenced intravenously for 48 h or until the pyrexia subsides, together with appropriate analgesics. Oral doxycycline 100 mg b.d. for 2 weeks and metronidazole 400 mg b.d. for 1 week are advisable. A stat dose of ampicillin 3 g with probenicid 1 g are given if swabs are positive for *Gonococcus*. Genito-urinary follow-up is essential for contact tracing, patient education, and test of cure when *Chlamydia* or gonorrhoea have been isolated. Sexual abstinence is mandatory until the partner has been evaluated and treated. The commonest causative organism of PID is *Chlamydia* (at least 60% of cases), and the risk of tubal damage and resulting infertility is high—a 40% risk of tubal occlusion after three episodes of infection. The other common exogenous or sexually acquired cause of PID is *Neisseria gonorrhoeae*. *Mycoplasma hominis* and anaerobes are possible endogenous causative agents present in vaginal flora. Laparoscopy may be necessary to confirm the diagnosis where doubt exists, and surgical drainage of abscesses may be required. Apart from subfertility, other possible sequelae of PID are chronic pelvic inflammation (20%) and a sixfold increased risk of ectopic pregnancy. It is important to emphasize that most cases of acute PID will resolve with antibiotic treatment alone, without recourse to surgery. This contrasts with the majority of general surgical abscesses, where drainage is usually required. Operative gynaecological procedures such as cervical dilatation and curettage, hysterosalpingography, IUCD insertion, and surgical termination of pregnancy carry a risk of ascending infection and iatrogenic PID. This is preventable by screening these women and treating any infection before the surgical procedure. The huge importance of PID in terms of adequate microbiological screening, appropriate therapy, partner notification and treatment, and sexual health education in a genito-urinary medicine clinic setting was recently addressed by guidelines from the Royal College of Obstetricians and Gynaecologists.

Toxic shock syndrome

Toxic shock syndrome is a rare, but potentially fatal, infection where a woman with a tampon in place for a period presents with pyrexia, hypotension, and an erythematous rash. The diagnosis is made by finding any three of the following criteria: profound diarrhoea, hypotension, multi-organ failure, disseminated intravascular coagulation, or neurological changes. The tampon should be removed, vaginal swabs taken for culture, and intravenous flucloxacillin commenced. The usual cause is an exotoxin produced by *Staphylococcus aureus*.

Genital trauma

Blunt trauma from a straddle injury or aggressive sexual activity can result in a vulval haematoma or vaginal laceration. Large haematomata require evacuation under general anaesthesia, while small collections resolve with compression by ice packs. Vaginal lacerations can bleed quite profusely, and often require suturing in theatre. Similar injuries can result from violence: rape, sexual assault, or domestic aggression. In such cases meticulous documentation of injuries sustained, collection of forensic specimens and swabs, and emergency postcoital contraception if pregnancy is a risk are vital aspects of care. A photographic record of lacerations and bruises should be made after obtaining written consent. Ideally these patients should receive attention from a female doctor in a dedicated sexual assault unit. Victims require long-term psychological support, involvement of social services in cases of domestic dispute, and frequently advice on available legal options. Follow-up at a genito-urinary disease clinic should be arranged.

Gynaecological emergency procedures

Resuscitation/management of massive haemorrhage

Extra staff should be summoned, such as anaesthetists, porters, and laboratory personnel. Early involvement of senior staff is important. Blood (20 ml) should be taken for blood grouping, crossmatching of 4–6 units of blood, and a coagulation profile and full blood count. Generally, haemaccel colloid solution is infused while awaiting type-specific red cell concentrate (usually about 20 min). Only if immediate transfusion is required should uncrossmatched Group O RhD negative blood be used. Abnormal platelet counts or coagulation studies dictate the necessity for replacement therapy (i.e. fresh frozen plasma (FFP) or platelet concentrates). Vascular lines to be set up include: two peripheral 14 gauge cannulae, a central venous pressure monitor via an internal jugular or subclavian line, and an arterial line to record blood pressure and allow serial blood assays. A urinary catheter with an hourly filling chamber should be inserted. Compression cuffs aid the rapid administration of fluids intravenously. Blood must be given through blood warming equipment. Monitoring of pulse rate, blood pressure, central venous pressure (CVP), blood gases, acid–base status, and urinary output in an intensive care setting is optimal.

Laparoscopy

Since the initial description of celioscopy by Kelling in 1902 the procedure has been widely accepted for diagnosis and treatment by gynaecologists, urologists, and general surgeons. The recent trend toward minimal access techniques in all surgical fields has led to a considerably expanded role for laparoscopy in both emergency and elective settings. Laparoscopy carries a relatively low operative mortality of 1.8 per 100 000 procedures, and an operative morbidity of 0.6–2.5%, related chiefly to modes of access, the pneumoperitoneum created, and anaesthetic problems. As more difficult surgical procedures are tackled laparoscopically there has been a corresponding increase in iatrogenic injuries caused by either trocar placement, dissection techniques, or various suturing or stapling devices. The guidelines issued by the working party of the Royal College of Obstetricians and Gynaecologists in June 1994 relating to endoscopic surgery was a welcome dictat. A structured, supervised/proctored training programme is essential to ensure that advanced laparoscopic techniques are only practised by adequately accredited surgeons. Even among experienced laparoscopists the incidence of laparotomy for complications ranges from 1 in 2000 for minor laparoscopic procedures to approximately 1 in 120 for major procedures such as extensive pelvic adhesiolysis. This small, but definite, risk of laparotomy should be mentioned to patients prior to surgery, as they commonly regard endoscopy and 'key-hole' surgery as minor, no-risk procedures.

Principles of trocar placement/minimizing trauma

The patient is paced in a Trendelenburg position after emptying the bladder. The abdominal wall should be elevated and the Veress insufflation needle inserted subumbilically at an angle of 45° without any lateral deviation in order to reduce the risk of injury to major blood vessels. A 2-ml syringe of saline should be attached to the Veress needle and aspirated to exclude vessel trauma. The 2 ml of saline is then injected and if it returns on re-aspiration is suggestive of loculation of the saline within the anterior abdominal wall and consequently that the peritoneal cavity has not been reached. Finally a drop of saline is left to rest on the Veress needle and should be drawn into the peritoneal cavity on elevating the anterior abdominal wall ('hanging drop test'; Fig. 32.1). These simple measures help to confirm correct

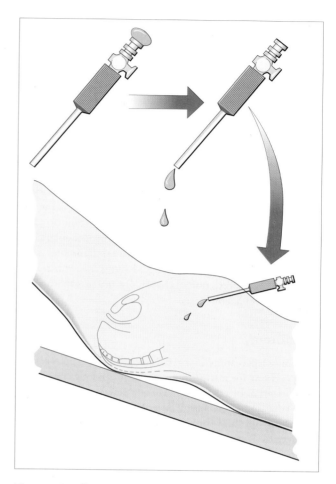

Fig. 32.1 Insufflation needle insertion—the hanging drop test.

intra-peritoneal placement of the insufflation needle. Alternative sites of Veress needle insertion are midline suprapubically, or in the left upper quadrant just below the subcostal margin in the midclavicular line. The subcostal placement of both insufflation needle and indeed laparoscopic viewing port is particularly useful in patients with lower midline surgical scars. A 3-L pneumoperitoneum is usually adequate to ensure safe placement of the subumbilical trocar. This trocar should be rotated during insertion and again directed in the midline.

Open trocar placement is used by many surgeons during laparoscopy to avoid some of the potential complications of Veress needle and sharp trocar insertion. Peritoneal cutdown and trocar insertion under direct vision has been found to be safer than blind insertion of the Veress needle and primary trocar. The open access technique carries less risk of serious visceral or vascular complications than a blind approach, and is particularly useful in patients with previous lower mid-line scars. However, bowel injury can also rarely occur in the open technique of laparoscopic cannula placement.

Abdominal wall blood vessels can be injured during placement of accessory ports for laparoscopic surgery. The inferior epigastric, superficial epigastric, and superficial circumflex iliac arteries are most at risk. The vascular anatomy is somewhat variable, but not apparently influenced by obesity. Transilluminating the anterior abdominal wall from within may help to define these superficial vessels, but if landmarks are not visible then lateral trocars should be placed approximately 8 cm from the midline and at least 5 cm above the symphysis pubis to minimize the risk of vessel injury. If an anterior abdominal wall vessel is hit by a trocar, it can be recognized internally by persistant dripping of blood from the port site. Often, diathermy coagulation of the parietal peritoneum, cranial and caudal to the site, is sufficient to control the haemorrhage. Failing this, suture ligatures can be placed transabdominally under laparoscopic vision to effect haemostasis.

Laparotomy

Generally laparotomy in a gynaecological emergency setting is carried out for a ruptured ectopic pregnancy, an ovarian cyst torsion or bleed, or drainage of a pelvic abscess. A transverse suprapubic incision is prefered in most cases for cosmetic reasons and because of a lower risk of wound dehiscence. If access proves difficult during the operation it can be improved by incising the medial one third of the rectus abdominis muscle on either side, or dividing the muscles in their full width after ligating the inferior epigastric vessels (Maylard), or by dividing the aponeurosis of the recti 0.5 cm above the pubic symphysis (DeCherney). Where more extensive exposure is necessary from the outset, e.g. with a pelvi-abdominal mass, a vertical midline incision is recommended. In patients with an uncertain diagnosis or if ovarian malignancy is a possibility, the surgeon should not hesitate to use a midline approach. For people with significant pathology cosmesis is not a consideration. Rectus sheath closure is generally with No 1 Vicryl, although Maxon and Prolene have become popular for full thickness closure of vertical incisions. Prophylactic peri-operative antibiotics are suggested for cases of pelvic infection, uterine or visceral perforation, and whenever the vaginal vault is opened as in total hysterectomy.

General surgical problems for the gynaecologist

Surgical emergencies can arise during a planned elective procedure as a result of trauma to adjacent vessels or viscera. Early recognition and repair of such iatrogenic injuries yields the best results. Even experienced gynaecologists must know their limitations in dealing with vascular, urological,

and intestinal damage. In the litigous climate of today and in order to produce the optimal repair, it is prudent to call on the assistance of a specialist colleague as soon as significant trauma is noticed. Certain injuries may fall within the realm of the gynaecologist's own surgical experience, and these can be adequately dealt with alone. If a surgical complication should arise the patient must be made aware of the events in the early post-operative period and afforded the opportunity to ask questions.

Uterine perforation

The uterine fundus is the usual site of perforation, and the softer uterus of early pregnancy is easier to puncture with instruments at the time of uterine curettage following a miscarriage. The uterine sound, Hegar's cervical dilators, polyp forceps, or endometrial curettes can perforate the uterus and, in the case of forceps or curette especially, damage the adjacent bowel lying in the pelvis. With the advent of hysteroscopy and endometrial ablation/resection a further set of instruments entering the uterine cavity can occasionally also enter the peritoneal cavity by mistake. Uterine perforation is the most frequent complication of hysteroscopy, occurring at a rate of 13 per 1000 procedures. Generally, if a blunt instrument such as a uterine sound, cervical dilator, or diagnostic hysteroscope breaches the uterus the procedure should be abandoned and the patient closely observed on the ward for a period of 24–48 h. The development of signs of peritonism or significant haemorrhage merits laparotomy. A broad-spectrum intravenous antibiotic in a single or triple dose is advisable. A thorough explanation of events should be given to the patient. If a sharp instrument such as a curette or polyp forceps punctures the uterus a laparoscopy is required to rule out visceral damage in the pelvis. In cases where a resectoscope or endometrial ablation technique is being used a thermal injury to bowel may be missed by laparoscopy, and an exploratory laparotomy is essential.

Bowel injury

Gynaecological surgery for cancer, severe pelvic infection, or advanced endometriosis are most likely to involve bowel adhesions to pelvic organs. Serosal damage can be easily reconstituted using interrupted 2/0 catgut or Vicryl sutures. An obstructed or devitalized segment of bowel requires

Potential injuries
• Uterine perforation
• Colon/small bowel perforation
• Ureteric/bladder trauma
• Major vessel trauma

resection and end-to-end anastomosis. Where necessary, the assistance of a general surgical colleague should be sought. A nasogastric tube ought to be passed by the anaesthetist and the position checked by the surgeon just prior to closure. Intestinal injury associated with laparoscopic surgery can result from instrument insertion or operative dissection. Insufflation needle injuries to bowel are usually self-limiting and require no specific treatment. Bowel damage associated with trocar insertion or operative dissection require direct suture repair. For colonic injury primary repair seems as good as defunctioning colostomy in terms of mortality and infectious morbidity and is the preferred method of treatment. Irrigation of the peritoneal cavity reduces contamination and broad-spectrum, short duration, intravenous antibiotics to cover principally coliforms and *Bacteroides* are advisable, e.g. cephradine 500 mg q.d.s. and metronidazole 500 mg t.d.s. Drains are not generally required as their use has been associated with increased infectious morbidity. If the wound is contaminated to any significant degree it may be left open to heal by secondary intention, or a delayed primary closure may be carried out if there is no evidence of infection. As laparoscopic skills advance and endoscopic stapling and suture techniques are perfected, it should be possible to manage many such injuries without needing to convert to laparotomy.

Urological trauma

The most important risk factors for urological injuries during gynaecological procedures are infiltrating cervical or ovarian carcinoma and pelvic adhesions. If the bladder is holed it can be oversewn with a double layer of 2/0 catgut or Vicryl, and an indwelling urinary catheter left in for 5 days postoperatively. A ureteric injury should be repaired with the assistance of a urology colleague as procedures such as tunnelled re-insertion of a ureter or construction of a Boari flap are outside the realm of most gynaecologists. Identifying and isolating the ureter extraperitoneally during difficult pelvic operations decreases the incidence of injury. For laparoscopic work in the region of the ureters identification can be aided by initially cannulating the ureters with illuminated stents via the cystoscope. End-to-end anastomosis of the transected ureter at the time of injury achieves better results than delayed diagnosis and treatment. In the hands of expert laparoscopists it may be possible to repair a damaged ureter endoscopically without recourse to laparotomy. Traditionally delayed repair of vesicovaginal fistulae has been the standard approach to posthysterectomy bladder injury. However, early repair also achieves a high rate of primary healing.

Vascular injury

Major vessel injury can occur while dissecting pelvic and

para-aortic lymph nodes or during insertion of laparoscopic insufflation needles or trocars. To date 24 cases of major vessel damage following laparoscopic procedures have been reported in the literature. Characteristically the terminal aorta, inferior vena cava, and iliac vessels are involved. Most injuries were sutured directly, and with immediate recognition recovery was the rule. Once a large vessel tear is noticed immediate conversion to an open procedure is essential, unless an endoclip can be swiftly applied after securing the vessel wall with a grasping forceps. The tear can be repaired at laparotomy with a running 4/0 Prolene suture. Occasionally, prosthetic bypass grafts may be necessary to restore vascular continuity.

Gynaecological surgical problems for the general surgeon

Surgery in the pregnant patient

Any woman who is sexually active and unsure of her last menstrual period, or whose last menstrual period (LMP) is more than 4 weeks prior to admission, should have a pregnancy test performed prior to surgery. Elective procedures should be postponed until at least 6 weeks after delivery. Semi-elective surgery, such as ovarian cystectomy, is best carried out during the second trimester of pregnancy when the risk of miscarriage is less than in the first 13 weeks and yet the gravid uterus is not too large to impede access. The first 13 weeks of pregnancy are avoided because of the small but definite risk of miscarriage, and the theoretical teratogenic risk of anaesthetic and analgesic agents used during the period of embryo organogenesis (primarily the initial 56 days following conception). For patients whose pregnancy has advanced beyond 24 weeks gestation the fetal well-being can be monitored peri-operatively by recording the fetal heart rate using a Doppler probe. The normal fetal heart rate is between 120–160 beats/min in the last trimester. An obstetric opinion should be sought prior to any elective surgery on a pregnant patient, and because of the additional thrombo-embolic risk of the pregnancy itself it is wise to use compression stockings and to encourage early mobilization following their surgery. If a gravid uterus is encountered unexpectedly during a laparotomy it should be disturbed as little as possible, and a pelvic ultrasound can be ordered postoperatively.

Ectopic pregnancy

If a bleeding ectopic pregnancy is encountered by a general surgeon the safest and the standard approach is salpingectomy. The ipsilateral ovary is preserved, except in the rare cases of ruptured ovarian ectopic. If an unruptured ectopic pregnancy is discovered it may be possible to preserve the involved uterine tube by milking a distal ectopic from the

> **Considerations for general surgeon**
>
> - ?Need for pregnancy test
> - Elective procedures postparturition
> - Semiurgent procedures in second trimester
> - Salpingectomy for ruptured ectopic
> - Ovarian preservation where possible

end of the tube, or by a linear incision along the antimesenteric border of the tube (salpingostomy). In such cases where there is no significant haemorrhage a gynaecological opinion can be sought if the involved surgeon is unsure about the optimal management or unskilled in laparoscopic salpingectomy/salpingostomy.

Ovarian pathology

When a general surgeon incidentally encounters an ovarian cyst of < 5 cm in diameter in a woman of reproductive age it should generally be left alone, unless torsion or bleeding have occurred or there are suspicious surface features on the cyst, such as abnormal vascularity or papillary growths. Cysts of > 6 cm in size should be shelled out by incising the ovarian capsule and using a small gauze swab to dissect the cyst free. The ovarian tissue can be reconstituted using a fine internal purse-string suture of 4/0 Prolene. It is important to visualize and document that the other ovary is healthy. In the postmenopausal woman an ovarian cyst can be dealt with by oophorectomy, but if suspicious of carcinoma a gynaecological colleague should be contacted. A bleeding ovarian follicle or ruptured corpus luteum, which may be found in a young woman presenting with acute lower abdominal pain, is simply diathermied or oversewn.

Tubo-ovarian abscess

If a pelvic abscess is encountered by a general surgeon the pus should be drained and loculi broken down digitally, followed by the usual peritoneal toilet using antiseptic or antibiotic wash-out. As with any infective focus, microbiological swabs of the pus are sent for culture. It must be remembered that, unlike many general surgical abscesses, there is no perforated viscus and no need to resect tissue even though the patient may be extremely toxic and the pelvic contents indurated. Tetracycline and metronidazole antibiotics intravenously in the postoperative period are recommended.

Sequelae of surgical termination of pregnancy

Approximately 165 000 legal abortions are carried out annually in the UK. Modern techniques of vacuum aspiration, including priming agents which facilitate cervical dilatation, have contributed to the overall safety and efficacy of this method so that major morbidity occurs in < 1% of cases, and the complete abortion rate approaches 98%. Medical abortion in the first 9 weeks of pregnancy using the antiprogestin mifepristone (RU486) with a suitable prostaglandin analogue has been shown to be an effective, safe, and acceptable alternative and is likely to be more widely adopted in the future. Complications resulting from uterine curettage can be categorized as being either immediate or delayed.

Immediate complications

These include haemorrhage and uterine perforation. Postabortal haemorrhage may result from cervical laceration, uterine perforation, or uterine atony. A perforation in the uterine fundus may go undetected as there is likely to be minimal bleeding, whereas a lateral uterine perforation may lacerate uterine blood vessels, resulting in immediate and profuse haemorrhage. In addition, a broad ligament haematoma may also develop as a delayed complication manifest by diffuse lower abdominal pain, pelvic mass, or maternal fever.

The evaluation of a patient in whom uterine perforation is suspected depends on the presenting symptoms and the instruments used at the time of suspected perforation. If the perforation occurred before the application of suction curettage, the patient should be observed for 24 h for signs of haemorrhage, characterized by either profuse bleeding per vagina, change in vital signs (tachycardia, hypotension), or the development of a broad ligament haematoma. If the potential perforation occurred after the application of suction curettage exploration is usually warranted, by laparoscopy if the patient is stable or by laparotomy if dictated by more severe symptoms or signs.

Immediate postoperative pain without overt bleeding via the vagina may indicate development of haematometra as the uterus distends with trapped blood. The onset is usually within the first hour after completion of the procedure, and pelvic examination reveals a large globular uterus that is tense and tender. Treatment requires immediate uterine evacuation and ergometrine 500 μg i.m. to maintain tissue contraction.

Delayed complications

These are defined as complications occuring more than 72 h after the procedure. They occur in approximately 1% of cases and include fever, haemorrhage, and retained products of conception. The latter may present as postabortal bleeding, fever, midline pelvic mass, or pelvi-abdominal pain, and if retained products are confirmed on pelvic ultrasound a repeat curettage is advisable. If no products are present on the uterine scan the likely diagnosis is endometritis, and oral doxycycline 100 mg b.d. for 2 weeks with metronidazole 400 mg b.d. for 1 week should be prescribed after taking the relevant high vaginal, endocervical, and urethral swabs. PID has been reported in up to 13% of women following first trimester termination of pregnancy. Partners must be seen and treated at a genito-urinary medicine clinic to prevent reinfection.

Further reading

HMSO (1996) *Triennial Report on Maternal Mortalities 1991–1993.* HMSO, London.

Nordestgaard, A.G., Bodily, K.C., Osborne, R.W. & Buttorff, J.D. (1995) Major vascular injuries during laparoscopic procedures. *American Journal of Surgery* **169** 543–545.

Penfield, A.J. (1977) Trocar and needle injury. In: *Laparoscopy.* (ed. J.M. Phillips), pp. 236–241. Williams and Wilkins, Baltimore.

Querleu, D., Chapron, C., Chevallier, L. & Bruhat, M.A. (1993) Complications of gynaecologic laparoscopic surgery — a French multicenter collaborative study (letter). *New England Journal of Medicine* **328**(18) 1355.

Stevens, L. & Kenney, A. (1994) *Emergencies in Obstetrics and Gynaecology.* Oxford University Press, Oxford.

Templeton, A. (ed.) *The Prevention of Pelvic Infection.* RCOG Press, London.

CHAPTER 33

The acute abdomen in pregnancy

Colm O'Herlihy

Introduction

When it is realized that virtually every pregnancy ends with abdominal pain, whether associated with labour or abortion or ectopic pregnancy, it is not surprising that this symptom very commonly prompts pregnant women to seek medical advice. In most instances, the problem is not serious or is easily explained, but if the onset of pain is sudden, severe or associated with other symptoms, such as nausea and vomiting, the patient may often present out of hours in a non-obstetric setting and may pose urgent diagnostic questions. As a general rule, the worse the woman's general condition, the more difficult is this differential diagnosis.

Added to a woman's understandable concern as to the cause of her acute abdominal discomfort, is the additional fear that it may predispose to loss of, or damage to, her pregnancy. Whenever possible, reassurance should be provided in this regard but, of course, only when the cause has been ascertained with reasonable certainty. With more serious conditions, diagnostic delay undoubtedly increases the risk of pregnancy loss. It is, therefore, most important to emphasize the imperative of reaching an early, accurate diagnosis based on an understanding of the likely pathology, a reliable clinical assessment and a modicum of readily and rapidly available investigations.

It is a truism, but important nonetheless, that the possibility of pregnancy should always be considered in any female presenting during her reproductive years, even if she is herself hitherto unaware of conception. Once the possibility of co-existent pregnancy has been raised, consultation with obstetric colleagues will usually accelerate the diagnostic process. Similarly, the relatively younger age group of the obstetric population makes some potential non-obstetric causes of abdominal pain, such as diverticular disease, very unlikely, while others, like appendicitis, are not uncommon. A history of abdominal or general disorders antedating pregnancy should always be sought, even when an obstetric cause seems likely.

Abdominal pain in early pregnancy

The principal causes of acute abdominal pain during the first trimester, together with their approximate respective incidences during pregnancy, are listed in Tables 33.1 & 33.2. The division between early and later pregnancy is most practically adopted at about 14 weeks' gestation, when the uterus becomes easily palpable in the suprapubic area. During the first trimester problems chiefly arise in the pelvic organs, urinary or gastrointestinal tracts. Differentiation between potentially serious disorders, which may require early surgical intervention, and less important ones, such as irritable bowel syndrome, will be aided by the identification of specific clinical clues at the initial examination.

In addition to abdominal palpation, bimanual pelvic examination is a mandatory component of the diagnostic process. This can provide invaluable information on (i) uterine enlargement and position; (ii) adnexal swellings or tenderness; and (iii) 'excitation' discomfort when the cervix is moved gently from side to side. Care should be taken when palpating the adnexa if ectopic pregnancy is suspected, because anything more than gentle examination may precipitate tubal rupture and sudden intraperitoneal haemorrhage and collapse.

A simple protocol of investigation is outlined in Table 33.3. Anaemia may be a feature of incomplete abortion or ectopic pregnancy, while examination of a blood film may identify a rare sickling crisis. Although the white cell count increases physiologically in pregnancy, values in excess of 18 × 10^9/L indicate a leucocytosis consistent with acute appendicitis, pyolonephritis or ovarian torsion. Direct urinary microscopy may immediately identify bacteriuria or haematuria, prior to the inevitable delay while awaiting culture of any pathogenic organisms present. The excess vomiting of hyperemesis gravidarum may lead to considerable electrolyte disturbance prior to clinical presentation with epigastric pain in a minority of cases. Modern urinary pregnancy tests are highly specific for human chorionic gonadotrophin (HCG), are sensitive enough to provide a positive result soon after conception and are very easily performed. They can prove invaluable in the assessment of abdominal pain associated with little, if any, delay in menstruation, as might be found in early ectopic pregnancy. In combination with an absent intrauterine gestation sac on ultrasound examination, a positive HCG result is strongly suggestive of tubal

Table 33.1 Acute abdominal pain in early pregnancy: pregnancy-related conditions.

		Incidence in pregnancy	Clinical clues
Common	1 Spontaneous abortion	1:5–7	Vaginal bleeding/uterus enlarged
	2 Ectopic pregnancy	1:100–300	Vaginal bleeding/cervical excitation/peritonism /adnexal mass
	3 Torsion/bleeding/ovarian cyst	1:2000	Adnexal mass/no vaginal bleeding
	4 Acute urinary retention	1:1000	At 12–14 weeks, distorted/retroverted uterus
	5 Hyperemesis gravidarium	1:200	Excess vomiting → oesophageal tears
Uncommon	Angular pregnancy		
	Rupture rudimentary uterine horn		Vaginal bleeding, septic abortion
	Pelvic infection		

Table 33.2 Acute abdominal pain in early pregnancy: incidental abdominal disorders.

		Incidence in pregnancy	Clinical clues
Common	Appendicitis	1:2000	Associated vomiting, no vaginal bleeding, peritonism
	Urinary infection	1:100	Dysuria/loin pain, right-sided preponderance.
	Urolithiasis	1:1500	Colicky/antecedent history
	Irritable bowel syndrome	1:200	Antecedent history, iliac fossa tenderness
Uncommon	Peptic ulcer		Antecedent history/dyspepsia
	Inflammatory bowel disease		Antecedent history/diarrhoea
	Sickle cell crisis		Antecedent history/homozygous SS,SC
	Porphyria		Dark urine on standing

Table 33.3 Acute abdomen in pregnancy: suggested investigative protocol.

Investigation	Significance
1 FBC, including white cell differential, platelets	Infection, porphyria, haematuria
2 Urine analysis—culture, microscopy, inspection	?Intrauterine, ?continuing gestation, ?extrauterine/ adnexal swelling/cyst
3 Ultrasound examination of pelvis	?Free peritoneal fluid behind uterus
	Early pregnancy pain
4 Urinary pregnancy test	
5 Urea/electrolytes	
6 Serum amylase/liver function tests	

pregnancy and mandates further investigation, such as laparoscopy.

The increased sophistication and ease of usage of modern ultrasound apparatus has greatly improved the speed and facility of accurate diagnosis in early pregnancy. Transvaginal probes offer superior imaging to abdominal transducers before the uterus becomes palpable suprapubically and obviate the need for a full bladder. Transabdominal scanners can, however, provide very useful data in cases of abdominal pain or bleeding during the first trimester. In any event, early access to skilled pelvic ultrasound examination is essential in confirming the continuing well-being of any early pregnancy, whether pain is a feature or not.

Pregnancy-related disorders

Spontaneous abortion

Because it is an indicator of imminent or actual expulsion of the intra-uterine contents, pain usually only becomes a feature of abortion once miscarriage is inevitable, when it will have been preceded by an interval of amenorrhoea and vaginal bleeding. Vaginal examination may then reveal tissue dilating the cervical os or already expelled from the uterus. Ectopic pregnancy co-exists with intra-uterine gestations only very rarely (except perhaps following *in-vitro* fertilization) and so can be virtually discounted once products of conception have been passed vaginally. Spontaneous abortion is often complete before 7 and after 14 weeks' gestation, but if it occurs in the intervening period, evacuation of the uterus either surgically or more recently using antiprogestogens, will usually be required.

Ectopic pregnancy

Extrauterine pregnancy remains a potential cause of maternal death, because of intraperitoneal bleeding when its diagnosis is delayed; its exclusion must be a primary objective in any woman presenting with abdominal pain at an early gestation. An adnexal gestation sac is not always visualized on ultrasound scanning but the presence of an empty uterus, combined with a positive pregnancy test, usually requires laparoscopic examination of the pelvis to exclude ectopic pregnancy. In contrast to spontaneous abortion, symptoms in ectopic pregnancies usually follow the sequence: amenorrhoea, then pain, followed by vaginal bleeding (often scanty); fainting and shoulder-tip pain, secondary to intraperitoneal bleeding, are other potential features but some women may remain remarkably well up to 12 weeks' gestation, despite the development of an increasing pelvic haematocoele. Laparoscopic surgical management is now preferred, especially for early and unruptured cases, where tubal conservation is usually possible but massive haemorrhage following tubal rupture may only be dealt with by laparotomy and salpingectomy.

Abdominal pain	Exclude
Positive pregnancy test	ectopic
Empty uterus (on U/S)	pregnancy

Ovarian torsion

Torsion of the ovary (also involving the adjacent fallopian tube) usually occurs when it is cystically enlarged. This is usually caused by a corpus luteum or benign cystic teratoma (dermoid) and is much commoner in early pregnancy, because of the rapidly altering intrapelvic anatomical relationships secondary to the enlarging uterus. The resulting pain is usually colicky at first but may become constant with time as ovarian ischaemia progresses. A tender lower abdominal or adnexal mass is palpable and can be confirmed with ultrasound, which may also reveal retro-uterine intraperitoneal fluid. The differential diagnosis from ectopic pregnancy prior to laparoscopy or laparotomy can thus be very difficult, although leucocytosis in subacute cases is more suggestive of ovarian torsion. At operation, the tube and ovary, if healthy, may be untwisted and conserved, permitting cystectomy alone, but should be removed if ischaemic signs persist after relocation. It is essential to provide appropriate progesterone supplementation until 12 weeks' gestation to prevent abortion if a corpus luteum cyst is excised before that gestation.

Acute urinary retention

Anterior displacement of the cervix so that it protrudes into the bladder base may occur secondary to acute retroversion or distortion of the uterus due to leiomyomata (fibroids). As the uterus enlarges to fill the pelvic brim at about 12 weeks, the cervix may obstruct urinary outflow causing retention. The bladder becomes massively distended causing acute abdominal discomfort and vaginal examination reveals the cervix protruding into the anterior fornix. Continuous catheter drainage is required for some days but the problem is self-limiting once the uterus enlarges through the pelvic brim to become an abdominal organ early in the second trimester.

Hyperemesis gravidarum

Excess nausea and vomiting are well-recognized features of a large minority of otherwise normal gestations. The symptoms are usually self-limiting by about 14 weeks' gestation but if vomiting is particularly frequent, oesophageal tears and cramping of the anterior abdominal musculature may sometimes occur. The symptom complex is readily recognizable, especially if mild haematemesis coexists and management is aimed at symptomatic relief, combined with correction of any fluid and electrolyte imbalance.

Uncommon first trimester disorders

Unusual obstetric causes of early abdominal pain include *pregnancy in a rudimentary uterine horn* and *angular pregnancy* which can be considered, in practice, as variants of ectopic gestation. Both are likely to cause marked uterine tenderness and cervical excitation, with associated scanty vaginal bleeding; if undiagnosed, the uterine wall may rupture during the middle trimester, leading to massive intraperitoneal bleeding and collapse. Following diagnosis, (often via the laparoscope), and resuscitation, surgical excision and repair of the damaged segment is usually possible.

In the absence of septic abortion, *pelvic inflammatory disease* (PID) is most unusual in pregnancy, because ascending infection is generally blocked by the presence of an intact intrauterine gestation sac. Salpingitis may rarely antedate conception and cause local pain and tenderness, sometimes extending to peritonism, pyrexia and generalized symptoms. The latter manifestations help differentiate acute PID from ectopic pregnancy, which may otherwise prove to be clinically very difficult.

Extrapelvic non-reproductive disorders in early pregnancy

Acute appendicitis

Appendicitis is the most common surgical emergency encountered during pregnancy, although its incidence, at 1 : 2000, is no greater than in non-pregnant women. The inci-

> Displacement of the appendix during later pregnancy often delays the diagnosis.

dence is probably constant throughout gestation but diagnosis is relatively easier and earlier during the first trimester because the location of the appendix, and thus the site of maximal tenderness, remains anatomically similar to prepregnancy. Appendicitis is no more fulminant in pregnancy but the upward and lateral migration of the appendix after 12 weeks' gestation, as it is progressively displaced by the enlarging uterus, frequently leads to a degree of diagnostic delay which increases the incidence of complications and, indeed, mortality from the condition, especially in the third trimester.

In early pregnancy, despite the frequency of nausea and vomiting, the classic clinical presenting sequence of periumbilical pain shifting to the right iliac fossa and culminating in persistent guarding and tenderness with peritonism localized to McBurney's point, is rarely ignored for long. Despite the relative leucocytosis of pregnancy, a white cell count exceeding 18×10^9/L is corroborative and should support surgical intervention. Early, localized disease and prompt appendicectomy carry minimal risks to the continuing pregnancy; general anaesthesia does not pose any demonstrable teratogenic jeopardy. Peritonitis, however, leads to a high incidence of abortion and premature labour. The commonest differential diagnoses in early pregnancy include: (i) urinary infection or calculus, which can usually be discounted following negative urine analysis and microscopy; or (ii) ovarian torsion, where the offending ovarian cyst is usually readily visible on transabdominal or especially, transvaginal ultrasound.

Urinary tract infection and stones

Because of a combination of progesterone-induced laxity of the urinary tract, together with anatomical compression of the ureters in later pregnancy, bacterial urinary infection is much commoner in pregnant than non-pregnant women. A previous history of clinical infection or asymptomatic bacteriuria is frequently elicited. In the absence of acute retention, symptoms may be vague and poorly localized when only the lower urinary tract is involved, as is usually the case in early pregnancy. It is only with progressive ureteric compression, secondary to uterine enlargement into the abdomen, that the frequency of typical pyelonephritis increases. Midstream urine microscopy and culture, should, therefore, be part of every assessment of abdominal pain in pregnancy even in the absence of localizing signs. Gradual dextrorotation of the uterus causes a preponderance of right-sided upper urinary infection and symptoms as gestation advances.

Urinary calculi cause symptoms more often in women who have a prepregnancy history of stone or pelvi-ureteric obstruction. Stones become more mobile as a result of relaxation of ureteric muscle and are usually passed spontaneously without the need for surgical intervention. Diagnostic features include the typical colicky characteristic and location and radiation of the pain which, unlike upper urinary infection, is just as likely to be felt on the left as the right side, and the invariable finding of haematuria. Plain abdominal radiography is best avoided until 12 weeks' gestation but may be useful thereafter.

Irritable bowel syndrome

Recurrent abdominal pain caused by spastic colon is common in women of reproductive age, whether pregnant or not, and recurrences sometimes cause an acute discomfort in one or other iliac fossae, associated with a palpable tender colon at the site. Episodes are less common as pregnancy advances because of the smooth muscle-relaxant effect of progesterone and have invariably been preceded by similar symptoms before conception in affected individuals. The general absence of other symptoms or signs usually points to the diagnosis but severe spasm may necessitate a period of observation before pathological intra-abdominal disorders can be excluded.

Other non-gestational conditions

Several other rare but serious conditions may occasionally require consideration in the pregnant woman with acute abdominal symptoms. Like peptic ulcer, *inflammatory bowel disorders* (IBD) such as Crohn's disease and ulcerative colitis almost never present for the first time in pregnant women; in exacerbations, symptoms of altered bowel habit provide the necessary diagnostic clues and medical treatment is not significantly affected by pregnancy, although the fetal loss rate is high. Women who have previously undergone bowel resection are at a markedly increased risk of developing *bowel obstruction* as pregnancy progresses. Puerperal relapses are not uncommon in IBD.

Acute intermittent *porphyria* can be precipitated for the first time by pregnancy, when abdominal pain co-exists with autonomic and psychiatric symptoms; associated labile hypertension, fever and leucocytosis may cause confusion but darkening of the standing urine sample is diagnostic. With supportive fluid, electrolyte and analgesic therapy in the acute phase, the prognosis is quite good; causative drugs, including ergometrine and anaesthetic agents, should thereafter be strictly avoided.

Abdominal pain crises may be a feature of *homozygous sickle cell disease* (SS, SC) which are often precipitated by infection. The patient is almost always aware of her haemoglobinopathy and the fetal prognosis is generally poor.

Key points in assessment of early abdominal pain
• Always specifically confirm/exclude pregnancy in women of menstrual age. • Pelvic examination is mandatory to evaluate, e.g. uterine enlargement, cervical excitation, adnexal swelling. • Always enquire about previous abdominal disorders or surgery. • Ultrasound examination of the uterus and pelvis can prove invaluable.

Acute abdominal pain in later pregnancy

Once gestation has progressed into the second trimester and the uterus becomes palpable above the pelvic brim, many disorders which require consideration before 14 weeks can be virtually discounted. Some which have been already discussed can still enter the differential diagnosis of abdominal pain; ovarian cysts may tort and intra-uterine pregnancy may abort, but much less frequently, while the incidences of appendicitis and urinary tract infection do not diminish. Causative conditions are best considered under three categories: (i) those directly related to the advancing pregnancy; (ii) those involving the uterus, ovaries or abdominal wall; and (iii) those incidental diseases which occur with varying frequency (Table 33.4).

In attempting to differentiate major complications of pregnancy from incidental abdominal conditions presenting in later pregnancy, *Alder's sign* may be very helpful. This is elicited by first localizing the site of tenderness while the patient lies supine and then turning her onto her left side while keeping the examining hand in position; if the pain and/or tenderness shift to the left, the cause is probably arising from the uterus or its adnexa but if the location remains unchanged, an extragenital source, such as appendicitis, should be suspected.

Pregnancy-related conditions

Painful uterine contractions

Uterine contractions can begin at any time and herald the onset of abortion or labour, either premature or at term. These pains are periodic and associated with palpable tightening of the uterine muscle, lasting less than a minute in duration. Pelvic examination may reveal effacement or dilatation of the cervix but it is worth remembering that intermittent painless but palpable uterine contractions (Braxton–Hicks) are a feature of all normal pregnancies.

Pre-eclampsia

Right upper quadrant pain may be a late feature of pre-eclampsia (PE), and is thought to be caused by subcapsular oedema and haemorrhage on the liver surface secondary to disordered coagulation and thrombocytopenia; blood pressure measurement and urine analysis for protein are integral

Table 33.4 Acute abdominal pain in later pregnancy.

Conditions related to pregnancy	Uterine contractions/labour		Intermittent signs of labour: dilated cervix, ruptured membranes
	Placental abruption		Bleeding, tense uterus, ?dead fetus
	Pre-eclampsia		Epigastric site + ↑BP, proteinuria uterine
	Uterine rupture		Previous uterine scar
Uterine disorders, ovarian and abdominal wall	Round ligament pain	1:10	Rarely acute or severe, exertional
	Uterine fibroids	1:500	Irregular uterus, localized
	Uterine torsion	1:20000	Very rare
	Ovarian tumours	1:1000	Usually benign
	Rectus abdominis, haematoma	1:10000	Localized, superficial painful swelling
	Spontaneous symphysiotomy	1:800	Localized tenderness on exertion
Incidental abdominal disorders	Reflux oesophagitis	1:2000	Rarely acute, postural exacerbation
	Appendicitis	1:200	Site displaced laterally, Alders' sign
	Cholecystitis	1:2000	Typical location unaltered
	Intestinal obstruction	1:3000	Usually previous abdominal surgery
	Urinary infection and urolithiasis	1:100 1:1500	
	Acute pancreatitis	1:5000	Nausea, vomiting; shock later
	Abdominal vascular accidents	Rare	Early severe shock
	Malignant neoplasms	Very rare	Associated gastrointestinal bleeding, obstruction

parts of all clinical examinations performed in later pregnancy. Nausea, vomiting and visual symptoms may co-exist and a diagnosis of severe PE in these circumstances necessitates early delivery while simultaneously taking steps to prevent eclamptic convulsions.

Placental abruption

Concealed intra-uterine haemorrhage between the fetal and maternal surfaces of the placenta (abruption) can result from the coagulopathy of PE or secondary to direct abdominal trauma, although in most cases no cause is apparent. Vaginal bleeding may be scanty or non-existent in the early stages of abruption despite severe abdominal discomfort, which is usually constant and associated with a tense, tender uterus, secondary to myometrial spasm. The fetus usually succumbs early in severe abruption but if the fetal heart is detectable, consideration should be given to prompt delivery by Caesarean section. Following fetal death, induction of labour should be combined with ample blood replacement and correction of any associated coagulopathy. Blood loss is notoriously underestimated in cases of abruption, so transfusion should be monitored through central venous pressure and urinary output.

Uterine rupture

Rupture of the intact gravid uterus is a disastrous, but rare, complication which almost always occurs during labour and always in multiparous women. The associated perinatal mortality is very high and there is also significant risk of maternal death from intraperitoneal haemorrhage if the diagnosis and subsequent laparotomy is delayed. Rupture before labour is, however, only likely to occur in the presence of pre-existing upper uterine segment scar, as may follow uterine reconstructive surgery or classical Caesarean section, and so does not figure prominently in the differential diagnosis of antepartum abdominal pain.

Uterine, ovarian and musculoskeletal conditions

Uterine fibroids

The uterus is not normally tender in later pregnancy, unless uterine leiomyomata (fibroids) are palpated. Fibroids are common but generally asymptomatic. They may, however, give rise to pain and tenderness during pregnancy in 10% of cases, especially if they undergo haemorrhagic infarction or 'red degeneration'. This complication can cause severe pain, localized to the uterine surface irregularity caused by the fibroid, but posteriorly-located tumours may be difficult to diagnose and may induce low-grade fever and local peritonism. Ultrasound can reliably locate fibroids, even if they are degenerating and management should invariably be

conservative (analgesia, hydration) until the pain resolves after a few days.

Ovarian tumours

Although torsion of a cystic ovary is much more likely to occur during early pregnancy, this complication may need to be considered during the second trimester, when palpation of an adnexal tumour becomes more difficult. Ovarian cysts at this gestation are more likely to be asymptomatic and found coincidentally during ultrasound examination of the pregnant uterus. Even when large cysts occur in the pregnant age group, they are most likely to be benign or, at worst, of borderline malignant potential. Surgical removal should be considered if cysts are causing symptoms, are larger than 5 cm in diameter and especially if there are ultrasound features suggestive of malignancy, such as mixed cystic and solid internal echoes within the tumour.

> Large ovarian cysts in this age group are likely to be benign.

Uterine torsion

Much less frequent than ovarian torsion is uterine torsion, which represents an exaggeration of the normal axial rotation of the gravid uterus. Predisposing factors include fibroids, uterine anomalies or previous pelvic surgery. Torsion leads to severe pain but does not always require surgical correction (by replacement or Caesarean section), unless maternal shock ensues.

Musculoskeletal conditions

Musculoskeletal conditions are much commoner causes of abdominal discomfort in pregnancy but rarely enter the differential diagnosis of the acute abdomen. At least 10% of pregnant women will complain of cramp-like lower abdominal discomfort on exertion on either side of the midline; this is allegedly due to *stretching of the round ligaments* and invariably resolves during the third trimester without intervention; local tenderness cannot usually be elicited. On the other hand, a large, unilateral, tender swelling may occasionally develop behind the rectus abdominis muscle, representing haematoma formation which can occur spontaneously or follow local trauma or coughing. Although such a *rectus abdominis haematoma* may be managed conservatively, surgical evacuation will relieve persistent discomfort.

Spontaneous separation of the symphysis pubis occurs during about 1 : 800 vaginal deliveries, giving rise to localized discomfort on walking in the early puerperium. Rarely, spontaneous symphysiotomy can present antepartum, usually as an exacerbation of an earlier obstetric separation and is recognizable by the typical localized pain and pubic tenderness and difficulty with gait.

Incidental causes of abdominal pain in later pregnancy

Acute appendicitis

The increasing difficulty encountered in the diagnosis of acute appendicitis as pregnancy progresses has already been discussed. At later gestations, otherwise helpful associated symptoms such as anorexia, vomiting, fever and rigors may be less evident than when the condition occurs in early pregnancy but the significance of increasing leucocytosis should not be underestimated. Lateral and upward displacement of the appendix in the third trimester means that appendicectomy through a laparotomy incision at the site of maximal tenderness in a woman with unresolving right-sided abdominal symptoms is a safer option for mother and fetus than continued expectancy.

Bowel obstruction

Intestinal obstruction, characterized by colicky pain, nausea, vomiting, constipation and abdominal distension represents another incidental abdominal disorder in which early surgical intervention is generally preferable to expectancy for more than 24 h. Cases tend to cluster in the second half of pregnancy, typically in women whose previous abdominal operations have left residual adhesions; much less often volvulus, hernias and neoplasms may obstruct. An erect abdominal radiograph demonstrating distended bowel loops with fluid levels will be diagnostic in established cases; bowel sounds are increased in the early stages but disappear if secondary paralytic ileus supervenes. Because the affected bowel may strangulate or perforate after undue delay, early laparotomy can greatly reduce morbidity; this should be performed jointly by a surgeon and obstetrician because Caesarean section may be necessary to provide appropriate abdominal access close to term.

Cholelithiasis and liver disorders

Because pregnancy alters both gall bladder motility and the accretion rate of stones, cholecystitis and obstructive jaundice are more common in pregnancy, with a frequency of almost 1 : 2000 women, some of whom will have no prior history of disease.

> Pregnancy is not an excuse for delay when appendicitis, bowel obstruction or other causes of 'acute abdomen' are suspected.

Ultrasound of the urinary tract can usually clearly demonstrate stones or duct dilatation to corroborate the typical clinical picture. The approach to management should then be conservative if possible, with analgesia, hydration and even antibiotics used in preference to surgery. When medical therapy proves ineffective, open cholecystectomy in pregnancy carries a relatively low morbidity, provided the maternal condition is good; laparoscopic procedures are preferable but are technically less feasible when the uterus has enlarged towards the umbilicus.

Hepatitis is rarely difficult to differentiate from gall bladder disease because pain is not an important feature but the nausea, vomiting, right upper quadrant pain and jaundice caused by the *HELLP* (haemolysis-elevated liver enzymes–low platelets) syndrome of pre-eclampsia, or the very rare *acute fatty hepatic necrosis* of pregnancy, may cause initial confusion until the latter conditions evolve. HELLP will be associated with hypertension, proteinuria and other signs of severe pre-eclampsia and may precede eclamptic seizures by only a short interval.

Acute pancreatitis

Acute pancreatitis is rare in pregnancy but occurs more commonly than in non-pregnant women of similar age. It clusters particularly in later gestations in association with biliary stones but the associated vomiting induced may delay the diagnosis if serum amylase measurement is not considered at the initial presentation with pain. Prompt correction of shock, pain relief, prophylactic antibiotics and suppression of pancreatic activity can avert fetal loss and serious maternal morbidity, which is otherwise significant in neglected cases. Surgical treatment is best avoided until after delivery.

Peptic ulcer and reflux oesophagitis

Gastric and duodenal ulceration can be virtually excluded from the differential diagnosis of pain in pregnancy in the absence of pre-existing disease, although puerperal relapse is not uncommon. Symptomatic exacerbations can usually be controlled with H_2 antagonists but most ulcer patients improve during pregnancy and acute exacerbations are rare. On the other hand, reflux oesophagitis tends to deteriorate with increasing gestation, but rarely presents as an acute diagnostic problem.

Abdominal vascular accidents

Vascular accidents are rare in the abdomen but remain significant causes of maternal mortality. Arterial ruptures of, for example, aortic or splenic artery aneurysms, are commonest in the third trimester and usually occur without a pre-existing vascular history. In addition to severe abdominal pain without uterine tenderness, increasing shock

---

Key points in assessment of later abdominal pain

- In the absence of shock, a brief period of observation and investigation safely improves diagnostic accuracy.
- Alders' sign can usefully differentiate uterine and extra-uterine causes of pain.
- Laparotomy (jointly with surgeon and obstetrician) is preferable to prolonged expectancy if the clinical condition fails to resolve.

Table 33.5 Abdominal pain in the puerperium.

Disorders related to pregnancy	Uterine/adnexal infection
	Urinary tract infection
	Caesarean section pain
	Spontaneous symphysiotomy
Incidental conditions at increased frequency	Bowel obstruction
	Appendicitis
	Inflammatory bowel disease
	Peptic ulceration

secondary to intraperitoneal haemorrhage predicates early surgical intervention coincident with resuscitation and coincident caesarean delivery may be needed to permit adequate exploration of the upper abdomen.

Abdominal pain in the puerperium

Following delivery the uterus rapidly involutes towards the pelvis, so that it usually becomes impalpable by 2 weeks postpartum. This rapid alteration in anatomical relationships may precipitate bowel obstruction secondary to adhesions but, in general, surgical diagnosis is much easier than during the third trimester. Several conditions may undergo puerperal exacerbation, such as peptic ulceration, inflammatory bowel disease or fibroid degeneration, while some pregnancy-related complications may also cause abdominal pain (Table 33.5). Spontaneous symphysiotomy is usually symptomatic for the first time after delivery and pelvic infection, which is rare antepartum, can frequently present with tenderness localized over the uterus and adnexa.

Thrombosis of the pelvic and ovarian veins and broad ligament haematomas are other pelvic conditions which predominantly occur postpartum and lead to painful pelvic masses. Early puerperal appendicitis may prove difficult to locate and distinguish from uterine discomfort, so that its morbidity is often increased at this time.

In general, observation of an investigative sequence comparable to that followed during pregnancy, but with greater consideration of an infective contribution, will lead to the appropriate diagnosis.

Further reading

Chamberlain, G.V.P. (1994) Abdominal pain in pregnancy. In: *ABC of Antenatal Care*, pp. 47–51. BMJ Publications, London.
Clewell, W.H. (1994) In: *Abdominal pain in: High Risk Pregnancy* (eds D.K. James, P.J. Steer, C.P. Weiner & B. Gonik), pp. 605–22. W.B. Saunders, London.

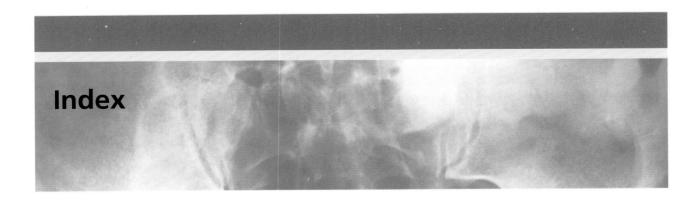

Index

Page numbers in *italics* refer to figures; those in **bold** to tables. The index entries are arranged in letter-by-letter alphabetical order.